M. Hansmann   B.-J. Hackelöer   A. Staudach

Ultrasound Diagnosis in Obstetrics and Gynecology

Coeditor: B.K. Wittmann

With the Collaboration of
D.N. Cox, V. Duda, W. Feichtinger, U. Gembruch,
P. Jeanty, G. Kossoff, R. Romero, A.G. Ross, H.D. Rott,
H. Schuhmacher, R. Terinde and U. Voigt

With 589 Figures

Springer-Verlag
Berlin Heidelberg New York Tokyo

Prof. Dr. Manfred Hansmann

Abteilung für Pränatale Diagnostik und Therapie, Universitäts-Frauenklinik, Sigmund-Freud-Straße 25, D-5300 Bonn

Prof. Dr. Bernhard-Joachim Hackelöer

Medizinisches Zentrum für Frauenheilkunde und Geburtshilfe, Philipps-Universität, Pilgrimstraße 3, D-3550 Marburg

Dr. med. Alfons Staudach

Landesfrauenklinik, Landeskrankenhaus Salzburg, Müllner Hauptstraße 48, A-5020 Salzburg

Coeditor:

Dr. Bernd K. Wittmann, Associate Professor,

Obstetrics and Gynecology. Director, Department of Diagnostic Ultrasound, Grace Hospital, 4490 Oak Street, Vancouver, B.C. Canada, VGH3V5

Translator:

Terry C. Telger, 6112 Waco Way, Ft. Worth, TX 67133, USA

Title of the German Edition:
Ultraschalldiagnostik in Geburtshilfe und Gynäkologie
© Springer-Verlag Berlin Heidelberg 1985

ISBN 3-540-15348-9 Springer-Verlag Berlin Heidelberg New York Tokyo
ISBN 0-387-15348-9 Springer-Verlag New York Heidelberg Berlin Tokyo

Library of Congress Cataloging-in-Publication Data

Hansmann, Manfred. Ultrasound diagnosis in obstetrics and gynecology.
Translation of: Ultraschalldiagnostik in Geburtshilfe und Gynäkologie.
Includes bibliographies and index. 1. Ultrasonics in obstetrics. 2. Generative organs, Female – Diseases – Diagnosis. 3. Diagnosis, Ultrasonic. I. Hackelöer, B.-J. (Bernhard-Joachim), 1945. II. Staudach, A. (Alfons) III. Wittmann, B.K. (Bernd K.) IV. Title. [DNLM: 1. Genital Diseases, Female – diagnosis. 2. Obstetrics. 3. Ultrasonic Diagnosis – in pregnancy. WP 141 H249u]   RG107.5.U4H3613 1985   618.2'07543   85-22197

Typesetting, printing, and bookbinding: Universitätsdruckerei H. Stürtz AG, Würzburg.
2121/3130-543210

TO IAN DONALD

Foreword

It will be a long time before the quality of this profusely illustrated book is overtaken and the present spate of books on the subject of obstetric ultrasound may, as a result, suffer a numerical set-back – especially with translation into English which will "deliver the milk on everyone's doorstep".

Two of the authors studied in our department in Glasgow and worked like demons. If there are any rewards for teaching, then we humble Scots who have had the privilege have had more than our share as a result of the pride with which we regard our pupils.

In my own old age and looking back over the last thirty years, the innumerable difficulties, set-backs and disappointments have been more than compensated for by those who have turned the subject from a laughable eccentricity (as I have at one time experienced) into a science of increasing exactitude. This transformation has come about, not by any efforts of mine, but by the enthusiasm and ingenuity of those who would probably have achieved as much on their own if given the encouragement which I ultimately received in Glasgow University life.

Limbo must be the expected lot of most of us ordinary mortals but the work lives on.

And so, in this reminiscent and philosophical mood I beg leave to quote a little poem which I wrote at an age when young men do that sort of thing. It was prompted by a love of the sea and the ships that used to sail them. It is applicable to my friends, the authors of this lovely book.

Up channel

The breeze is fair off Ushant and the Eastern sky's aglow
To greet the dawn of this, your landfall's day
As you wear the ship to starboard and you call the watch below
Ploughing your way up-channel through the spray.

To Eastward of the Lizard and on to Portland Bill,
The scene of many a tall ship's last distress,
With royal and skysail billowing from the yards aloft until
You've logged it all the way to Dungeness.

While I far out to Westward in the Doldrums' lazy roll
Whistle for wind to give me steerage way,
I'll think of you up-channel as you romp towards your goal
And wish you luck from yonder faraway.

Ian Donald

Preface

More than 25 years ago Ian Donald and his colleagues introduced the use of ultrasound diagnosis into obstetrics and gynecology. When reading their famous Lancet article "Investigation of Abdominal Masses by Pulsed Ultrasound", only a few may have foreseen the significance it would achieve in medical diagnosis. In some European countries, particularly in the Federal Republic of Germany, where ultrasound diagnosis has been adopted in prenatal screening in the past five years, the list of special indications has grown constantly.

It is today practically impossible for the ultrasound user in the hospital or his own practice to sift out from the flood of publications the information he needs to enable him to employ the technique to full advantage. This book is thus deliberately designed as a textbook and atlas to help solve this problem. It shows the reader what possibilities are offered by ultrasound diagnosis and how they are best applied. In light of the tremendous technical advances in recent years, the illustrations consist almost exclusively of real-time images, which hardly need accompanying sketches even for the less experienced diagnostician. Where we want to draw attention to particular details, we have indicated them on the original image. This should make it easier for the reader to draw comparisons with his findings in daily practice.

In writing this volume we had the benefit of over 15 years in ultrasound diagnosis. We thus see the book in one sense as a topical look at the current position in a process of ongoing development, to which we have contributed and whose end is not yet in sight. The major topics are presented with practice in mind, but due space is also devoted to discussion of the possibilities and limitations of the newer advances in diagnosis. We are aware that many of the specialist applications cannot and should not be exploited fully by less experienced users, but it is nonetheless essential for every diagnostician to appreciate the full potential of the technique.

We are especially indebted to our friends Philip Jeanty and R. Romero for supplying to this book a chapter on biometry based on the "outer-to-inner-method" as is widely used in North America. This special chapter and the relating nomograms in the appendix have been marked with a shade margin for easy reference.

We hope that this book will help our colleagues in hospitals and in their own practices to familiarize themselves even further with ultrasound diagnosis and to apply it even more selectively.

Like every new and rapidly developing technique, ultrasound diagnosis has had to face some severe criticism. The question of whether there are side effects involved in this method has not yet been solved. However, there is increasing evidence that ultrasound diagnosis, applied skillfully and selectively, is only to the benefit of the patients. This has been confirmed recently by the World Federation of Ultrasound in Medicine and Biology during the 4th Meeting in Sydney (July 1985) where its president stated: "The Federation holds the view that up to the present time no independently confirmed study has demonstrated any deleterious effect following in vivo diagnostic examination, and that there is no reason to withhold ultrasonic examinations when these are indicated on clinical grounds."

November 1985   M. Hansmann
                                                          B.-J. Hackelöer
                                                          A. Staudach
                                                          B.K. Wittmann

Acknowledgments

We would like to thank all the colleagues whose criticism and encouragement helped us in writing this volume and who willingly shared their experience with us: Prof. E.J. PLOTZ, Prof. R. BUCHHOLZ, Prof. G. REIFFENSTUHL, Prof. N. LANG, and Dr. T.T.S. CHOW for their long years of support.

We also express our gratitude to Prof. D. KREBS, Prof. K.D. SCHULZ, Prof. S. KOWALEWSKI, Dr. M. NIESEN, Prof. H.J. FÖDISCH, Prof. H. REHDER, Prof. D. REDEL, Priv.-Doz. U. CLAUSSEN, Prof. E. SCHWINGER, Prof. G. SCHWANITZ, Prof. J. THURNER, Prof. W. ROSENKRANZ, Prof. J. FRICK, Prof. E. HUBER, Dr. H. HENKEL, Dr. R. LASSMANN, Priv.-Doz. Dr. H. SCHMOLLER, Dr. G. KUNIT, Dr. M. ENGELS, Dr. B. MC GILLIVRAY, and Dr. G. SANDOR.

We are grateful to Ms. M. PRZYBILKA, Ms. U. VIANDEN, and Ms. H. WENZ for their help in preparing the manuscript, and owe our thanks to a great number of members of the staff of our respective clinics, in particular Ms. G. GEMBRUCH, Ms. G. HENDRICH-SCHMELZ, Sister G. WOLF, Sister R. BORNE-MANN, Sister M.L. KERP, and Sister A. MEINCKE.

Contributors

Cox, D.N., Grace Hospital, 4490 Oak Street, Vancouver BC, Canada

Duda, V., Universitäts-Frauenklinik und Hebammenlehranstalt, Pilgrimstein 3, D-3550 Marburg

Feichtinger, W., Arbeitsgemeinschaft extrakorporale Fertilierung und Fertilitätsdiagnostik, Trauttmannsdorffgasse 3a, A-1130 Wien

Gembruch, U., Universitäts-Frauenklinik, Abt. für Pränatale Diagnostik, Venusberg, D-5300 Bonn 1

Jeanty, P., Department of Diagnostic Radiology, Yale University, Connecticut, USA

Kossoff, G., O.H.M.S., Commonwealth of Australia, Ultrasonics Institute, 5 Hickson Road, Millers Point N.S.W. 2000, Australia

Romero R., Department of Obstetrics and Gynecology, Yale University, New Haven, Connecticut, USA

Ross, A.G., Grace Hospital, 4490 Oak Street, Vancouver BC, Canada

Rott, H.D., Institut für Humangenetik, Universität Erlangen-Nürnberg, Schwabachanlage 10, D-8520 Erlangen

Schumacher, H., Nonnepfad 8, 5300 Bonn-Beuel

Terinde, R., Universitäts-Frauenklinik, Moorenstraße 5, D-4000 Düsseldorf

Voigt, U., Institut für Medizinische Statistik, Dokumentation und Datenverarbeitung, Universitätskliniken, Venusberg, D-5300 Bonn

Contents

Contents

1 Physics and Instrumentation in Diagnostic Ultrasound

G. Kossoff

The principle of imaging by ultrasound is well known (Shirley et al. 1978; McDicken 1981). An ultrasound transducer is energised by a short electric pulse which is converted into an ultrasound pulse. This pulse propagates along the line of sight of the transducer with a velocity which is characteristic of the medium. When the pulse strikes an interface some of the energy is reflected, and that portion which returns to the transducer is reconverted into electric form. Being of low magnitude, the echo must be amplified by a receiver before being displayed in its appropriate position on the trace of a display unit, the direction of the trace representing the line of sight of the transducer. A cross-sectional image is obtained by moving the ultrasound line of sight (either by mechanical or electrical means) and having the trace on the display follow synchronously.

1.1 Propagating Properties of Ultrasound

When the ultrasound energy propagates from one semi-infinite medium of acoustic impedance Z_1 into a second medium of impedance Z_2, some of the energy is reflected back whilst the rest is transmitted into the second medium. The acoustic impedance (Z) of the medium is defined as a product of the density of the medium (p) times the velocity of propagation of ultrasound in that medium (c):

$$Z = pc$$

As long as the interface is larger than the ultrasound beam it may be considered to be semi-infinite, and the features of propagation of ultrasound waves apply to the larger interfaces encountered in obstetrical and gynecological examinations.

The laws of reflection and refraction which govern the propagation of ultrasound waves are similar to those that apply to optics. Thus, as shown in Fig. 1.1, the reflected angle θ_r is equal to the incident angle θ_i, whilst the refracted angle θ_t is given by Snellius' law:

$$\frac{\sin \theta_i}{c_1} = \frac{\sin \theta_t}{c_2}.$$

When the ultrasound energy passes from a faster medium into a slower medium, the angle of refraction is reduced, i.e. the energy is deflected closer to the vertical. Inversely, when the energy passes from a slower medium into a faster medium, the angle of refraction is increased. When the refracted angle equals 90°, total reflection occurs, i.e. no energy is transmitted into the second medium. The critical angle of incidence at which total reflection occurs is given by:

$$\sin \theta_i = \frac{c_1}{c_2}.$$

Of specific interest in water-path scanning is the nature of propagation through a relatively thin, parallel, fast velocity medium such as skin. At vertical incidence no deviation of energy

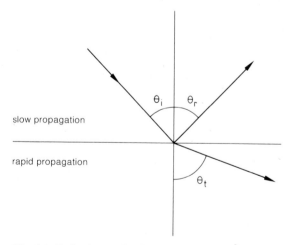

Fig. 1.1. Reflection and refraction of ultrasound at the interface between two media

Table 1.1. Acoustic properties of biological media at 37° C

Medium	Density $(kg/m^3 \times 10^3)$	Velocity (m/s)	Acoustic impedance $(kg/m^2\ s \times 10^6)$	Attenuation (dB/cm) at 1 MHz
Air	0.00129	345	0.00042	1.7
Water	1.0	1,520	1.52	0.002
Blood	1.0	1,560	1.56	0.1
Urine	1.02	1,535	1.57	0.0025
Fat	0.97	1,450	1.41	0.4
Muscle	1.07	1,570	1.68	0.7
Liver	1.06	1,560	1.65	0.6
Kidney	1.04	1,555	1.61	0.5
Brain	1.03	1,520	1.56	0.5
Skin	1.1	1,950	2.15	1
Bone	3,200	2,200	7.3	5

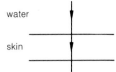

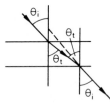

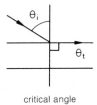

Fig. 1.2. Propagation of ultrasound through a thin, fast-conducting medium

on the posterior surface, which, being parallel to the front surface, refracts the beam back to the original incident angle. Thus the ultrasound beam may be considered to propagate along the same line of sight as the incident beam. Finally, at the critical angle of incidence total reflection occurs and there is no penetration of energy into the skin and deeper tissues.

Table 1.1 lists the acoustic properties at 37° C in the various media encountered in clinical examinations. Skin is a medium in which the velocity is significantly higher than in the other soft tissues, a fact not frequently appreciated by echographers. Refraction phenomena must therefore be considered in the water-path examinations. The most important of these is associated with total reflection, which from the values given in Table 1.1 occurs at an angle of:

$$\sin \theta_i = \frac{1525}{1950} = 0.78 \quad \text{i.e. } \theta_i \simeq 50°.$$

The propagating characteristics of ultrasound are illustrated in Fig. 1.2

1.2 Grey-Scale Sonography

In grey-scale sonography the magnitude of echoes is displayed on the echogram (Kossoff et al. 1976). The magnitude is determined by four factors:

1. Degree of acoustic impedance mismatch
2. Attenuation by tissue

takes place. This is the situation which occurs in contact scanning, because the pressure of the transducer makes the skin conform to the surface of the transducer. As the incident angle is increased the beam is refracted according to Snellius's law. Because the skin is thin, the beam is deviated only slightly before it impinges

3. Ultrasound pattern
4. Geometry of reflecting interfaces

1.2.1 Acoustic Impedance Mismatch

Echoes originate at interfaces between media with different acoustic impedances. The amount of energy that is reflected back is called the intensity reflection coefficient R. For a large interface it is given by

$$R = \left[\frac{Z_2 \cos\theta_i - Z_1 \cos\theta_t}{Z_2 \cos\theta_i + Z_1 \cos\theta_t} \right]^2.$$

At vertical incidence the expression reduces to

$$R = \left[\frac{Z_2 - Z_1}{Z_2 + Z_1} \right]^2.$$

The simple equation also applies at oblique angles of incidence if the velocities in the two media are equal.

As shown in Table 1.1, the greatest impedance mismatch occurs at a liquid or soft tissue–air interface. Because of the very large impedance mismatch all of the incident energy is reflected back, giving rise to a very strong echo, and as no energy crosses the interface it is not possible to examine posterior detail. Bowel and structures posterior to it are therefore not amenable to examination by ultrasound techniques. Bony interfaces and calcifications arising from various pathological processes also give rise to strong echoes and strongly shadow posterior detail.

The velocity in liquids and soft tissue is approximately constant. The simple equation is therefore employed in calculations of reflection coefficient from liquid and soft tissue interfaces. Because the acoustic impedances are also approximately equal relatively weak echoes are obtained from liquid and soft tissue interfaces and most of the energy propagates further into the tissues, allowing the visualisation of deeper detail.

Calculation of intensity reflection coefficient from skin–liquid or soft tissue interface must be based on the more complex equation. For example, for a density of skin of 1.1, the reflection coefficient at normal incidence of a water–skin interface is 3%. At an angle of incidence of 30°, the angle of refraction is 39°, and the use of the complex equation shows that the

value of the reflection coefficient is increased to 6°.

The intensity reflection coefficient from small interfaces is proportional to the degree of acoustic impedance mismatch. The value also depends on the geometry of the interface. The relationship is complex and outside the scope of this chapter.

1.2.2 Attenuation by Tissue

As the ultrasound wave propagates through a medium the energy content of the wave is gradually diminished. Several mechanisms are responsible for the reduction, the main ones being absorption, beam divergence and scattering. All mechanisms which contribute to the reduction of the intensity come under the term attenuation.

Absorption mechanisms convert the vibration energy content of the ultrasound wave ultimately into heat and are important in considerations involving biological effects of ultrasound. Beam divergence is determined by diffraction, which dictates that after a certain distance the ultrasound beam must begin to diverge. The beam is widened by a redistribution of energy from the axis towards the edges, thus reducing the central intensity. In propagation in a non-homogeneous medium, the energy is reflected or scattered in directions different to the incident wave, and this also reduces the intensity of the incident beam.

The value of attenuation is specified in terms of the decibel (dB) notation:

$$dB = 20 \log \frac{V_{out}}{V_{in}}$$

where V_{out} and V_{in} are parameters corresponding to the voltage at the output and input of a system.

Where a system has gain, the output is greater than the input and the ratio $\frac{V_{out}}{V_{in}}$ is greater than 1. The logarithm of a number greater than 1 is positive, and a positive dB number is obtained. If the system has a loss, then the output is less than the input and a negative dB number is obtained. As the dB notation simply represents a ratio, in cases where a system has a loss, it is customary to alter the definition to

$$dB = 20 \log \frac{V_{in}}{V_{out}}.$$

A positive dB number is then obtained which is qualified by the term loss.

Consider a situation where the output voltage is ten times the input voltage. The gain of the system in dB is

$$20 \log \frac{V_{out}}{V_{in}} = 20 \log \frac{10\,V_{in}}{V_{in}} = 20 \log 10 = 20 \text{ dB}.$$

Thus the dB notation, being based on logarithms, reduces multiplications to additions, i.e. a gain or an attenuation of $100 = 10 \times 10$ is equivalent to an attenuation of $40 \text{ dB} = 20 \text{ dB} + 20 \text{ dB}$.

The commonly employed voltage dB figures are as follows:

dB	Corresponding gain/attenuation
1	1.1
2	1.3
3	1.4
6	2.0
10	3.2
20	10

The value of attenuation at 1 MHz in various biological liquids at a temperature of 37° C is set out in Table 1.1. It may be seen that biological liquids do not significantly attenuate the ultrasound energy. This property is clinically useful, as the enhancement of detail posterior to liquid-filled lesions may be used as one of the criteria for diagnosing the liquid nature of the lesion.

Soft tissue absorbs ultrasound at an average rate of 0.5 dB/cm MHz on a "there-and-return" basis. Thus less energy impinges on deeper tissues and the same interface lying deeper in the body returns a weaker echo. Most modern instruments employ time gain compensation (TGC), i.e. increase the gain of the equipment for deeper structures. Unfortunately this compensation allows only for the average attenuation. This is adequate in the examination of homogeneous organs such as the liver, but is not sufficient in the general case of the simultaneous examination of several structures with different attenuations. In obstetrics, for example, the head and the trunk of the fetus attenuate the energy at different rates, and it is difficult to set the TGC controls to compensate for both attenuations simultaneously.

The attenuation by soft tissues is linearly proportional to frequency, and this determines the highest frequency and thus the resolution with which one may examine deeply located structures. Frequencies of the order of 3.5 MHz are generally employed in obstetrical studies, allowing a resolution of the order of 1–2 mm.

1.3 Transducer Beam Pattern

The ultrasound energy emanating from the transducer is not uniformly distributed across the beam, nor does the beam remain of the same width over the examining depth.

The beam pattern of a flat transducer consists of two regions known as the near and the far field. The transition distance T between the two regions is given by

$$T = 1.6\, d^2 f.$$

where d is the diameter of the transducer in cm and f is the frequency in MHz. In the near field the beam propagates within the cylindrical confine equal to the diameter of the transducer. The energy distribution across the beam is not uniform, and pronounced axial maxima and minima occur at various distances. In the far field the beam diverges conically at an angle θ given by

$$\sin \theta = \frac{0.19}{df}.$$

Within this conical confine the beam profile is regular, the intensity being maximum on axis and gradually reducing off axis.

Flat transducers are not commonly used in modern examinations, as the ultrasound beam may be narrowed by focusing to improve the lateral resolution. Currently, three types of transducers are used with the articulated arm manually scanned equipment: the 3.5-MHz, 1.9-cm-diameter long-focus transducer, the 3.5-MHz, 1.3-cm-diameter medium-focus transducer and the 5-MHz, 1.3-cm-diameter medium-focus transducer. The beam width and focal zone of these transducers as functions of distance are shown in Fig. 1.3. As can be seen, the 5-MHz medium-focus transducer has the best resolution, but because of the close position of focus and the short focal zone, it is suitable only for the examination of relatively small structures lying close to the skin, e.g. an early

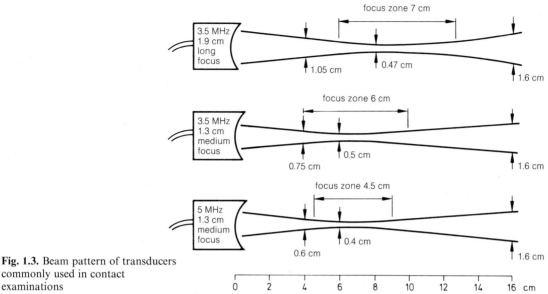

Fig. 1.3. Beam pattern of transducers commonly used in contact examinations

pregnancy. The 3.5-MHz long-focus transducer has the best performance for the examination of large structures, e.g. in late pregnancy, whilst the 3.5-MHz medium-focus transducer bridges these two beam patterns.

The echo from an interface is proportional to the beam pattern and therefore varies as a function of distance. In general, the strongest echo is obtained when the interface is located at the transition distance of a flat transducer or at the focus of a focused transducer. Some instruments have built-in receiver gain characteristics to compensate for this variation. Unfortunately, the geometry of the interface also has an influence on the variation, large interfaces having a different dependence than small ones, and only partial compensation is possible by this technique.

1.3.1 Geometry of Reflecting Interfaces

The geometry of the reflecting interface has a major effect on the magnitude of the echo received from the interface. In the analysis it is helpful to separate the interfaces into two classes, those that are much bigger and those that are much smaller than the ultrasound beam. Boundaries of organs are examples of interfaces that are much larger than the ultrasound beam and therefore fall into the first class, whereas the stromal organisation of tissue is an example of an interface which is much smaller than the ultrasound beam and falls into the second class.

Because a large interface intercepts the whole ultrasound beam, the echo is reflected in a specular or mirror-like manner. Thus, when a large flat interface is vertical to the ultrasound beam, all of the energy is reflected back to the transducer and a large echo is obtained. However, as illustrated in Fig. 1.4, a small degree of inclination reflects a considerable portion of the energy away from the transducer, and only a small echo is obtained. For a typical transducer this inclination dependence is quite dramatic and a reduction in the size of an echo by a factor of ten for each 5° inclination is not uncommon. Similarly, a small change in shape from flat to concave or convex significantly affects the size of the echo. This dependence on geometry is often much greater than the differences in acoustic impedance mismatch. For this reason it is unwise to attach much clinical significance to the magnitude of an echo from a large interface, and it is better to simply note whether a boundary echo is present or not. This is clinically relevant, since the presence of a smooth boundary echo from a mass is indicative that the mass is encapsulated and therefore probably benign, whereas the absence of boundary echoes or the presence of a jagged border is indicative of an invasive and therefore probably malignant process.

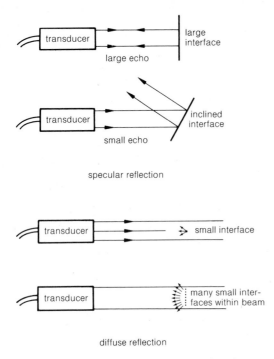

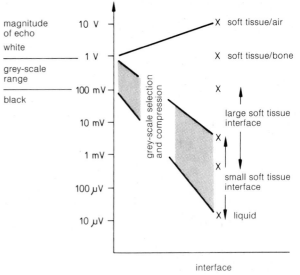

Fig. 1.5. Magnitude of echo and grey scale of display unit. The *diagonal lines* illustrate the compression of echoes from small interfaces into major portion of grey scale of display unit

Fig. 1.4. Specular reflection from large interfaces and diffuse reflection from small interfaces

A small interface intercepts only a small portion of the ultrasound beam and gives rise to a small echo. As illustrated in Fig. 1.4, the energy is reflected diffusely, i.e. in all directions. As the inclination dependence factor is not present, the magnitude of the echo is related to the impedance mismatch and the position of the interface within the ultrasound beam. In general, many such small interfaces lie within the ultrasound beam, all contributing to the overall echo. The pattern of the internal echoes is specific to the type of tissue, and many normal tissues, as well as localised and diffuse pathological processes, may be distinguished by their characteristic internal texture appearance.

Liquid-filled structures are internally homogeneous. They do not return any internal echoes and are readily identified by this feature.

1.3.2 Principle of Grey-Scale Sonography

The range of amplitudes of echoes encountered in a diagnostic examination is quite vast. As illustrated in Fig. 1.5, the largest echo is obtained from a large, flat soft tissue–air interface such as that present in air-containing bowel.

With current equipment, the amplitude of this echo is on the order of 10 V. The next largest echo is obtained from a soft tissue–bone interface, the amplitude typically being of the order of 1 V. Large, flat soft tissue interfaces give echoes that range from a maximum value of 100 mV down to noise level, depending on the degree of impedance mismatch and the inclination. Echoes from the structural organisation of tissue range from a maximum value of 1 mV down to noise level, the strongest internal echoes being obtained from the parenchyma of the placenta, the weakest from the white matter of brain.

The vertical scale of Fig. 1.5 also shows a typical grey-scale range of a display unit. As shown, a voltage of greater than 100 mV is required to make an echo just visible, whilst voltages above 1 V saturate the display. The grey scale of the device is distributed between these two voltages, and generally ranges from 10 to 20 shades. With this restricted grey-scale range, it is not possible to display the whole range of amplitudes of echoes, and some form of selection and compression must be employed to display the range of magnitudes that is considered to be of maximum clinical significance.

Since the amplitude of echoes from large interfaces is highly dependent on their geometry, it is unwise to allocate much of the available grey-scale range to their portrayal. It is more effective to utilise most of the range to display the amplitude of echoes received from the structural organisation of tissue. This selecting process forms the fundamental principle of grey-scale sonography and is illustrated by the diagonal lines in Fig. 1.5 which show the selection and compression of the range of magnitudes of internal echoes for display over the major portion of the grey scale, whilst only a small portion is allocated for the portrayal of echoes from large interfaces. The selecting process varies between instruments, and this to a large extent determines the characteristics of the grey-scale sonograms obtained on different equipment.

1.4 Quality of Image and Frame Rate

An ideal ultrasound instrument would provide high-resolution sonograms at rapid frame rates permitting detailed study of the most rapid dynamic movements which occur in the body. Unfortunately, the relatively low speed with which ultrasound propagates in soft tissue forces a compromise between the quality of a sonogram and the frame rate.

The quality of an image is determined by the number of resolvable elements which it contains. Under normal viewing conditions, the human eye is unable to perceive the substructure of an image consisting of 500×500 pixels. For this reason images containing this number of pixels are said to be of high quality. Sonograms are formed by laying down lines of sight, each line representing the direction travelled by the ultrasound pulse. Using the same argument, a high-quality echogram needs to contain at least 500 lines of sight.

The average velocity of ultrasound in tissue is 1530 m/s. It therefore takes ultrasound 13 μs to propagate through 1 cm of tissue on a "there-and-return" basis. If a penetration distance of P cm is required, then the time taken to traverse this distance is $13\,P$ μs, whilst the minimum time necessary to form a sonogram consisting of N number of lines of sight is $13\,PN$ μs. Frame rate F is defined as the number of times a sonogram may be formed in 1 s. It is therefore equal to the inverse of

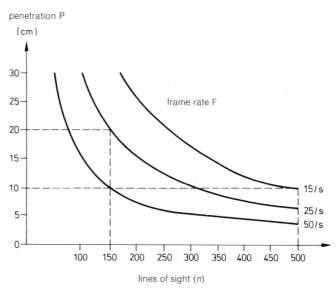

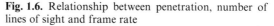

Fig. 1.6. Relationship between penetration, number of lines of sight and frame rate

the time taken to form one sonogram and is given by

$$F = \frac{1}{13\,PN\ \mu s}$$

Rearranging this equation gives the following fundamental relationship between penetration, number of lines of sight and frame rate:

$$PNF = 77 \times 10^3.$$

This relationship is illustrated in Fig. 1.6, which shows for instance that if a sonogram representing a penetration of 10 cm is required and this sonogram contains 500 lines, the frame rate cannot be faster than 15 echograms/s.

1.5 Real-Time Scanning

"Real-time" is the term given to ultrasound techniques that provide sonograms at rates faster than the flicker rate of the human eye, namely 15 frames/s. To simplify the design of the equipment and to make it TV-compatible, most real-time instruments present their images at rates equal to half the mains voltage frequency. In Europe the mains frequency is 50 cycles/s and real-time instruments generally present their images at 25 frames/s. Fig. 1.6 shows that at this frame rate a sonogram representing a penetration of 20 cm can consist of no greater than 150 lines. Thus images obtained on real-time instruments are of lower quality than those obtained with static equipment. Real-time is also generally restricted to operation in the simple scan mode and provides a limited view of the anatomy. Despite these limitations, the ease of use of real-time equipment and the importance of the dynamic information which it provides has made real-time an indispensable part of ultrasound obstetrical and gynecological examinations (Garrett et al. 1980).

1.6 Simple and Compound Scanning

Simple scanning is defined as a form of scanning in which the transducer is moved in such a manner that the lines of sight which form the sonogram never intersect, i.e. no tissue is ever examined from two different directions. Single-pass scanning in which the transducer is kept vertical to the patient's skin line is an example of simple scanning, used with the articulated arm scanner, whilst sector and linear scanning are the most common forms of simple scanning used with real-time equipment.

Compound scanning is a more general form of scanning in which the transducer is moved so that the lines of sight originate from many different directions. With manual equipment, compound scanning is achieved by superimposing a rocking motion on the single-pass scan, whilst in mechanised equipment it is usually achieved by combining two simple scan motions, such as a sector and a linear scan. Compound scanning was originally developed to ensure that all outlines of organs are examined at the same time during the scanning period at vertical incidence when they return large echoes.

The features of simple and compound scanning (illustrated schematically in Fig. 1.7) are as follows:

1. Because of generally less favourable inclinations, the boundary echoes are less readily visualised on simple scans. Compound scanning gives a more complete display and is the best method of scanning to provide whole-body scan sonograms.

2. Simple scanning gives single line of sight textural information whilst compound scanning gives an integrated line of sight textural representation. These two forms of textural representation are complementary.

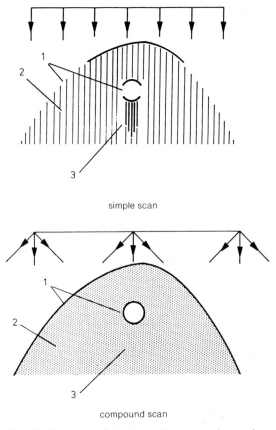

simple scan

compound scan

Fig. 1.7. Features of simple and compound scanning. *Numbers* refer to items in list, Sect. 1.6

3. Simple scanning is superior in portraying changes such as shadowing and enhancement behind areas in which the attenuation is higher or lower than that in the surrounding tissues. This difference in attenuation affects the amount of energy incident on posterior tissues, and on simple scans these are displayed by echoes of reduced or enhanced intensity. In compound scanning the posterior tissues are also examined by lines of sight that do not traverse the areas with different attenuation and therefore shadowing or enhancement effects are not as obvious.

Thus the two methods of scanning are complementary, and both should be employed to attain the full information that may be obtained from an ultrasound examination.

To obtain the features characteristic of compound scanning it is necessary to examine tissues from many different directions. Compound scan sonograms therefore contain a larger number of lines of sight and cannot be formed as rapidly as simple scan sonograms (Fig. 1.6).

1.7 Contact and Water-Path Coupling

The ultrasound energy may be coupled into the patient either by placing the transducer in contact with the skin or by immersing the transducer in a water tank and coupling the energy into the patient through a membrane.

Contact coupling has the advantage that the transducer is easily applied and its position relative to the patient's anatomical landmarks is obvious. The equipment is less bulky and more portable. The transducer may be pressed deep into the skin to get highly inclined views below the symphysis pubis. The pressure of the transducer makes the skin conform to the surface of the transducer ensuring that the scanning is always performed at vertical angle of incidence. Finally, the technique is effective in utilising a limited access window and is ideally suited for needle biopsy studies. On the other hand, contact coupling is limited with regard to the maximum diameter of transducer that may be applied to the patient. The resolution of the ultrasound technique is proportional to the transducer aperture, and this limitation means that contact coupling has an upper limit on the resolution that may be achieved at any one frequency. Contact scanning also provides inferior subcutaneous detail due to overload of the receiver by the transmit pulse.

The water-path coupling method also has both limitations and advantages. The equipment is more bulky, and to avoid the display of multiple reflections between the transducer and the coupling membrane, the transducer must be kept at a distance equal to the total penetration. The need to traverse this water distance is a significant limitation, as it slows down by a factor of two the speed with which the echograms may be acquired. The membrane of the tank generally conforms to the shape of the patient. It is therefore not possible to indent the skin to obtain a vertical angle of incidence for deeply inclined views, and total reflection at angles of incidence beyond the critical angle precludes the acquisition of these views. This method does not, however, impose any limitation on the size of the transducer which is used for the scanning, and is therefore capable of

higher resolution. The scanning motions of the equipment are more readily mechanised and a multiple widely spaced transducer construction may be employed to allow rapid acquisition of whole-body compound-scan sonograms. Water-path equipment is more easily designed to operate in an automated mode to provide a series of sonograms stepped by a selected interval. Accurate comparison of results obtained in orthogonal planes is also more practical on water-path equipment.

1.8 Current Instrumentation

No current equipment allows independent selection of the described operational features, and as these impose conflicting design requirements it is unlikely that such an instrument will ever be produced. Instead, it has become common to use several instruments to perform a complete examination. Analysis of the characteristics of these instruments show that they may be grouped into four categories.

1.8.1 Articulated Arm Manual Contact Scanner

The first category encompasses the conventional articulated arm manual contact scanners. These are versatile instruments which are able to perform most examinations well. They provide the highest quality images in either the simple or the compound scan mode, the high quality being the result of extensive research into the construction of the single transducer used in the instrument. Technically, the performance of the equipment has reached a plateau, and all of the available instruments provide about the same level of performance.

The major disadvantage is the manual nature of the scanning. Despite considerable improvements, the quality of the results is still dependent on the scanning skill of the operator and the equipment is incapable of operating in the real-time mode.

1.8.2 Linear Array Scanner

Linear array scanners represent a very popular category of equipment used today. A multi-element transducer is employed, and the ultrasound beam is generated by energising a group

Table 1.2. Operational features of ultrasound equipment

Operational feature	Equipment			
	Articulated arm scanner	Linear array scanner	Mechanical sector scanner	Multiple-transducer water-path scanner
Scanning mode	Manual	Automated electronic	Automated mechanical	Automated mechanical
Coupling	Contact	Contact	Contact	Water path
Quality of image	High	Good	High	High
Acquisition speed	Slow	Real time	Real time	Slow or real time
Image format	Simple or compound scan	Simple linear scan	Simple sector scan	Simple or compound scan
Application	General purpose	Simpler examinations	General purpose	General purpose
Cost	Medium to high	Low to medium	Medium	High

of the elements. Scanning of the beam is performed electronically at real-time rates by sequentially energising adjacent groups of elements and moving in the line of sight synchronously along the length of the transducer. The scanning is thus performed automatically, eliminating the dependence of image quality on the scanning skill of the operator. As the scanning is performed along the length of the transducer, there is no need for an expensive articulated arm. This significantly reduces the cost of the equipment and makes it considerably more manoeuvrable.

The linear simple scan provides a rectangular image format which gives a relatively wide view of the anatomy. The resolution of the image is somewhat inferior to that obtained with the conventional single-transducer scanner because of the poorer echo response and beam pattern of the multi-element transducer and the smaller number of lines of sight used to form the image. The main disadvantage of the equipment is the need for a relatively large flat surface for the contact, and because of the length of the transducer it is difficult to obtain deeply inclined views. Linear arrays have now been available for several years and their performance is beginning to plateau.

1.8.3 Mechanical Sector Scanner

Mechanical sector scanners are rapidly attracting considerable interest. In these instruments

either one or several transducers are rapidly oscillated or rotated about a point to provide a simple scan sector or "keyhole" image format. They represent a simple extension of the conventional single-transducer scanner, and as the same transducer technology is employed, they provide high-quality images. The point contact transducer head of this equipment is highly manoeuvrable and allows the acquisition of deeply indented views. The main disadvantage is the keyhole image format, which gives limited visualisation requiring more scanning and good knowledge of anatomical relationships, necessary for the mental superposition of images obtained in the examination of large structures. The cost of the equipment is in the same range as that of linear array scanners, and as the equipment has been available for several years its performance is also starting to plateau.

1.8.4 Water-Path Scanners

Water-path scanners represent a new category of ultrasound equipment which employs automated mechanical scanning to provide the best quality images. With single-transducer instruments these are usually real-time simple linear scans. On multiple-transducer scanners, such as the U.I. Octoson (Carpenter et al. 1977), it is also possible to acquire static compound scans using any combination of the transducers to provide whole body scans.

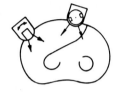

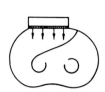

articulated arm scanner   linear array scanner

mechanical sector scanner

Fig. 1.8. Current equipment

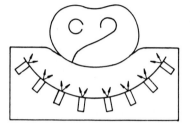

multiple-transducer water-path scanner

Water-path scanners are general-purpose instruments in the medium to high cost range. Being relatively new, the performance of the equipment is likely to continue to improve and to extend into other areas, such as the combined imaging and pulsed Doppler technique for quantitative measurement of blood flow in deep vessels (Gill et al. 1981) and tissue characterisation studies.

A summary of the performance characteristics of these four categories of equipment is given in Table 1.2, and their construction is shown schematically in Fig. 1.8.

1.9 Future Developments

One of the features characteristic of the development of ultrasound in the 1970s was the great improvement in the technical performance of the equipment. New generations of instruments were introduced on the average every 3 years and the equipment was generally obsolete in 5 years. The field has now passed from this stage of rapid evolution to a stage of consolidation during which it is unlikely that major advances in imaging will be made at the same rate.

Modern ultrasound departments are requested to perform a wide variety of examinations, and ideally should be capable of providing the following services:

1. Real-time examinations for demonstration of dynamic events, delineation of normal anatomical relationships and diagnosis of simpler pathological processes
2. Whole-body examination for high quality visualisation of anatomical detail and determination of complex pathological processes
3. Guided needle biopsy studies
4. Examinations for deformable organs.

Analysis of the operational characteristics of current equipment shows that it is possible to provide all of these services by using only two instruments, namely, a mechanical sector scanner and a multiple-transducer water-path scanner. The former provides the highest quality real-time scans. Its point contact area allows it to be used to obtain highly indented views, whilst the contact method of coupling permits it to be used for biopsy investigations. The latter provides the highest quality whole-body scan images and may be used to examine deformable organs. Because of the low cost and wide image format, linear array scanners also have an important role in ultrasound departments. They allow the most rapid examinations of simpler conditions, and their use is in many ways a natural extension of the conventional techniques of inspection, palpation, percussion and auscultation for the clinical work-up of the patient. The use of the articulated arm scanner is on the decline, however, and it is likely that this instrument will gradually become obsolete (Kossoff 1980).

As diagnostic ultrasound is still a relatively new science, major advances will undoubtedly continue to occur. It is likely, however, that the emphasis will shift from morphological examinations to functional studies. The combined use of B-mode and pulsed Doppler imaging, which allows the quantitative measurement of blood flow in the fetal umbilical vein and aorta, is one example of such advances beginning to appear in the literature.

References

Carpenter D, Kossoff G, Daniel K, Boele P (1977) The UI Octoson. A new class of ultrasonic echoscope. Australas Radiol 21:85–89

Garrett WJ (1980) The place of real time and static B-mode scanning in obstetric practice. Ultrasound Med Biol 6:59–61

Gill RW, Trudinger BJ, Garrett WJ, Kossoff G, Warren PS (1981) Fetal umbilical venous flow measured in utero by pulsed doppler and B-mode ultrasound in normal pregnancies. Am J Obstet Gynecol 139:720–725

Kossoff, G (1980) The king is dead – long live the king. Austral Radiol 24:220–222

Kossoff G, Garrett WJ, Carpenter DA, Jellins J, Dadd MJ (1976) Principles and classifications of soft tissues by grey scale echography. Ultrasound Med Biol 2:89–105

McDicken WN (1981) Diagnostic ultrasonics: principles and use of instruments, 2nd edn. Wiley, New York

Shirley I, Blackwell R, Cusick G, Forman D, Vicary F (1978) A users guide to diagnostic ultrasound. Pitman Medical, Kent

2 Safety of Diagnostic Ultrasound

H.D. ROTT

The question of possible adverse effects associated with the use of diagnostic ultrasound is as old as the modality itself. Since 1964, when Sunden conducted extensive experiments in this area, a tremendous volume of material has been published on the biologic effects of ultrasound. On the basis of these investigations, it is now generally agreed that diagnostic ultrasound, unlike modalities that use ionizing radiation, does not pose a significant health risk to the patient or examiner.

However, it must be remembered that safety is a quality that can be judged only from the absence of deleterious effects, i.e., it cannot be proved in a positive sense. Since adverse effects that are subtle or rare are difficult to detect experimentally and statistically, one is forced to develop increasingly sensitive experimental methods and to conduct investigations on an ever broader scale. Thus, we are justified in reviewing recent experimental and epidemiological findings as a means of testing the hypothesis that ultrasound is innocuous (Rott 1981).

Data on ultrasound intensity are basic to the evaluation of experimental findings. With pulsed ultrasound as used for diagnostic imaging, the intensity may be described and measured in four different ways in terms of its spatial and temporal characteristics:

I_{SATA} spatial average – temporal average intensity.

I_{SATP} spatial average – temporal peak intensity.

I_{SPTA} spatial peak – temporal average intensity.

I_{SPTP} spatial peak – temporal peak intensity. This parameter presumes a constant level of emission throughout the duration of the pulse, though this is not the case in reality. The problems involved in the measurement of intensity parameters are discussed by Haerten (1980).

To avoid confusion, intensity data should always be stated in terms of these parameters. Unfortunately, this point has frequently been neglected in the references cited below, particularly in the older literature.

2.1 Primary Effects

The various biologic effects of ultrasound are the product of a few primary physical and chemical actions. Because a knowledge of these primary actions is important in understanding the effects of ultrasound on tissues, we shall review them briefly.

2.1.1 Heat Production

Ultrasound is a mechanical form of energy that is converted to thermal energy when absorbed. Whether this raises the temperature of tissues depends on the intensity and frequency of the ultrasound, the type of tissue exposed, and the capacity of the bloodstream for heat removal. The occurrence of thermal injury will likewise depend on the heat tolerance of the tissue. Thus, for example, while liver tissue may be completely unaffected by ultrasound at a given frequency and intensity, the same radiation may cause painful thermal irritation at bone surfaces due to the greater absorption of energy and the limited blood flow.

By and large, diagnostic ultrasound is applied at I_{SATA} levels below 0.01 W/cm² (Zweifel 1979). This is far too low to cause measurable temperature elevation in tissues, even if we disregard thermal convection by the circulation (Ter Haar and Williams 1981).

2.1.2 Pseudocavitation and Microstreaming

When degassed fluids are exposed to high intensities of ultrasound, small areas of true vacuum can form in the low-pressure phase (cavitation). When these areas subsequently collapse in the pressure phase, extremely high pressures and temperatures are created. A similar phenomenon, called pseudocavitation, occurs in biologic tissues and involves the formation of small bubbles that contain gas. These bubbles may collapse almost immediately after formation, they may remain stable and undergo synchronous oscillations in a continuous ultrasound field, or they may expand, causing the disruption of tissues. The occurrence of this phenomenon depends on the intensity and frequency of the ultrasound, the length of exposure, the texture of the tissue, the gas content of the tissue, and the external pressure.

Persistent bubbles oscillating in a sound field generally do not oscillate in a spherically symmetric fashion. This causes pressure gradients to develop at the surface of the bubbles. These in turn cause a localized movement of the ambient fluid known as "microstreaming." This phenomenon produces gravitational forces that are potentially damaging to membranes or organelles. With diagnostic Doppler ultrasound, the intensities are too low for pseudocavitation to occur. With pulsed ultrasound imaging, the intensity would be sufficient to cause bubble formation, but the duration of the pulse, which lasts only a few microseconds, is too short. In any case, this phenomenon has not yet been observed under the exposure conditions used in pulsed ultrasound at diagnostic levels (Hill and Ter Haar 1982).

2.1.3 Chemical Effects

The cavitational effects associated with ultrasound are capable of initiating a number of chemical reactions. For example, ultrasound is known to cause oxidation through the formation of H_2O_2 and to reduce nitrate to nitrite. The local temperature elevations that are possible with pseudocavitation can probably also precipitate chemical reactions or increase their rate. On the other hand, the depolymerization of macromolecules appears to be independent of cavitation and pseudocavitation. This effect has been observed in polysaccharides, polyglycols, various proteins, and in isolated DNA, but not in intracellular DNA. Besides the reparative capacity of the intact cell, this is presum-

ably due to differences in the spatial configuration of the DNA molecule. Because the wavelength of diagnostic ultrasound is on the order of 1 mm, the molecule must cover an area at least 1 mm in diameter if all the energy of a wave phase is to act upon it. This is possible only with isolated DNA, since the DNA in intact cells is far too compact.

2.2 Biologic Effects

Discussion of all biologic effects of ultrasound that have been reported to date would exceed the scope of this survey. We will therefore discuss only the effects that are potentially injurious. These include tissue damage (inflammation, hemorrhage, necrosis), teratogenicity, and mutagenicity.

2.2.1 Tissue Lesions and Ultrastructural Changes in Cells

The potential for gross and ultrastructural damage from ultrasound has been studied since the 1950s, when ultrasound was introduced as a therapeutic modality for the application of heat. In some cases the intensities used in animal experiments greatly exceeded accepted therapeutic ranges. These experiments proved the existence of thermal effects ranging from hyperemia to necrosis and hemorrhage due to tissue disruption, depending on the experimental setup and the duration and intensity of the exposure (Taylor and Pond 1972; survey: Holländer 1972; Sunden 1964). Prerequisites for tissue lesions were continuous ultrasound intensities in the upper therapeutic range and above and a stationary sound field. The intensities continuous ultrasound used in diagnostic Doppler instruments and the pulsed ultrasound used in imaging equipment are not sufficient to produce such lesions.

Besides gross lesions, ultrastructural changes have been described in various cell structures. Electron microscopic investigations following ultrasound exposure have shown changes even in cells that survived the exposure. These included swollen and rounded mitochondria, damaged outer and inner mitochondrial membranes, and degeneration of the cristae (Harvey et al. 1975; Hrazdira 1980; Webster et al. 1978). Hrazdira (1980) states, however, that these alterations are nonspecific and may also result from exposure to other physical or chemical agents. Saclike evaginations have been observed in the granular endoplasmic reticulum, and chromatin aggregation and the formation of DNA-free interspaces have been observed in the nucleus. It is not known whether these changes are reversible or whether they are lethal for the cell. Webster et al. (1978) were able to prevent these changes by raising the ambient pressure to 203 kPa before exposing the cell. This led them to conclude that cavitation was the predominant pathogenic mechanism.

2.2.2 Teratogenicity

An effect is teratogenic if it damages developing or differentiating embryonic tissues in such a way that fetal death or malformation ensues. Thus, teratogenicity can be manifested only in pregnant females. It is distinguished from mutagenicity, in which similar damage is produced by entirely different mechanisms.

The possibility of teratogenic effects from ultrasound has been studied for more than three decades (survey: Holländer 1972; Sunden 1964). Therapeutic ultrasound was the first modality to be investigated, with experimental animals (rats, mice, rabbits, hamsters) exposed to intensities of 0.5–5 W/cm^2 at frequencies of 0.8–1 MHz. On the whole, the experiments did not provide evidence of teratogenicity. While there were a few reports of increased rates of abortion and fetal resorption, these could be satisfactorily explained on the basis of local hyperthermia.

With the advent of diagnostic ultrasound, investigations were done using pulsed ultrasound of higher frequency, but no adverse affects of any kind were demonstrated (survey: Holländer 1972; Sunden 1964). However, when continuous ultrasound was applied in the same frequency range, increased rates of malformations, fetal resorption and low birthweight were recorded at intensities exceeding 1 W/cm^2. The observed dependence of these effects on the length of exposure (Mannor et al. 1972) points to hyperthermia as the most probable terato-

genic mechanism. This is further supported by the findings of Hara (1980), who measured the rectal temperature of gravid mice exposed to ultrasound. When the body temperature rose above 41° C (this occurred after about 3 min exposure to 3 W/cm^2), there was a rise in the incidence of facial clefts, skeletal anomalies, and neural tube defects. The same malformations have been observed in hyperthermia experiments without ultrasound (Hellmann 1980). Curto (1976) and O'Brien (1976) noted an increased rate of early neonatal death and reduced birthweight in animals exposed to only 1.5 mW/cm^2; no malformations were reported. Similar observations were made by Shoji et al. (1975), but in only one of two strains of mice exposed to 40 mW/cm^2, and by Pizarello et al. (1978), who applied 1.5 mW/cm^2 directly to one uterine horn of laparotomized pregnant rats, using the opposite side as a control. Unfortunately, these observations, which can no longer be attributed to thermal injury, have not been checked by other investigators. The groups of Shoji and Pizarello did not report an increased incidence of malformations.

Besides animal experiments, several studies have been done in which the physical and mental development of children exposed to ultrasound in utero was followed for up to 3 years post partum (Bernstine 1969; Hellman et al. 1970; Koranyi et al. 1972).

A total of 2452 children were followed up in these studies, 1732 of whom had been exposed to pulsed ultrasound and 720 to continuous ultrasound. There was no apparent increase in the incidence of malformations or spontaneous abortions. The attempts of Kamocsay and Gy (1958) to induce abortion with ultrasound are particularly interesting in this context: 150 women who had elected to have their pregnancies terminated were exposed to ultrasound at an intensity of 0.5–1 W/cm^2. *The ultrasound failed to induce abortion in any of the women treated.* Following termination by conventional methods, the aborted fetuses exhibited no morphologic abnormalities. Two women who declined to have their pregnancies terminated following the ultrasound treatment subsequently bore apparently normal children. On the basis of these findings and the animal studies discussed above, it is reasonable to assume that diagnostic ultrasound in the form currently used does not pose a teratogenic risk.

2.2.3 Mutagenicity

Mutations are changes in genetic information, usually deletions or changes in base structure of DNA, whose quality is later manifested in the process of natural selection. Mutations are cellular events which may have relevance to the organism as a whole. If they affect somatic cells, the mutated cells may retain the ability to replicate, but their division and growth may proceed in an uncontrolled fashion, leading to malignant change. Mutations in germ cells can lead to abortion, malformation, or genetic disease – effects that may be expressed generations later if a recessive gene is involved.

The detection of mutations is a relatively difficult task. Structural and numerical chromosome aberrations are directly observable with light microscopy following the application of cytogenetic techniques. The situation is more difficult with smaller lesions, which may simply involve the exchange or loss of individual bases (gene or point mutations). In these cases the mutation can be recognized only by a change in genetic behavior, i.e., altered metabolic activity in unicellular organisms, or genetically changed offspring in higher organisms and man. In animal studies on mutations, the experimental animals are first exposed to the suspected mutagen and afterward are mated. Based on the results of previous mutagenic research, it appears that known mutagenic agents cause both chromosomal and point mutations. Thus, once the induction of chromosome aberrations has been established, it is likely that point mutations have also been produced.

Because mutations are irreversible, are not directly perceived by the organism, and cause effects that may be expressed only after a prolonged latent period, the question of mutagenic effects from ultrasound is of considerable interest and has been a subject of scientific research for more than 30 years.

The important studies on point mutations are listed in Table 2.1. In the experiments on unicellular organisms, a major question was whether bacteria that survived ultrasound cleaning and sterilization underwent potentially dangerous mutation. Thus, higher levels of ultrasound were utilized in some studies in which cavitation was desired (Ausländer et al. 1966). None of these experiments succeeded in producing bacterial mutations. It should be added, however, that some authors (Abel et al. 1981; Combes 1975a, b) worked with test organisms whose mutability was unknown. Thus, Abel et al. (1981) noted that not only ultrasound but also x-irradiation exceeding 100 Gy failed to increase mutation rates in their test system. On the other hand, Barnett et al. (1982) and Wegner et al. (in preparation) performed the Ames test using a *Salmonella* strain of precisely known molecular structure and mutagen sensitivity; this makes the negative outcome of their study all the more persuasive.

In experiments with laboratory mammals, some authors found that exposure to ultrasound at high therapeutic levels elicited defensive movements (Loch 1971), produced thermal ulcerations of the scrotal skin (Brüschke 1955), or induced temporary sterility (Brüschke 1955; Friedli 1951). Again, no evidence of mutagenicity was observed.

On the other hand, there is growing evidence that ultrasound can cause mutations in insects. It is suspected that the susceptibility of these animals to ultrasound derives from the peculiar anatomy of the insect respiratory system. Specifically, the insect body is completely permeated by air-filled cavities. On exposure to ultrasound, these cavities vibrate by a pseudo-cavitation-like mechanism, and mechanical or thermal lesions are produced. These findings are not applicable to man.

Numerous studies have also been published on the possibility of ultrasound-induced chromosomal damage. In vivo studies in humans, which included children exposed to ultrasound in utero and examined postpartum (Abdulla et al. 1971; Boyd et al. 1971; Lucas et al. 1972), as well as fetuses exposed to ultrasound prior to elective abortion, did not show any increase in the rate of aberrations. Levi et al. (1974), who analyzed the bone marrow cells of live mice exposed to 1.5 W/cm² at 0.81 MHz, came to the same conclusions. In vitro experiments are considered to be more informative, because the ultrasound intensity can be increased as desired, and the length of exposure greatly extended. A disadvantage of these experiments is the greater likelihood of artifactual errors. In vitro studies have been performed using various types of cells and ultrasound. They are reviewed in Table 2.2. The findings of Macintosh and Davey (1970, 1972) are noteworthy. Initially these authors reported chromosome breaks at

Table 2.1. Studies[a] on the induction of mutations by ultrasound. (Modified from Rott 1981; q.v. for references)

Authors	Test system	Intensity[b] (W/cm^2)	Frequency (MHz)	Length of exposure[c]	Result (negativ −, positive +)
		Unicellular organisms			
Ausländer (1966)	*Bact. tuberculosis*	?	1	5 min–3 h	−
Thacker (1974)	Yeast	11.3	0.02	5–30 min	−
Combes (1975)	*Bact. subtilis*	4	0.02	5–60 min	−
Combes (1975)	*Bact. subtilis*	10–60	1; 1,5; 2	5–60 min	−
Abel et al. (1981)	*Chlamydomonas*	15.5[d]; 193[e]	3.5	30 min	−
Barnett et al. (1982)	*Salmonella typhimur.*	100	3	5 min; 30 min	−
Wegner et al. (in preparation)	*Salmonella typhimur.*	0.01[d]; 33.5[e]	2.2; 1	30 min; 90 min	−
		Mammals			
Friedli (1951)	Rat	2; 4	0.8	1 min	−
Mohr and Reiter (1952)	Guinea pig	1.5–4.5	0.8	5–15 min	−
Kamocsay et al. (1955)	Rat	4	0.8; 2.8	0.5–4 min	−
Brüschke (1955)	Rabbit	3.5	1	5–15 min	−
Kirsten et al. (1963)	Mouse	0.14–4	1	5 min	−
Sunden (1964)	Rat	0.001–0.002[f]	1.5; 2.5	3 min	−
Smyth (1966)	Mouse	0.01	2.25	20 min	−
Loch (1969)	Rabbit	0.5; 3	0.87	5; 10; 15 min	−
		0.01[f]	0.87	5; 10; 15 min	−
Mannor et al. (1972)	Mouse	0.164–1.05	2.28	5 min; 60 min	−
Muranaka et al. (1972)	Mouse	0.02	2.3	6 h	−
Lyon et al. (1974)	Mouse	1.6	1.5	15 min	−
		6.4[g]; 45[g]	1.5	15 min	−
		Insects			
Wallace et al. (1948)	*Drosophila*	?[h]	0.4	?	+
Fritz-Niggli et al. (1950)	*Drosophila*	0.3–1.75	0.8	0.6–25 min	−
Kato (1966)	*Drosophila*	up to 30	0.56	5 min; 30 min	+
Grubbs et al. (1976)	Wasp	0.26–1.46	0.02	3–10 min	+

[a] Some studies were done primarily to detect teratogenic effects; however subsequent generations were followed up

[b] Spatial average continuous ultrasound, unless stated otherwise

[c] With multiple exposures, the length of individual exposure

[d] Continuous ultrasound, spatial peak

[e] Pulsed ultrasound, SPTP

[f] Pulsed ultrasound, SATA

[g] Pulsed ultrasound, SATP

[h] Only a total output of 150 W was indicated

intensities of above 8 mW/cm², but later they were unable to reproduce their findings and had to retract them (Macintosh et al. 1975). It is possible that their experimental arrangement gave rise to higher-intensity standing waves as a result of resonance, which may have been responsible for the effects observed. Interestingly, the author's retraction did not gain the same level of attention as their earlier publications and is frequently omitted even in recent literature surveys. The reasons for the increased rate of aberrations noted in the studies of Bugnon et al. (1972) are not apparent. Other authors were unable to produce aberrations even by short-term exposure to levels above 300 W/cm² (Coakley et al. 1972) and 35 W/cm² spatial peak intensity (Rott and Soldner 1973). In these experiments cellular suspensions were exposed to ultrasound with plastic films used as boundary surfaces. On the other hand, Fishman et al. (1972) exposed human lymphocytes to ultrasound in Petri dishes and found increased chromosomal aberrations at levels of 22 W/cm² or more; at 40 W/cm² most cells were destroyed.

Table 2.2. Studies on the induction of chromosome anomalies by ultrasound in vitro. (After Rott 1981; references listed chronologically)

Authors	Test system[a]	Intensity[b] (W/cm^2)	Frequency (MHz)	Length of exposure	Result (negative −)
Fischer et al. (1967)	Blood	3	0.81	10 min	−
Bernstine (1969)	Lymphocytes	0.02–0.03	6	18 h	−
Macintosh et al. (1970–75)	Lymphocytes	0.008–0.017	2	1 h; 2 h	Breaks/−
Bobrow et al. (1971)	Lymphocytes	0.014–2.77	1.5	1 min–1 h	−
Boyd et al. (1971)	Lymphocytes	0.03	2	13 h	−
	Lymphocytes	diagnostic[c]	1.5	13 h	−
Abdulla et al. (1972)	Lymphocytes	0.023–3.5	2	2 h–8 h	−
Bucton et al. (1972)	Lymphocytes, blood	0.03–3	1	1 h	−
Bugnon et al. (1972)	Lymphocytes	0.003	2.5	3 min; 5 min	Breaks
Coakley et al. (1972)	Lymphocytes, blood	1–350	1; 2.5; 3	20 s–30 min	−
Fischman et al. (1972)	Lymphocytes	5–90	1.3	2 min	Breaks beyond 22 W/cm^2
Hill et al. (1972)	CHO cells	150[c,d]	1	1 h; 2 h	−
Kunze-Mühl et al. (1972)	Blood	0.02; 3	2; 1	1 h; 10 min	−
Mannor et al. (1972)	Fetal mouse[e]	0.164–1.05	2.28	5 min–1 h	−
Watts et al. (1972)	Lymphocytes, blood	0.009–7.7	1; 2	2 h; 20 h	−
	Lymphocytes, blood	6.5–64[c,d]	1.5; 2; 2.5	2 h; 20 h	−
Brock et al. (1973)	Human and marsupial blood	0.4–425[f]	2.25	several sec–1 h	−
Mermut et al. (1973)	Lymphocytes, blood	0.003[c]	2.25	72 h; 90 h	−
Rott et al. (1973)	Lymphocytes, blood	0.002–35[f]	2; 0.87	5 min–24 h	−
	Lymphocytes, blood	10[c,d]	2	1 h–9 h	−
Sperling et al. (1973)	Lymphocytes	0.025	2.3	15 min–90 min	−
Braeman et al. (1974)	Lymphocytes	0.0064–0.08	1; 2.5	2 min–1 h	−
Lyon et al. (1974)	Mouse spermatocytes[g]	1.6	1.5	15	−
		1.6[c]	1.5	15	−
Thacker et al. (1976)	Drosophila	0.05–2	1	1–5	−
Roseboro et al. (1978)	Lymphocytes, HeLa cells	0.12–2.24	0.065	1	−
Harkanyi et al. (1978)	Mouse bone marrow[g]	0.1–1	0.8	5 min	−

[a] Human cells, unless stated otherwise
[b] Continuous ultrasound, unless stated otherwise
[c] Pulsed ultrasound
[d] Intensity (I_{SATP})
[e] Exposed in utero
[f] Continuous ultrasound, spatial peak
[g] Exposed in vivo in a study on comutagenesis with X-rays

These findings can be satisfactorily explained in terms of local thermal effects. Available studies indicate that ultrasound does not cause chromosomal damage when applied in the diagnostic range of frequencies and intensities.

Besides the mutagenicity tests cited above, sister chromatid exchanges (SCEs) have been used for some time as an indicator of mutagenic effects. SCE refers to the exchange of sister chromatids at homologous sites within a chromosome. These exchanges are detected by means of differential chromatid staining with 5-bromodeoxyuridine (BrdU). When this metabolite is introduced into cell cultures, it is incorporated in place of thymidine and thus alters the staining behavior of the substituted DNA. Because the DNA replicates in a semiconservative manner, after two cell divisions a chromosomal structure develops in which the two sister chromatids are differentially substituted and therefore stain differently (Figs. 2.1 and 2.2). This method enables the visualization of SCEs that have ocurred one cell cycle previously (see Wolff 1977 for technical details). Today SCEs are considered to be an expression of specific changes in the DNA. Some authors interpret them as the result of a successful cellular repair and compare the process to crossing-over in meiosis. A number of known mutagenic chemicals can induce SCEs, but ionizing radiation

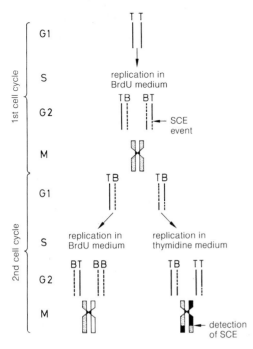

Fig. 2.1. Principle of differential chromatid staining for the detection of SCEs (T ——, thymidine-DNA strand; B -----, BrdU-DNA strand; $G1$, S, $G2$, M, phases of cell cycle). (After Rott 1982)

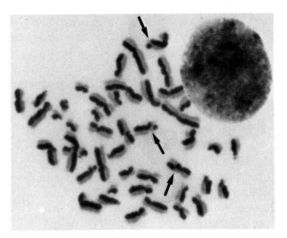

Fig. 2.2. Differential chromatid staining and SCEs (*arrows*) in human chromosomes. (Photo: G. Abel, Erlangen)

increases the SCE rate very little. Thus, the significance of SECs as an indicator of mutagenicity is controversial (Gebhart 1981). The biologic significance of SCEs is unknown.

Studies on the induction of SCEs by ultrasound are listed in Table 2.3. The findings of Liebeskind et al. (1979b) in lymphocytes were interpreted very cautiously by the authors

themselves, but their study was quickly cited in the lay press as evidence of chromosome damage by ultrasound and became a cause of general concern. A notable feature of this study was the fact that the increase in SCE rates fluctuated greatly in eight identical experiments, ranging from 20% to 100%. In addition, the findings with HeLa cells were not reproducible (Liebeskind et al. 1979a). Light, which is known to produce SCEs in BrdU-substituted DNA, could have caused the observed increases; it was not stated whether the experiments were conducted in light or darkness. The groups of Wegner and of Barnett were unable to confirm these findings, even though they used comparable exposure conditions. Haupt

Table 2.3. Studies on the induction of SCEs by ultrasound

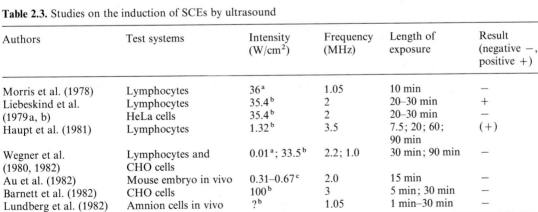

Authors	Test systems	Intensity (W/cm^2)	Frequency (MHz)	Length of exposure	Result (negative −, positive +)
Morris et al. (1978)	Lymphocytes	36[a]	1.05	10 min	−
Liebeskind et al. (1979a, b)	Lymphocytes	35.4[b]	2	20–30 min	+
	HeLa cells	35.4[b]	2	20–30 min	−
Haupt et al. (1981)	Lymphocytes	1.32[b]	3.5	7.5; 20; 60; 90 min	(+)
Wegner et al. (1980, 1982)	Lymphocytes and CHO cells	0.01[a]; 33.5[b]	2.2; 1.0	30 min; 90 min	−
Au et al. (1982)	Mouse embryo in vivo	0.31–0.67[c]	2.0	15 min	−
Barnett et al. (1982)	CHO cells	100[b]	3	5 min; 30 min	−
Lundberg et al. (1982)	Amnion cells in vivo	?[b]	1.05	1 min–30 min	−

[a] Continuous ultrasound (SP)
[b] Pulsed ultrasound (SPTP)
[c] Not stated whether continuous or pulsed ultrasound was used

et al. (1981) recorded average SCE increases of 5.1–6.8 SCEs/cell in their experiments. However, because this test system is highly susceptible to disturbance, rate increases of 100%–500% would be required to prove the induction of SCEs, and so these findings cannot be considered evidence of an adverse effect. Finally, we should comment on the study of Lundberg et al. (1982), which is included in Table 2.3 only for the sake of completeness. In this study amniotic fluid cells were exposed to ultrasound for 2–3 weeks in utero and then cultured before being substituted with BrdU. With this procedure, a positive result would be extremely unlikely even if the ultrasound did in fact increase SCE rates. Hence, this study should not be cited as evidence for the innocuousness of diagnostic ultrasound.

On the whole, available findings refute the notion that ultrasound induces sister chromatid exchanges. Whether ultrasound is capable of producing such an effect at all, and under which specific conditions it can be observed, remains to be determined.

2.2.4 Comutagenicity

An absence of mutagenicity does not necessarily mean that ultrasound does not enhance the effect of a known mutagen. To date, ultrasound has been investigated for comutagenicity only in connection with ionizing radiation. The potentiation of the bioeffects of ionizing radiation by ultrasound has been documented by a range of methodologies, including the monitoring of growth in cell cultures, plant growth, and the inhibition of tumor growth. An increase in X-ray-induced mutation rates on concomitant exposure to X-rays and ultrasound (9000 Hz) was demonstrated as early as 1948 by Conger in spores of *Tradescantia*, a tropical flowering plant. The first cytogenetic studies were performed by Kim (1968) and Kunze-Mühl (1975). The former found increased X-ray-induced chromosome aberrations, including exchange events, in lymphocyte cultures treated with X-rays at 50 R (12,900 μC/kg) combined with ultrasound (3 W/cm² at 0.8 MHz). Kunze-Mühl confirmed these findings for the 3 W/cm² level and also discovered that exposure to 0.02 W/cm² of continuous ultrasound at 2 MHz de-

creased the rate of X-ray-induced aberrations compared with X-irradiation alone. The author speculated that cellular repair systems became activated in this intensity range. If true, this would mean that ultrasound exposure at that level protects against the mutagenic effect of ionizing radiation. Ultrasound exposure before or more than 2 h after the X-irradiation had no impact on X-ray-induced aberration rates. Burr et al. (1978) treated human lymphocytes with a combination of ^{60}Co and ultrasound (3 W/cm² at 1 MHz) and found the same aberration-enhancing effect. On the other hand, Harkanyi et al. (1978) were unable to influence aberration rates in mouse bone marrow cells exposed in vivo to X-rays and ultrasound (0.1 and 1 W/cm² at 0.8 MHz), presumably due to absorption of the ultrasound at the body surface.

No other systematic studies on this question are available. For the present, it will have to be assumed that ultrasound intensities above 1 W/cm² can have a comutagenic effect if the exposure follows X-irradiation. Prior ultrasound exposure does not appear to have this effect. The comutagenic properties of diagnostic pulsed ultrasound having a low average intensity but a high peak intensity have not yet been investigated.

2.2.5 Other Effects

In addition to the studies cited above, a large volume of material has been published dealing with various other biologic effects of ultrasound. While these effects must of course be considered potentially deleterious, they should not automatically be interpreted as being injurious to health. Some of these findings will be reviewed briefly.

The proliferative behavior of cell cultures can be inhibited or stimulated by ultrasound. Temperature elevation appears to be the basic mechanism for these effects (Bleanley et al. 1972). Presumably the same mechanism underlies the ability of ultrasound to stimulate the in vitro protein synthesis of fibroblasts (Harvey et al. 1975), to promote the regeneration of tissue defects in the rabbit ear (Dyson et al. 1970), and to accelerate the healing of varicose ulcers (Dyson et al. 1976).

When the testis is directly exposed to continuous ultrasound at therapeutic levels, an arrest of spermatogenesis, probably thermally induced, is obtained both in experimental animals and in man (Fahim et al. 1981). A diminished immune response was found in mice whose spleens had previously been treated with diagnostic ultrasound (Anderson and Barrett 1979). In the chicken embryo, a stationary, continuous ultrasound field produced a hematologic disturbance in which the erythrocytes became aggregated into bands spaced one-half wavelength apart (Dyson et al. 1974). All these effects were reversible.

In vitro erythrocytes were found to release ATP on ultrasound exposure when plastic film containing air bubbles had previously been placed into the cell suspension. In a similar experimental arrangement the release of β-thromboglobin from blood platelets was observed (Williams et al. 1981; Williams and Miller 1980). It is unclear whether this was a result of membrane alterations or cytolysis. Similar effects could not be demonstrated in vivo. While these findings are relevant to the understanding of the biologic effects of ultrasound, they offer no evidence of adverse effects in vivo.

2.3 The Problem of Safe Levels

Because higher ultrasound intensities apparently have the ability to cause lesions, there has been much interest in defining what constitutes a "safe" level of exposure. The recommendations made by Ulrich and Wells in 1974 are not only questionable from a methodologic standpoint (they evaluated a wide range of published findings), but are also antiquated and no longer suitable as a basis for discussion (see critique in Rott 1981). Moreover, because the establishment of "safe levels" without sufficient knowledge and data might create an unjustified sense of security on the one hand, while also implying dangers that may not exist, the American Institute of Ultrasound in Medicine (AIUM) has taken a more pragmatic approach. Its Bioeffects Committee formulated a statement in 1976 which was slightly revised in 1978 (AIUM Bioeffects Committee 1979) and currently reads as follows:

Statement on the Biologic Effects of Ultrasound in Mammals In Vivo

As of October, 1978, no definite, confirmed biologic effects have occurred in mammals exposed to ultrasound intensities[1] below 100 mW/cm² in the frequency range of several megahertz. Even at higher intensities, no such effects were found when, in exposure times[2] of more than 1 s and less than 500 s, the product of intensity and exposure time was less than 50 J/cm².

[1] Spatial peak-temporal average intensity measured in the free field in water
[2] Total time spanning the interval between activation and deactivation of the pulsed beam

---

This represents a policy statement and a summary of evidence presently available on the bioeffects of ultrasound; it is not intended to define safe levels of exposure. It pertains exclusively to in vivo effects and is entirely consistent with the findings in recent publications. It does not state that ultrasound is definitely harmless within the limits indicated, or that adverse effects are inevitable if those limits are exceeded. When petitioned by the U.S. Food and Drug Administration to define safe exposure limits, the AIUM declined, stating that it was unable to do so on the basis of available evidence. For the present, the statement of the AIUM may be regarded as the best available guide in matters relating to ultrasound safety.

Another question that is relevant to the safety issue concerns the possibility of a cumulative effect from prolonged exposure to low levels of ultrasound, like those associated with the monitoring of fetal heart activity. This seems extremely unlikely on physical and theoretical grounds, and no such effect has yet been reported. An analogy with ionizing radiation is misleading, because it is an entirely different form of energy with a different pattern of spatial distribution.

2.4 Concluding Remarks

After surveying the available literature on the bioeffects of ultrasound, one must conclude that the use of diagnostic ultrasound does not pose a significant health risk to the patient or the user. If a potential for injury does exist, it is apparently so small that years of laboratory and clinical investigation have failed to disclose it.

The objection of some authors that the status of medical ultrasound is comparable to that of X-rays 50 years ago may be correct with regard to its potential for future development, but it cannot be validly applied to questions of safety. Fifty years ago the mutagenic effect of X-rays was first demonstrated in experiments on *Drosophila*. Since then, mutagenic research has become an established discipline in its own right, and a number of effective test methods have been developed, most of which were available when diagnostic ultrasound was introduced. Similar advances have been witnessed in teratology. Thus, the foregoing objection implies an unjustified level of uncertainty in the assumption that diagnostic ultrasound is innocuous.

A second objection, that animal experiments and studies in isolated cellular material are not applicable to humans and therefore irrelevant, is likewise unsound. It may have some validity in studies of chemical mutagenesis, because species-specific differences in hepatic metabolism may cause test substances to be metabolized differently. But in the case of ultrasound, adverse effects would involve a direct action on genetic information, whose carrier in all living organisms is DNA, and which is present in the form of chromosomes in countless organisms from protozoans to man. This explains why it has been possible to derive the basic principles of human genetics from studies of organisms like *Drosophila* and the pea. It also explains why laboratory mammals and their cells make excellent objects for studying the genetic effects of ultrasound.

Given the current trend toward the use of higher ultrasound frequencies as a means of enhancing image quality, which also requires that the pulse intensity be increased to obtain adequate penetration, there is a definite need for further investigations – particularly experiments using very high peak intensities administered in pulsed form.

Because no persuasive evidence of potential adverse health effects from diagnostic ultrasound has yet been produced, and a cumulative effect seems extremely unlikely, there is no reason why diagnostic ultrasound cannot be utilized for a wide range of indications. It is partic-ularly reommended in situations where it could reduce exposure to ionizing radiation.

References

Abdulla U, Campbell S, Dewhurst CJ, Talbert D, Lucas M, Mullarkey M (1971) Effect of diagnostic ultrasound on maternal and fetal chromosomes. Lancet II:829–831

Abel G, Rott H-D, Soldner R (1981) Safety of ultrasound: Genetic studies with Chlamydomonas as test object. In: Kurjak A, Kratochwil A (eds) Recent advances in ultrasound diagnosis 3. Excerpta Med Internat Congr Series Nr 553. Excerpta Medica, Amsterdam Oxford Princeton, pp 39–41

AIUM Bioeffects Committee (1979) AIUM responds to EDA notice of intent for diagnostic ultrasound. Reflections 5:299

Anderson DW, Barret JT (1979) Ultrasound: A new immunosuppressant. Clin Immunol Immunpathol 14:18–29

Au WW, Obergoenner N, Goldenthal KL, Corry PM, Willingham V (1982) Sister-chromatid exchanges in mouse embryos after exposure to ultrasound in utero. Mutat Res 103:315–320

Ausländer D, Pop E, Buzila A, Veress A, Ardevan A (1966) The action of ultrasound on Koch's Bacillus. Microbiol Parazitol Epidemiol 11:9–14

Barnett SB, Bonin A, Mitchell G, Meher-Homji KM, Baker RSU (1982) An investigation of the mutagenic potential of pulsed ultrasound. Br J Radiol 55:501–504

Bernstine RL (1969) Safety studies with ultrasonic Doppler technique. A clinical follow-up of patients and tissue culture study. Obstet Gynecol 34:707–709

Bleanley BI, Blackbourn P, Kirley J (1972) Resistance of CHLF hamster cells to ultrasonic radiation of 1,5 MHz frequency. Br J Radiol 45:354–357

Boyd E, Abdulla U, Donald I, Fleming JEE, Hall AJ, Ferguson-Smith MA (1971) Chromosome breakage and ultrasound. Br Med J 2:501–502

Brüschke G (1955) Tierexperimentelle Untersuchungen zur Frage der Schädigung von Testis, Ovar und gravidem Uterus durch Ultraschall. Z gesamte Inn Med 10:895

Bugnon C, Cottin Y, Kraehenbuhl J, Weill F (1972) Aberrations chromosomiques provoquées par des ultrasons diagnostiqués sur des lymphocytes humains en culture. J Radiol 53:750–755

Burr JG, Wald N, Pan S, Preston K jun (1978) The synergistic effect of ultrasound and ionising radiation on human lymphocytes. In: Evans HJ, Lloyd DC (eds) Mutagen induced chromosome damage in man. Edinburgh University Press, Edinburgh, pp 120–128

Coakley WT, Slade JS, Braeman JM, Moore JL (1972) Examination of lymphocytes for chromosome aberrations after ultrasonic irradiation. Br J Radiol 45:328–332

Combes RD (1975a) Inability of genetic systems of Bacillus subtilis to detect a mutagenic effect of low frequency ultrasound. J Appl Bact 39:219–226

Combes RD (1975b) Absence of mutation following ultrasonic treatment of Bacillus subtilis cells and transforming deoxyribonucleic acid. Br J Radiol 48:306–311

Conger AD (1948) The cytogenetic effect of sonic energy applied simultaneously with X-rays. Proc Natl Acad Sci USA 34:470–474

Curto KA (1976) Early post partum mortality following ultrasound radiation. In: White DN, Barnes R (eds) Ultrasound in medicine, vol 2. Plenum, New York, pp 535–536

Dewhurst CJ (1971) The safety of ultrasound. Proc Roy Soc Med 64:996–997

Dyson M, Pond JB, Joseph J, Warwick R (1970) Stimulation of tissue regeneration by pulsed plane wave ultrasound. IEEE Transact Son Ultrason SU-17:133–140

Dyson M, Pond JB, Woodward B, Broatbent J (1974) The production of blood cell stasis and endothelial damage in the blood vessels of chick embryos treated with ultrasound in a stationary wave field. Ultrasound Med Biol 1:133–148

Dyson M, Franks C, Suckling J (1976) Stimulation of healing of varicose ulcers by ultrasound. Ultrasonics 14:232–236

Fahim MS, Fahim S, Der R, Hall DG, Harman J (1981) Heat in male contraception (hot water 60°, infrared, microwave and ultrasound) Contraception 1:235–254

Fishman HK, Coleman DJ, Lizzi FL (1972) Effects of ultrasound on human chromosomes. J Cell Biol 55:74a

Friedli P (1951) Ultraschall und Ovar. Gynaecol (Basel) 131:97

Gebhart E (1981) Sister chromatid exchange (SCE) and structural chromosome aberration in mutagenicity testing. Hum Genet 58:235–254

Haerten R (1980) Technische Kenngrößen von Ultraschalldiagnosegeräten und ihre Bestimmung. Ultraschall 1:1–11

Hara K (1980) Effects of ultrasonic irradiation on chromosomes, cell division and developing embryos. Acta Obstet Gynecol Jpn 32:61–68

Harkanyi Z, Szollar J, Vigvari Z (1978) A search for an effect of ultrasound alone and in combination with X-rays on chromosomes in vivo. Br J Radiol 51:46–49

Harvey W, Dyson M, Pond JB, Grahame R (1976) The in-vitro stimulation of protein synthesis in human fibroblasts by therapeutic levels of ultrasound. In: Excerpta Medica International Congress Series No 363. Proc 2nd European Congress on Ultrasonics in Medicine. Munich, May 1975. Excerpta Medica, Amsterdam Oxford

Haupt M, Martin AO, Simpson JL, Iqbal MA, Elias S, Dyer A, Sabbagha RE (1981) Ultrasonic induction of sister chromatid exchanges in human lymphocytes. Hum Genet 59:221–226

Hellmann W (1980) Embryotoxische Wirkungen durch erhöhte mütterliche Körpertemperaturen und E. Coli Endotoxin beim Kaninchen Oryctolagus cuniculus L. Habilitationsschrift, Wuppertal

Hellman LM, Duffus GM, Donald I, Sunden B (1970) Safety of diagnostic ultrasound in obstetrics. Lancet I:1133–1134

Hill Cr, Ter Haar G (1982) Ultrasound. In: Suess MJ (ed) Nonionizing radiation protection. WHO Europa, Copenhagen, pp 199–228

Holländer H-J (1972) Die Ultraschalldiagnostik in der Schwangerschaft. Urban & Schwarzenberg, München Berlin Wien

Hrazdira I (1980) Ultrastructural changes caused by ultrasound. In: Kurjak A (ed) Recent advances in ultrasound diagnosis 2. Excerpta Medica, International Congress Series 498. Excerpta Medica, Amsterdam Oxford Princeton, pp 108–110

Ikeuchi T, Sasaki M, Oshimura M, Azumi J, Tsuji K, Shimizu T (1973) Ultrasound and embryonic chromosomes. Br Med J 1:112

Kamocsay D, Gy DO (1958) Ultrasound in gynecology. Am J Phys Med 37:196

Kim AM (1968) Chromosomenanalysen nach Behandlung von menschlichem Venenblut mit Röntgenstrahlen und Ultraschall. Phil. Dissertation, Wien

Koranyi G, Falus M, Sobel M, Pesti E, Van Bao T (1972) Follow-up examination of children exposed to ultrasound in utero. Acta Paediatr Acad Sci Hung 13:231–238

Kunze-Mühl E (1975) Chromosome damage in human lymphocytes after different combinations of X-ray and ultrasonic treatment. Proc 2nd Europ Congr on Ultrasonics in Medicine, München 1975. Excerpta Medica, Amsterdam Oxford

Levi S, Gustot P, Galperin-Lemaitre H (1974) In vivo effect of ultrasound at human therapeutic doses on marrow cell chromosomes of golden hamster. Humangenetik 25:133–141

Liebeskind D, Bases R, Elequin F, Neubert S, Leiter R, Goldberg R, Koenigsberg M (1979a) Diagnostic ultrasound: effects on the DNA and growth patterns of animal cells. Radiology 131:177–184

Liebeskind D, Bases R, Mendez F, Elequin F, Koenigsberg M (1979b) Sister chromatid exchange in human lymphocytes after exposure to diagnostic ultrasound. Science 205:1273–1275

Loch EG (1971) Experimentelle Untersuchungen mit Ultraschall am Kaninchenovar. In: Böck J et al. (Hrsg) Ultrasonographica Medica. 1. Weltkongreß über Ultraschalldiagnostik in der Medizin und SIDUO III, Wien 1969. Verlag der Wiener Med Akademie, Wien, S. 503–511

Lucas M, Mullarkey M, Abdulla U (1972) Study of chromosomes in the newborn after ultrasonic fetal heart monitoring in labour. Br Med J 3:795–796

Lundberg M, Jerominski L, Livingston G, Kochenour N, Lee T, Fineman R (1982) Failure to demonstrate an effect of in vivo diagnostic ultrasound on sister chromatid exchange in amniotic fluid cells. Am J Med Genet 11:31–35

Macintosh IJC, Davey DA (1970) Chromosome aberrations induced by an ultrasonic fetal pulse detector. Br Med J 4:92–93

Macintosh IJC, Davey DA (1972) Relationship between intensity of ultrasound and induction of chromosome aberrations. Br J Radiol 45:320–327

Macintosh IJC, Brown RC, Coakley WT (1975) Ultrasound and 'in vitro' chromosome aberrations. Br J Radiol 48:230–232

Mannor SM, Serr DM, Tamari I, Meshorer A, Frei E (1972) The safety of ultrasound in fetal monitoring. Am J Obstet Gynecol 113:653–661

Morris SM, Palmer CG, Fry FJ, Johnson LK (1978)

Effect of ultrasound on human leucocytes. Sister chromatid exchange analysis. Ultrasound Med Biol 4:253–258

O'Brien WD (1976) Ultrasonically induced fetal weight reduction in mice. In: White DN, Barnes R (eds) Ultrasound in medicine, vol 2. Plenum, New York, pp 531–532

Pizzarello DJ, Vivino A, Madden B, Wolsky A, Keegan AF, Becker M (1978) Effect of pulsed low-power ultrasound on growing tissues. I. Developing mammalian and insect tissue. Exp Cell Biol 46:179–191

Rott H-D (1981) Zur Frage der Schädigungsmöglichkeit durch diagnostischen Ultraschall. Ultraschall 2:56–64

Rott H-D (1982) Sicherheitsaspekte der Ultraschalldiagnostik. Swiss Med 4:11–15

Rott H-D, Soldner R (1973) The effect of ultrasound on human chromosomes in vitro. Humangenetik 20:100–112

Scheidt PC, Stanley F, Bryla DA (1978) One-year follow-up of infants exposed to ultrasound in utero. Am J Obstet Gynecol 131:743–748

Serr DM, Padeh B, Zakut HJ, Shaki R, Mannor SM, Kalner B (1970) Studies on the effects of ultrasonic waves in the fetus. Second Europ Congr of Perinatal Medicine, London

Shoji R, Murakami U, Shimizu T (1975) Influence of low intensity ultrasonic irradiation on prenatal development of two inbred mouse strains. Teratology 12:227–231

Sunden B (1964) On the diagnostic value of ultrasound in obstetrics and gynecology. Acta Obstet Gynecol Scand XLIII [Suppl 6]

Taylor KJW, Pond JB (1972) A study of the production of haemorrhagic injury and paraplegia in spinal rat cord by pulsed ultrasound of low mega Hertz frequencies in the context of the safety for clinical usage. Br J Radiol 45:343–353

Ter Haar GR, Williams AR (1981) Biophysical and physiological consequences of ultrasonic irradiation of tissue. In: Kurjak A, Kratochwil A (eds) Recent advances in ultrasound diagnosis 3. Excerpta Med Internat Congr Series Nr 553. Excerpta Medica, Amsterdam Oxford Princeton, pp 33–36

Ulrich WD (1974) Ultrasound dosage for nontherapeutic use on human beings. Extrapolation from a literature survey. IEEE Trans Biomechan Eng BM 21:48–51

Webster D, Pond JB, Dyson M, Harvey W (1978) The role of cavitation in the vitro stimulation of protein synthesis in human fibroblasts by ultrasound. Ultrasound Med Biol 4:343

Wegner R-D, Meyenburg M (1982) The effects of diagnostic ultrasonography on the frequencies of sister chromatid exchange in Chinese hamster cells and human lymphocytes. J Ultrasound Med 1:355–358

Wegner R-D, Obe G, Meyenburg M (1980) Has diagnostic ultrasound mutagenic effects? Hum Genet 56:95–98

Wells PNT (1974) The possibility of harmful biological effects in ultrasonic diagnosis. In: Reneman RS (ed) Cardiovascular application of ultrasound. North-Holland, Amsterdam London, pp 1–17

Williams AR, Miller DL (1980) Photometric detection of ATP release from human erythrocytes exposed to ultrasonically activated gas-filled pores. Ultrasound Med Biol 6:251–256

Williams AR, Chater BV, Allen KA, Sanderson KH (1981) The use of β-thromboglobin to detect platelet damage by therapeutic ultrasound in vivo. J Clin Ultrasound 9:145–151

Wolff S (1977) Sister chromatid exchange. Ann Rev Genet 11:183–201

Zweifel HJ (1979) Ultraschall in der Medizin: Eine aktuelle Anwendung von elektronischer Diagnosetechnik. Bull SEV/VSE 70:917–923

AIUM Statement on Clinical Safety

At the October 18–19, 1983 meeting of the Board of Governors, the following slightly revised statement on the clinical safety of ultrasound was approved.

Diagnostic ultrasound has been in use for over 25 years. Given its known benefits and recognized efficacy for medical diagnosis, including use during human pregnancy, the American Institute of Ultrasound in Medicine herein addresses the clinical safety of such use:

No confirmed biological effects on patients or instrument operators caused by exposure at intensities typical of present diagnostic ultrasound instruments have ever been reported. Although the possibility exists that such biological effects may be identified in the future, current data indicate that the benefits to patients of the prudent use of diagnostic ultrasound outweigh the risks, if any, that may be present.

October 1982, revised March 1983 and October 1983

3 Examination of the Female Pelvis

3.1 General

The pioneering work of Donald et al. (1958) dealt with the possibility of visualizing lower abdominal structures by ultrasound. Today all modern ultrasound instruments can demonstrate normal anatomic structures in the pelvis, a knowledge of which is fundamental to diagnosis.

Generally, scans are performed with a full urinary bladder. This is accomplished either by having the patient drink about a liter of fluid an hour before the examination or, rarely, by retrograde filling. With the bladder adequately distended, it is possible to visualize the uterus, ovaries, pelvic blood vessels, and occasionally the fallopian tubes. The main purpose of a full bladder is to displace gas-filled bowel loops that might otherwise obstruct visualization of the pelvis. A full bladder also creates an acoustic window which, with most transducers, will permit the uterus and adnexa to be imaged in the optimum focal region of the ultrasound beam (Fig. 3.1 a, b).

Excessive filling of the urinary bladder is undesirable, because an overdistended bladder may displace organs of interest out of the focal zone and limit evaluation.

In contrast to the bladder, the distal bowel should be as empty as possible for ultrasound scanning. This particularly applies to the sigmoid colon, which can obstruct visualization of the left adnexa. Preliminary evacuation of the bowel should be considered and the patient prepared accordingly.

3.1.1 Selection of Equipment

At one time the compound scanner was the instrument of choice owing to its excellent resolution and depth of penetration. Modern real-time scanners also provide excellent resolution and depth, and their image quality equals or surpasses that of many compound instruments. The disadvantage of real-time scanners is their relatively narrow image field.

Sector scanners are generally preferred to the linear-array types, as their smaller contact area allows greater freedom in the selection of scanning angles.

3.1.2 Examination Procedure

Normally the patient is examined in the supine position. The first scan is made in the sagittal plane through the umbilicus, and then parallel scans are made by shifting the transducer to the right and left of the midline. Transverse scans complete the examination. Women after the 20th week of pregnancy should be examined in a position with slight left lateral tilt to prevent supine hypotensive syndrome.

3.1.3 Findings

The uterus appears as a pear-shaped organ situated between the urinary bladder and rectum. The fundus, body, and cervix of the uterus are easily identified on the sonographic image (Figs. 3.2–3.5). The length of the body and fundus can be measured and ranges between 4 and 8 cm. The width of the body is about 3–5 cm. The myometrium is approximately 8–14 mm thick. The normal uterine position is anteverted and anteflexed (Figs. 3.2, 3.3), but a retroflexed uterus can also be demonstrated (Fig. 3.4). Because the retroflexed uterus projects posteriorly, especially when the bladder is very distended, the fundus may not be depicted in its entirety by linear-array scanners having a 14- to 16-cm depth of penetration. Sector and compound scanners are advantageous in such cases.

The typical trumpet-shaped contour of the fallopian tube is generally not depicted even in transverse scans, because the tube is seldom in one plane for its entire length (Fig. 3.6). The same is true of the uterine ligaments (round ligaments, parametria), which are rarely visualized (Fig. 3.7).

Using the scanning procedure described, one can shift the transducer farther laterally to demonstrate the ovary on a longitudinal scan (Figs. 3.8–3.10). Often the ovary presents as a relatively echo-poor mass exhibiting both cystic and solid components. The average ovarian diameter is 2–2.5 cm. In some cases ovarian diameters may appear increased owing to an elongation of ovarian shape; generally, however, it is safe to assume that ovaries with diameters of 4 cm or more are significantly enlarged. The normal measurable volume is 15 cm³ or less.

The ovary is subject to cyclic physiologic changes that can be monitored sonographically on the basis of follicular growth. Early in the ovarian cycle the follicles commonly present as multiple cystic structures, one appearing notably larger than the rest (Figs. 3.8, 3.10). Follicles larger than 5–8 mm in diameter can usually be resolved with good-quality equipment (see Chap. 15).

Ultrasound consistently demonstrates blood vessels along the pelvic side wall, especially the vessels of the infundibulopelvic ligament (ovarian artery and vein), which show a constant relationship to the ovaries (Figs. 3.10, 3.11) and thus provide a useful reference plane for locating these structures (Hackelöer and Nitschke-Dabelstein 1981).

Another useful landmark is the internal iliac artery (Fig. 3.9). This vessel courses superior to the ovary and is easily identified in real-time scans by its obvious pulsation. However, only about 80% of scans will depict both the artery and the ovary on the same image.

All these blood vessels vary appreciably in size during the course of the normal menstrual cycle, often reaching as much as 10 mm in diameter (Fig. 3.12). The iliac bifurcation may be visualized in some cases.

Transverse scans sometimes show two well-defined, echogenic structures located some distance lateral to the uterus (Fig. 3.13). These structures, which may be mistaken for the ovaries, represent portions of the os coxae with their surrounding connective tissue and muscles. Frequently the ovaries can be seen in the same scan and identified by their associated blood vessels.

A transverse scan performed too far cranially may demonstrate the psoas muscles located immediately adjacent to the spine (Fig. 3.14). These also may be confused with the ovaries.

Longitudinal scans frequently show an elongated, complex structure situated behind the uterus that may mimic the uterus itself or a retrouterine mass (Figs. 3.15, 3.16). Usually this is a fluid-filled segment of rectum or small bowel. Real-time scans will often show peristaltic movement within the "mass", disclosing its true nature. The same applies to smaller cystic areas. Adnexal varicosis, or pelvic congestion syndrome, is a condition that may mimic the appearance of follicular structures (Fig. 3.17).

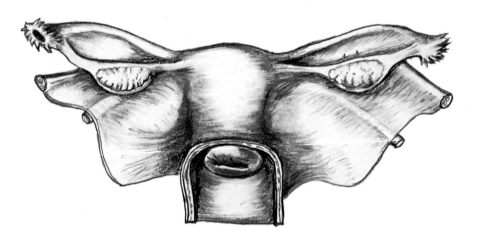

Fig. 3.1a

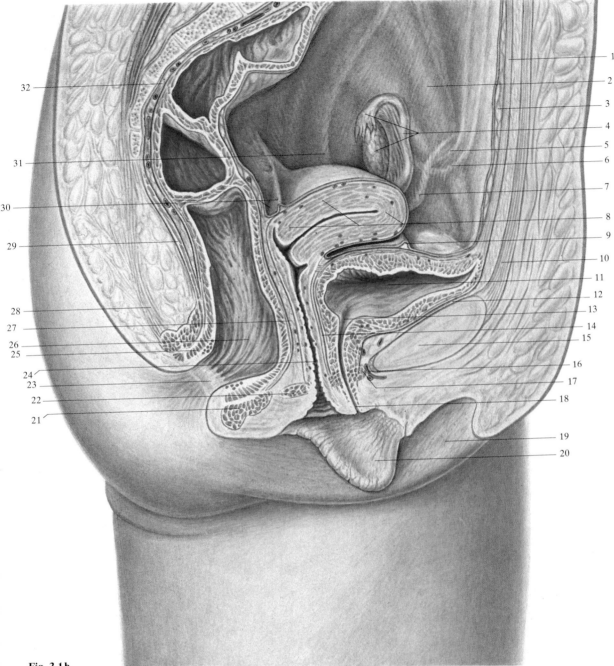

32
31
30
29
28
27
26
25
24
23
22
21

1
2
3
4
5
6
7
8
9
10
11
12
13
14
15
16
17
18
19
20

Fig. 3.1 b

Fig. 3.1. a Uterus and adnexa, anterior view. **b** Female pelvis, sagittal view: *1* Median umbilical ligament; *2* external iliac artery; *3* preperitoneal connective tissue; *4* fallopian tube, ovary, infundibulum; *5* lateral umbilical fold; *6* medial umbilical fold; *7* round ligament; *8* cervix, corpus, fundus uteri; *9* transverse vesical fold; *10* linea alba; *11* urinary bladder; *12* prevesical space; *13* bladder neck; *14* vesicovaginal space; *15* symphysis pubis; *16* clitoral vein; *17* pubovesical muscle; *18* urethra; *19* labium majus; *20* labium minus; *21* external anal sphincter; *22* deep transverse perineal muscle; *23* anal canal; *24* vagina; *25* internal anal sphincter; *26* rectal ampulla; *27* rectovaginal space; *28* rectal sling; *29* rectococcygeus muscle; *30* rectouterine fold, rectouterine pouch (cul-de-sac); *31* ureter; *32* presacral space

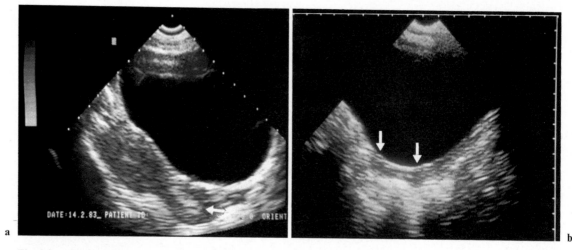

Fig. 3.2. a Median longitudinal scan of pelvis with full bladder. Uterine fundus on left, cervix on right (*arrow*).
b Prepubertal uterus, length 19 mm

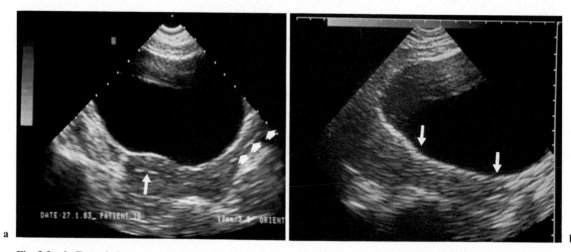

Fig. 3.3a, b. Extended uterus with endometrial and vaginal echoes (**a**, *arrows*), elongated cervix (**b**, *arrows*)

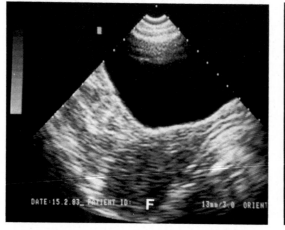

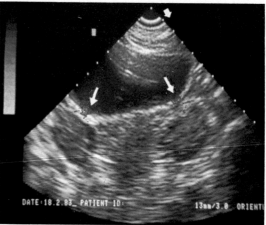

Fig. 3.4. Retroverted and retroflexed uterus, fundus (*F*)   **Fig. 3.5.** Transverse scan of uterus and ovaries (*arrows*)

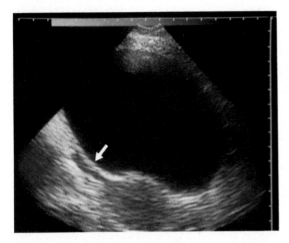

Fig. 3.6. Right fallopian tube (*arrow*)

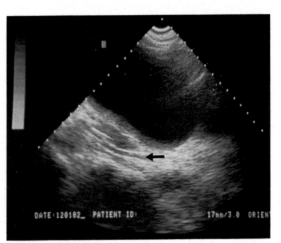

Fig. 3.9. Lateral longitudinal scan of pelvic wall (*arrow*, internal iliac artery)

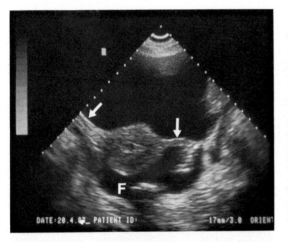

Fig. 3.7. Uterus with round ligament (*arrows*); fluid in cul-de-sac (*F*)

Fig. 3.10. Ovary with maturing follicle (15 mm) and blood vessels of pelvic side wall (*arrows*)

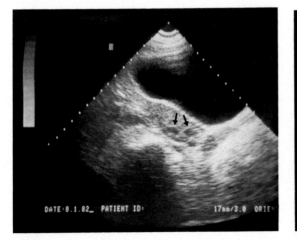

Fig. 3.8. Longitudinal scan of ovary; follicle diameter less than 5 mm (*arrows*)

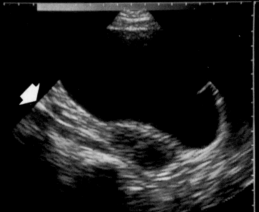

Fig. 3.11. Infundibulopelvic ligament (suspensory ligament of the ovary) with blood vessels (*arrow*)

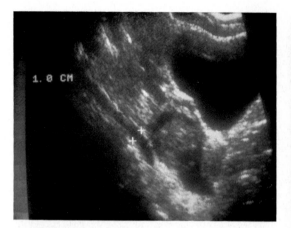

Fig. 3.12. Periovulatory dilatation of the ovarian blood vessels (10 mm)

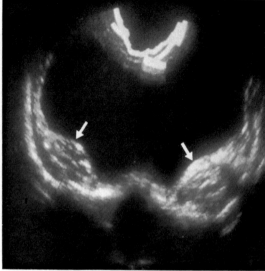

Fig. 3.14. Transverse scan depicting iliopsoas muscles (*arrows*). The bladder is overdistended

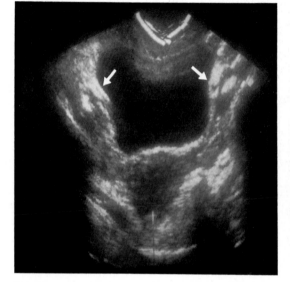

Fig. 3.13. Transverse scan of uterus showing iliac crests (*arrows*). These should not be mistaken for ovaries

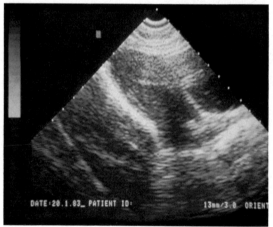

Fig. 3.15. Longitudinal scan showing full bowel posterior to uterus

The normal uterine and ovarian dimensions are as follows (modified from von Lanz and Wachsmuth 1984, pp. 272 and 283):

a) Uterus

Length (cm)

Before puberty	1.5–3
Nullipara	6–8
Multipara	7.5–9
Gravida (term)	37.5

Width (cm)

Body

Before puberty	0.5–1
Nullipara	3–5.5
Multipara	5–6
Gravida (term)	26

Cervix

Nullipara	1.5–3
Multipara	2.7–3.2

Anterior-posterior diameter (cm)

Fundus	2.2–4
Cervix	1.5–2.5

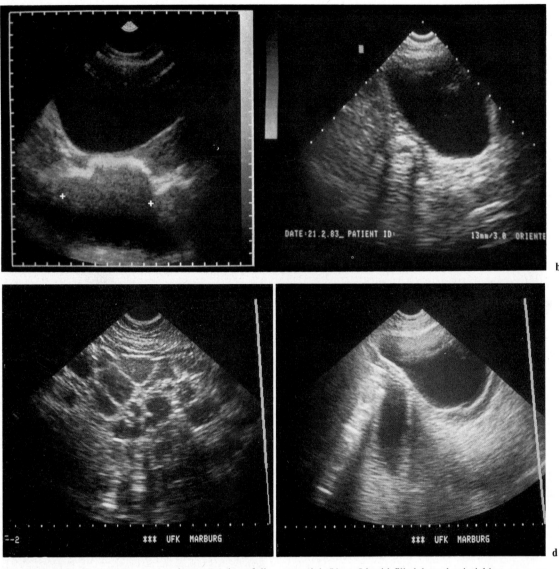

Fig. 3.16. a–d. Transverse scans demonstrating full bowel posterior to uterus (**a**) with shadowing from fecal material (**b**). **c** Liquid-filled bowel mimicking cysts or follicles. **d** Gas-filled bowel over adnexal area

Wall thickness (cm)			**b) Ovary**	
Nullipara	1–1.5		Size variable	
Multipara	2.0		*Length* (cm)	
Anterior wall	0.5–1		Neonate	2
Posterior wall	1.2–1.6		Child	2.5
Gravida (term)	1.4		Adult	3–5
			Weight (g)	
Relative lengths (cm)			Neonate	0.5
Body:cervix	4.2:2.5 (nullipara)		Child	2–3
	5.5:2.5 (multipara)		Adult	6–8

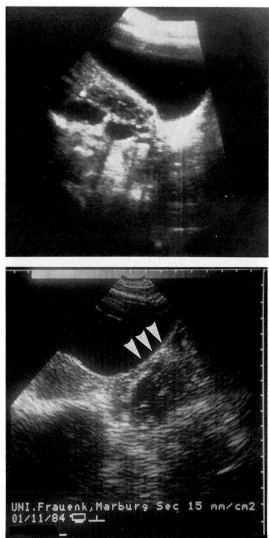

Kurtz AB, Rifkin MD (1983) Normal anatomy of the female pelvis. In: Callen PW (ed) Ultrasonography in obstetrics and gynecology. Saunders, Philadelphia, p 193

Lanz T von, Wachsmuth W (1984) Praktische Anatomie, 2. Bd: Teil 8A Becken. Springer, Berlin Heidelberg New York Tokyo

Sample WF (1980) Gray scale ultrasonography of the normal female pelvis. In: Saunders RC, James AE (eds) The principles and practice of ultrasonography in obstetrics and gynecology, 2nd edn. Appleton-Century-Crafts, New York, p 75

3.2 Pelvimetry

The sonographic measurement of pelvic dimensions was described some years ago by Kratochwil (1972), but pertained exclusively to the

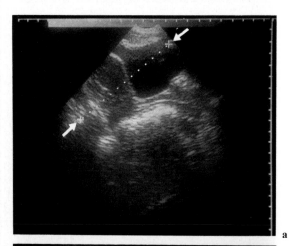

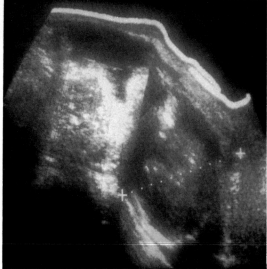

Fig. 3.17. a Longitudinal scan demonstrating cystic structures posterior to ovary (varicose veins!). **b** Large varicose vein over left adnexal area (*arrows*)

References

Callen PW, De Martini WJ, Filly RA (1979) The central uterine cavity echo: A useful anatomic sign in the ultrasonographic evaluation of the female pelvis. Am J Obstet Gynecol 131:187

Donald I (1965) Ultrasonic echo sounding in obstetrical and gynecological diagnosis. Am J Obstet Gynecol 93:935

Donald I, MacVicar J, Brown TG (1958) Investigation of abdominal masses by pulsed ultrasound. Lancet I:1188

Hackelöer BJ, Nitschke-Dabelstein S (1980) Ovarian imaging by ultrasound: An attempt to define a reference plane. JCU 9:275

Kratochwil A, Urban G, Friedrich F (1972) Ultrasonic tomography of the ovaries. Ann Chir Gynaecol 61:211

Fig. 3.18. a Sector scan showing true conjugate from posterior wall of symphysis to sacral promontory (10.6 cm). **b** Compound scan (12.1 cm)

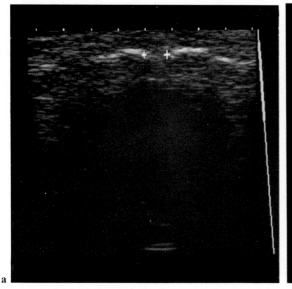

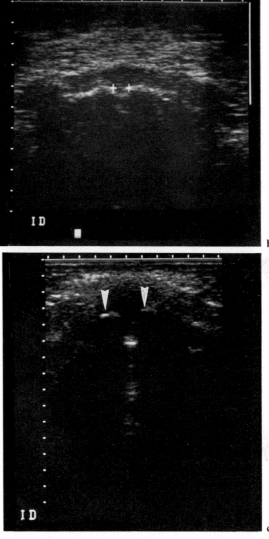

Fig. 3.19. a Normal distance of symphysis tissue of 7 mm. **b** Symphysiolysis of 12 mm (*arrows*). **c** Slightly enlarged distance of 8.5 mm after therapy

use of compound scanners and has not been widely applied. Nevertheless, we were able to show in a series of over 100 pelvimetries that high-resolution compound scanning is as accurate as X-ray pelvimetry in measuring the true conjugate of the pelvis.

A longitudinal scan is made between the umbilicus and symphysis in an attempt to outline the pelvic contour and to visualize the symphysis and sacral promontory on one image. When the correct points of measurement are selected on the posterior surface of the symphysis and sacral promontory, the true conjugate can be determined to an accuracy of 3 mm (Fig. 3.18).

It should be emphasized that this technique

requires a considerable amount of experience, and that a compound scanner must be used to obtain consistently accurate measurements. Real-time scanners (sector scanners) will accurately measure the true conjugate in only a small percentage of cases. Schlensker (1979) measured the true conjugate in 776 women and found the sonographic measurement to be about 2 mm less than the value measured intraoperatively and about 2 mm greater than that measured radiographically. The discrepancy between sonographic and intraoperative measurements was no more than 1 cm in 85% of cases (range of +19 to −18 mm).

X-ray pelvimetry is unquestionably more in-

34

formative than sonographic pelvimetry owing to its ability to diagnose abnormalities of pelvic shape. As an aid to decision-making in the management of breech presentations, we recommend that X-ray pelvimetry be combined with sonographic assessment of fetal head size (biparietal and occipitofrontal diameters: BPD and OFD).

Based on a series of 50 measurements of the symphysis pubis where we compared ultrasound and X-ray technique, we believe that ultrasound is as valuable as X-ray for the measurement of the symphysis fissure (Fig. 3.19). Normal distance is 5–8 mm (± 1 mm;

Fig. 3.19a); pathological findings (Fig. 3.19b) can be established, and changes following physiotherapy monitored (Fig. 3.19c).

References

Holländer DJ (1984) Die Ultraschalldiagnostik in der Schwangerschaft, 3. Aufl. Urban & Schwarzenberg, München, p 157

Kratochwil A, Zeibekis N (1972) Ultraschall-Pelvimetrie. Acta Obstet Gynecol Scand 51:357

Schlensker KH (1979) Ultraschallmessungen der Conjugata vera obstetrica. Geburtshilfe Frauenheilkd 39:333

4 Pregnancy (First Trimester)

In the first trimester ultrasound is not yet generally accepted as a screening procedure, and in many countries used only where specific indications exist. One such indication is to monitor the outcome of therapy in infertile patients (see Chap. 15).

Other candidates for ultrasound are women who show symptoms suggestive of an abnormal pregnancy. In these cases the following inquiries should be made:

1. Has implantation occurred?
2. Is implantation in the uterus?
3. Has the conceptus developed into a live embryo?
4. Where is the site of implantation?
5. Is fetal development appropriate for gestational age?
6. What is the gestational age based on early biometry of the fetus?
7. Is fetal morphology normal?

For didactic reasons we shall treat these questions separately (Sects. 4.1–4.5), and begin with a discussion of embryologic terms and principles that are relevant to obstetric ultrasound.

4.1 Normal Development

4.1.1 Definition of Terms, Basic Embryology

Gestational Age

When we speak of the gestational age of an embryo or fetus, confusion may result unless we specify the reference points being used.

While most obstetricians use the last normal menstrual period (LMP) as their reference point and thus speak of the "menstrual age" of a pregnancy, embryologists speak in terms of "conception age," meaning the time elapsed since fertilization of the ovum. In the present book, all gestational ages will be stated in terms of menstrual age unless the fertilization age is specifically given. The use of the term "week" should also be clarified, as it may lead to confusion. It is the European custom to state the current week of fetal development, rather than the completed week, and with a range of gestational age from $31+1$ to $31+7$ a fetus would be in its 32nd week. In this volume the concept of the completed week will be used when stating gestational age. Thus a 31-week fetus is one that has completed 31 weeks gestation.

Twenty-four weeks of pregnancy are the legal time limit in Western Germany as well as in some other countries for medical abortion. As long as malformations of the fetus are considered, all efforts are made to establish diagnosis before 24 weeks are completed.

Orientation. In describing position and direction, we shall draw upon the nomenclature of descriptive anatomy. Thus, "cranial" and "caudal" will always mean toward and away from the head respectively, and "anterior" and "posterior" will designate respectively the front and rear body surfaces. When viewing a sonogram or an image on a monitor screen, the caudal part of the image is always on the right side in longitudinal scans. In transverse scans, the maternal left side corresponds to the right side of the image (see Chap. 7). Standard obstetric terms relating to fetal presentation will not be discussed in this section, because these features are transitory at this stage of gestation.

The embryonic period begins at 5 weeks gestation (3 weeks after fertilization) and continues until 10 weeks, at which time the embryo becomes a fetus and remains so until parturition.

Basic Embryology. To aid in understanding the structures that are accessible to ultrasound visualization in early pregnancy, an outline of early embryologic changes is presented in

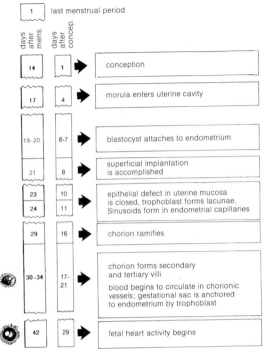

Fig. 4.1. Summary of pertinent aspects of embryologic development

Fig. 4.1. The gestational sac (chorionic cavity) has reached a size by about 34 days gestation which theoretically can be resolved with ultrasound. According to Lyons and Levi (1983), the earliest that an implanted gestational sac has been identified is within a few days after the expected date of the next menstrual period. In identifying these early structures, it must be remembered that only the gestational sac is visible at this stage, and not the amniotic cavity (Fig. 4.2). The changes occurring in the decidua (chorion), amnion, and embryo between 5 and 10 weeks gestation are shown schematically in Fig. 4.3. It is not until 10 weeks that the amniotic sac attains sufficient relative growth to fill the gestational sac. As a result of this growth, the chorionic villi come into contact with the decidua capsularis and form the chorion laeve. Sac growth causes the decidua capsularis to be pressed against the decidua parietalis, with subsequent degeneration from deficient blood supply at about 21 weeks.

4.1.2 Earliest Detection of Intrauterine Pregnancy

The pivotal question is: How early is a gestational sac visible, and what criteria can be used to identify it as such? Because the normal gestational sac is larger than 5 mm in diameter at 4 weeks gestation, and this is within the resolving power of most conventional ultrasound equipment, it should be possible to visualize the gestational sac at that time. It is important, however, to be able to differentiate it from other ring-like structures, particularly the "pseudogestational sac" of ectopic pregnancy (see Sect. 4.3) and the ring-shaped features that may be observed at midcycle (Chap. 15). Specific sonographic criteria are required for differentiation.

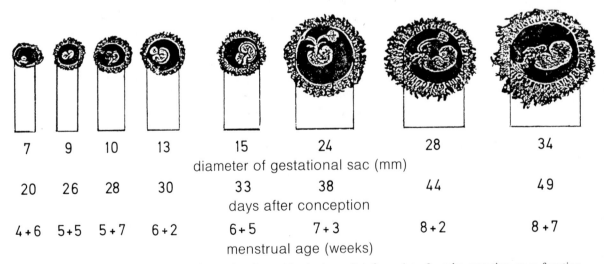

Fig. 4.2. Morphology and size of gestational sac (chorionic cavity) from 4 to 8 weeks gestation as a function of menstrual age and conceptional age

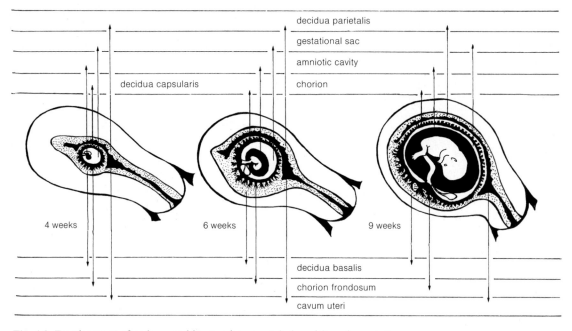

Fig. 4.3. Development of embryo and its membranes at 4, 6, and 9 weeks gestation

The example shown in Fig. 4.4a–i illustrates how these questions can be resolved. In this patient we were unable to establish a gestational or fertilization age. It was largely by chance that a β-HCG assay was performed and followed immediately by the first sonographic examination. At that time the β-HCG value was 216. Besides a cystic structure in the region of the left ovary, sonograms revealed an area of increased echogenicity within the endometrium and a distinct echo-free ring-like structure about 2 mm in diameter (arrow, Fig. 4.4a). One day later the β-HCG value had risen to 712, and ultrasound showed definite enlargement of the ring (Fig. 4.4b). Two days later (β-HCG 1024) the ring had reached 5 mm in diameter and featured a bright, asymmetrical border. This border showed echo-enhancement-type features at its base, and small, rounded, honeycomb-like structures were visible within the asymmetrical hyperechoic area (Fig. 4.4c). Two days later we were able to diagnose intrauterine pregnancy with complete confidence. The sonographic picture corresponded well to the structures shown schematically in Fig. 4.4f, representing 4 weeks gestation. Six days later (β-HCG 4950) the gestational sac had reached a mean diameter of 11 mm (5 weeks; Fig. 4.5i).

The ability to accurately detect pregnancy be-tween the 30th and 34th days of gestation (16th–20th day of development), assuming a normal cycle with conception on the 14th post-menstrual day, depends on the success with which the following changes can be demon-strated:

On the 15th day of development (29th post-menstrual day), ramification of the chorion be-gins. Between the 16th and 20th days of devel-opment (30th–34th postmenstrual day), second-ary and tertiary villi form in the chorion (Moore 1980). These villi cover the entire sur-face of the chorion but are particularly well de-veloped at the implantation site. When we com-pare the morphology at the base of the gesta-tional sac in Fig. 4.4e (β-HCG 1024) following magnification (Fig. 4.4g) with a histologic sec-tion of endometrium taken on day 30 of the menstrual cycle, we find that the sonogram ac-curately depicts the structural asymmetry in the implantation region. This distinguishes normal pregnancy from ectopic gestation and from hormone-induced changes associated with the normal menstrual cycle, in which endometrial changes are always symmetrical. A pseudoges-tational sac of ectopic pregnancy is pictured in Fig. 4.5. Given the size of the sac, the peripheral ring should be considerably more echogenic and should show a definite asymmetry. In the

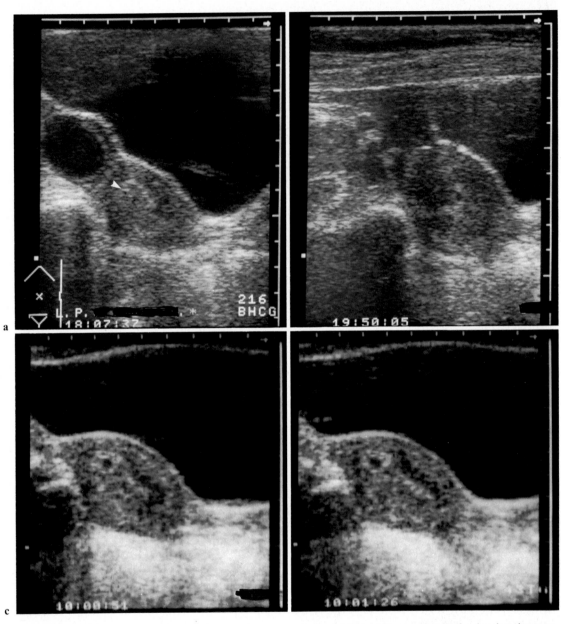

Fig. 4.4a–i. Early diagnosis of intrauterine pregnancy. **a** A tiny ring-shaped structure is visible (*arrow*), and the endometrium shows increased echogenicity (*β*-HCG = 216 mU/ml). **b** One day later the ring is 3 mm in diameter (*β*-HCG = 712 mU/ml). **c** The gestational sac is clearly seen (5 mm); the endometrium shows a bright, asymmetrical ring with "honeycomb" appearance (*β*-HCG = 1024 mU/ml). **d** Two days later the gestational sac is well outlined (6 mm) and there is an asymmetrical ring corresponding to 4 weeks gestation. **e** Uterus at 4 weeks gestation (*β*-HCG = 1024 mU/ml). *Inset:* area enlarged in **g**. **f** Schematic drawing of the pregnant uterus at 4 weeks gestation. **g** Detail of **e** showing the gestational sac and implantation site. A thin, echogenic ring surrounds the chorionic cavity from 8 to 2 o'clock; irregular "honeycomb" appearance is seen from 3 to 7 o'clock. **h** Histologic section through the endometrium on the 29th postmenstrual day (15th day of development; magnification 15 ×). Secondary villi are abundant at the embryonic pole. (After Moore 1980, modified from Leeson and Leeson 1976). **i** The gestational sac is 10 mm in diameter. This pattern is characteristic of a 5-week pregnancy. The echogenic ring around the gestational sac is thickened and asymmetrical

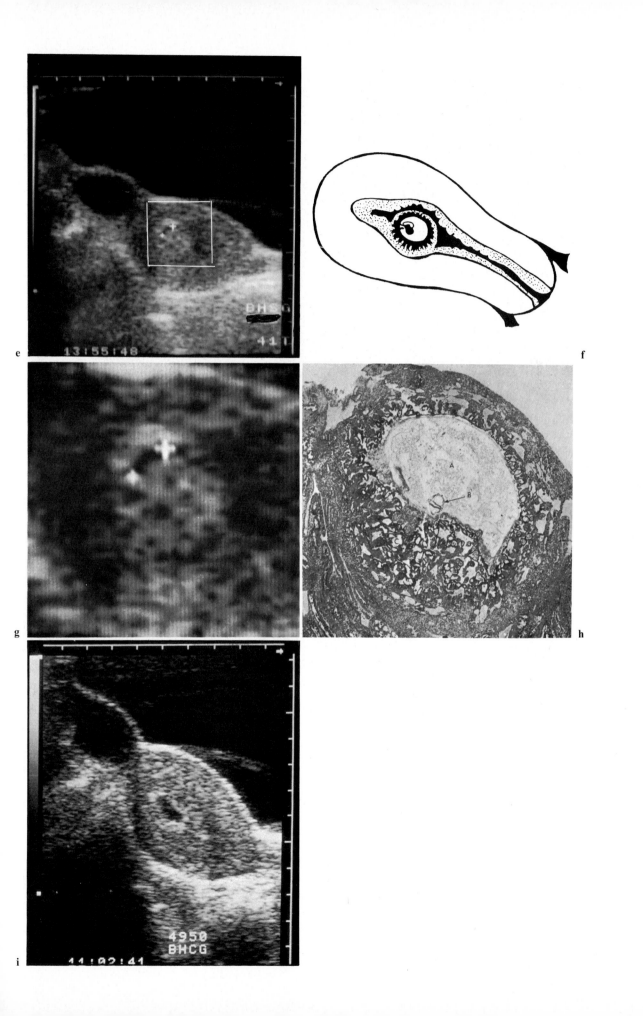

e

f

g

h

i

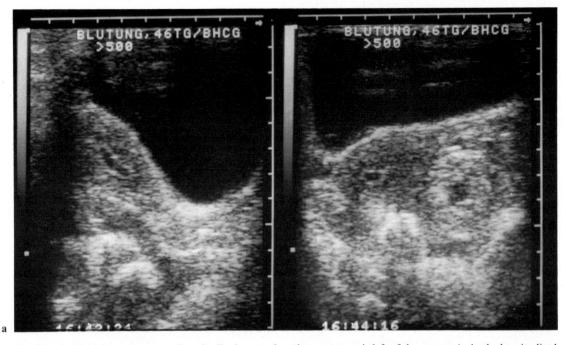

Fig. 4.5a, b. Ectopic pregnancy. **a** Longitudinal scan of uterus illustrating a pseudogestational sac. The uterine cavity is relatively large (20 mm long), but the sac is symmetrical and not very echogenic. **b** Transverse scan: the pregnancy is left of the uterus. As in the longitudinal scan, the pseudogestational sac does not show the asymmetric echogenic ring characteristic of a true sac (cf. normal pregnancy in Fig. 4.7)

transverse scan (the ectopic pregnancy is seen to the left of the uterus), we again note the absence of a bright ring around the pseudosac.

4.1.3 Five Weeks: Morphology and Biometry of the Gestational Sac

The drawings in Fig. 4.3 illustrate the development of the amniotic cavity and gestational sac. While the amniotic cavity still cannot be demonstrated in isolation at 4 weeks gestation, its continuous growth causes it to approach the decidua capsularis. The amniotic border is sometimes visible as a streak-like feature in the gestational sac especially when a high gain setting is used (Figs. 4.13b, 4.14b, arrow). This is not possible before 6–7 weeks, however, and the amniotic border is not considered an important landmark during the period relevant for measurement of the gestational sac. Because the outer border of the decidua cannot be clearly identified, the reference points for measuring the gestational sac must lie on its well-defined inner border (Fig. 4.6, 4.7). One should not attempt to measure the gestational sac after

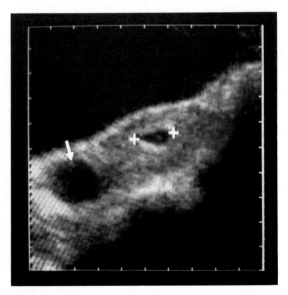

Fig. 4.6. Pregnancy, 5 weeks: measurement of gestational sac (16 mm). *Arrow:* adnexal cyst

11 weeks gestation, both for morphologic reasons (poorly defined borders) and because other criteria – crown-rump length (CRL) and biparietal diameter (BPD) – take precedence

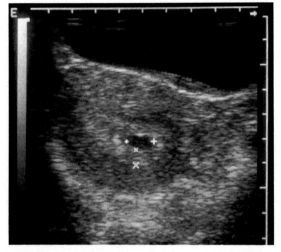

Fig. 4.7. Pregnancy, 5 weeks: transverse scan. Asymmetry of gestational sac is apparent

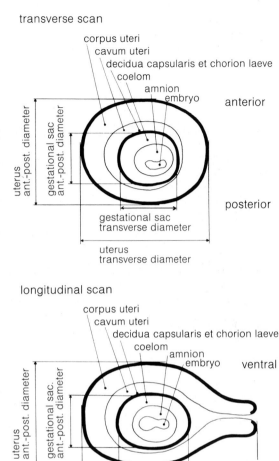

Fig. 4.8. Schematic drawings showing structures relevant to biometry of gestational sac. (After Reinold 1976)

after 8 weeks. A number of authors have published normal growth curves for the gestational sac (Hellmann et al. 1969; Holländer 1972; Jouppila 1971; Kossoff et al. 1974; Reinold et al. 1975; Stein et al. 1972; Troostwijk 1972). It must be stressed, however, that these growth curves show only the relationship of sac size to known gestational age, and that gestational age cannot be accurately deduced from these charts simply by switching the coordinates.

This problem was first addressed by Holländer (1972), who used methods of statistical analysis to calculate a regression for the dependence of gestational age on the arithmetic mean of individual sac diameters. He found that the mean deviation from the regression lines was 0.93 weeks. This means that the age of an intact gestation can be determined to an accuracy of a week with a confidence limit of 68%. Haller et al. (1976) confirmed this in a prospective study. They found that gestational age can be most accurately determined from the arithmetic mean of the sac diameter, with a standard deviation of 1.1 weeks. This is consistent with our own experience.

Figure 4.8 shows the anatomic borders that are relevant to measurements of the gestational sac (Reinold 1976). External factors limit the accuracy with which the gestational sac can be measured. These include deformation of the sac by an overdistended bladder, local contractions, and fibroids. Figure 4.2 illustrates the growth of the gestational sac from 4 to 8 weeks

gestation. Prior to 8 weeks it is not possible to diagnose a blighted ovum on the basis of mean gestational sac diameter. On the other hand, if the mean gestational sac diameter is greater than 3 cm (8 weeks) and no fetal structures can be visualized, a diagnosis of blighted ovum is justified. However, we recommend that a repeat study be performed whenever possible to obtain confirmation. Embryonic structures cannot be identified before 6 weeks.

To summarize findings at 5 weeks:

1. A gestational sac should be visible.
2. The gestational sac should be surrounded by a broad, echo-dense ring.
3. This ring should show asymmetry.

4. The gestational sac is measurable, but a prognosis cannot yet be made as to the outcome of the pregnancy.
5. Embryonic structures are usually not identifiable with conventional scanners at this stage.

4.1.4 Six Weeks: Embryonic Structures, Viability

Between 6 and 7 weeks the embryo passes the 5-mm limit, thus enabling the depiction of embryonic structures. Figure 4.9 compares the ul-

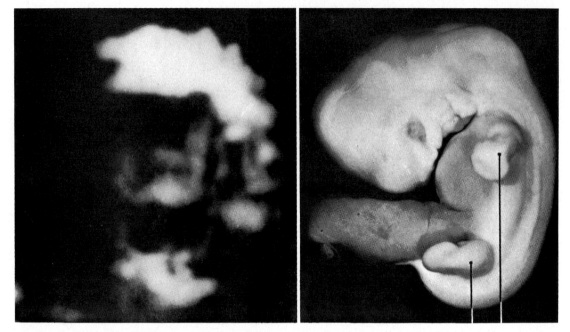

Fig. 4.9. Embryonic morphology in an ultrasound zoom image (*left*) and anatomic correlation (*right*) at 6 weeks gestation

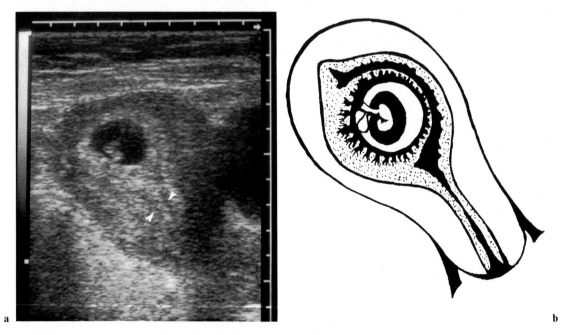

a   b

Fig. 4.10. a. Pregnancy, 6 weeks. Embryo is clearly visible. Brightness differences are apparent between decidua and uterine cavity. **b** Schematic drawing of uterus at 6 weeks gestation

trasound image of an embryo at 6 weeks with an actual specimen.

Consistent visualization of the embryo at this stage requires proper preparation, patience and a meticulous technique. This is particularly true in patients with a retroverted uterus. A full bladder is helpful in such cases, and vaginal manipulation may be necessary to place the uterus beneath the acoustic window of the bladder or move it away from the bowel shadow (Fig. 4.11 a, b). The embryo can be clearly identified only if it is floating freely in the amniotic cavity. An embryo that lies in a corner on the bottom of the gestational sac is easily overlooked (Fig. 4.13 c), and is best demonstrated by making a series of closely-spaced parallel scans using a very slow transducer motion in all planes.

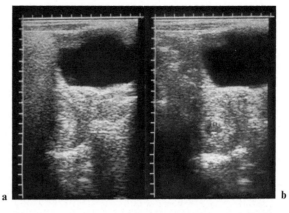

Fig. 4.11. a Retroversion and retroflexion of pregnant uterus. Bowel loops overlying fundus prevent visualization of intrauterine structures. **b** With increased bladder distension, pregnancy can be detected

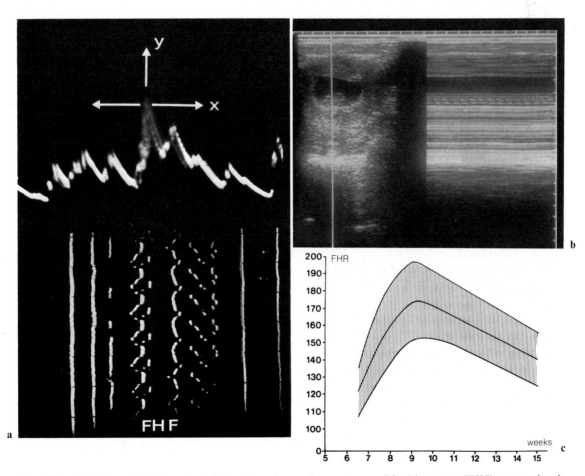

Fig. 4.12. a Detection of fetal heart activity by A-mode and time-motion display. **b** Combined use of real-time B-scan and time-motion to document heart activity.

c Normal range of fetal heart rate (*FHR*) vs gestational age (± 2 SD). (After Robinson and Shaw-Dunn 1973)

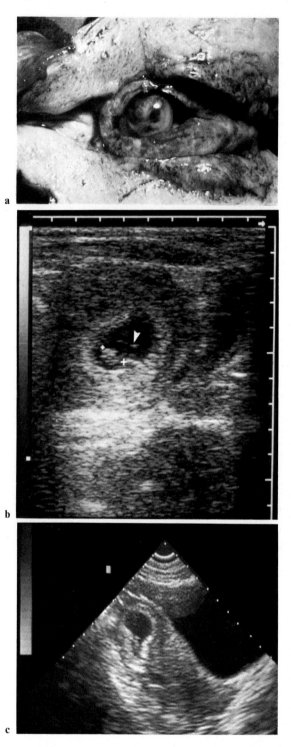

Fig. 4.13a–c.7 weeks gestation. **a** The decidua parietalis is seen at the edge of the uterus. The decidua capsularis and gestational sac are opened to reveal the embryo within the amnion, which does not yet fill the chorionic cavity. **b** The wall of the amnion appears as a streak-like feature within the gestational sac (*arrow*). **c** The embryo is seen in a corner at the base of the gestational sac

Detection of Life. An intact intrauterine pregnancy may be diagnosed only if fetal viability is confirmed.

Fetal heart motion has been detected as early as the 42nd postmenstrual day by Hackelöer and Hansmann (1976), the 44th day by Piiroinen (1974, 1975), the 45th day by Robinson et al. (1973), and the 46th day by Kratochwil et al. (1967). However, the last-named authors used the pulsed-echo method with an intravaginal transducer and an A-mode display, a technique that was not acceptable to patients for routine examinations.

Hackelöer and Hansmann (1976) used a combination of B-scan, A-mode, and time-position display for their investigations (Fig. 4.12a).

With the improved resolution of modern ultrasound equipment, it is easier to observe fetal heart activity, especially with instruments which have a zoom capability. The combined use of real-time B-scan and time-motion is illustrated in Fig. 4.12b. This is useful mainly for purposes of demonstration and documentation. It should be noted that the average fetal heart rate is only 123 bpm at 6 weeks, increasing to 171 bpm at 8 weeks and then gradually decreasing until term (Robinson 1973; Fig. 4.12c). Thus, the relatively slow heart rate at 6 weeks does not represent a pathologic finding. Also, in the presence of maternal tachycardia, the rapid pulse wave that may be transmitted should not be misinterpreted as a fetal heart rate abnormality.

The detection of fetal heart activity confirms the presence of fetal life. Of course, if body movements are observed, detection of heart activity is not needed to confirm viability. Embryonic structures at rest will usually show brisk, active movements when the maternal abdomen is lightly percussed. With a missed abortion, percussion will elicit only a passive, swaying motion of the dead embryo.

Another important and controversial theme relates to the structure of the uterine cavity (Fig. 4.10a). Lyons and Levi (1982) found that in 60% of their patients between 4 and 7 weeks, the uterine cavity was not sonographically empty. They interpreted the echo-poor area partially surrounding the gestational sac as the residue of a physiologic "implantation bleed" which did not reach the external cervical os. Nelson et al. (1983) used the presence of this

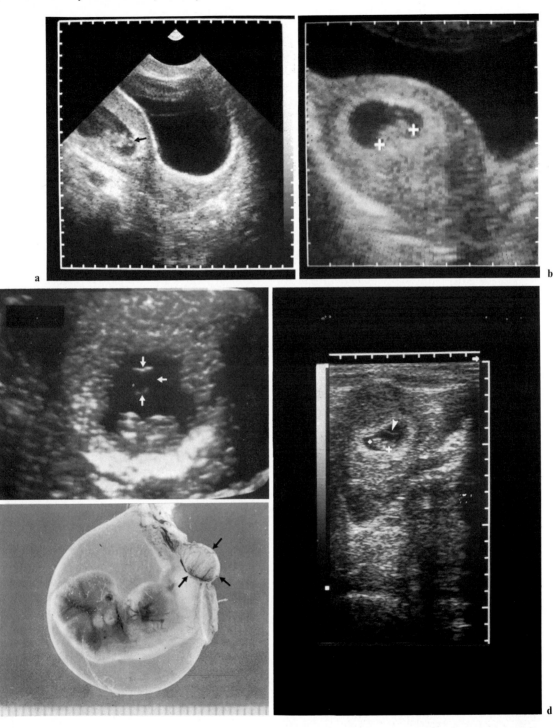

Fig. 4.14. a, b 7 weeks gestation. **a** Embryo and yolk sac (*arrow*). **b** Measurement of CRL. The fetal head and trunk can now be differentiated. **c, d** 8 weeks gestation. **c** *Top:* ultrasound image; *arrows* indicate yolk sac. *Bot-* *tom:* 8-week embryo; note yolk sac on outer surface of amniotic sac (*arrows*). **d** Embryo: measurement of CRL. *Arrow* marks amniotic sac, which still does not fill gestational sac

structure as a criterion for differentiating intrauterine from ectopic pregnancy, pointing out that the structures disappear when compressed by an overdistended bladder. The degree to which decidua-altering hormonal factors are responsible for this phenomenon remains unclear. Nevertheless, it appears important that implantation bleeding is observed only in association with intrauterine pregnancy (Nelson et al. 1983).

To summarize the situation at 6 weeks:

1. Embryonic structures are almost always visible.
2. Doubtful cases are resolved by filling of the urinary bladder, vaginal manipulation, or percussion.
3. Heart activity can usually be demonstrated.
4. The heart rate at this stage is relatively low.
5. The presence of a prominent ring around the gestational sac aids exclusion of ectopic pregnancy.

4.1.5 Seven Weeks

The embryo exceeds 10 mm in length and thus can be visualized in 100% of intact pregnancies. The same applies to heart activity. The anatomy at 7 weeks is shown in Fig. 4.13a, and sonographic morphology is shown in Fig. 4.13b. With a high-quality instrument, the experienced examiner can measure the embryo at this time.

4.1.6 Eight Weeks: Yolk Sac

Fetal structures are now clearly discernible, and the longitudinal body axis can be identified and measured (Fig. 4.14b). The technique of CRL

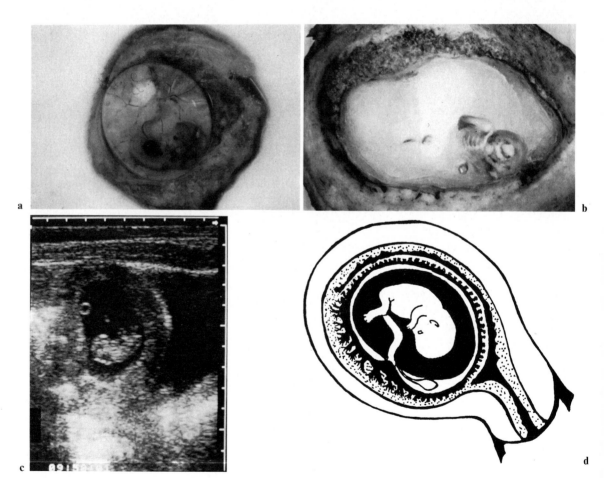

Fig. 4.15a–d. 9 weeks gestation. **a** Embryo and membranes: gestational sac has been opened, revealing intact amniotic sac. **b** Frozen section traversing head, thorax, and trunk of embryo; ossification zones can be recognized. Placenta visible at 11 and 12 o'clock. **c** Sonogram of embryo. **d** Schematic drawing of uterus

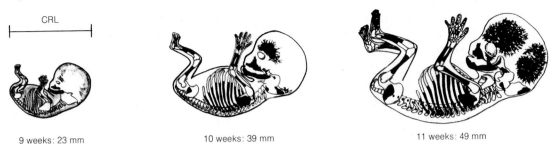

Fig. 4.16. Formation of ossification centers at 9, 10, and 11 weeks gestation: fetuses shown actual size. (Modified from Patten 1948)

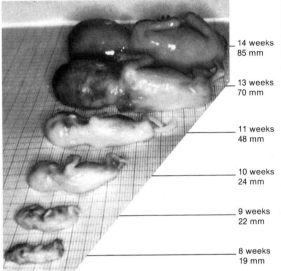

Fig. 4.17. Demonstration of the growth in CRL from 8 to 14 weeks gestation

measurement is described in Sect. 4.1.7 (9–11 weeks).

Frequently a circular echo about 5 mm in diameter is visible within the gestational sac (Fig. 4.14c). The top picture in Fig. 4.14a shows the real-time zoom image of an embryo and yolk sac (arrows). The bottom picture shows an 8-week embryo in the amniotic cavity with the yolk sac adherent to its outer surface (arrows). Sauerbrei et al. (1980) have investigated the sonographic visualization of this structure and its significance. The yolk sac may be located some distance from the embryo, but must not be mistaken for a twin gestation. Also, a yolk sac in close proximity to the embryo must not be included in the measurements of CRL (Fig. 4.21a, b). Finally, the detection of a yolk sac precludes the diagnosis of a blighted ovum, because without a developing embryo, there is no yolk sac.

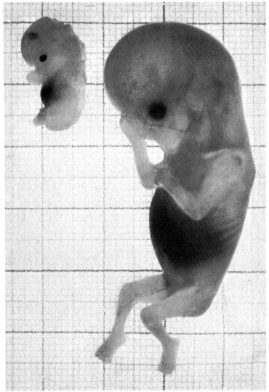

Fig. 4.18. A error of one cycle in estimating gestational age is not possible when the CRL is measured, as this comparison of fetuses at 8 weeks (*left*) and 11 weeks (*right*) illustrates

To summarize the situation at 7 and 8 weeks:

1. Fetal structures and heart activity are always demonstrable in an intact pregnancy.
2. An empty gestational sac larger than 3 cm (mean diameter) and the absence of visible embryonic structures justify a diagnosis of blighted ovum.
3. The yolk sac frequently presents as a circular structure 5 mm in diameter.

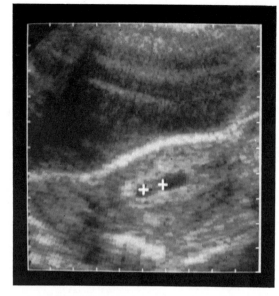

Fig. 4.19. Earliest possible measurement of CRL, at 6 weeks (8 mm)

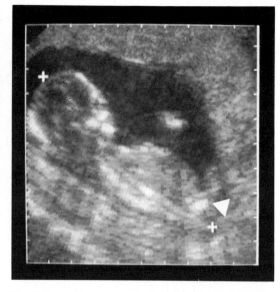

Fig. 4.20. Accurate measurement of CRL on extended fetus at 15 weeks. *Arrow* indicates ossification center in ilium ($+$—$+$ = 93 mm)

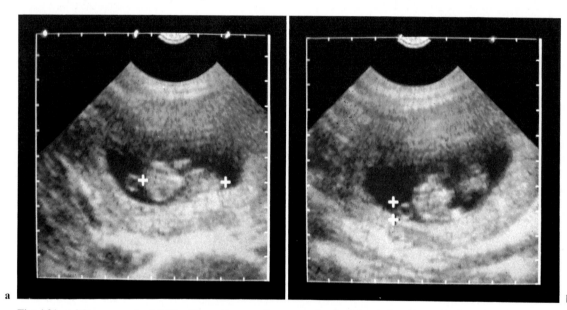

Fig. 4.21. a Measurement of CRL. The yolk sac adjacent to the fetal head should not be included in the CRL measurement ($+$—$+$ = 37 mm). **b** Measurement of the yolk sac at 10 weeks (7 mm)

4. The yolk sac must not be mistaken for a twin gestation, and its presence precludes the diagnosis of blighted ovum.

4.1.7 Nine to Eleven Weeks: Biometry, Embryofetal Structures

Figure 4.15a shows the gross anatomy of the embryo at 9 weeks. The frozen section in Fig. 4.15b illustrates the already marked differences in the density of embryonic structures. The section traverses the head, thorax, and upper arm, and early ossification is evident in the skull, clavicle, humerus, and ribs. The placenta can be observed at the margin of the gestational sac. The details of placentation are discussed in Chap. 11. The increasing differentiation of the fetus explains why fetal biometry becomes

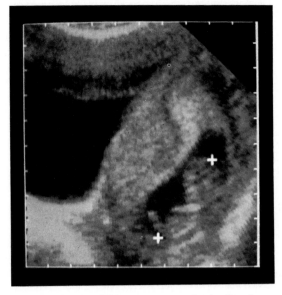

Fig. 4.22. Correct CRL measurement in the flexed embryo (11 weeks). The entire longitudinal axis is demonstrated (+ —— + = 38 mm)

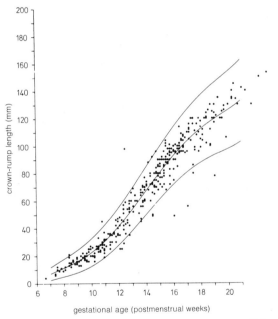

Fig. 4.23. Gestational age as a function of CRL. Fifth-degree polynomial with 2 SD range. (From Hansmann et al. 1979)

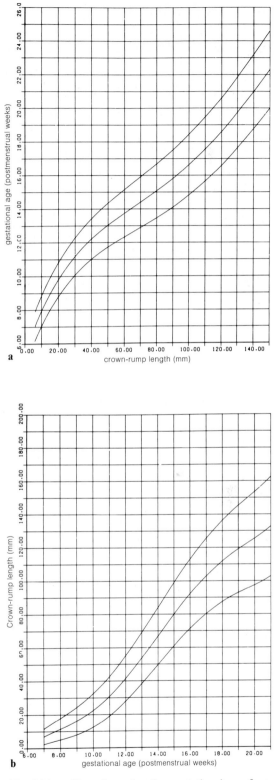

easier at this stage. Ultrasound differentiation is made possible by the rapid growth of the embryo, which is accompanied by an increase in the density of fetal tissues relative to the amniotic fluid. It is noteworthy that the weight of the embryo increases from 1 g at the end

Fig. 4.24. a Chart for estimating gestational age from sonographically measured CRL. **b** Chart for assessing individual growth of sonographic CRL. (From Hansmann et al. 1979)

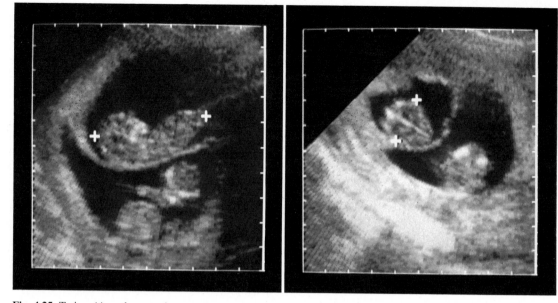

Fig. 4.25. Twins, 11 weeks gestation: measurement of CRL ($+$——$+$ = 48 mm) and BPD ($+$——$+$ = 17 mm)

of the 2nd month to 14.2 g by the end of the 3rd month (Streeter 1920).

Another important feature during this period is progressive ossification. Figure 4.16 shows the rapid progression of ossification from 9 weeks to 12 weeks gestation.

The major ossification centers in the fetus are located in the calvarium and in the pelvic region (ilium). They provide important landmarks for measuring CRL. It was Robinson, from the school of I. Donald, who developed the technique of CRL measurement. He showed that with this new parameter, gestational age could be estimated with a standard deviation of only 1.6 days. In other words, the age of a pregnancy could be estimated to an accuracy of ±3 days at the 96% confidence limit. The initial reaction to this report was astonishment. Later, Robinson and Fleming (1975) conducted a series of in vivo and in vitro experiments to determine accurately the limits of the method. They found that gestational age could be estimated to an accuracy of ±4.7 days by a single CRL measurement and to ±2.7 days by three independent CRL measurements at the 95% confidence limit. While this was somewhat less optimistic than the original report, the results were still unparalleled. The high accuracy of the method is based on the fact that the embryo and later the fetus grow more rapidly in length than in any other direction, showing an average longitudinal growth rate of 1.6 mm/day between 8 and 14 weeks. Growth dynamics during this period are illustrated in Fig. 4.17. Figure 4.18 shows that even if an inaccurate measurement is made the error can never amount to several weeks. This is obvious when we compare the 16-mm CRL of the smaller, 8-week embryo with the 48-mm CRL of the larger, 11-week fetus.

The basis of gestational age assessment with CRL is the good correlation that exists between age and body length in the first trimester (Foebus 1981).

Measuring Technique. Measurement of CRL has been greatly simplified by the introduction of real-time equipment. Nevertheless, the following points are important in obtaining an accurate measurement:

1. The embryofetus must be displayed along its longest axis.
2. The measurement should be made with the fetus in an extended position if at all possible. Usually an inactive fetus can be made to extend by tapping the maternal abdomen.
3. At the moment of maximum extension, the image should be frozen and also magnified if possible.
4. The points of the caliper should be applied to the outer margins of the head and trunk.

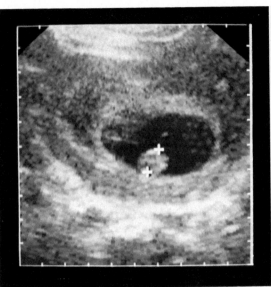

a

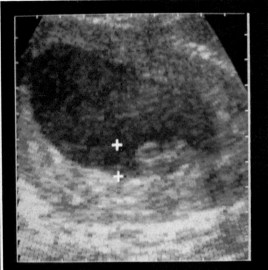

b

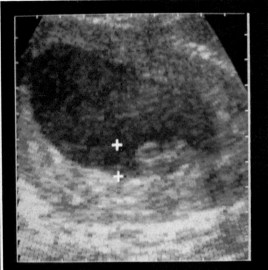

c

Fig. 4.26. a Measurement of BPD at 9 weeks ($+$———$+ = 10$ mm). **b** Measurement of BPD at 10 weeks ($+$———$+ = 13$ mm). **c** Chart for estimating gestational age from sonographic BPD

5. The yolk sac and extremities should not be included in CRL measurements.
6. If the fetus remains flexed, 5% of the measured length should be added as a correction (e.g., measured length of flexed fetus = 60 mm, corrected length = 63 mm).

A detailed discussion of the importance of CRL measurement was presented by Foebus (1981). Practical examples of CRL measurements are shown in Figs. 4.19–4.22.

Measurement and evaluation of the CRL may be done for one of two reasons: (1) to learn whether the CRL is appropriate for a known gestational age, or (2) as a means of estimating an unknown gestational age.

In answering the first question (whether fetal length is appropriate for a known gestational age), the chart in Fig. 4.24b should be used. The corresponding scattergram in Fig. 4.23 shows the data from the Foebus study (1981) on which the chart is based.

If the intent is to estimate gestational age from CRL, the chart in Fig. 4.24 a is used. Because the accuracy of the estimate decreases as the pregnancy progesses, the measurement should be performed at the earliest possible opportunity.

The BPD can be measured from 8 weeks on (Fig. 4.26a, b). Gestational age is derived from BPD by referring to the chart in Fig. 4.26c. For practical applications it is best to use both CRL and BPD measurements (Fig. 4.25).

By the end of the first trimester, fetal development has progressed far enough for fetal anatomic detail to be evaluated by ultrasound (Fig. 4.27a). The extremities are also examined more easily. The increasing difference in the tissue appearance and outline of fetal organs forms the basis for these evaluations. The similarity between the fetus in Fig. 4.27a and a pho-

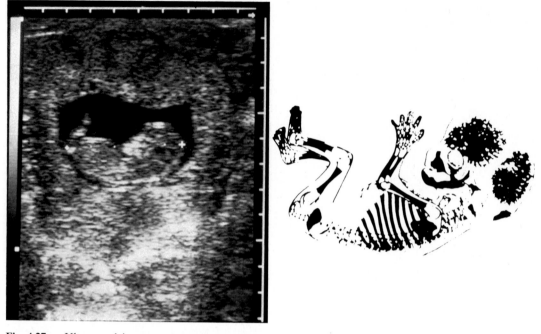

Fig. 4.27. a Ultrasound image at 11 weeks: flexed position of fetus results in underestimation of CRL by 5%.
b Ossification centers at 11 weeks

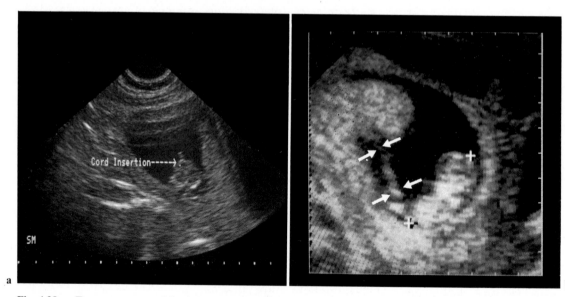

Fig. 4.28. a Transverse scan of fetal trunk at 12 weeks: umbilical cord can be recognized. **b** At 11 weeks: CRL
37 mm. *Arrows,* umbilical cord

tomechanical drawing showing the status of fetal ossification at 11 weeks (Fig. 4.27b) clearly
illustrates this point. It should also be noted
that the umbilical cord is frequently visible at
the end of the first trimester (Fig. 4.28), and
that a short cord length is perfectly normal at
this stage.

References

Foebus J (1981) Die Bedeutung der Scheitelsteißlänge
    und des biparietalen Durchmessers für die Schätzung
    des Gestationsalters in der Frühgravidität. Med Diss,
    Bonn
Hackelöer BJ, Hansmann M (1976) Ultraschalldiagno-
    stik in der Frühschwangerschaft. Gynäkologe 9:108

Haller U, Liebchen C, Henner H, Wesch H, Kubli F (1976) Assessment of gestational age by means of sonar biometry of amniotic sac during early pregnancy. Vortrag: No. 284, 5. Europäischer Kongreß für Perinatale Medizin, Uppsala

Hansmann M (1981) Sonar biometry in early pregnancy. J Perinat Med 9 (Suppl 1):20

Hansmann M, Schuhmacher M, Foebus J (1979) Ultraschallbiometrie der fetalen Scheitel-Steiß-Länge in der ersten Schwangerschaftshälfte. Geburtshilfe Frauenheilkd 39:656

Hellmann LM, Kobayashi M, Fillisti L, Lavenhar M, Cromb E (1969) Growth and development of the human fetus prior to the twentieth week of gestation. Am J Obstet Gynecol 103:798

Holländer HJ (1972) Die Ultraschalldiagnostik in der Schwangerschaft. Urban & Schwarzenberg, München Berlin Wien

Jouppila D (1971) Ultrasound in the diagnosis of early pregnancy and its complications. Acta Obstet Gynecol Scand [Suppl 15] 50

Kossoff G, Garrett WJ, Radavanovich G (1974) Grey scale echography in obstetrics and gynecology. Australas Radiol 18:62

Kratochwil A, Eisenhut L (1967) Der früheste Nachweis der fetalen Herzaktion durch Ultraschall. Geburtshilfe Frauenheilkd 27:176

Leeson CR, Leeson TS (1976) Histology, 3rd edn. Saunders, Philadelphia

Lyons EA, Levi CS (1983) Ultrasound in the first trimester of pregnancy. In: Callen PW (ed) Ultrasonography in obstetrics and gynecology. Saunders, Philadelphia London Toronto, p 1–19

Moore KL (1980) Embryologie, Lehrbuch und Atlas der Entwicklungsgeschichte des Menschen. Schattauer, Stuttgart New York

Nelson P, Bowie JD, Rosenberg ER (1983) Early intrauterine Pregnancy or decidual cast: An anatomic-sonographic approach. J Ultrasound Med 2: 543

Patten BM (1948) Human embryology. Blakiston, Philadelphia Toronto

Piiroinen O (1974) Detection of fetal heart activity during early pregnancy by combined B-scan and Doppler examination: A new application. Acta Obstet Gynecol Scand 53:231

Reinold E (1976) Ultrasonics in early pregnancy. Karger, Basel

Reinold E, Kucera H (1975) Ultraschallmessungen in der Frühschwangerschaft. Wien Klin Wochenschr 87:62

Robinson HP, Fleming JEE (1975) A critical evaluation of sonar "crown-rump-length" measurements. Br J Obstet Gynecol 82:707

Robinson HP, Shaw-Dunn J (1973) Fetal heart rates as determined by sonar in early pregnancy. Br J Obstet Gynecol 80:805

Sauerbrei E, Cooperberg PL, Poland BJ (1980) Ultrasound demonstration of the normal fetal yolk sac. J Clin Ultrasound 8:217

Stein WW, Kuhl H, Halberstadt E, Taubert HD (1972) Frühschwangerschaft: Ultraschalldiagnostik. Diagnostik 5:647

Streeter GL (1920) Weight, sitting height, head size, foot length and menstrual age of the human embryo. Embryolog 11:143

Troostwiik AL (1972) MD: Thesis. Free Univ of Amsterdam

4.2 Abnormalities in the First Trimester

Bleeding in the first trimester is among the most frequent complications of gestation and always raises the question of whether the pregnancy is normal or abnormal. Clinical and laboratory investigations are frequently unable to resolve the vague diagnosis of "threatened abortion". In previous chapters we have described the capabilities of ultrasound imaging in early pregnancy and demonstrated its reliability. When applied clinically, ultrasound can aid greatly in the evaluation of patients whose symptoms have traditionally been grouped under the heading of "threatened abortion" and open up new approaches to management.

Preparation for the examination is the same as in a normal pregnancy, i.e., the bladder is filled by having the patient drink about 1 liter of fluid 1 h prior to examination. In many cases the examination is a prelude to a planned curettage, and the necessary fluid volume can be infused.

Retrograde filling of the bladder is rarely indicated, and the administration of furosemide (Lasix) for this purpose is not recommended.

The procedure is as follows:

1. The topographic location and shape of the uterus are determined. *Note:* This is difficult with a retroflexed uterus; vaginal manipulation may be helpful.
2. An intrauterine ring-like structure, if present, is identified and measured. *Note:* Ring-like structures up to 1 cm in diameter or more may be seen in ectopic pregnancy (Nelson et al. 1983) and following normal ovulation.
3. The embryo or fetus is visualized. *Note:* A sac may appear empty if the embryo is lying in a corner at the bottom.
4. Fetal viability is confirmed by cardiac activity and/or body movement. *Note:* Vascular pulsations in the adnexal region can mimic cardiac activity and movement.

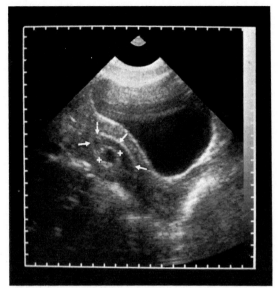

Fig. 4.29. Threatened abortion: subchorionic hemorrhage (*arrows*) at 5 weeks gestation

The great majority of findings in the group of patients with threatened abortion can be assigned to one of the following categories:

1. Intact intrauterine pregnancy (about 50% of cases)
2. Blighted ovum (20%–25%)
3. Missed abortion (25%–30%)
4. Incomplete abortion (2%–5%)
5. Ectopic pregnancy (1%–3%)
6. Hydatidiform mole (<1%)

The most fundamental classification, and one that is basic to further differentiation, rests upon the detection of fetal life. There is only a 10% likelihood that the live fetus will abort (Hackelöer and Hansmann 1976).

When a patient with symptoms of imminent abortion presents for examination, it is often possible to see subchorionic hematomas on ultrasound. An example is given in Fig. 4.29. These hematomas (Fig. 4.30a, b) appear as a second cavity within the uterus and are not easily distinguished from a pregnancy, especially in twin gestations where one pregnancy is normal and the other abnormal (see Chap. 5).

The different stages of the abortion process can also be documented by ultrasound (Fig. 4.31a–c). However, the diagnosis of incomplete abortion should be based on clinical criteria in addition to sonographic findings (Fig. 4.31b; cf. Fig. 12.3a, b).

4.2.1 Blighted Ovum

In approximately half of all abortions an embryo can be identified neither in sonograms nor on uterine evacuation. Donald (1972) coined the term "blighted ovum" for this type of gestation. Typically, the sonogram shows an echo-free gestational sac which is often irregular in outline, poorly defined, and too small for the gestational age. On repeat examinations the sac shows little or no growth or may even diminish in size (Figs. 4.32 and 4.33).

Differential diagnosis is made by excluding an earlier intact pregnancy in which the embryo is still too small to be detected. Here we must caution the sonographer not to perform the examination too hurriedly, for a gestational sac which appears empty on first examination may well contain an embryo that is obscured by an irregularly contoured sac or is situated peripherally, making it difficult to distinguish the embryo from its surroundings. Moreover, real-time scanners are often unable to demonstrate the entire sac in a retroflexed uterus, and the embryo may be missed. These problems underscore the necessity of repeat examinations! Even the most experienced examiner is not immune to misinterpretations, especially if examining conditions are not ideal (patient obesity, inadequately filled bladder).

We agree with Robinson's suggestion that the menstrual history and all clinical information be ignored, and that the final diagnosis be based entirely on sonographic criteria.

The blighted ovum may be regarded as the typical abnormality of early pregnancy, because chromosome abnormalities are present in approximately 50% of cases (Bone et al. 1976). The diagnostic criteria are as follows:

1. Absence of an embryo or fetus
2. Discrepancy between uterine size and gestational sac
3. Irregular outline of the gestational sac
4. Mean gestational sac diameter 3 cm or more without a fetus (beware of retroflexion!)

4.2.2 Missed Abortion

Missed abortion is relatively easy to diagnose in cases where an embryo or fetus can be demonstrated. If there is visible movement or cardi-

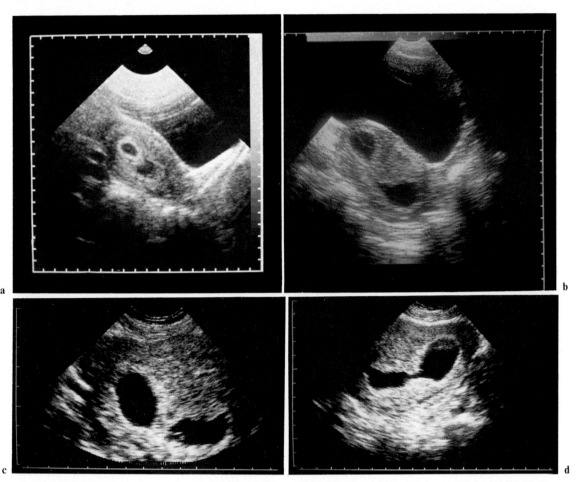

Fig. 4.30. a Longitudinal scan: hematoma caudal to gestational sac. Confusion with a second gestational sac possible. **b** Further caudal migration of hematoma in presence of blighted ovum, 8 weeks. **c** Transverse scan: double sac configuration of a blighted ovum at 8 weeks.

d More cranial transverse scan in same case: hourglass pattern of one gestational sac. (The wall in **c** resulted from a low-set septum in the uterus arcuatus, proven by hysteroscopy.)

ac activity, a viable pregnancy is diagnosed. We feel that further hormonal evaluations in such cases are unnecessary, since they will not make a live fetus any more viable, and because even a "negative" assay would not justify intervention (uterine evacuation) in the presence of positive sonographic findings. It is far more rational and cost-effective to perform hormonal assays only when sonographic findings are inconclusive.

If evidence of fetal life cannot be detected, and the presumption of fetal death is supported by clinical and hormonal parameters, menstrual history, and a discrepancy between fetal size and gestational age, repeat examinations may be dispensed with, and evacuation may be performed (Fig. 4.34a, b).

As a general rule, however, we would caution against hasty intervention and would recommend repeat examination 1–2 weeks later. In a retrospective study of patients with threatened abortion treated at our center, we found that the traditional 30- to 40-day waiting period prior to uterine evacuation (Levi 1973) could be significantly shortened with the help of ultrasound. Besides lowering costs, this greatly reduced psychologic stress on the patient and physician. Most instances of prolonged bedrest occurred when high HCG levels appeared to conflict with ultrasound findings. However, there were a number of cases in which a severely macerated fetus was found on curettage, while all or most of the trophoblastic tissue appeared healthy.

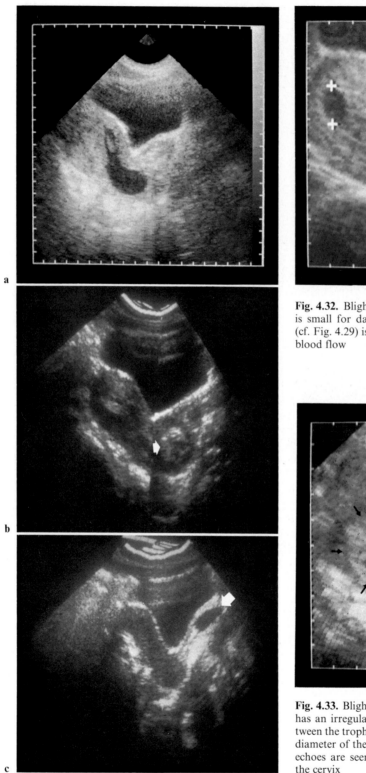

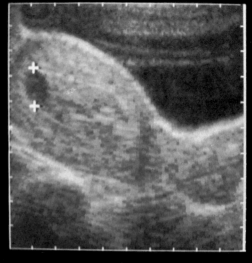

Fig. 4.32. Blighted ovum, 8 weeks. The gestational sac is small for dates and the echogenic chorionic border (cf. Fig. 4.29) is absent, probably as a result of impaired blood flow

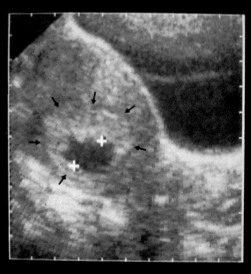

Fig. 4.33. Blighted ovum, 12 weeks. The gestational sac has an irregular outline, and there is little contrast between the trophoblast and its surroundings (*arrows*). The diameter of the gestational sac is 13 mm. No embryonic echoes are seen. The gestational products are close to the cervix

Fig. 4.31 a–c. Sonographic visualization of progress of abortion, 8 weeks. Products of conception are in lower uterus and distending cervical canal (CRL 17 mm = 8 weeks). **b** Gestational products have passed into cervical canal (*arrow*). **c** Uterus is empty. There is still a small amount of blood in vagina (*arrow*)

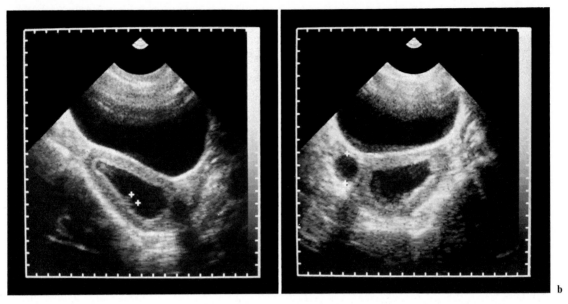

a   b

Fig. 4.34a, b. Missed abortion, 14 weeks. There is marked disproportion between the embryonic echo (7 mm, no heart motion) and the size of the gestational sac. **a** Longitudinal scan. **b** Transverse scan with right adnexal cyst

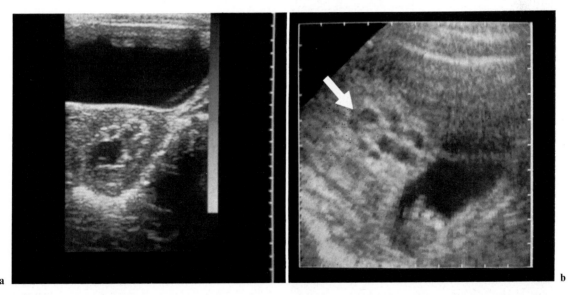

a   b

Fig. 4.35. a Pregnancy with molar changes, 9 weeks: gestational sac still visible. **b** Hydatidiform degeneration, 14 weeks

The diagnostic criteria are:

1. Demonstrable fetus
2. Absence of heart activity
3. Size discrepancy between fetus and gestational sac
4. Passive motion in response to percussion

4.2.3 Hydatidiform Mole

A diagnosis of hydatidiform mole is made relatively easily from its characteristic "snowstorm-like" sonographic appearance, which is considered to be pathognomonic for this disorder. With modern real-time scanners, there should

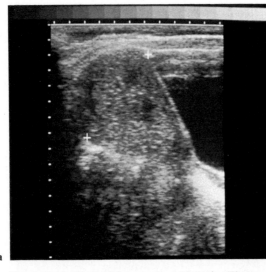 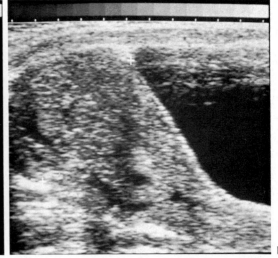

a   b

Fig. 4.36a, b. Hydatidiform mole at 15 weeks. The uterus is filled with trophoblastic tissue that has undergone cystic changes. Neither gestational sac nor fetus is seen. Acoustic enhancement at the posterior uterine wall indicates the presence of tissue with a high fluid content (differentiation from uterine fibroids. **a** Longitudinal scan; **b** magnified view

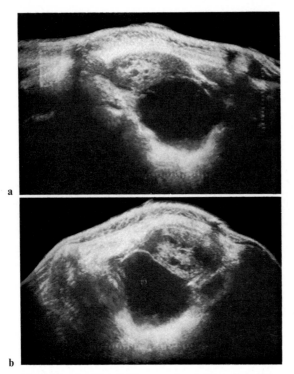

a

b

Fig. 4.37a, b. Hydatidiform mole at 15 weeks with a large theca-lutein cyst. **a** longitudinal scan. **b** transverse scan

no longer be a danger of confusion with uterine fibroids. Doubtful cases are quickly resolved by HCG radioimmunoassay, although HCG levels are not necessarily elevated in molar pregnancies.

As early as 1976 we reported that serial studies had demonstrated the transformation of intact 8-week pregnancies into hydatidiform moles with death of the embryo. In each case there was a marked discrepancy between embryonic size, sac size, and the volume of trophoblastic tissue, which showed a disproportionately rapid proliferation.

Various stages can be recognized in the formation of a hydatidiform mole (Figs. 4.35–4.37). The coexistence of lutein cysts may indicate a progression to choriocarcinoma, but this is not inevitable. To date we have observed 90 hydatidiform moles, only 10 of which had coexisting lutein cysts; choriocarcinoma developed in three. Specific sonographic criteria for malignancy are not available.

Also interesting is the observation, confirmed by other investigators, of a marked decline in the incidence of hydatidiform moles in recent years. This is attributed mainly to the early use of ultrasound in threatened abortions, enabling blighted ova and missed abortions to be evacuated at an earlier date. As a result, there is insufficient time for the complete picture of a hydatidiform mole to evolve. This declining trend represents one of the great triumphs of modern diagnostic ultrasound.

The diagnostic criteria are:

1. Small gestational sac surrounded by excessive amount of trophoblastic tissue

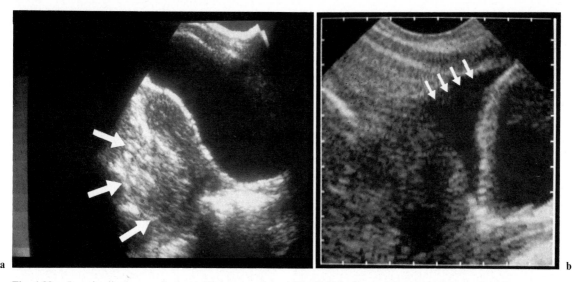

a

b

Fig. 4.38. a Longitudinal scan of uterus. No intrauterine pregnancy is seen. The solid mass lateral to and behind the uterus represents a collection of clot and blood associated with tubal rupture (*arrows*). **b** Longitudinal scan. The fluid in front of the bladder (*arrows*) indicates massive hemorrhage from an ectopic pregnancy that ruptured during the ultrasound examination

2. Uterine cavity filled with small cystic structures
3. Uterus apparently too large for dates
4. Coexistence of lutein cysts

4.3 Ectopic Pregnancy

Sonography has not yet attained the degree of accuracy hoped for in the diagnosis of ectopic pregnancy, despite many exaggerated reports to the contrary. Of course, it is useful in excluding a suspected ectopic pregnancy by confirming intrauterine gestation. This question is raised in about 20%–30% of early pregnancy examinations and is usually based on the concurrent presence of adnexal cysts (see also Fig. 4.34).

It is not uncommon for an intramural or cornual ectopic pregnancy to be misdiagnosed as an intrauterine pregnancy, with potentially tragic consequences, as Donald pointed out in 1965. The direct visualization of an ectopic pregnancy is often not possible, because the gestational products tend to deteriorate quickly outside the uterus, and may present sonographically as a solid mass with cystic components (Figs. 4.38 and 4.39). In some instances a rupture has been observed during the course of the ultrasound examination (Fig. 4.38b). Evidently the combined pressure from the distended urinary bladder and the ultrasound

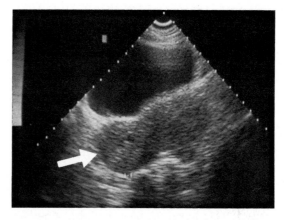

Fig. 4.39. Transverse scan of uterus showing a solid adnexal mass associated with a tubal rupture (*arrow*)

transducer was enough to precipitate a rupture. Although Kobayashi's 1969 report of a 29% failure rate in the diagnosis of ectopic pregnancy may be overstated, it is likely that at least 5%–10% of extrauterine pregnancies cannot be directly diagnosed by ultrasound. This applies specifically to chronic ectopic pregnancies.

4.3.1 Detection of an Intact Intrauterine Pregnancy

At first sight detection of an intact intrauterine pregnancy would appear simple enough, and

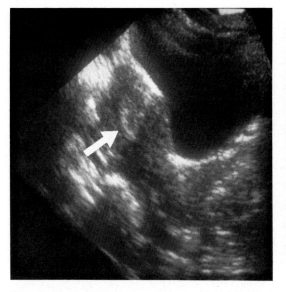

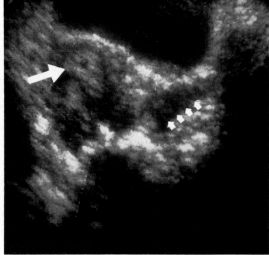

Fig. 4.40. Longitudinal scan of uterus showing a pseudo-gestational sac (decidual reaction, *arrow*) associated with ectopic pregnancy

Fig. 4.41. Transverse scan of uterus showing a pseudo-gestational sac (*arrow*) associated with left ectopic pregnancy (*small arrows*)

this is, in fact, the most common finding in patients suspected of having an ectopic pregnancy. However, two significant problems are encountered:

a) There may be a decidual reaction in ectopic pregnancy, producing an intrauterine ring-like structure that mimics the appearance of a gestational sac. A similar phenomenon may be produced by hormonal stimulation in the normal cycle immediately following ovulation (Figs. 4.40 and 4.41; cf. Fig. 15.4). Several authors (Bradley et al. 1982; Laing and Brooke-Jefrey 1983) have claimed that this ring-like structure can be differentiated from a true gestational sac by the presence of double lines around the sac in an early intrauterine pregnancy – the "double sac" sign. These double lines represent the adjacent borders of the decidua and trophoblast.

It is our opinion (Staudach 1984, personal communication) that intrauterine gestations are clearly distinguished by their asymmetrical sonographic pattern (cf. Figs. 4.1, 4.2), as opposed to the circular decidual sac that is associated with ectopic pregnancy and postovulation (Figs. 4.40, 4.41, 15.7). Nelson et al. (1983) state that the uterine cavity must be delineated in order to differentiate intrauterine from ectopic pregnancy, because normal implantations always occur outside the endometrial canal,

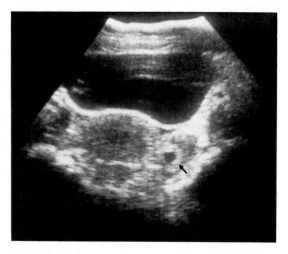

Fig. 4.42. Transverse sonogram of a pregnancy at 6 weeks showing an unruptured left tubal pregnancy with prominent chorion (*arrow*). Uterus contains no gestational products

while the decidual sac of ectopic pregnancy forms within this canal.

b) An intact ectopic pregnancy may be found in the midline, displacing the small, undistended uterus. In such cases serial longitudinal scans are needed to establish the relationship of the gestational sac to the cervix and the vagina and confirm that the pregnancy is in fact intrauterine.

Evaluation becomes more difficult in cases

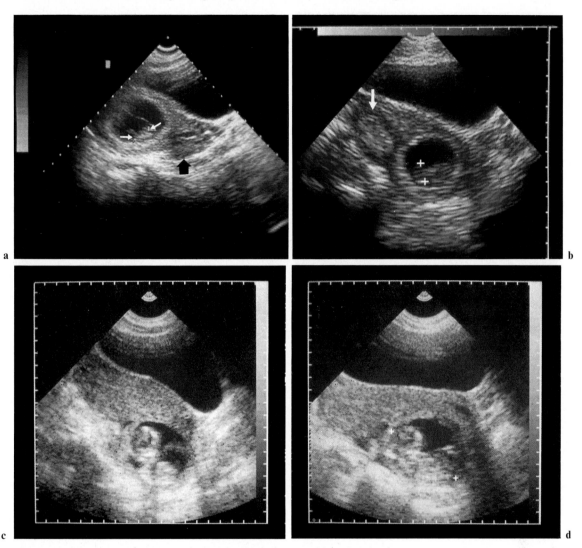

Fig. 4.43. a Transverse scan, 8 weeks. The uterine cavity contains a pseudogestational sac (*black arrow*); there is an intact tubal pregnancy with a live embryo of appropriate size (CRL = 19 mm, *white arrows*). **b** Intact tubal pregnancy at 10 weeks, also with a dilated uterine cavity and normal-size fetus (BPD 12 mm). **c** Intact tubal pregnancy located in cul-de-sac at 13 weeks. **d** Same case, displaying CRL of 66 mm

of intrauterine abortion with retained products and abnormal findings in the adnexal region, which are not uncommon (e.g., corpus luteum cysts). As before, close attention should be paid to the symmetry or asymmetry of the intrauterine "ring."

4.3.2 Demonstration of an Intact Ectopic Pregnancy in the Cul-de-Sac or Adnexal Region

In our experience, an intact ectopic pregnancy is demonstrable in about 1%–5% of all extrauterine pregnancies and thus is a relatively rare

occurrence. A clear differentiation cannot always be made between tubal, ovarian, and abdominal pregnancies. If an intact gestational sac can be visualized in the adnexal region with the uterus also well defined, an early diagnosis of ectopic pregnancy may be made (Fig. 4.42). If the fetus is alive, vital signs should also be demonstrable (Fig. 4.43).

If sonograms disclose an adnexal cyst in the presence of positive adnexal palpatory findings and a positive pregnancy test, this is not sufficient to exclude an ectopic pregnancy, because corpus luteum cysts may also be present in ectopic gestations (Fig. 4.44).

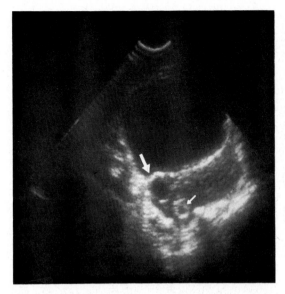

Fig. 4.44. Transverse scan of ectopic pregnancy, 6 weeks. The right tubal pregnancy is unruptured and shows a prominent chorion (*small arrow*). There is an adnexal cyst on the right side

Diagnosis may be aided by the presence of fluid in the cul-de-sac, which is seen in a high percentage of tubal ruptures (Fig. 4.46) and tubal abortions. Although concurrent intrauterine and ectopic pregnancies are reported to have a prevalence of only 1 in 30000, we have observed two such cases during 10 years sonographic practice at our center. The personal communications of other investigators appear to substantiate a higher incidence. On the other hand, the incidental finding of a twin ovarian pregnancy (Fig. 4.45b) is an extremely rare oc-

currence, although development to a live, fullterm infant has been reported (Williams et al. 1982).

It is quite possible for intact ectopic pregnancies to persist into the 5th month. Hansmann (1982) observed the case of a cornual pregnancy at 25 weeks gestation (Fig. 4.47). While the pregnancy was readily accessible to ultrasound visualization, the patient had no significant complaints, and even experienced clinicians failed to appreciate the true nature of the pregnancy or the magnitude of the risk. Referral for sonography in this case was life-saving.

4.3.3 Complex Adnexal Masses

Complex masses, which differ from corpus luteum cysts in their elongated shape and their greater content of solid material, are seen in association with tubal ruptures as well as tubal abortions. These masses vary in shape and cannot be differentiated sonographically from inflammatory adnexal lesions (cf. Fig. 16.8).

4.3.4 Fluid in the Abdomen or Cul-de-Sac

With tubal rupture, a large amount of fluid may be visible in the abdomen and in the flanks (Fig. 4.46). These fluid collections may present as free fluid or organized blood clots in the cul-de-sac lateral and cranial to the uterus. The clots exhibit the sonographic features of solid masses, appearing homogeneous and contrast-

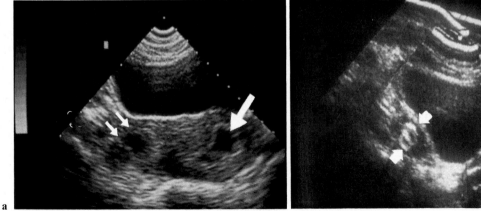

a   b

Fig. 4.45. a Transverse scan of coexisting intrauterine and ectopic pregnancy, 7 weeks. Besides the intrauterine gestational sac with fetus (*arrow*), there is a right tubal

pregnancy with an irregularly shaped sac (*small arrows*). **b** Longitudinal scan at 7 weeks showing a twin ovarian pregnancy (two gestational sacs, *arrows*)

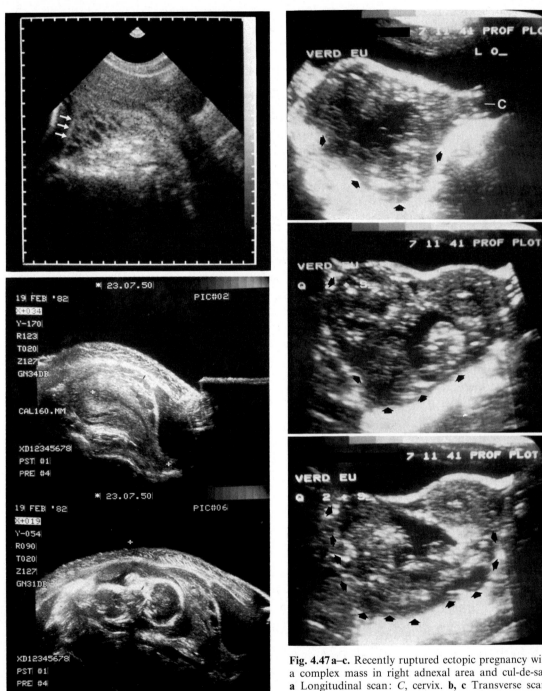

Fig. 4.46a–c. Cornual pregnancy, 25 weeks. **a** The patient was referred for examination with a suspected partial hydatidiform mole. *Small arrows:* vascular structures. **b** Longitudinal scan of uterus: cervicofundal distance 16 cm, pregnancy not intrauterine. **c** A longitudinal scan farther to the right demonstrates the fetus in a sac extending from the right border of the fundus. The patient was asymptomatic at this time. At surgery, uterus and adnexa could be preserved

Fig. 4.47a–c. Recently ruptured ectopic pregnancy with a complex mass in right adnexal area and cul-de-sac. **a** Longitudinal scan: *C*, cervix. **b, c** Transverse scans show a mass behind and to right of uterus. Note irregular outline and mixed internal pattern of mass

ing poorly with surrounding tissues (Fig. 4.47). The tube may present sonographically as an intact solid or cystic mass, and fluid will be present in the cul-de-sac in at least 80% of cases. Small collections of free fluid may be seen under normal conditions in the nongravid patient, especially during the immediate postovulatory period (see Figs. 15.10–15.12).

4.3.5 Principal Sources of Misdiagnosis in Patients with a Positive Pregnancy Test, No Visible Gestational Sac, and Suspected Ectopic Pregnancy

False-positive diagnosis	*False-negative diagnosis*
Early pregnancy and corpus luteum cyst prior to 5 weeks	"Decidual sac" misinterpreted as intrauterine pregnancy
Early pregnancy, corpus luteum cyst with retroflexed uterus, inability to demonstrate gestational sac	Concurrent intrauterine and ectopic pregnancy
Pregnancy in one horn of a bicornuate uterus	Cornual or abdominal pregnancy with a small uterus that is difficult to visualize

Today a negative β-HCG pregnancy test excludes ectopic pregnancy in virtually 100% of cases. Earlier tests on urine specimens had a false-positive or false-negative rate of up to 10%. This may lead to a wrong diagnosis, and unnecessary intervention in patients with adnexitis, a ruptured ovarian cyst or endometriosis. Given the prevalence of repeat ectopic pregnancies, this diagnosis should always be considered in patients with a prior ectopic gestation (Hallatt 1975). Because ectopic pregnancy is difficult to diagnose, and because of the associated morbidity and mortality, all available information must be used to make the diagnosis. Even then, ultrasound may be unable to provide definitive results. The sonographer should personally perform a gynecologic examination, if possible, so that he can better interpret the ultrasound findings. Although frequently sonography can only suggest a range of diagnoses

and aid selection of candidates for laparoscopy, it should always be performed as long as the patient is well enough to tolerate it.

References

Allibone GW, Fagan CJ, Porter SC (1981) The sonographic features of intraabdominal pregnancy. J Clin Ultrasound 9:383

Bradley WG, Fiske CE, Filly RA (1982) The double sac sign of early intrauterine pregnancy: use in exclusion of ectopit pregnancy. Radiology 143:223

Donald I (1965) Ultrasonic echo sounding in obstetrical and gynecological diagnosis. Am J Obstet Gynecol 93:935

Hallatt IG (1975) Repeat ectopic pregnancy: A study of 123 consecutive cases. Am J Obstet Gynecol 122:520

Kobayashi M, Hellmann LJ, Fillisti LP (1969) Ultrasound: An aid in the diagnosis of ectopic pregnancy. Am J Obstet Gynecol 103:1131

Laing FC, Brooke-Jefrey R (1983) Ultrasound Evaluation of Ectopic pregnancy. In: Callen PW (ed) Ultrasonography in obstetrics and gynecology. Saunders, Philadelphia, p 291

Langhlin CL, Lee TG, Richards RG (1983) Ultrasonographic diagnosis of cervical ectopic pregnancy. J Ultrasound Med 2:137

Müller E, Leucht W (1981) Ultraschalldiagnostik bei ektopen Schwangerschaften. Ultraschall 2:158

Nelson P, Bowie JD, Rosenberg E (1983) Early intrauterine pregnancy or decidual cast: An anatomic-sonographic approach. J Ultrasound Med 2:543

Schaffer RM, Stein K, Shih JH, Goodman JD (1983) The echoic pseudogestational sac of ectopic pregnancy simulating early intrauterine pregnancy. J Ultrasound Med 2:215

Williams PC, Malvar TC, Krafft JR (1982) Term ovarian pregnancy with delivery of a live female infant. Am J Obstet Gynecol 142:589

4.4 Tumors Associated with Pregnancy

Tumors coexisting with pregnancy may be of the physiologic or the neoplastic type. Functional cysts may develop as a result of stimulation therapy, signifying hyperstimulation (Fig. 4.48) or may occur as cystic corpora lutea in normal pregnancies. In our experience, corpus luteum cysts of varying size are present in about 20% of all pregnancies, often lead to a presumptive diagnosis of ectopic pregnancy, and usually disappear completely by 15 weeks. With hyperstimulation these cysts may enlarge to more than 10 cm in diameter, while in normal pregnancy they rarely exceed 6–8 cm. They

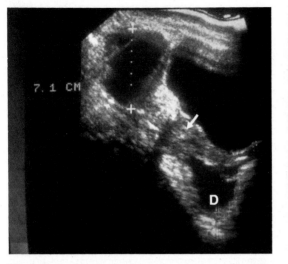

Fig. 4.48. Longitudinal scan at 4 weeks (*arrow*): ovulation induction. There is a 7.1-cm adnexal cyst and fluid in cul-de-sac (D)

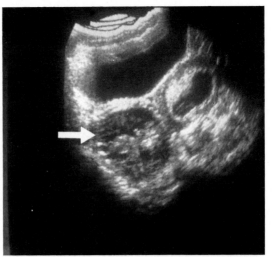

Fig. 4.49. Transverse scan at 8 weeks showing dermoid cyst of right ovary (*arrow*)

are usually asymptomatic, detected incidentally on palpation, and require no treatment. Corpus luteum cysts are relatively uncommon in abnormal intrauterine pregnancies, but we have seen several cases where they coexisted with ectopic pregnancy, making diagnosis more difficult (cf. Sect. 4.3).

Bleeding corpus luteum cysts can produce the same symptoms as ruptured ectopic pregnancy. No clear differentiation can be made on clinical or sonographic grounds.

Even nonbleeding corpus luteum cysts may have areas which appear solid. However, masses that seem more solid than cystic and are also highly echogenic are frequently dermoid cysts, and must be viewed differently (Fig. 4.49). In rare cases large ovarian cystadenomas may also coexist with pregnancy. We have observed an ovarian cystadenoma extending to the costal margin that obscured visualization of the coexisting pregnancy until 15 weeks. Initial sonograms even raised the suspicion of a hydatidiform mole coexisting with pregnancy. Following operative removal of the tumor, the gestation progressed normally and the fetus was carried to term. However, such cases are rare (Fig. 4.50). It is far more common for fibroids to coexist with pregnancy, in which case the location, growth tendency, and spread of the tumor will determine the type of problems that arise (Fig. 4.51 a–d). Repeat examinations may be scheduled throughout the pregnancy, depending on the severity of complaints, the ini-

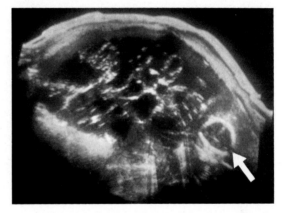

Fig. 4.50. An ovarian cystadenoma completely fills abdominal cavity at 15 weeks. *Arrow:* fetal skull. Pregnancy remained intact after surgery

tial size of the neoplasm, and the increase in size which can be seen in some fibroids. In cases where the location of the fibroid might compromise the pregnancy, sonography is useful in defining the exact location of the tumor and deciding whether it could be enucleated without harming the pregnancy (Fig. 4.51 c) or whether an intervention of this type would compromise the gestational sac (Fig. 4.51 b). It has been our experience that fibroids observed close to the cervix in early pregnancy do not necessarily interfere with delivery of the infant. As in migration of the placenta, growth of the lower uterine segment and uterine rotation can cause fibroids to alter their location.

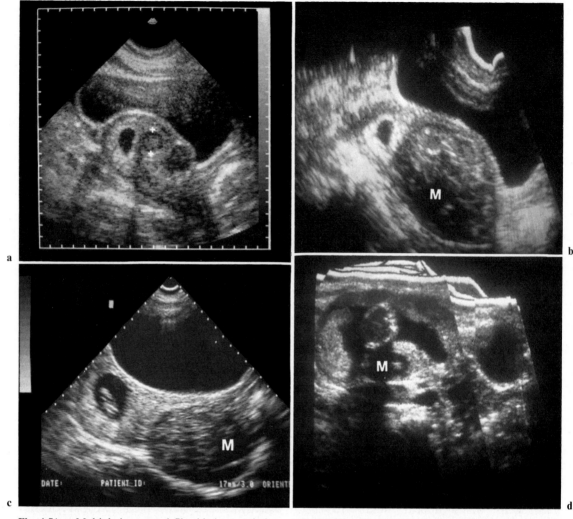

Fig. 4.51. a Multiple intramural fibroids in association with pregnancy 6 weeks). **b** Longitudinal scan showing large intramural fibroid (*M*) and gestational sac. **c** Lon-gitudinal scan at 8 weeks showing cervical subserous fi-broid (*M*). **d** Scan at 13 weeks showing submucous fi-broid (*M*) protruding into amniotic cavity

Muran et al. (1980) report that a large per-centage of fibroids located within the corpus uteri are not detected clinically. These authors state further that the size of the fibroids is not necessarily related to the ultimate mode of de-livery, since even large fibroids may be compati-ble with a normal vaginal delivery.

With regard to the growth tendency of fi-broids there is general agreement that approxi-mately 80%–90% show no appreciable growth (Stein et al. 1975; Muran et al. 1980; Fleischer et al. 1980). Size increases of up to 30% have been observed in some cases, but size reductions have also been noted. This is consistent with our own experience. Statistics show no increase in the incidence of fetal growth retardation. Se-rious complications have developed in cases where the fibroid was in direct contact with the site of placental implantation (Muran et al. 1980), leading to premature rupture of the membranes with antepartum and postpartum bleeding. However, all these patients had un-complicated deliveries.

Malignant neoplasms occur, but are extreme-ly rare. The principle followed in these cases is similar to that applied in general gynecology – that solid or cystic tumors (excluding fibroids and corpus luteum cysts) should be managed surgically even during pregnancy.

The ultrasound appearance of a bicornuate uterus is not always easy to interpret and is apt to be mistaken for a tumor, especially a

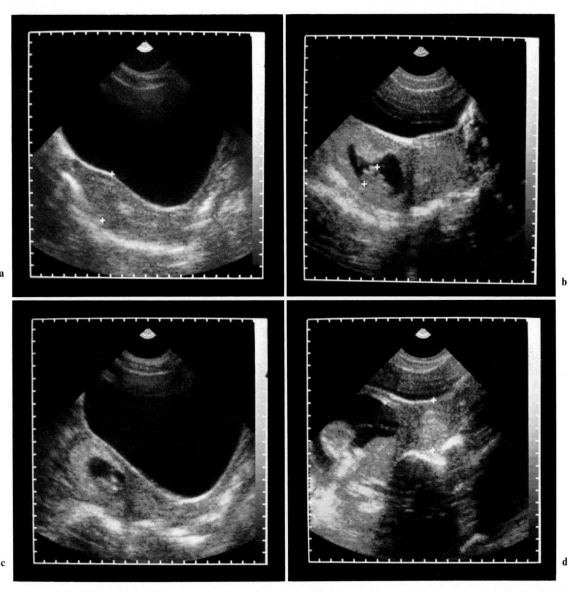

Fig. 4.52a–d. Gravid bicornuate uterus. **a** Longitudinal scan, 11 weeks: left uterine horn empty. **b** Transverse scan: left horn empty, intact pregnancy in right horn. **c** Longitudinal scan: fundal placenta and fetus in right horn. **d** Transverse scan: empty left horn, right horn at 15 weeks

fibroid (Fig. 4.52a–d). In such cases it is important to demonstrate the second uterine cavity, which will show little or no growth on consecutive examinations. Differentiation from ectopic pregnancy may be difficult.

References

Blarr RG (1960) Pregnancy associated with congenital malformations of the reproductive tract. J Obstet Gynaecol Br 67:36

Buttery BW (1972) Spontaneous haemoperitoneum complicating uterine fibromyoma. Aust NZJ Obstet Gynaecol 12:210

Creen WM, Berry S, Wilkinson G (1979) Twin pregnancy in a bicornuate uterus. JCU 7:303

Fleischer AC, Boehm FH, Everette James A (1980) Sonographic evaluation of pelvic masses occurring during pregnancy. In: Saunders R, James E (eds) The principles and practive of ultrasonography in obstetrics and gynecology. Appleton-Century-Crofts Medical, New York, p 263

Muran D, Gillieson M, Walters JH (1980) Myomas of the uterus in pregnancy: Ultrasonographic follow up. Am J Obstet Gynecol 138:16

Stein W, Halberstadt E, Leppien G, Eckert H (1975)
    Ultraschallkriterien zur Beurteilung der Gravidität bei
    Uterus myomatosus. Arch Gynecol 219:398

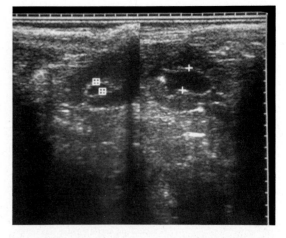

4.5 The Kidney in Pregnancy

Dilatation of the urinary tract in pregnant
women is a well documented phenomenon. As
early as 1842 Cruvelhier found hydronephrosis
and hydroureter, usually on the right side, at
autopsy of pregnant women. For many years
this observation could not be further evaluated
since it would have required excessive irradiation of pregnant patients.

In 1933 Kretschmar et al. were able to demonstrate the dilatation by several X-ray examinations, and in recent years several authors
have confirmed these findings by means of ultrasound (Braasch 1978; Bernascheck and Kratochwil 1981; Spernol et al. 1982). We have
found that dilatation of the urinary tract is
present in about 40% of pregnant women, with
the right kidney more severely affected than the
left in over 80% of cases (Figs. 4.53, 4.54). The
incidence of bilateral hydronephrosis is about
15%. Interestingly, there appears to be no correlation between hydronephrosis and gestational age, although hydronephrosis developing
in a kidney with preexisting disease tends to
worsen as term approaches. These changes are
twice as frequent in women who have a history
of renal disease (Braasch 1978). Many cases are
asymptomatic.

Generally, we assume that dilatation of the
renal pelvis up to 3 cm in diameter is within
normal limits. Dilatation beyond that point
warrants close supervision of urinary findings
during the pregnancy and serial ultrasound examinations. If on the other hand the urinary
findings are abnormal and the patient is symptomatic, a renal ultrasound evaluation is always
indicated. Spernol et al. (1982) drew the following conclusions from studies of pregnant wom-
en with confirmed pyelonephritis:

1. Tenderness at percussion of the renal area
and a dilated renal pelvis on sonography are
associated with urinary tract infection more frequently than tenderness to percussion alone.

2. Simultaneous dilatation of the renal pelvis
and urinary tract infection are associated with
a high incidence of recurrence. In these risk pa-

Fig. 4.53. Longitudinal scan of maternal kidneys in pregnancy: distension of left renal pelvis minimal but right
renal pelvis dilated to 2.1 cm

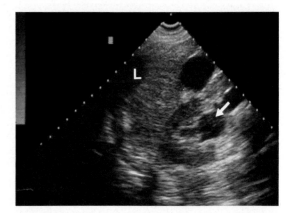

Fig. 4.54. Scan along right costal margin showing dilatation of proximal ureter in pregnancy (*arrow*). *L,* liver

tients it is appropriate to monitor renal findings
during the pregnancy (Fig. 4.54).

We prefer to examine patients in the prone
position up to the 7th month, keeping the examination time as brief as possible. Thereafter
we visualize the kidneys in the supine position,
which can usually be done without much difficulty.

If cystic changes are seen in the kidney, it
may be that the hydronephrosis of pregnancy
is accompanied by a more serious, possibly inherited renal disease (e.g., polycystic kidneys).
In this situation it is appropriate to visualize
the fetal kidneys as well, which can usually be
done during the maternal examination. The
maternal liver and gallbladder can be demonstrated concurrently with the kidneys. Gall-

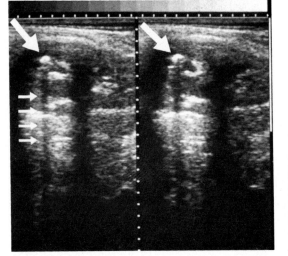

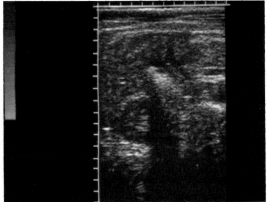

Fig. 4.55. Longitudinal scans of left kidney: only mild dilatation of renal pelvis, but obvious calculus and associated acoustic shadow (*arrows*)

Fig. 4.56. Transverse scan through upper abdomen: liver, gallbladder with stones, associated acoustic shadow

stones, which are not uncommon, are easily identified (Fig. 4.56).

Renal calculi, which also cause pain, abnormal urinalysis, and dilatation of the urinary tract, are common but may be difficult to detect (Fig. 4.55).

References

Bernaschek G, Kratochwil A (1981) Graviditätsbedingte Erweiterungen am Nierenhohlraumsystem. Sonographische Diagnose und Verlaufskontrollen. Geburtshilfe Frauenheilkd 41:208

Braasch M (1978) Ultraschalldarstellung mütterlicher Nierenveränderungen mit Ultraschall. Med Diss Marburg

Fochem K, Wagenbichler P (1969) Beitrag zur Problematik der Veränderungen am Ureter und Nierenhohlsystem in der Schwangerschaft. Geburtshilfe Frauenheilkd 29:278

Harrow BR, Sloane JA, Salhanick L (1964) Etiology of the hydronephrosis of pregnancy. Surg Gynecol Obstet 119:1042

Kretschmer HL, Heaney NS, Ockuly EA (1933) Dilatation of the kidneys, pelvis and ureter during pregnancy and puerperium. JAMA 101:2025

Spernol R, Riss P, Bernaschek G (1982) Echographische Untersuchung des Nierenbeckens bei klinischer Diagnose Pyelitis gravidarium. Geburtshilfe Frauenheilkd 42:717

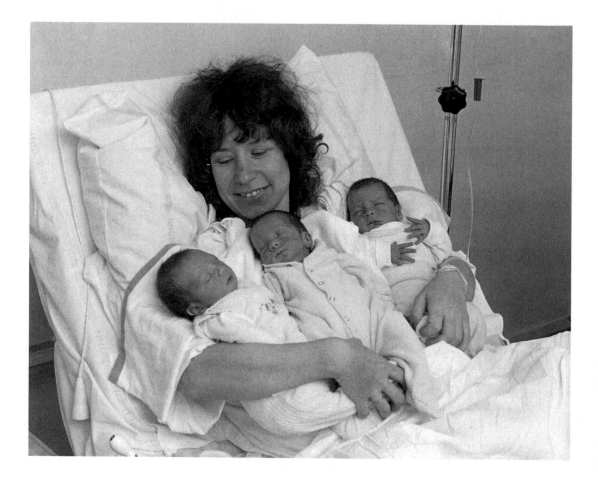

5 Multiple Pregnancy

The early diagnosis of multiple pregnancy is based on the demonstration of two or more gestational sacs, and can be made as early as 5 weeks gestation. By 1976, Campbell et al. were able to diagnose quintuplets by ultrasound at 8 weeks. The earliest we have been able to detect a multiple pregnancy was at 5 weeks.

However, we have suspected multiple pregnancy within 15–20 days after conception, especially in cases where ovarian stimulation was monitored. It should be emphasized that a definite diagnosis of multiple pregnancy should only be made when fetal heart activity can be demonstrated (Figs. 5.1–5.6).

Fig. 5.1.a Longitudinal scan of a quintuplet pregnancy at 8 weeks: four sacs and the anterior wall placenta can be distinguished. **b** A more lateral longitudinal scan: very early growth retardation of one embryo (CRL 12 mm). **c** Oblique section: all five sacs seen

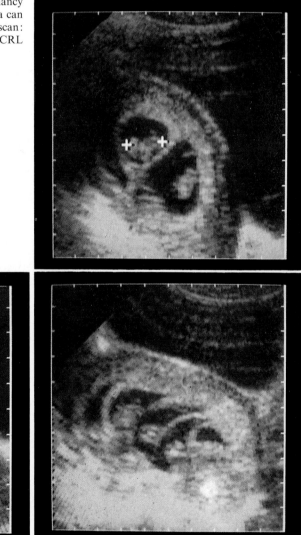

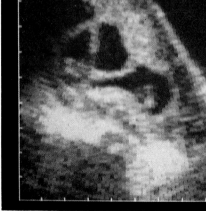

a

b

c

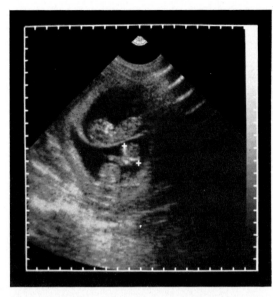

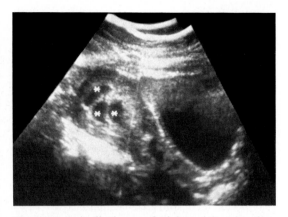

Fig. 5.4. Longitudinal scan of triplets at 6 weeks: three gestational sacs (*asterisks*)

Fig. 5.2. Transverse scan of twin pregnancy at 12 weeks: BPD 17 mm

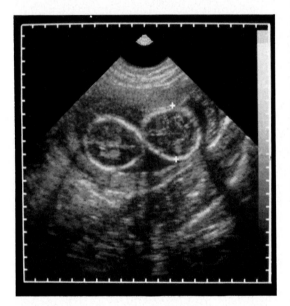

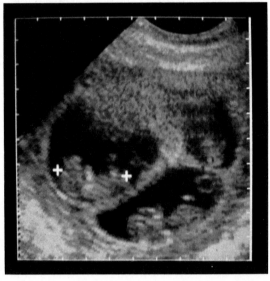

Fig. 5.5. Triplets at 10 weeks: three gestational sacs with three fetuses

Fig. 5.3. Twins at 17 weeks: BPD 40 mm

Hoffbauer (1974) and Levi (1976) were able to confirm the observation of Verschuer in Stökkel's *Textbook of Obstetrics* (1945) that in up to 70% of multiple pregnancies, one or more of the fetuses perish in the first trimester. This estimate may be somewhat high due to the difficulty of differentiating gestational sacs from other intrauterine cystic structures on sonograms. We have seen many cases where the initial scans revealed several gestational sacs which were subsequently expelled (Fig. 5.7a, b). However, we have observed no case in which an embryo or fetus of established viability has "disappeared" without a trace. In the interest of the patient, we refrain from informing her of the diagnosis of multiple fetuses until their viability has been confirmed.

As a general rule, we do not inform our patients of multiple pregnancies prior to 12 weeks. Based on many years of experience with monitoring of follicles and ovulation induction, we believe that the number of empty gestational sacs may correlate with the number of immature follicles that rupture concurrently with a mature follicle.

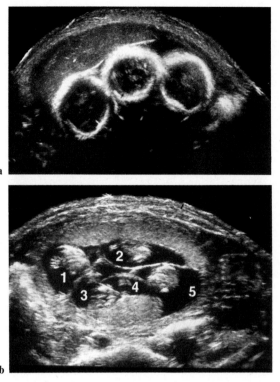

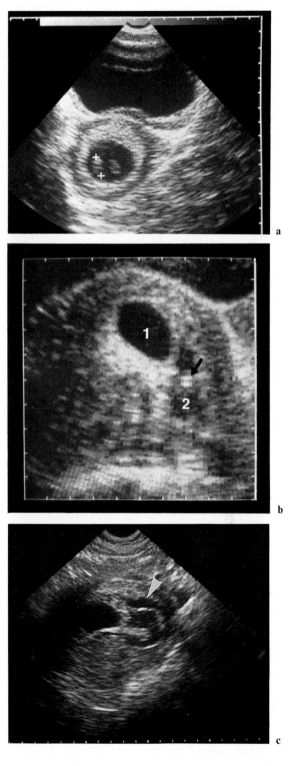

Fig. 5.6. a Triplets at 19 weeks. **b** Multiple pregnancy: five gestational sacs with fetal parts

A similar picture to that shown in Fig. 5.7 may result from therapeutic reduction of multiple pregnancies, which was performed at our center in Bonn in three cases. Induction of ovulation by means of gonadotropin stimulation (HMG/HCG) had been carried out (in other hospitals) and had resulted in two quintuplet pregnancies and one sextuplet pregnancy. After early ultrasound diagnosis, the parents and their physicians insisted on therapeutic abortion, but accepted as an alternative an attempt of "reduction." This was then accomplished by sonar-guided transabdominal aspiration of the fluid from two or three of the sacs followed

Fig. 5.7. a Abnormal twin pregnancy at 6 weeks and 5 days (ovulation induction). There is a live, normal-sized embryo (CRL 13 mm) and a smaller, less well defined structure representing a second, dead embryo. **b** Abnormal twin pregnancy at 9 weeks and 2 days. One sac appears normal and appropriate for dates (*1*); the second is smaller, irregular, and contains an embryonic structure (*arrow*; *2*). **c** Twin pregnancy at 7 weeks: *left*, normal gestational sac; *right* collapsed sac and retrochorionic bleeding (arrow)

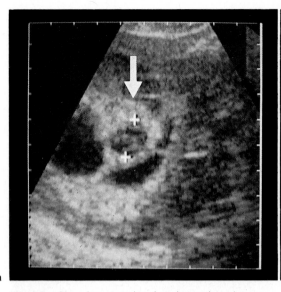

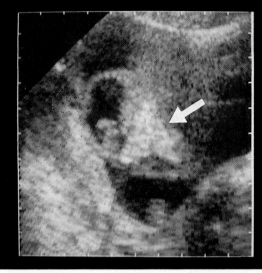

a

b

Fig. 5.8. a Shrunken gestational sac in a quintuplet pregnancy 3 days after aspiration of fluid (20 ml) followed by injection of 5 ml 8.9% NaCl solution. **b** Same case, longitudinal scan: echogenic chorion (*arrow*) of a "reduced" sac, two "untouched" embryos in their fluid-containing sacs

by injection of 5 ml 8.9% NaCl solution (Fig. 5.8a, b). None of the mothers showed any ill effects from this "embryocide". In one case, reduced to a triplet pregnancy, abortion followed 10 weeks later after performance of cerclage in another hospital. In the other two cases healthy twins were born.

If one fetus of a twin pregnancy dies, it may become compressed and mummified (fetus papyraceus; Fig. 5.9a–d). This does not automatically lead to complications, although the death of a twin after 20 weeks is associated with an increased risk of premature labor and delivery. Litschgi and Stucki (1980) report the death of one twin in almost 7% of their twin pregnancies, usually in the second and third trimester. The major cause of these deaths was twin-to-twin transfusion (Holländer and Backmann 1974), which is discussed in greater detail in Sect. 9.1.

Twin pregnancies also have a higher rate of fetal anomalies. In this chapter we shall consider only thoracopagus (twins conjoined at the chest). Until recently, this malformation was not recognized sonographically until the third trimester of pregnancy (Hansmann et al. 1979; Fig. 5.11a–e). However, Schmidt et al. (1981) and we have been able to identify conjoined twins at 11 weeks (Fig. 5.10). It is conceivable that an accurate anatomic evaluation of con-

joined twins in the antepartum state might help in deciding between termination and continuation of the pregnancy with postpartum separation. To the best of our knowledge, however, the early diagnosis of thoracopagus has always led to elective termination.

Fig. 5.9. a Twin pregnancy at 19 weeks: in front of head of normally developed fetus, a recently expired, severely growth-retarded fetus (CRL 68 mm) is shown in longitudinal axis (*arrows*). **b** Longitudinal scan of fetus papyraceus: skull is flattened and compressed. **c** Abnormal twin pregnancy at 25 weeks: compressed head of fetus papyraceus (*arrow*) presents as spindle-shaped structure in front of head of live fetus. **d** Fetus papyraceus with placenta after delivery. **e** Fetofetal transfusion syndrome at 16 weeks: left, sitting fetus has a cystic hygroma 17 mm in diameter. **f** Fetofetal transfusion syndrome at 24 weeks: smaller twin seems to be fixed at anterior placenta resulting from anhydramnios (TTD 48 mm), larger fetus shows marked ascites in this longitudinal scan. **g** Longitudinal scan of twin pregnancy at 19 weeks: one fetus appears normal, one is an acephalus (+——+ = 96 mm). **h** Same pregnancy at 22 weeks: acephalus shows considerable growth and hydrops, healthy fetus is threatened by onset of preterm labor. **i** Abnormal twin pregnancy at 29 weeks: dead fetus with BPD of 40 mm (17 weeks); live fetus with BPD of 68 mm showing early growth retardation

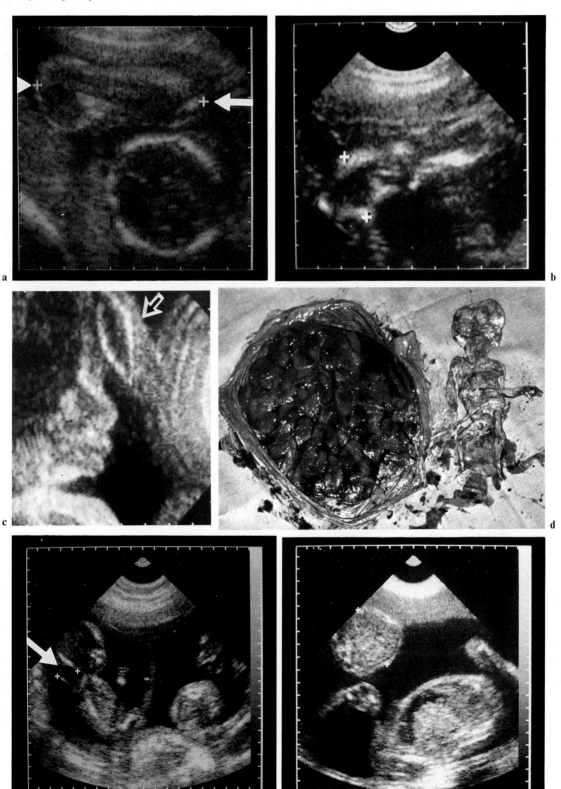

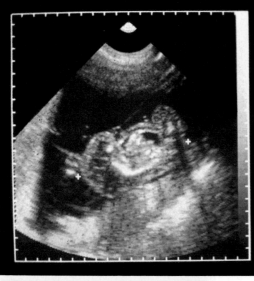

g

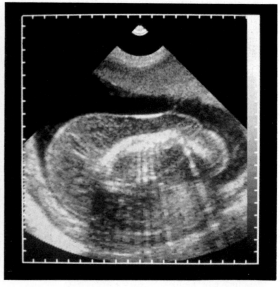

h

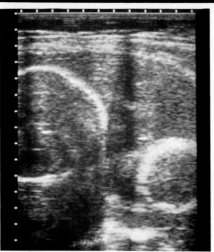

i

Fig. 5.9
g–i

Signs suggestive of thoracopagus are:

1. The absence of a membrane between the fetuses
2. A fixed position of the fetuses relative to each other in motion over a period of several examinations
3. Inability to separate the trunks in transverse scans
4. Inability to detect two different heart rates

Twin pregnancies are considered to represent a high-risk group, and it may be neccessary to monitor them sonographically at 4-week intervals initially, with an increase in frequency to 2 weeks in the third trimester. This may be nec-essary to ensure the early recognition of discordant growth.

Twin pregnancies are associated with a 3–4 times higher rate of perinatal mortality than singleton pregnancies. This is due mainly to the high incidence of preterm delivery (approximately 50%), malpresentation, growth retardation, malformations, and maternal preeclampsia.

A number of authors, most notably Grennert et al. (1978), have pointed to the substantial value of routine sonograms for twin gestations. Through early diagnosis, it has been possible to institute specific intensive prenatal care measures, with a reduction of perinatal mortality from 6% to 0.6% and a reduction of preterm births from 33% to 10%. These results are confirmed by Kucera et al. (1980) and by Goeschen (1980).

Even when ultrasound is used, however, it is possible for twins to be missed, at least on initial examination. The period from 16 to 20 weeks gestation is the time when multiple fetuses are most clearly discerned. This actually becomes more difficult in the third trimester, and a thorough, systematic examination is necessary if a multiple pregnancy is to be disclosed at that stage.

Because the biometry of multiple fetuses should commence either in the first trimester or between 16 and 20 weeks gestation, the ta-

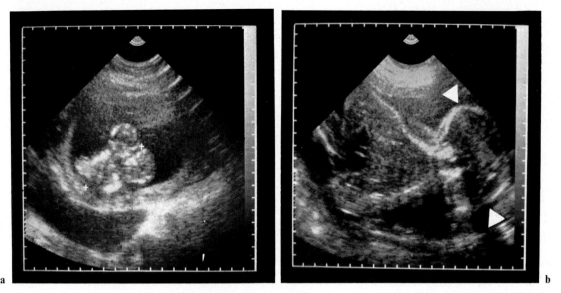

Fig. 5.10. a Thoracopagus at 13 weeks: fetuses facing each other (+——+ = 56 mm). **b** Thoracopagus at 21 weeks: position of fetuses unchanged (*arrows* indicate occiputs)

bles used for singletons will apply. This is not true of weight estimates in the third trimester, when conventional charts and tables will yield erroneously high values. In this case one can subtract 10% from the value for singletons to obtain a satisfactory weight estimate. It is important to use ultrasound not only in labour to check lie and presentation of the fetuses, but also during the course of delivery. Immediately after the first twin is delivered, it is easy to assess lie and presentation of the second twin and recognize any unexpected changes in the position so that appropriate obstetric action can be taken. With a transverse lie, ultrasound can even be used to monitor the internal version of the fetus.

Ultrasound is also used in the antepartum period as a means of localizing both fetal hearts for CTG monitoring. We feel that an ultrasound instrument should be available at every labor-delivery facility for twin pregnancies, especially in instances where vaginal delivery is planned.

References

Berkowitz RL (1979) Ultrasound in the antenatal management of multiple gestations. In: Hobbins JC (ed) Diagnostic ultrasound in obstetrics. Churchill Livingstone, New York

Campbell S, Dewhurst CJ (1970) Quintuplet pregnancy diagnosed and assessed by ultrasonic compound scanning. Lancet 17:101

Campbell S, Grundy M, Singer J-D (1976) Early antenatal diagnosis of spina bifida in a twin fetus by ultrasonic examination and alpha-feto-protein determination. Br Med J 2:676

Goeschen K (1980) Sonographische Befunde bei Mehrlingen und ihre Konsequenzen. Geburtshilfe Frauenheilkd 40:836

Grennert I, Persson P-H, Gennser G (1978) Benefits of ultrasonic screening of a pregnant population. Acta Obstet Gynecol Scand [Suppl] 8:5

Hansmann M, Schlächter H, Födisch HJ, Plotz EJ (1979) Präpartale Diagnose eines Thoracopagus mittels Ultrasonographie. Gynäkologe 12:64

Hellmann LM, Kobayski M, Cromb E (1973) Ultrasonic diagnosis of embryonic malformations. Am J Obstet Gynecol 115:615

Hoffbauer H (1974) Problematik der Ultraschalldiagnose von normalen und anormalen Mehrlingsschwangerschaften. 2. Jahrestagung der DAUD, Hannover

Holländer HJ (1969) Monoamniotische Zwillinge. Z Geburtshilfe 171:292

Holländer HJ, Backmann R (1974) Das Transfusionssyndrom bei Zwillingen. Geburtshilfe Frauenheilkd 34:931

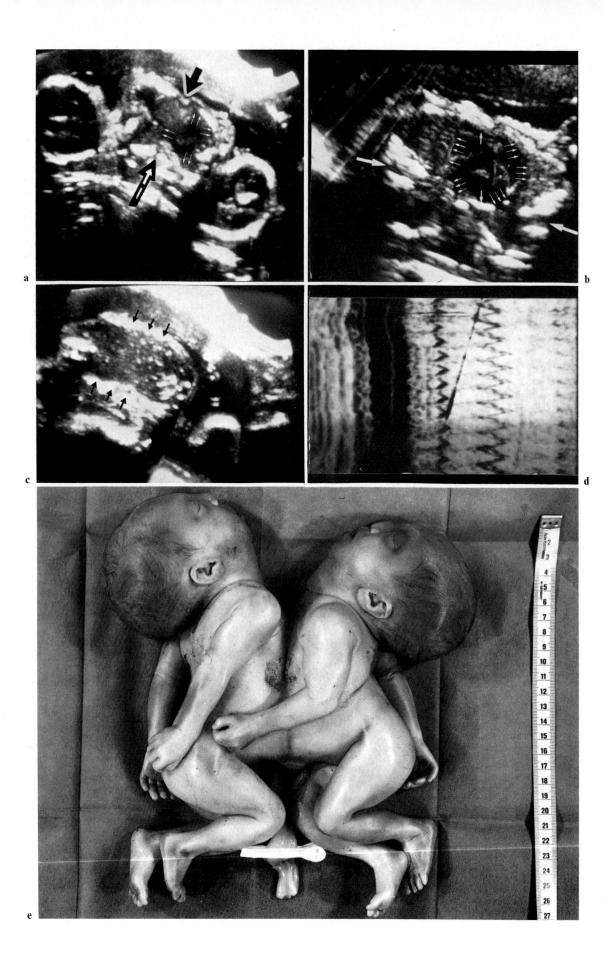

a

b

c

d

e

Houlton MCC (1977) Divergent biparietal diameter growth rates in twin pregnancies. Obstet Gynecol 49:542

Kucera H, Reinold E, Schönswetter P (1980) Zur Bedeutung der Ultraschalldiagnostik für das perinatale Schicksal von Mehrlingsschwangerschaften. In: Hinselmann M, Anliker M, Mendt R (eds) Ultraschalldiagnostik in der Medizin. Drei-Länder-Treffen Davos. Thieme, Stuttgart New York, p 157

Leveno KJ, Santos-Ramos R, Duenhoelter JH, Reisch J-S, Whalley PJ (1979) Sonor cephalometry in twins: A table of biparietal diameters for normal twin fetuses and a comparison with singletons. Am J Obstet Gynecol 135:727

Leveno KJ, Santos-Ramos R, Duenhoelter JH, Reisch J-S, Whalley J (1980) Sonar cephalometry in twin pregnancy: Discordancy of the biparietal diameter after 28 weeks gestation. Am J Obstet Gynecol 138:615

Levi S (1976) Ultrasonic assessment of the high rate of human multiple pregnancy in the first trimester. J Clin Ultrasound 4:3

Litschgi M, Stucki D (1980) Verlauf von Zwillingsschwangerschaften nach intrauterinem Fruchttod eines Föten. Z Geburtshilfe Perinatol 184:227

Morgan CL, Trought WS, Sheldon G, Barton TK (1978) B-scan und real-time ultrasound in the antepartum diagnosis of conjoined twins and pericardial effusion. Am J Roentgenol 130:578

Ottow B (1945) Die Mehrlingsschwangerschaft und die Mehrlingsgeburt. In: Stoeckel W (ed) Lehrbuch der Geburtshilfe, 8. edn. Fischer, Jena

Schmidt W, Kubli D, Heberling D (1981) Diagnose von siamesischen Zwillingen in der 12. Schwangerschaftswoche. Geburtshilfe Frauenheilkd 41:227

Walter HM (1982) Zur Diagnose eines Acardius in der Schwangerschaft durch Ultraschall. Geburtshilfe Frauenheilkd 42:551

Wilson DA, Young GZ, Crumley CS (1983) Antepartum ultrasonographic diagnosis of ischiopagus. J Ultrasound Med 2:281

Wilson RL, Cetrulo CJ, Shaub MS (1976) The prepartum diagnosis of conjoined twins by the use of diagnostic ultrasound. Am J Obstet Gynecol 126:737

◁ **Fig. 5.11 a–e.** Thoracopagus at 27 weeks. **a** Longitudinal scan shows both heads in frontal section. Between them are fetal trunks, facing each other and cross-sectioned level of upper thorax. *Small arrows* indicate heart, also seen in cross-section. Lateral chest walls are joined (*large arrows*). **b** Transverse scan through the upper thorax: *larger arrows* indicate fetal spines, which show excessive lordosis. Common heart, sectioned at level of valves, is seen as oval feature between spines (*small arrows*). **c** Longitudinal scan to right shows cross-sections of fused trunks at level of liver. *Small arrows* mark lateral trunk walls. Spine of superior fetus is at 10 o'clock, that of inferior fetus at 4 o'clock. **d** Time-motion display at this and various other angles and levels shows only one fetal heart rate (Hansmann et al. 1979)

6 Amniocentesis

Amniocentesis for prenatal diagnosis of genetic disease has become a universally practiced technique. Owing to improvements in methodology, it is no longer reserved for high-risk cases.

Amniocentesis for prenatal genetic diagnosis is usually performed between 15 and 17 weeks gestation. This period is favored because by then the amniotic fluid contains an adequate number of cells, and there is still time to consider an elective termination within legal limits.

Amniocentesis for evaluation of Rh incompatibility or lung maturity is not discussed here, but the technique is the same. The goal of genetic amniocentesis includes the determination of karyotype from cell cultures, α-fetoprotein assay, and possibly metabolic studies if indicated by the patient's history. The role of ultrasound in amniocentesis is both to increase the safety and accuracy of the procedure and to supplement the finding of fluid analysis by providing a detailed anatomic profile of the fetus. Today we consider ultrasound to be an indispensable adjunct to amniocentesis.

Although indications for amniocentesis have been clearly defined in collaboration between obstetricians and geneticists, every candidate for amniocentesis should be given individual preliminary counseling. In the Federal Republic of Germany, amniocentesis is considered in the following situations: patient age over 35 years at time of delivery or husband age over 45 years (about 75%); history of trisomy 21 or other chromosome anomalies (about 7%); neural tube defects (about 8%) or multiple malformations (3%); heterozygosity for Duchenne-type muscular dystrophy (about 1%) or hemophilia (about 1%); and the presence of stress factors (radiation, drugs), including psychologic stress (about 6%).

At one time transvaginal amniocentesis and blind transabdominal punctures were performed solely on the basis of clinical palpatory findings; this practice is no longer justified.

According to studies by Jonatha (1974), Schmidt et al. (1980), Romero et al. (1985), and a recent survey by Holzgreve and Hansmann (1984), the optimum technique for amniocentesis should not rely either on fixed ultrasound guidance alone or on blind puncture, but should consist of ultrasound-guided, freehanded needle insertion.

Immediately following a preliminary sonographic examination (both to establish the puncture site and for detailed fetal anatomic evaluation), the site of needle insertion is marked on the maternal abdomen. The area is then aseptically prepared and draped with a sterile towel or slit drape.

Since visualization of the needle has become much easier and risk of contamination less with the advent of new high-resolution scanners with small sector heads, we monitor most needle insertions continuously. The transducer is held perpendicular to the needle and the needle tip is visualized (Figs. 6.1 and 6.3). With this technique it is nearly always possible to find the most direct path to the gestational sac, thus enabling the use of relatively short and small gauge needles (less than 1 mm outer diameter; Fig. 6.2). Although they are useful in other areas, we feel that special biopsy transducers are not necessary for amniocentesis.

In our experience local anesthesia is unnecessary, because most pain is felt as the needle perforates the peritoneum, and this is not prevented by local anesthesia. We always use stylet-armed needles, and routinely discard the initial 1–2 ml amniotic fluid before drawing 12–20 ml for analysis.

General recommendations:

1. It is essential that ultrasound be used to localize the placenta and determine the site of needle insertion.
2. The aspiration should be performed under direct guidance whenever possible.

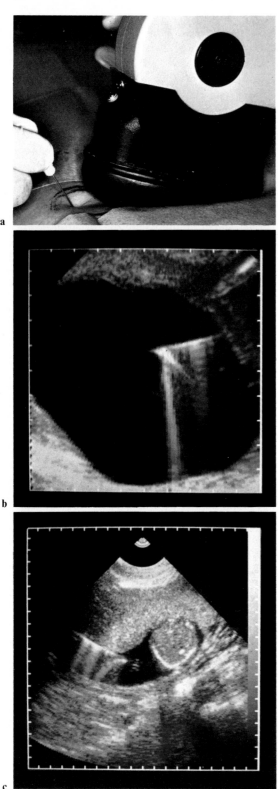

3. The operator should be experienced in amniocentesis. Even at larger centers, amniocenteses should be done by a limited number of physicians who are well versed in the technique.

4. The operator should have expertise in ultrasound.

5. The needle should not exceed 1.0 mm in outer diameter.

It follows from these recommendations that amniocentesis should be practiced only in centers where significant numbers of procedures are performed on a regular basis by experienced personnel.

The recommended needle size is also important for transplacental aspirations, which are sometimes necessary. We believe that it is safer to insert a 0.7-mm needle transplacentally, if that is the most direct route, than to bypass the placenta by inserting a larger gauge needle over a greater distance from a more lateral site and thus increasing the risk of bowel trauma and infection. This opinion is shared by Harvey and Levine (1983), who found no increase in abortion rates with small-gauge needles inserted transplacentally.

Following the aspiration, fetal viability is reassessed. Rh prophylaxis with anti-D gamma globulin is indicated in patients at risk for isoimmunization (Golbus et al. 1982).

For amniocenteses in twin gestations, we collect the first fluid sample and then instill 1–3 ml of indigo carmine dye into the gestational sac (Fig. 6.4). We than draw fluid from the second sac (localized by ultrasound) and check the color of the sample to verify that the correct sac has been entered.

Potential complications are listed in Tables 6.1 through 6.3 (Holzgreve and Hansmann 1984).

Milunsky stated in a 1981 editorial in the *American Journal of Medicine* that the risk of fetal loss associated with amniocentesis was less than 0.5%, and that the procedure caused no significant maternal or fetal morbidity. Indeed, in the more than 100,000 amniocenteses that have been performed to date internationally, only one case of maternal death (in the Federal Republic of Germany) has been recorded. There still appears to be a small risk as far as the fetus is concerned (Harvey and Levine 1983), but independent of the various amnio-

Fig. 6.1. a Ultrasound-guided amniocentesis using a sector scanner with water coupling. **b** Needle in place. **c** Needle in place, avoiding an anterior placenta

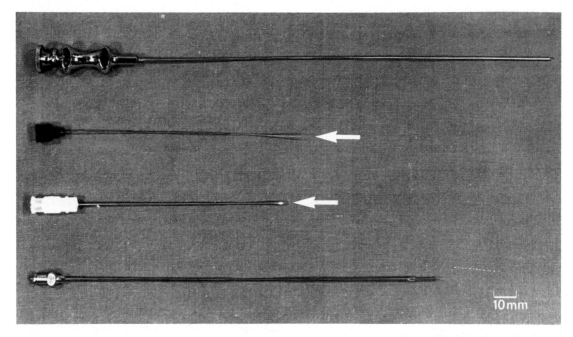

Fig. 6.2. Amniocentesis needles. *Arrows:* the 22G3 needle used by the authors. Stylet, black head; needle, white head

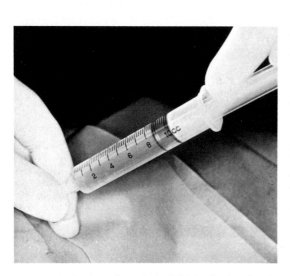

Fig. 6.3. Collection of amniotic fluid by freehand technique. Important: needle is stabilized using one hand as sample is drawn

Fig. 6.4. Amniocentesis needle in place with contrast medium dripping from needle tip

centesis techniques used, it is always less than 1% (Simpson et al. 1980).

Few data are yet available on a new prenatal diagnostic procedure, first-trimester chorion biopsy, but several centers have already started to conduct the procedure under ultrasound guidance (Fig. 6.5). Most examiners either aspirate the biopsy material with a Portex catheter or remove the specimen with biopsy forceps. Unfortunately, few data are yet available on associated abortion risks. For the foreseeable future this procedure will remain confined to

Table 6.1. Reasons for repeat amniocentesis

Reasons	Patients	
	Bonn (n = 2,000)	Münster (n = 1,215)
Dry tap	1	5
Poor growth of cell culture	40	9
Pathology found on initial amniocentesis (chromosome abnormality or elevated AFP with no sonographic evidence of pathology)	–	27
Total	41 (2.1%)	41 (3.4%)

Table 6.2. Color of amniotic fluid samples

Color	Patients	
	Bonn (n = 2,000)	Münster (n = 1,215)
Clear	1,896 (94.8%)	1,148 (94.5%)
Red-tinged	40 (2.0%)	30 (2.5%)
Bloody	10 (0.5%)	10 (0.8%)
Discolored	54 (2.7%)	27 (2.3%)

Table 6.3. Complications associated with amniocentesis

Complications	Patients	
	Bonn (n = 2,000)	Münster (n = 1,215)
"Spontaneous" abortion (within 14 days following amniocentesis)	6 (0.3%)	6 (0.5%)
Amniotic fluid loss after amniocentesis	11 (0.6%)	9 (0.7%)

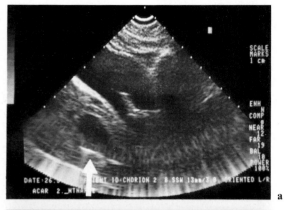

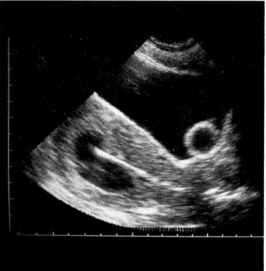

Fig. 6.5a, b. Chorion biopsy performed with a Portex catheter. **a** At 7 weeks gestation. **b** At 8 weeks: the tip of the catheter threatens to perforate the anterior wall of the sac

centers where a cytogeneticist or biologist and facilities for immediate sterile preparation of the specimen are available (Brambati and Simoni 1983; Gustavii et al. 1984; Tietung Hospital, Ansham, Dept. of Obstetrics 1975; Ward et al. 1983).

References

Berner HW, Seisler EP, Barlow J (1972) Fetal cardiac tamponade. Obstet Gynecol 599

Brambati B, Simoni G (1983) Diagnosis of fetal trisomy 21 in first trimester. Lancet 12:586

Broome DL, Wilson MG, Weiss B, Kellogg B (1976) Needle puncture of fetus: A complication of second-trimester amniocentesis. Am J Obstet Gynecol 126:257

Cross HE, Maumenee AE (1973) Ocular trauma during amniocentesis. Arch Ophthalmol 90:303

Deutsche Forschungsgemeinschaft (1982) 16. Informationsblatt über die Dokumentation der Untersuchungen im Rahmen des Schwerpunktprogramms „Pränatale Diagnostik genetisch bedingter Defekte". Stand 10431 dokumentierte Fälle. München

Gerbie AB, Elias S (1980) Amniocentesis for antenatal diagnosis of genetic defects. Semin Perinatol 4:159

Golbus MS, Loughman WD, Epstein CJ, Halbasch G, Stephens JD, Hall BD (1979) Prenatal genetic diagnosis in 3000 amniocentesis. N Engl J Med 300:157

Golbus MS, Stephens JD, Cann HM, Mann J, Hensleigh PA (1982) Rh-isoimmunization following genetic amniocentesis. Prenat Diagn 2:149

Gustavii, Chester BA, Edvall H, Iosif S, Kristofersson

U, Löfberg L, Mineur A, Mitelman F (1984) First-trimester diagnosis on chorionic villi obtained by direct vision technique. Hum Genet 65:373

Hackelöer BJ (1977) Unter-Sicht-Amniocentese mit neuem schnellen Ultraschall-B-Bild-Verfahren. In: Schmidt B, Dudenhausen JW, Saling E (eds) Perinatale Medizin, Bd VII. Thieme, Stuttgart

Hansmann M, Knoerr K (1978) Amniozentese in der Frühschwangerschaft – Technik, Probleme. In: Saling E, Dudenhausen J (eds) Perinatale Medizin, Bd 7. Thieme, Stuttgart New York, S 305

Harvey M, Levine RJ (1983) The risk of research procedures: Methodologic problems and proposed standards. Clin Res 31:126

Holzgreve W, Hansmann M (1984) Erfahrung mit der „Free-Hand-Needle"-Technik bei 3215 Amniocentesen im 2. Trimenon zur pränatalen Diagnostik. Gynäkologe 17:77–82

Jonatha W (1974) Amniozentese in der Frühschwangerschaft unter Sichtkontrolle mit Ultraschall. Electromedica 3:94

Lamb MP (1975) Gangrene of a fetal limb due to amniocentesis. Br J Obstet Gynaecol 82:829

Milunsky A (1981) Prenatal diagnosis of genetic disorders. Am J Med 70/7

Murken JD, Stengel-Rutkowski S (eds) (1979) Pränatale Diagnostik. Enke, Stuttgart

Nelson LH, Goodman HO, Brown SH (1977) Ultrasonography preceding diagnostic amniocentesis and its effect on amniotic fluid cell growth. Obstet Gynecol 50:65

NICHD – National Registry for Amniocentesis Study Group (1976) Midtrimester amniocentesis for prenatal diagnosis. JAMA 236:1471

Schmidt W, Gabelmann J, Mueller U, Voigtlaender T, Hager HD, Schroeder TM, Garoff L, Kubli F (1980) Pränatale Diagnostik. Technik und Ergebnisse von 1000 Fruchtwasserpunktionen. Geburtshilfe Frauenheilkd 40:761

Simpson NE, Turnbull AC, Alexander D, Bantock H, Czerski P, Doran TA, Kaback M, Liedgren S, Murken JD, Ogita S, Seigal D, Sutherland I (1980) Prenatal diagnosis – Past, present and future. Report of an International Workshop. Prenatal Diagnosis (Special Issue) 1:5

Stengel-Rutkowski (1980) Antenataldiagnostik: Resultate und Risiken. Erfahrung West-Deutschlands. J Genet Hum 28:73

Tettenborn U (1978) Amniozentesetechnik. Vorgetragen auf der 3. Konferenz für Prenataldiagnose, München

Tietung Hospital, Ansham, Dept. of Obs. Gynec. (1975) Fetal sex prediction by sexchromatin of chorionic villi cells during early pregnancy. Chin Med J 1(2):117

Ward RHT, Modell B, Karagozlie F, Douratsos E (1983) Method of sampling chorionic villi in first trimester of pregnancy under guidance of real time ultrasound. Br Med J 286:1542

Working party on Amniocentesis of the United Kingdom Medical Research Council (1978) An assessment of the hazards of amniocentesis. Br J Obstet Gynaecol 85 (Suppl 2):1

7 Normal Fetal Anatomy in the Second and Third Trimester

The key to successful ultrasound diagnosis lies in the ability to obtain a detailed image in which a maximum of anatomic information is presented. The examiner must know the complete spectrum of "normal" sonographic findings, and he must be able to demonstrate them adequately. Only in this way will he consistently be able to recognize fetal abnormalities and measure fetal structures with the necessary degree of accuracy.

There is no question that real-time techniques are far superior to static imaging in the depiction of anatomic details. Today the resolution, gray-scale reproduction, and high rate of image generation of real-time equipment closely approximate or even surpass the quality obtained with static scanners.

We decided to approach the subject of fetal anatomy from a practical standpoint, organizing our material on the basis of procedures that we routinely follow in the conduct of sonographic examinations.

7.1 Examination Procedure

Every ultrasound examination should be performed in two phases, regardless of whether it is a routine screening examination (level I) or a more detailed evaluation (level II or III; see Sect. 8.9).

Phase 1. This serves the purpose of general orientation. The goals of phase 1 are to determine:

1. Uterine location
2. Uterine shape
3. Uterine size
4. Placental location
5. Amniotic fluid volume
6. Number of fetuses
7. Fetal heart activity
8. Fetal movements
9. Fetal presentation and lie

For didactic reasons the examiner should check these points in logical sequence and make a mental note of each. Only then should he proceed to phase 2 – the detailed inspection and biometry of the fetus. If the examination is conducted without a plan, there is definite risk that important features will be missed. The examiner who confines himself to measuring the biparietal diameter (BPD) may well overlook multiple fetuses, fetal death, or the presence of a placenta praevia. The importance of ascertaining fetal position is again emphasized in this regard. Unless he knows the position of the fetus within the uterus, the examiner cannot be sure which side of the fetal body he is observing. It must be remembered that the maternal *right* side is on the *left* in the transverse scan, and the maternal *left* side is on the *right* (as in any anatomic atlas). In longitudinal scans, the *left* side of the sonogram is cranial, and the *right* side is caudal. These relationships are illustrated schematically in Figs. 7.1 and 7.2.

When real-time equipment is being used, even an experienced examiner may become con-

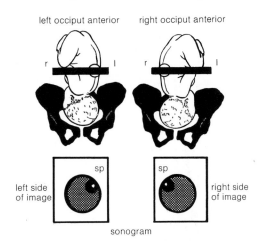
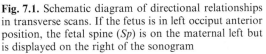

Fig. 7.1. Schematic diagram of directional relationships in transverse scans. If the fetus is in left occiput anterior position, the fetal spine (*Sp*) is on the maternal left but is displayed on the right of the sonogram

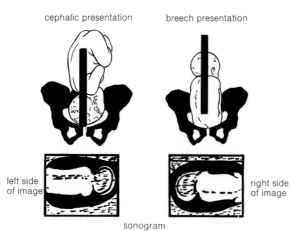

cephalic presentation   breech presentation

left side
of image   right side
                                                            of image

sonogram

Fig. 7.2. Directional relationship in longitudinal scans. In cephalic presentation the fetal head is on the right of the sonogram. In breech presentation the head is on the left

patient will the examiner be able to evaluate fetal lie, presentation, and position. We have found an almost foolproof way to maintain left/ right orientation during ultrasound examinations: The examiner determines the fetal position, noting whether the fetal spine is anterior, transverse or posterior, and then imagines himself assuming the same position in utero. From then on he will know at once which arm is left or right and will maintain his orientation even if the fetus changes position during the course of the examination.

Phase 2. The success of the phase 2 examination is determined essentially by two factors:

1. The ability of the examiner to extrapolate three dimensions from the two-dimensional images on the screen

2. The examiner's basic knowledge of fetal topographic anatomy

Even the best equipment cannot guarantee success unless both of these requirements are satisfied.

fused, since the transducer may be rotated 180° without the examiner being aware of it (this is especially common with small, hand-held sector scanners).

To avoid this loss of orientation, we recommend that the examiner check the scanning direction by slipping a finger in laterally between the transducer and the abdominal wall. Only by knowing which part of the image is left and right and which is up and down relative to the

To facilitate the learning process, we shall use a standard nomenclature consistently throughout this chapter. In cases where the isolated depiction of sonograms might be confusing topographically, frozen anatomic sections will be shown for clarity. The principal scanning planes are illustrated in Fig. 7.3. Experi-

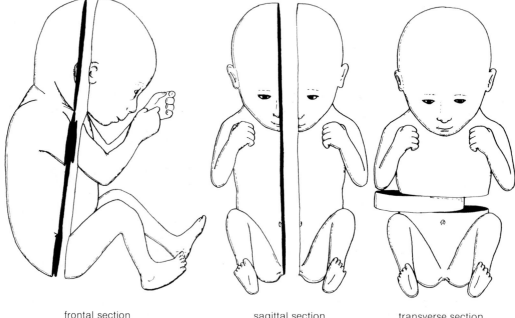

frontal section   sagittal section   transverse section

Fig. 7.3. Standard planes of section

a *Posterior sagittal section*
  Skull
  Neck region
  Spine
  Kidneys (paravertebral)

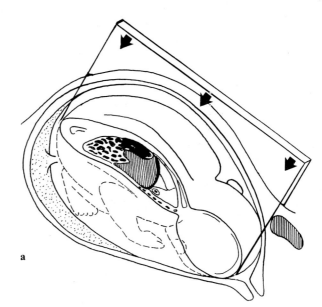

b *Anterior sagittal section*
  Facial profile
  Anterior body surface (look for defects
    of the thoracic and abdominal wall)
  Body shape (relationship of thorax
    to abdomen)
  Diaphragm
  Liver, umbilical vein
  Stomach
  Extremities

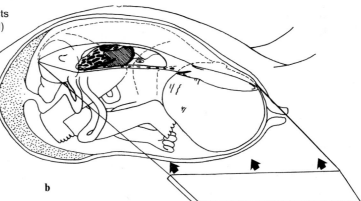

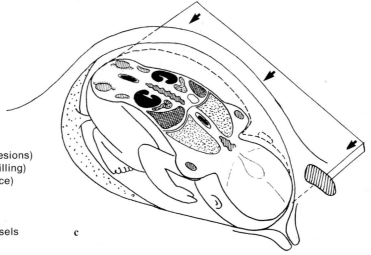

c *Frontal sections*
  Body symmetry
  Spine (check for asymmetry, lesions)
  Stomach (location, degree of filling)
  Kidneys (symmetry, appearance)
  Diaphragm, aorta
  Urinary bladder
  Extremities, genitalia
  Umbilical cord, number of vessels

Fig. 7.4a–c. Sectional anatomy in longitudinal scans. Objects of primary interest in each plane of section are listed

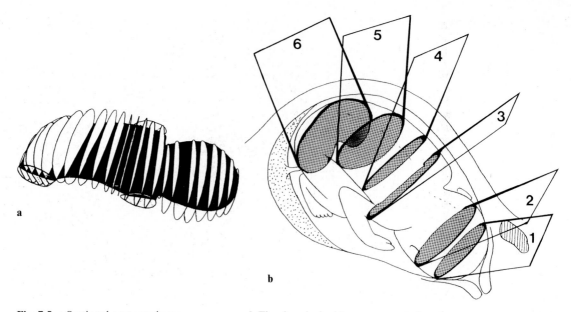

Fig. 7.5. a Sectional anatomy in transverse scans. **b** The six principal transverse scanning planes

ence has shown that fetal anatomy is demonstrated and evaluated most easily by locating the standard scanning planes at the start of the screening examination. While the examiner who is accustomed to three-dimensional thinking can modify these planes as needed during the examination, the less experienced operator should follow a strict schematic approach. To obtain a general appreciation of the fetal anatomy, the examiner should always begin by making a series of longitudinal scans. The standard longitudinal planes and the structures demonstrated in each are shown schematically in Fig. 7.4. After the fetal head has been located, the transducer is moved over the maternal abdomen until it is directly over the fetal spine. This is always possible except in the rare cases where the fetus is directly supine. The calvarium and the neck region are inspected, and then the spine is visualized down to and including the sacrum.

Because of shadowing from the vertebral bodies and ribs, there is little point in trying to evaluate fetal organs other than the kidneys, which can be visualized with a paravertebral sagittal scan (Fig. 7.4a).

The transducer is now rotated 180° about the same axis so that it is directly above and perpendicular to the anterior fetal body surface (Fig. 7.4b). The examiner is now able to inspect the anterior body surface and assess the relative sizes of the thorax and abdomen. After the fa-

cial profile is checked, the transducer is shifted farther along the sagittal plane to depict the neck and then the internal structures of the trunk: the diaphragm, liver, umbilical vein, urinary bladder, and, to the left of the midline, the stomach. The upper and lower extremities, also present in this section in front of the trunk, interfere with visualization. If the fetal limbs are flexed, then fetal movements should be elicited either by repositioning the mother or by percussing the maternal abdomen. The acoustic windows created by these movements will usually enable a thorough screening in this plane.

A frontal scanning plane between the anterior and posterior sagittal planes should also be used (Fig. 7.4c). This scan serves primarily to assess body symmetry in the facial region, while also delineating the orbits and facial prominences (nose, lips, chin). Within the fetal abdomen the diaphragm is usually well visualized in this plane, and the stomach and bladder contrast markedly with other intraabdominal structures. On scanning tangentially and anteriorly to the spine, the kidneys will present to the right and left of the pulsating aorta. The upper and lower extremities are visible in cross section, and frequently the fetal genitalia will be demonstrated.

The screening procedure concludes with serial transverse scans. These are performed both to provide a final check of fetal anatomy and to identify the reference planes for biometry.

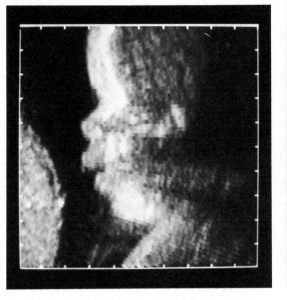

Fig. 7.6. Face in profile

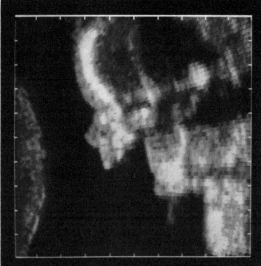

Fig. 7.7. Face in profile with mouth open

The examiner initiates the scans at the fetal head and proceeds caudally. He should not just "take in" the sectional anatomy as it appears, but should actively look for and confirm the anticipated structures by slowly advancing the transducer. In theory there is no limit to the number of transverse scans that can be performed (Fig. 7.5a). For level I screening, however, it is sufficient to image the six planes shown schematically in Fig. 7.5b. After the lateral ventricles are visualized (*plane 1*), the reference plane for fetal cephalometry is identified (*plane 2*). *Plane 3* traverses the upper extremities and the heart. By angling the transducer slightly, it is usually possible to obtain a classic four-chamber view of the heart. *Plane 4* is scanned to demonstrate the liver and stomach and to locate the reference plane for trunk measurements between the cardiac plane and the entry of the umbilical vein into the abdomen.

The kidneys are reexamined in *plane 5,* and *plane 6* visualizes the bladder, genitalia, and lower extremities. Screening concludes with a gross evaluation of each individual extremity.

We caution the examiner not to employ a disorganized examining technique. In particular, the habit of "lingering" on interesting or prominent details is a common cause of incomplete screening. The examiner is also cautioned against informing the patient of perfectly normal anatomic variants during the course of the

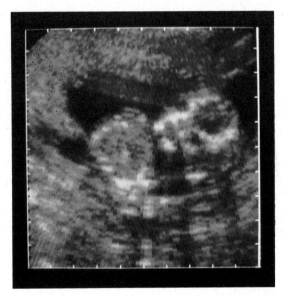

Fig. 7.8. Face: frontal scan through orbits, nose, and mouth

examination. Comments about small placental cysts or a transverse lie at 18 weeks gestation will only upset the patient unnecessarily. If these points are noted and the outlined examination procedure is consistently followed, it should be possible to recognize major developmental anomalies or detect signs suggestive of them within a relatively short period of time.

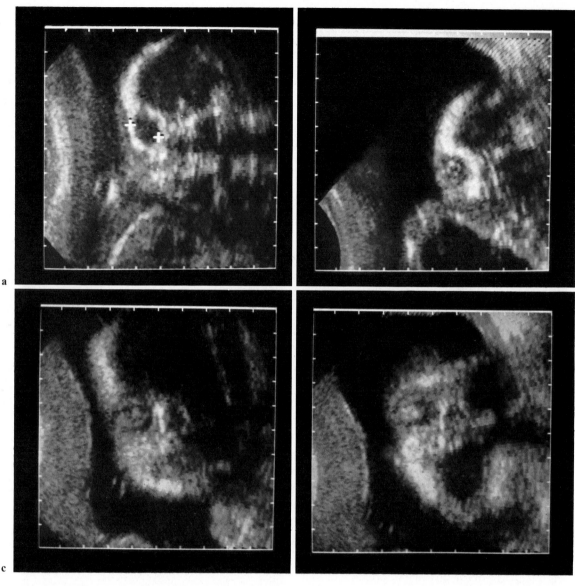

Fig. 7.9. a Frontal scan through face at 18 weeks with measurement of orbit (12 mm). **b** Frontal scan through face in a slightly more anterior plane than in **a**. Scan traverses eye within orbit, and ocular movements can be observed. **c** A more anterior scan demonstrates facial soft tissues: eyelids, cheeks, nose, and mouth. **d** Same plane as in **c,** with mouth wide open

7.1.1 Face

The face of the fetus provides an excellent example of what ultrasound can accomplish in the recognition of structural details. While detailed facial screening may seem overly ambitious for a level I examination, it is nevertheless true that increasing importance is being attached to structural details of this type (Figs. 7.6 and 7.7). The profile and frontal views of the face may exhibit definite anomalies, which are discussed further in Chap. 10. It requires considerable experience demonstrating "normal faces" frontally and in profile to have a chance of detecting cyclops, anophthalmia, arrhinia, or facial clefts.

Facial structures are identifiable by ultrasound as early as 10–11 weeks gestation. At 12–13 weeks, the impression of a human face becomes clearer as the orbits enlarge and separate

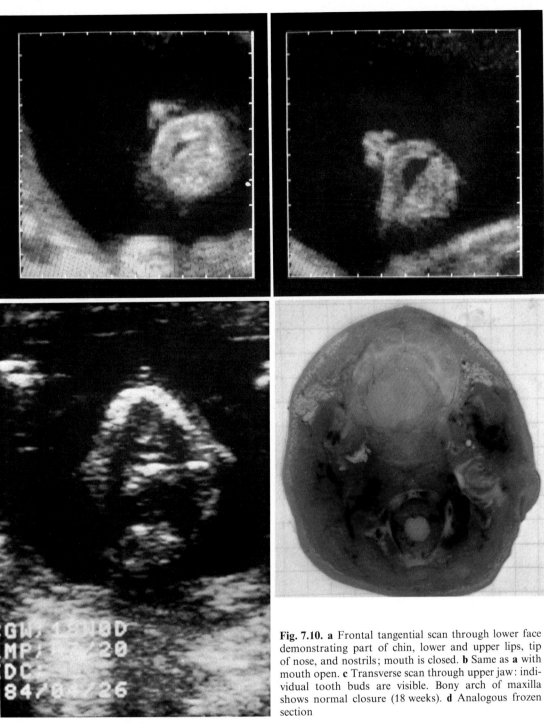

Fig. 7.10. a Frontal tangential scan through lower face demonstrating part of chin, lower and upper lips, tip of nose, and nostrils; mouth is closed. **b** Same as **a** with mouth open. **c** Transverse scan through upper jaw: individual tooth buds are visible. Bony arch of maxilla shows normal closure (18 weeks). **d** Analogous frozen section

and a mouth can be recognized. Usually the orbits are easily depicted and can be measured without difficulty (cf. Figs. 7.8, 7.9, 7.12).

It is more difficult to demonstrate the eyes themselves (Fig. 7.9b). According to Birnholz (1981), the eyes can always be seen by ultrasound except in the occiput anterior position. The eye is best depicted on a semioblique transverse scan. With a real-time unit, patterns of eye movements can also be studied. These

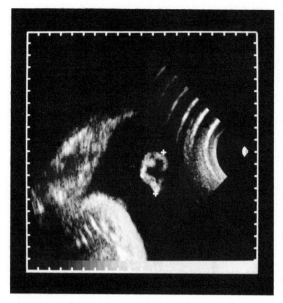

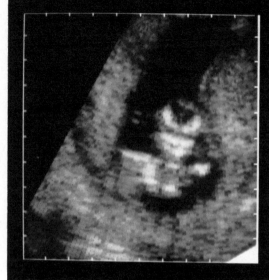

Fig. 7.11. Tangential scan of fetal head: structure of ear depicted with exceptional clarity

Fig. 7.12. Frontal scan through fetal skull and face at 12 weeks. Anterior horns visible above orbits; maxilla and mandible also visualized

movements begin with isolated, relatively slow excursions that are seen only sporadically prior to 16 weeks. Between 20 and 24 weeks, the movements become more brisk but still show no periodicity. As time passes they increase in frequency and duration.

These "rapid eye movements" (REMs), also called nystagmus, appear to decrease with progressive hypoxia. Birnholz (1983) states that REMs are considerably more common than "breathing" movements and thus provide a better indicator of fetal condition. Episodes of deep sleep, with an absence of REMs, reportedly appear after 35 weeks. According to Birnholz (1983), deep sleep occurring before 35 weeks is a sign of fetal distress. He goes so far as to rate the presence or absence of fetal REMs higher in diagnostic value than the nonstress test.

Besides ocular movements, the face exhibits additional dynamic processes that may have diagnostic significance. These include swallowing, belching, yawning, and in the future, perhaps even more subtle changes in facial expression will be recognizable. It is still too early to be definite about the value of these criteria for fetal assessment.

Phenotypic features are far easier to evaluate, and would include the eyes, mouth, nose, and ears (Figs. 7.6, 7.7, 7.9c, d, 7.10a, b, 7.11).

The mouth and lips have proved to be a particularly worthwhile object of ultrasound scrutiny. By directing a transverse scan through the upper jaw with a slightly anterior angulation of the beam (Fig. 7.10c, d), it is possible to exclude defects of the lip region (Fig. 7.10a, b) while also assessing the integrity of the bony arch of the maxilla. This would mainly be indicated for the exclusion of facial clefts or similar defects. In view of the risks involved, we no longer consider fetoscopy to be appropriate for this investigation.

7.1.2 Brain

With modern equipment it is possible to visualize the fetal skull at 7 weeks gestation. At this stage the ventricles almost completely fill the cranium. By 11 weeks the brain still consists mainly of ventricles surrounded by a thin cerebral mantle (Fig. 7.15a). The relatively large, echogenic choroid plexus is easily seen in transverse scans and appears to fill the interior of the skull almost completely (Fig. 7.15b; cf. schematic drawing in Fig. 7.14).

A frontal scan at 12 weeks (Fig. 7.12) shows the large, echo-poor anterior horns of the lateral ventricles. A paramedian sagittal scan through a fetus at 12 weeks (Fig. 7.13) demon-

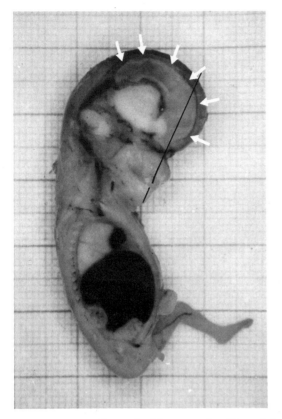

Fig. 7.13. Paramedian sagittal frozen section (12 weeks). Scanning plane in Fig. 7.12 is indicated (*line*)

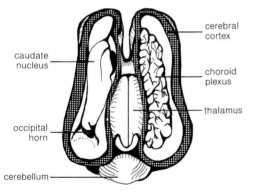

caudate nucleus

cerebral cortex

choroid plexus

thalamus

occipital horn

cerebellum

Fig. 7.14. Cross-section of brain at 12 weeks showing the cortex, size of ventricles, and choroid plexus

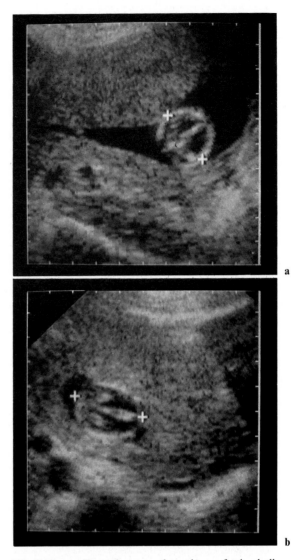

Fig. 7.15. a Frontal scan through a fetal skull (11 weeks): BPD 21 mm. Lateral ventricles still fill skull completely in cranial direction (*dark areas*). **b** Transverse scan of same skull showing measurement of the occipito-frontal diameter (OFD; 29 mm). The choroid plexuses appear as highly echogenic areas to the left of the image

strates the extent of the lateral ventricles (the line indicates the plane of Fig. 7.12). These relationships do not change significantly until 15–16 weeks at which time the lateral ventricular walls become progressively separated from the cortex and move inward as the cortex expands (Fig. 7.16a). The choroid plexus now fills the lateral ventricles in their transverse dimension, but generally does not extend into the anterior horns (Fig. 7.16a). After 20 weeks the ventricles, reduced in their relative size, appear progressively less prominent.

To review the main features of brain anatomy, the series of illustrations in Fig. 7.17 show the relationship between eight transverse scans and one midsagittal scan of the fetal brain at 19 weeks gestation. Some of the liquorfilled spaces in the left brain halves have been dissected free to show their relation to surrounding

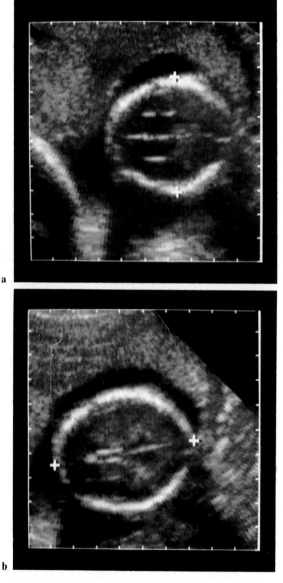

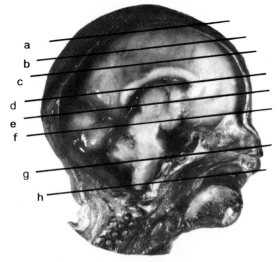

Fig. 7.17 a–h. Midsagittal section through fetal skull ▶ (frozen section), at 19 weeks. The bony structures of the face, the soft palate, and the tongue are seen anteriorly. Visible brain structures include the cerebral hemispheres, corpus callosum, brain stem, part of the cerebellum, and the ventricles (dark). The transverse sections (**a–h**) were cut parallel to the orbitomeatal line and progress serially in a cranial-to-caudal direction. **a** Both cerebral hemispheres with cranial portions of lateral ventricles. **b** Lateral ventricles (fluid was removed from upper ventricle to show its true size). **c** Section 5 mm lower, demonstrating anterior and posterior horns. **d** Section at level of greatest BPD and OFD. Anterior horns, cavum septi pellucidi, thalami, posterior horns, and insula are demonstrated. **e** Section through basal portion of anterior horns, aqueduct, and posterior horns, which are still large at this level. **f** This section just traverses the base of the frontal lobes anteriorly; the brain stem is visible centrally, and posterior to it the cisterna ambiens and posterior horns. **g** Section through base of skull. The choanae are visible anteriorly, and the posterior cranial fossa and spinal cord are seen posteriorly. **h** Section at level of maxillary arch, demonstrating tooth buds, tongue, bony structures of cranial base, and small portion of posterior cranial fossa

Fig. 7.16. a Transverse scan through fetal skull: cortex has expanded, causing inward displacement of ventricles (18 weeks). **b** Transverse scan through same skull at a slightly more caudal level: cavum septi pellucidi is seen frontally, and posterior horns with choroid plexus are visible occipitally. Measurement of OFD (18 weeks)

brain. At this stage the brain stem and cerebellum are easily recognized in both frontal and sagittal views (Fig. 7.18 a, b). It should be noted that transverse scans usually demonstrate a space interrupting the midline in the anterior third of the brain; this represents the cavum septi pellucidi (Fig. 7.16 b).

The anatomy of the reference plane for measuring the BPD and the occipitofrontal diame-

ter (OFD) is reviewed in detail in Sect. 7.2. In the older literature (up to 1980) the cavum septi pellucidi was erroneously identified by most authors as the third ventricle. The true third ventricle lies somewhat farther posteriorly between the thalami and is generally visible only as a midline streak. If marked enlargement of this area is noted, screening for hydrocephalus is indicated (see also Sects. 7.2, 8.3). Johnson et al. (1980) have also used the cerebral vasculature as an aid to orientation in the fetal skull. The pulsating cerebral arteries are easily identified, particularly in the area of the brain stem

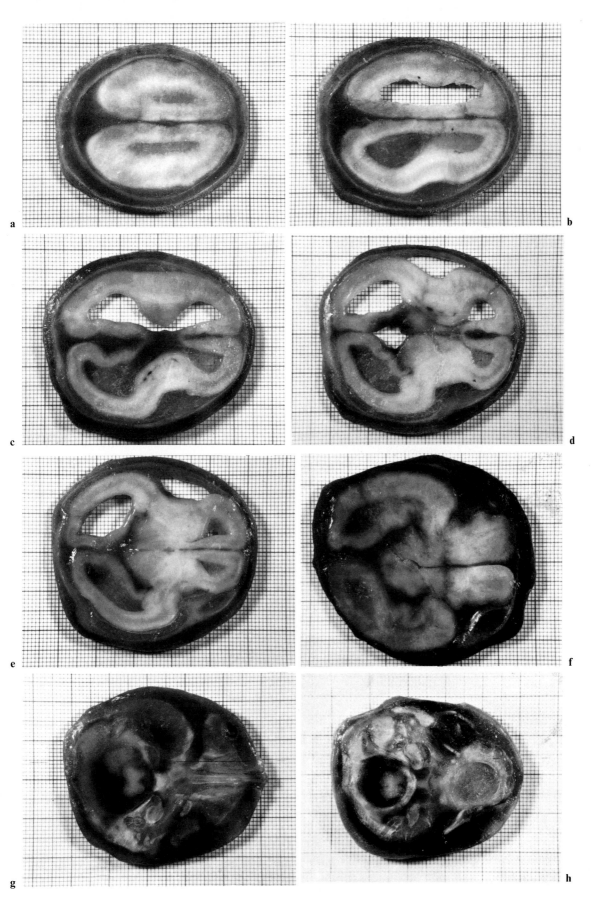

Fig. 7.17 a–h.

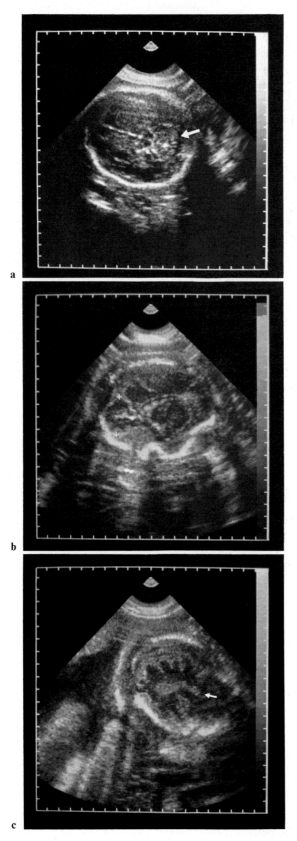

a

b

c

and basal cisterns. With regard to future research, it is apparent that a careful structural
analysis of the fetal brain will assume growing
importance in the immediate pre- and intrapar-
tum period. The clinical relevance of structural
analyses of the fetal brain has been demonstrated by Bliesener (1984) in relation to neonatology and pediatrics.

7.1.3 Spine

The fetal spine is clearly visible as two parallel,
echogenic lines from 12 weeks on. It is important to note the observation of Stark (1965)
that the ossification of the vertebrae begins in
the 3rd lunar month, but that dorsal closure
of the vertebral canal through union of the la-
minae does not occur until the 4th lunar month.
The development of the ossification centers of
the spine and the resulting progressive improvement in the sonographic depiction of the vertebrae, claviculae and ribs are illustrated in
Fig. 7.19–7.21. In Fig. 7.20a the top drawing
depicts a thoracic vertebra and developing ribs
of a fetus in the 3rd month, with ossification
centers shaded gray. The ribs have not yet fused
with the vertebral body. The bottom drawing
represents the same thoracic vertebra at
19 weeks. The areas of ossification in the vertebral body have increased markedly in size, and
the lateral ossification centers have almost
fused together. Advanced ossification of the
ribs and three ossification zones are illustrated
in Fig. 7.20b. On longitudinal scans (sagittal
or frontal) there may be a recognizable segmentation of the vertebral elements, depending on
the resolving power of the equipment
(Fig. 7.21a) The dark band between the echogenic vertebral structures represents the neural
tube. In the third trimester the caudal extremity
of the spinal cord in the neural tube can be
visualized with a midsagittal scan if the fetus
is supine (Fig. 7.22). The lumbar spine, a very

Fig. 7.18. a Transverse scan through fetal skull at level
of cerebellum (arrow). Internal brain structures are visible; the midline echo is from the falx cerebri. b Sagittal
scan. The cerebellum is indicated by the two crosses;
the craniocaudal distance is 30 mm. c Paramedian sagittal section through lateral ventricle. Arrow: choroid
plexus. Individual gyri shown at boundary of ventricle

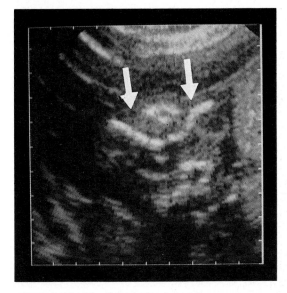

Fig. 7.19. Display of claviculae (*arrows*)

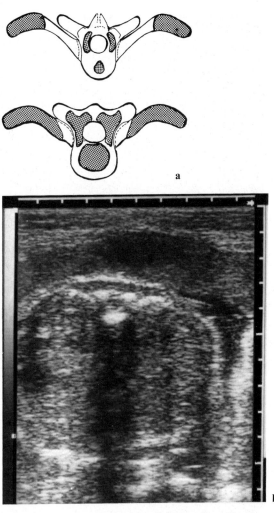

Fig. 7.20. a Schematic representation of ossification centers of thoracic vertebra in 3rd and 5th month. **b** Transverse scan through trunk: spine at 12 o'clock. Vertebral ossification centers shown in **a** and advanced ossification of ribs are clearly seen

common site for lesions, is most easily located by following the insertions of the ribs in the frontal plane (Fig. 7.21 b). The five segments of the lumbar spine will be found caudal to the 12th rib. Distal to the lumbar region the double contour of the spine is seen to taper like the tip of a pencil. This represents the os sacrum, which still shows some degree of segmentation (Fig. 7.21 c). The wings of the ilium are usually seen extending laterally and obliquely from the sacrum. Neural tube abnormalities will be discussed in Chap. 8.

7.1.4 Thorax

The external shape of the thorax is like that of a truncated cone whose narrow end is directed cephalad. The most obvious structure within the fetal thorax is the heart. The lungs are also easily seen and in the third trimester may appear more echogenic than the liver. This contrast indirectly delineates the diaphragm in both the frontal and sagittal planes (Figs. 7.23, 7.24 a). The outline of the diaphragm is most easily identified from movements associated with fetal "breathing". Studies by Benson et al. (1983) have shown that it may be possible in the future to use radiofrequency to detect subtle differences in tissue density and thus assessing fetal lung maturity. The most important intrathoracic organ is the heart. Basic views for

evaluating the fetal heart are obtained by angled transverse scans, which provide the classic four-chamber view (Fig. 7.25a, b). A satisfactory four-chamber view allows visualization of both ventricles, both atria, and the major valves from 15 weeks on. In normal circumstances the heart is located relatively close to the anterior chest wall and is displaced slightly to the left, with the apex directed downward and to the left (see drawing in Fig. 7.26). It is essential that the scan be performed through the anterior fetal chest. If the fetus is prone, acoustic shadowing from the spine and ribs will generally prevent detailed visualization of the heart. In a satisfactory four-chamber view the transverse diameter

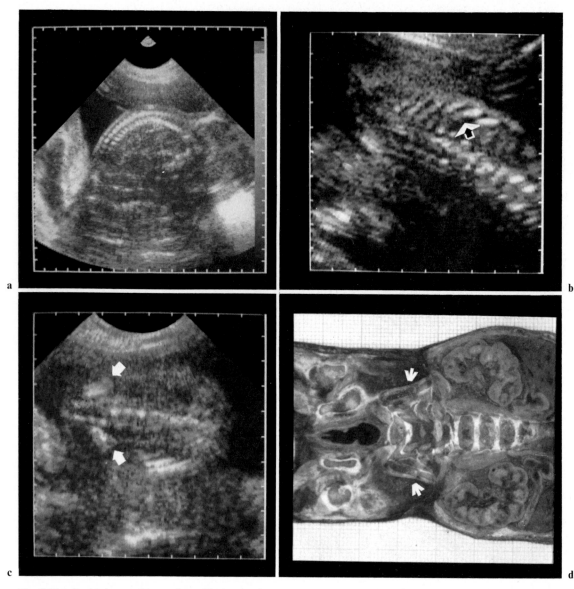

Fig. 7.21. a Sagittal scan of prone fetus. Shadowing from the spine prevents visualization of the trunk. The neural tube is demarcated as a dark band by the strong vertebral echoes. **b** Frontal scan through lower thorax and lumbar spine. The 12th rib is a helpful landmark (*arrow*). **c** Frontal scan through the lumbosacral region. *Arrows:* iliac wings. **d** Analogous frozen section (19 weeks). *Arrows:* iliac wings

of the heart in the plane of the major valves (the "short axis") is easily defined and measured, although this measurement can be made more accurately by time-motion imaging. The origin of the aorta can be demonstrated in the center of this view by tilting the transducer (Fig. 7.27). A useful additional landmark is the septum primum, a thin membrane on the left side of the foramen ovale which shows a left-directed, valve-like motion in accordance with

blood flow (Fig. 7.28). In the sagittal plane the right atrium is easily located by following the inferior vena cava to its junction with the atrium (Fig. 7.29a). The great vessels provide useful landmarks for a number of intrafetal structures. By locating the aorta in the sagittal scan, it is possible also to demonstrate the origin of the carotid arteries (Fig. 7.30); in the prevertebral frontal scan, the bifurcation of the aorta can be recognized distally (Fig. 7.31).

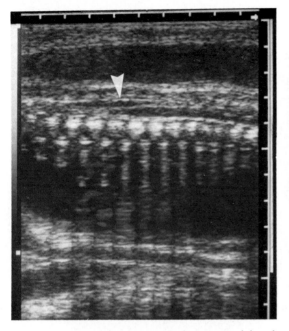

Fig. 7.22. Median, posterior sagittal scan: caudal end of spinal cord visible within neural tube (*arrow*)

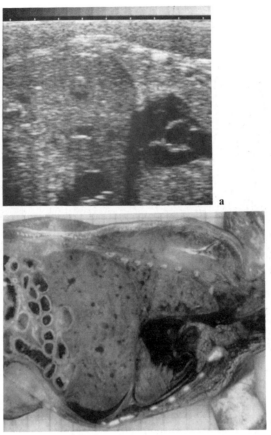

Fig. 7.24. a Frontal scan of fetal trunk: the echogenic lungs contrast markedly with the relatively hypoechoic liver (indirect demonstration of diaphragm; 21 weeks). **b** Analogous frozen section at 21 weeks: this contrast of tissue pattern is not evident in anatomic preparations

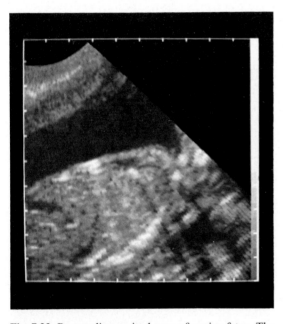

Fig. 7.23. Paramedian sagittal scan of supine fetus. The echo-poor liver tissue contrasts sharply with the echogenic lung, providing indirect delineation of the diaphragm

7.1.5 Abdomen

The main purpose of the examination of the fetal abdomen is to evaluate the anatomic relationship between fluid-filled structures (stomach, bladder) and the other organs (liver, kidney, spleen). It is noteworthy that the kidney (see below) is significantly less echogenic than the liver throughout gestation. Bowel loops show a wide range of variation, but generally cannot be visualized individually until the third trimester. The liver is the most prominent intraabdominal organ in all scanning planes owing to its size. The fetal diaphragm is elevated and is thus partly intrathoracic in location (Fig. 7.24a). The anatomy of the fetal intrahepatic structures is shown diagramatically in Fig. 7.32. The course of the umbilical vein is easily seen within the abdomen (especially in anterior sagittal scans). This vessel, which shows considerable variation, usually passes from its site of entry into the abdomen obliquely in a cranial direction into the liver parenchyma, terminating at the portal sinus (Fig. 7.33a).

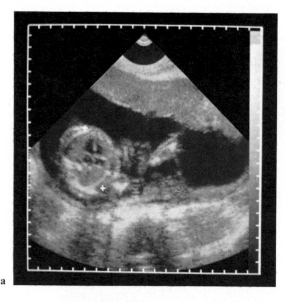

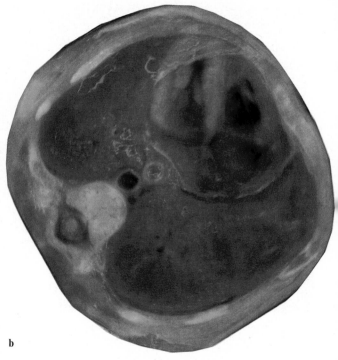

a   b

Fig. 7.25. a Four-chamber view at 21 weeks: spine at 8 o'clock. The atria, ventricles, and ventricular septum are easily identified. **b** Analogous frozen section of four-chamber view: spine at 8 o'clock with aorta anterior

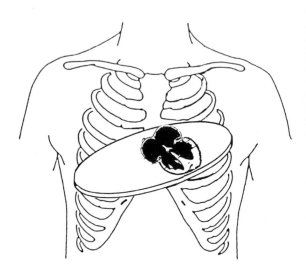

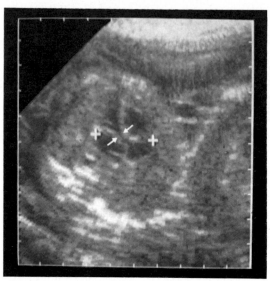

Fig. 7.26. Plane of section for four-chamber view of heart

Fig. 7.27. Transverse scan of thorax at 25 weeks: four-chamber view showing aortic root (*arrows*). Transverse cardiac diameter 24 mm, spine at 8 o'clock

From there the ductus venosus continues in a cranial direction and enters the inferior vena cava close to the right atrium. The hepatic veins also enter the inferior vena cava at that loca-

tion. Another structure that is frequently visible is the gallbladder (Fig. 7.33b). Beretsky and Lankin (1983) have noted gallstones in a fetus shortly before term. The gallbladder is variable

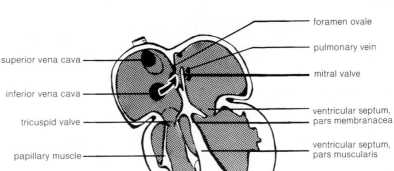

superior vena cava —

inferior vena cava —

tricuspid valve —

papillary muscle —

— foramen ovale

— pulmonary vein

— mitral valve

— ventricular septum, pars membranacea

— ventricular septum, pars muscularis

Fig. 7.28. Schematic representation of fetal heart in four-chamber view. Cardiac valves shown

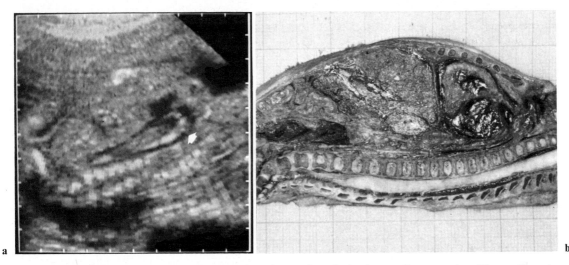

a   b

Fig. 7.29. a Anterior sagittal scan. The aorta and aortic arch are clearly seen anterior to the spine. The inferior vena cava is seen coursing obliquely upward to the right atrium. **b** Analogous frozen section. The aortic arch, the inferior vena cava entering the right atrium, and a portion of the right ventricle are shown (21 weeks)

in size and can commonly be visualized in an oblique scan parallel to the umbilical vein (Fig. 7.33b). On moving the scanning plane caudally, the gallbladder will disappear, while the umbilical vein can be traced caudally to its site of entry into the abdomen. From 12 weeks on the stomach usually contains fluid and thus presents as an echo-free space in the left upper abdomen (Fig. 7.34). Changes in the shape of the stomach associated with peristalsis are most obvious in the third trimester. At this time a tubular, partially haustrated, hypoechoic structure is frequently visible below the stomach. This is believed to represent fluid and meconi-

um in the descending colon and must be differentiated from the left kidney (Fig. 7.35).

7.1.6 Urogenital Tract

Estimation of amniotic fluid volume, sonographic visualization of the kidneys, and assessment of bladder filling are of major importance in evaluating the fetal urogenital tract. A systematic scanning technique is particularly important in demonstrating the kidneys (see table below).

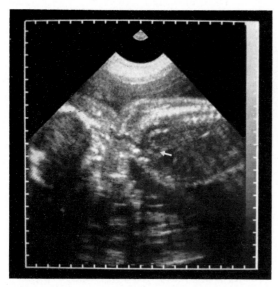

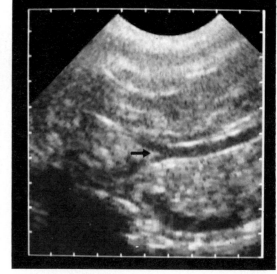

Fig. 7.30. Posterior paramedian sagittal scan. *Arrow:* origin of common carotid artery from aortic arch

Fig. 7.31. Prevertebral frontal scan: abdominal segment of aorta and aortic bifurcation (*arrow*) are depicted

Scanning Techniques for Examining the Urogenital Tract

12–17 weeks gestation
> *Transverse scan* (anterior or posterior)
> Visualization of kidneys and bladder

After 17 weeks
> *1. Transverse scan* (anterior or posterior)
> a) Assessment of renal size in relation to abdominal size
> b) Visualization and measurement of renal pelves
>
> *2. Paravertebral sagittal scans*
> Assessment of position, borders, number, and morphologic comparison
>
> *3. Prevertebral frontal scan*
> a) Concurrent visualization of both kidneys (comparison of structures and pelves)
> b) Evaluation of bladder and kidneys together, demonstration of dilated ureter

Bowie et al. (1983) have investigated the sonographic appearance of the fetal kidneys at different stages of gestation. They have found that up to 17 weeks gestation, the kidneys can usually be visualized only in transverse section, and that both kidneys can be depicted concurrently only if the fetus is in a precisely prone or supine position. The kidneys present as rounded masses that are considerably less echogenic than their surroundings (Fig. 7.36). A prevertebral frontal scan in the region where the scanning plane is just in front of the spine, and the aorta and usually the inferior vena cava are visible in their caudal portions, will allow simultaneous visualization of both kidneys, permitting their size, appearance and symmetry to be assessed. Bernaschek and Kratochwill (1980) and Grannum et al. (1980) have studied renal size throughout gestation and have confirmed a linear increase. It must be emphasized that the kidney and adrenal gland cannot at present be consistently separated by ultrasound. This problem is discussed further in Sect. 8.5. Figure 7.37 illustrates the relative sizes of the fetal kidneys and adrenal glands at 17 weeks gestation. Lewis et al. (1982) and Jeanty and Romero (1984) showed that the fetal adrenals can be demonstrated by ultrasound. The adrenals can be visualized by an anterior transverse scan angled in a caudal-to-cranial direction. Due to the anatomic relationship to the liver, which provides contrast, the right adrenal is more easily visualized below the diaphragm. Demonstration of the left adrenal is frequently limited by the colonic flexure and spleen. Since the adrenals are the most cranially situated paravertebral organs within the abdomen, they cannot be confused with other organs. It is important that the scanning plane passes through the adrenal superior to the kidney; otherwise differentiation can be difficult. Structurally, the adrenal

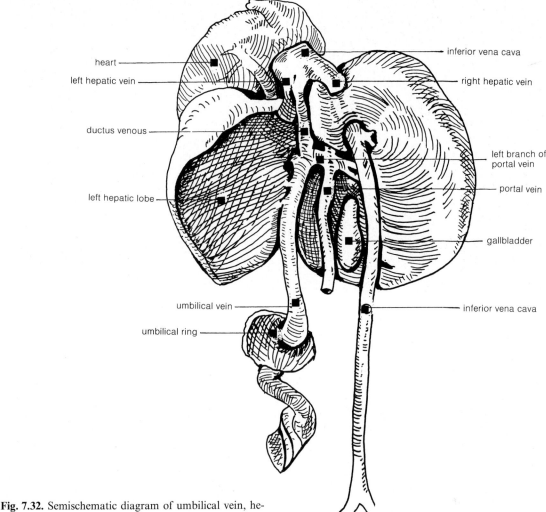

heart
left hepatic vein
ductus venous
left hepatic lobe
umbilical vein
umbilical ring

inferior vena cava
right hepatic vein
left branch of portal vein
portal vein
gallbladder
inferior vena cava

Fig. 7.32. Semischematic diagram of umbilical vein, hepatic veins, and gallbladder (posterior aspect)

consists of an echogenic inner ring surrounded by a hypoechoic outer ring (Fig. 7.39b). Jeanty and Romero (1984) have published measurements of the fetal adrenals after 20 weeks gestation.

By angling the frontal scanning plane slightly anteriorly in the caudal part of the body, the fetal bladder and kidney can be demonstrated together. This plane also allows visualization of the ureters, if they are pathologically dilated. A sagittal paravertebral scan will permit individual visualization of the kidneys and, after 17 weeks, the renal pelvis can be recognized (Fig. 7.38a).

After 19 weeks the kidney becomes easier to differentiate from its surroundings (Fig. 7.39a), probably due to the renal incorporation of fat that begins around this time (Bowie 1983). In the third trimester the kidney is always clearly defined in relation to surrounding tissues, particularly in longitudinal scans.

Assessment of the amniotic fluid volume is important for the evaluation of urogenital function. With a normal amniotic fluid volume and demonstrable kidneys, the presence of the bladder as a round, echo-free area in the lower abdomen is helpful, though not obligatory, in confirming intact function. Campbell et al. (1973) studied fetal bladder dynamics and determined hourly urine production at various stages of gestation. They measured an output of approxi-

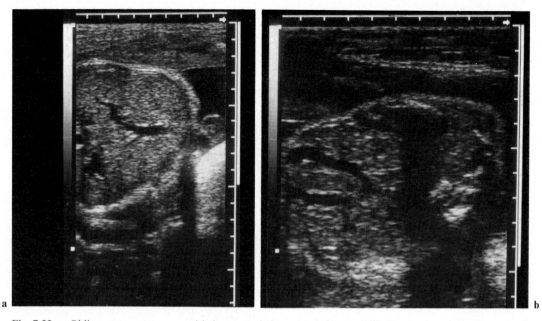

a   b

Fig. 7.33. a Oblique transverse scan with beam angled cranially: site of entry of umbilical vein into portal vein is demonstrated. **b** Oblique transverse scan: gallbladder seen below umbilical vein; its outline is more distinct than that of the vein

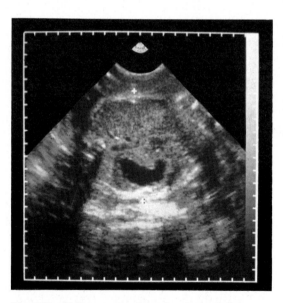

Fig. 7.34. Oblique scan through upper abdomen at 33 weeks: spine at 9 o'clock with aorta anterior to it. Outline of stomach seen below liver

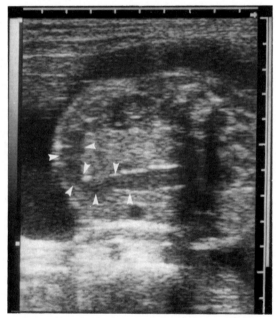

Fig. 7.35. Transverse scan through trunk: spine at 1 o'clock. Colon (*arrow*) curves along abdominal wall anterior to left kidney

mately 12 ml/h at 31 weeks and 26.4 ml/h at term. The importance of these values will be discussed later (Sect. 8.5). Figure 7.40, which is based on the data of Queenan and Thompson

(1972) and Abramovich (1970), shows the amniotic fluid volume (with its range of variation) as a function of gestational age and indicates the importance of fetal swallowing and urina-

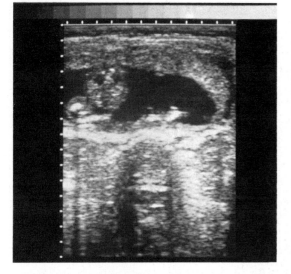

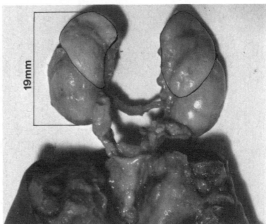

Fig. 7.36. Transverse scan through fetal trunk (prone) at 14 weeks: spine at 12 o'clock. Kidneys present as echo-poor structures lateral to spine

Fig. 7.37. Anatomic specimen at 17 weeks: both kidneys and adrenals demonstrated (adrenals almost as large as kidneys)

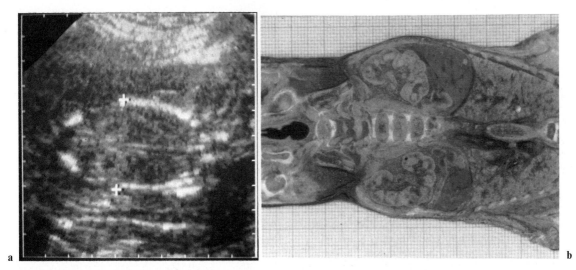

a   b

Fig. 7.38. a Prevertebral frontal scan at 17 weeks: kidneys seen parallel to longitudinal axis. **b** Analogous frozen section in a slightly more posterior plane, cutting the vertebrae tangentially

tion in the regulation of fluid volume. This will be discussed further in Sect. 8.5.

7.1.7 Genitalia

The visualization of fetal genitalia by ultrasound is well documented (Figs. 7.41–7.48), and there are definite indications for antenatal sex identification (e.g., sex-linked recessive dis-

eases, inappropriate hormonal therapy in early pregnancy, or urogenital malformations). It is wise to train the eye under optimal conditions during routine examinations so that anomalies can be recognized in complicated cases. The genitals can best by located by serial transverse scans starting from the urinary bladder and proceeding caudally. The male genitalia (scrotum, testes, and penis) are often visualized with this technique, though care must be taken not

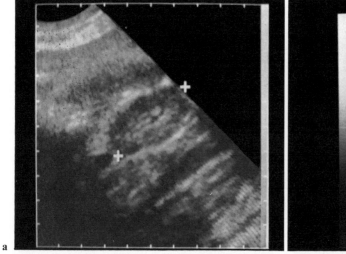

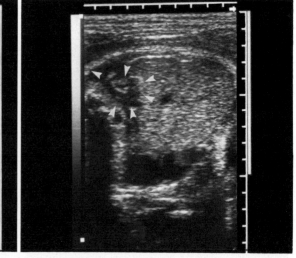

a

b

Fig. 7.39. a Magnified view of kidney at 25 weeks: the different echogenicities of the renal capsule and pelvis are helpful in identifying the kidney. **b** Oblique trans-verse scan: right adrenal (*arrows*) visible behind liver, cortex and medulla well defined

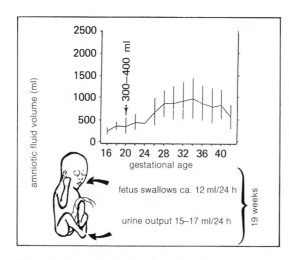

Fig. 7.40. Amniotic fluid volume in relation to gestational age (Queenan 1972) and fetal contribution at 19 weeks (Abramovich 1970)

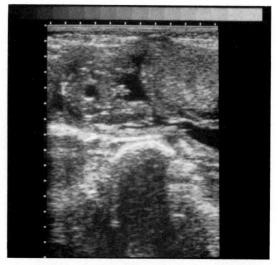

Fig. 7.41. Transverse scan through lower end of body at 17 weeks: spine at 9 o'clock. Bladder seen at center of trunk, penis visible between thighs (at 3 o'clock)

to mistake the umbilical cord between the legs for the male genitalia (Figs. 7.41, 7.42). With patience, one can even observe the act of urina-tion by the "jet phenomenon", probably created by fluid turbulence (Fig. 7.43). The demonstration of hydroceles is not uncommon, and they are usually not important (Fig. 7.44). The value of genital diagnosis as an additional aid in the diagnosis of fetal malformations is illustrated in Fig. 7.45 in a case of genital hy-poplasia in trisomy 18. The demonstration of female genitalia relies entirely on the detection of labia. This is most readily accomplished with the legs abducted or with a tangential scan (Fig. 7.46).

7.1.8 Extremities

Holländer (1972), and especially Hofbauer et al. (1978), were the earliest advocates of real-

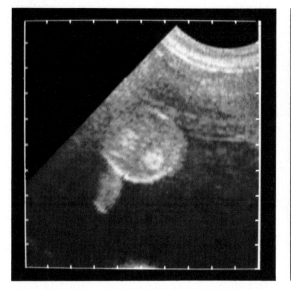

Fig. 7.42. Penis and scrotum at 33 weeks: testes have already descended

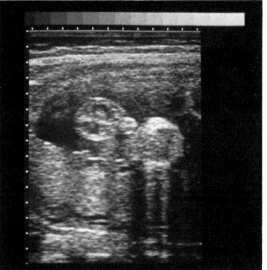

Fig. 7.44. Male fetus with mild hydrocele (no pathologic significance)

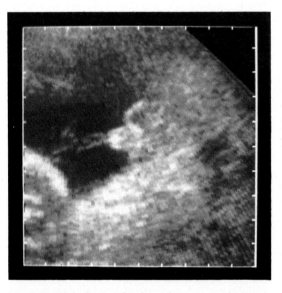

Fig. 7.43. Male fetus urinating: the stream of urine is made visible by amniotic fluid turbulence (jet phenomenon)

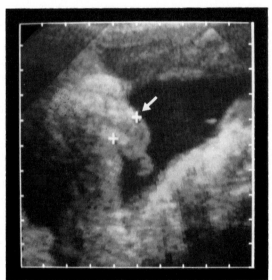

Fig. 7.45. Male fetus at 38 weeks with genital hypoplasia associated with trisomy 18: scrotal diameter (*crosses*) only 11 mm

time imaging and stressed the diagnostic importance of visualizing the fetal extremities by ultrasound. Hofbauer et al. (1978) and Arabin (1980) determined the length of the femoral and tibial diaphyses as well as overall femoral and tibial length in relation to gestational age (20 weeks to term). Hofbauer et al. (1978) also attempted to use the thigh diameter for the assessment of fetal weight by multiple parameters.

Later, numerous authors constructed growth curves for the fetal long bones (e.g., Campbell et al. 1981; Jeanty et al. 1981; Schlensker 1982). These values are useful for the diagnosis of fetal limb malformations (see Sect. 8.5) and evaluation of gestational age in cases where the usual parameters are inadequate.

Evidence of fetal extremities can be seen from 8 weeks on, and after 10 weeks complete

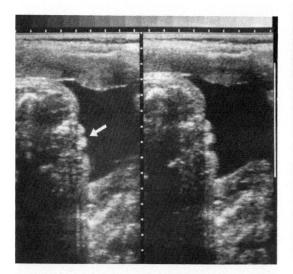

Fig. 7.46. Tangential scan through lower end of body of a female fetus: labia majora (*arrow*) seen between buttocks

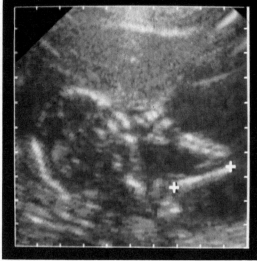

Fig. 7.48. Paramedial sagittal scan of "thumb-sucking" fetus at 17 weeks. *Crosses* mark humerus (24 mm). Face also seen

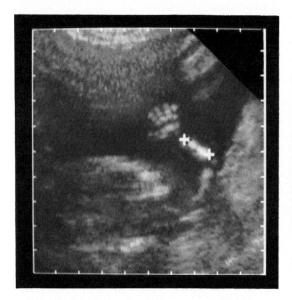

Fig. 7.47. Upper extremity with fingers spread at 13 weeks: humerus clearly defined, radioulnar complex seen (*crosses*, 11 mm)

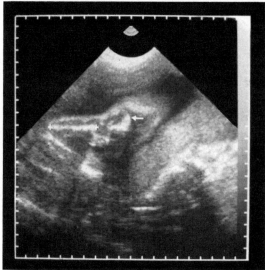

Fig. 7.49. Scan through shoulder girdle at 23 weeks: scapula indicated by *arrow*, humeral length 39 mm

limbs can be clearly identified (Figs. 7.47–7.49). Because usually only one or perhaps two extremities can be demonstrated concurrently in one plane, a complete evaluation of fetal limbs requires meticulous attention to right/left orientation. If an extremity is sectioned in a transverse plane, the presence of either one or two

bones will identify it as proximal or distal. There is usually no difficulty in distinguishing the tibia from the fibula; the fibula is the more lateral bone, and the diaphyses are always parallel. The situation in the forearm is more complex, since rotation can alter the relationship of the bones. This problem can be resolved by

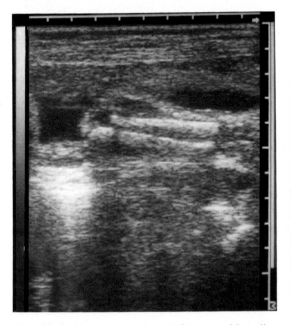

Fig. 7.50. Scan through supinated forearm with radius closer to transducer: radial head visible in elbow region, with ulna below it

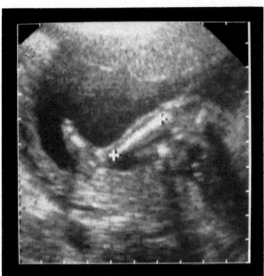

Fig. 7.52. Sagittal scan through lower leg and foot at 18 weeks: tibia (24 mm), calcaneus, metatarsals, and toes well defined

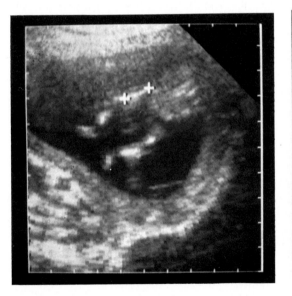

Fig. 7.51. Scan through both lower extremities at 12 weeks: femur can already be measured (10 mm)

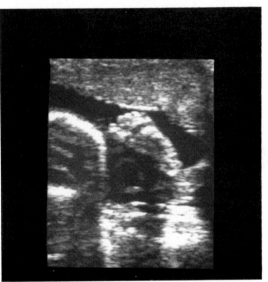

Fig. 7.53. Scan through sole of foot: metatarsals partially sectioned, toe well visualized

examining the hand, which can be visualized in detail after 13 weeks (Figs. 7.47 and 7.48). Because the fetal hands are usually partially closed, often only the proximal phalanges can be identified and the thumb is "missed." Percussion of the maternal abdomen or repositioning of the mother may result in activation of the fetus, with extension of the digits and visualization of the thumb.

If this does not succeed, repeat examinations are indicated. Clearly, a detailed examination of this type should be limited to selected

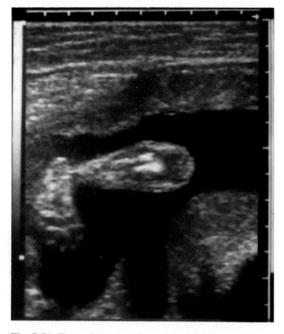

Fig. 7.54. Frontal scan at 22 weeks: clubfoot. Tibia and fibula both seen, sole visualized in same plane

patients with a genetic risk. If the scan cuts the forearm in supination, the radius and ulna can be identified by their characteristic appearances (Fig. 7.50). Visualization of the legs and feet (Fig. 7.52) generally poses fewer difficulties than that of the upper extremities. It is not surprising that the femur is the most frequently mentioned fetal long bone and is being used in biometry (Fig. 7.51). The feet can be seen in sagittal scans and occasionally in the plantar view (Figs. 7.53 and 7.54). If the axial relationship of the lower leg and foot is normal, a frontal scan that demonstrates both the tibia and fibula should cut the foot transversely. Visualization of the entire plantar view of the foot on such a scan is highly suggestive of clubfoot (Fig. 7.54). This aspect is important in assessing the prognosis of a recognized neural tube defect. This diagnosis may also be important as one aspect of a malformation syndrome.

References

Abramovich DR (1970) The volume of amniotic fluid in early pregnancy. Br J Obstet Gynaecol 77:865

Arabin B (1980) Fetale Ultraschallbiometrie im 2. und 3. Schwangerschaftstrimenon. Inaugural-Dissertation, Freie Universität Berlin

Benson DM, Waldroup LD, Kurtz AB, Rose JL, Rifkin MD, Goldberg BB (1983) Ultrasonic tissue characterization of fetal lung, liver and placenta for the purpose of assessing fetal maturity. J Ultrasound Med 2:489

Beretsky J, Lankin DH (1983) Diagnosis of fetal cholelithiasis using real-time high resolution imaging employing digital detection. J Ultrasound Med 2:381

Bernaschek G, Kratochwill A (1980) Echographische Studie über das Wachstum der fetalen Niere in der zweiten Schwangerschaftshälfte. Geburtshilfe Frauenheilkd 40:1059

Birnholz JC (1981) The development of human fetal eye movement patterns. Science 213:679

Birnholz JC (1983) Fetal behavior and condition. In: Callen PW (ed) Ultrasonography in obstetrics and gynecology. Saunders, Philadelphia

Bliesener JA (1984) Sonographie der normalen und pathologischen Hirnanatomie bei Neugeborenen und Säuglingen. Habilitationsschrift Köln

Bowie JD, Rosenberg ER, Andreotti RF, Fields SJ (1983) The changing sonographic appearance of fetal kidneys during pregnancy. J Ultrasound Med 2:505

Campbell S, Wladimiroff JW, Dewhurst CJ (1973) The antenatal measurement of fetal urine production. Br J Obstet Gynaecol 80:680

Filly RA, Golbus MS (1983) Ultrasonography of the normal and pathologic fetal skeleton. In: PW Callen (ed) Ultrasonography in obstetrics and gynecology. WB Saunders, Philadelphia

Grannum P, Bracken M, Silverman R, Hobbins JC (1980) Assessment of fetal kidney size in normal gestation by comparison of ratio or kidney circumference to abdominal circumference. Am J Obstet Gynecol 136:249

Hofbauer H, Pachaly I, Arabin B (1978) Fetale Ultraschall-Somatometrie, Ultraschalldiagnostik. Thieme, Stuttgart

Holländer HJ (1972) Die Ultraschalldiagnostik in der Schwangerschaft, 1. Aufl. Urban & Schwarzenberg, München Berlin Wien

Jeanty P, Romero R (1984) Obstetrical ultrasound. McGraw-Hill, New York

Jeanty P, Kirkpatrick C, Dremaix-Wilmet M (1981) Fetal limb growth. Radiology 140:165

Johnson ML, Dunne MG, Mack LA, Rashbaum CL (1980) Evaluation of fetal intracranial anatomy by static and real-time ultrasound. J Clin Ultrasound 8:311

Kratochwil A (1982, 6a) Sonographische Anatomie der normalen Schwangerschaft. Swiss Med 4:104

Lewis E, Kurtz AB, Dubbins PA et al. (1982) Real-time ultrasonographic evaluation of normal fetal adrenal glands. J Ultrasound Mes 1:265

Queenan JT, Thompson (1972) Amniotic fluid volumes in normal pregnancies. Am J Obstet Gynecol 114:34

Schlensker KH (1982, 6a) Biometrie der fetalen Extremitäten. Swiss Med 4:104

Stark D (1965) Embryologie. Thieme, Stuttgart

7.2 Ultrasound Biometry in the Second and Third Trimester

7.2.1 Introduction

The basic difference between simple ultrasound imaging and ultrasound biometry is that the former yields pictorial information that is essentially qualitative (e.g., fetal presentation, placental localization, presence of a mass), while the latter provides quantitative information relating to fetal age, weight, etc. The basic problem of fetal biometry is that the information of clinical interest (age and weight) cannot be directly obtained by ultrasound, but must be indirectly derived. To do this, it is necessary to know how a given measurable parameter correlates with the item that is to be determined. Three questions must be addressed:

1. What parameter should be measured?
2. How can it be measured?
3. How reliably can the item of interest be determined from the parameter measured?

Ideally, the fetal structure that is selected for measurement should correlate very closely with the desired item for all fetuses, and the measurement should be easily and quickly performed. Despite technical advances, however, these goals remain elusive since there is no fetal structure which displays a perfect relationship to the age or weight of the fetus (except for volume determinations, which are not feasible at the present time), and all measurements necessarily involve a certain degree of error.

These factors determine the limitations of the test, and the examiner must be aware of them if he wants to do more than just add one more "laboratory value" to many others.

7.2.2 Ultrasound Cephalometry

Donald and Brown (1961) were the first to describe the use of ultrasound for measuring the fetal biparietal diameter (BPD). Later Willocks (1963), of the same group, conducted studies that defined basic methodology. At one time the one-dimensional A-scan was the only mode utilized for BPD measurements. With this method it was necessary first to locate the fetal head by abdominal palpation before applying the ultrasound transducer at various angles.

The above authors based their technique on experiments indicating that deflections of maximum and equal amplitude, which form the typical A-scan of the skull, are observed only when the sound waves strike both the near and far walls of the skull at a perpendicular angle. According to their experiments, some of which were done in newborns, this kind of pattern could be obtained only from measurement of the BPD or the occipitofrontal diameter (OFD).

Willocks et al. (1964) measured a sound propagation velocity of 1,525 m/s in fetal brain, which showed good agreement with the value of 1,515 m/s reported by Ludwig (1950).

Initial tests of the reliability of this method were somewhat discouraging. When prenatal measurements with ultrasound were compared with direct caliper measurements after delivery, discrepancies of 5 mm or more were found in 35% of cases (Willocks 1963; Durkan and Russo 1966). Kohorn (1967) was able to improve results with his "triple spike echogram," which included the midline echo. But the real breakthrough came when Campbell (1968) introduced the combined A- and B-scan method, which still provides the greatest accuracy. With this technique the skull is first scanned longitudinally, and this view is used to determine the angle at which to place the transducer for the subsequent transverse scans. On a correct transverse scan the head should present as an oval with a streak-like midline echo (with proper gain setting). The examiner then moves the transducer over the largest transverse diameter, performs an A-scan across the fetal skull, and reads the distance between the amplitudes created by the leading edges of the parietal bones (Figs. 7.63, 7.64). Correct plane selection is indicated by the presence of skull echoes of equal amplitude and a midline echo at the lowest possible gain setting. Campbell (1970) found that this method was accurate to ±2 mm in 90% of his study population. A major advantage of the method is its independence of palpation. Hofmann and Holländer (1968) were the first to report results of fetal cephalometry with real-time equipment. Their results showed good agreement with those of other investigators (Kratochwil 1966; Thompson et al. 1965).

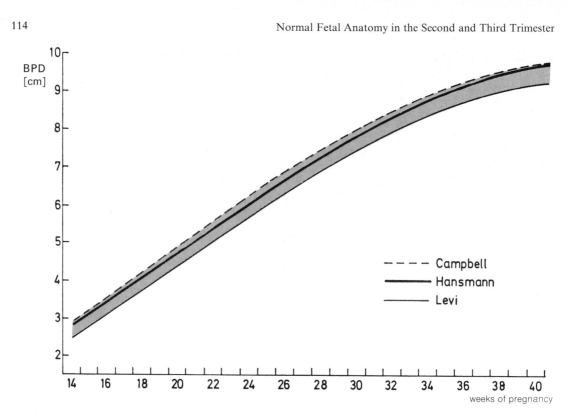

Fig. 7.55. Comparison of BPD growth curves for different velocity calibrations: Campbell 1,600 m/s, $n=1,029$; Hansmann 1,580 m/s, $n=2,628$; Levi 1,500 m/s, $n=2,000$ (see text)

Later Holländer (1972, 1975) described the details of the measurement technique and reported the results of extensive investigations. He found an error of ± 2 mm in 83% of a selected population, based on a comparison of pre- and postnatal measurements. The mean value of the deviations was 1.83 mm; the greatest deviation was 8 mm.

Numerous studies were published in the early 1970s relating the growth of the BPD to gestational age (Campbell 1969; Campbell and Newman 1971; Hansmann et al. 1972; Hellmann et al. 1967; Hinselmann 1968, 1969; Holländer 1972; Kratochwil 1966, 1968, 1971; Levi 1972, 1973; Levi and Erbsmann 1973; Schlensker 1972; Willocks et al. 1971). The graphs depicted in these studies all showed a similar trend – a decline in the growth rate of the BPD as pregnancy progressed (Fig. 7.55). However, large variations were noted in the absolute mean values of the BPDs measured for different weeks of gestation. We believe that the causes of these variations are essentially methodologic.

Determination of the BPD can have several objectives:

1. Assessment of gestational age
2. Monitoring of fetal growth in the second and third trimester in high risk pregnancies (hypertension, placental dysfunction, diabetes, Rh incompatibility, etc.)
3. Estimation of fetal weight
4. Detection of disproportion between head size and pelvic inlet

Technique. The BPD can be measured from 9 weeks gestation on throughout pregnancy. The standard plane for measuring the BPD is transverse, although an experienced examiner can get equally good readings from the frontal (coronal) plane (Fig. 7.56a). The transverse plane (Fig. 7.56b) is preferred because it makes orientation easier. The growth curves for the BPD in the first half of pregnancy are shown in Fig. 7.56c. It will be noted that the range of variation increases with gestational age, underscoring the importance of performing measurements early in pregnancy (see Sect. 4.1). On the transverse scan it is possible to identify both the BPD and the OFD, enabling the head circumference (HC) to be determined. The ana-

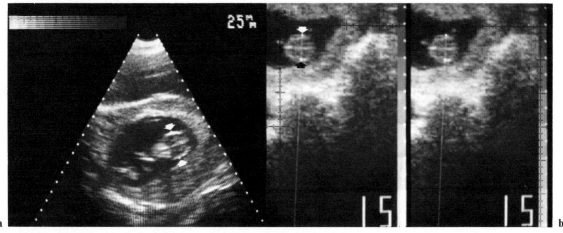

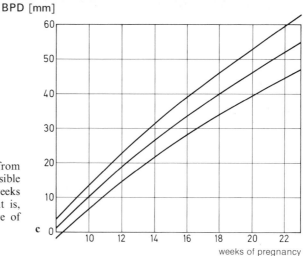

Fig. 7.56. a Measurement of BPD in frontal plane from outer table to outer table (*arrows*): facial skeleton visible below BPD. **b** Measurement of BPD at 11 weeks (15 mm): midline echo clearly visible (distal point is, incorrectly, within skull contour). **c** Growth curve of BPD in first half of pregnancy (8–22 weeks)

tomic reference plane for concurrent measurement of the BPD, OFD, and HC is shown in Fig. 7.58a–d. With high-resolution equipment, a scan in this plane will depict: (1) the less echogenic frontal and occipital horns of the lateral ventricles, the cavum septi pellucidi, and the insulae; (2) the somewhat more echogenic structures of the thalami, the basal ganglia, and the cerebral cortex; and (3) highly echogenic midline structures representing the borders of the third ventricle, as well as portions of the falx cerebri anteriorly and posteriorly. As gestation progresses, the less echogenic areas (ventricles, cavum septi pellucidi, insulae) are seen to decrease in size relative to the growing cerebrum.

The highly echogenic choroid plexus of the lateral ventricles provides another important anatomic landmark (cf. Fig. 7.57) up to

20 weeks gestation (Fig. 7.59a–c). Early in gestation the choroid plexus appears quite large and must not be mistaken for a "brain tumor" (Fig. 7.60a–c). The plane for measuring the BPD is too low if the bony base of the skull is visualized. In this case tilting the beam posteriorly will demonstrate the cerebellum in the posterior cranial fossa (Fig. 7.60c), and the orbits will be imaged when the plane is tilted anteriorly.

As long as the thalami remain in the image, the BPD can be measured without error from these planes. The OFD, however, will be too short, and so the HC cannot be measured accurately at this level (Fig. 7.59a–c).

Measurement Procedure. When a compound scanner is used, it is best to measure the BPD from an A-scan using a built-in ruler or elec-

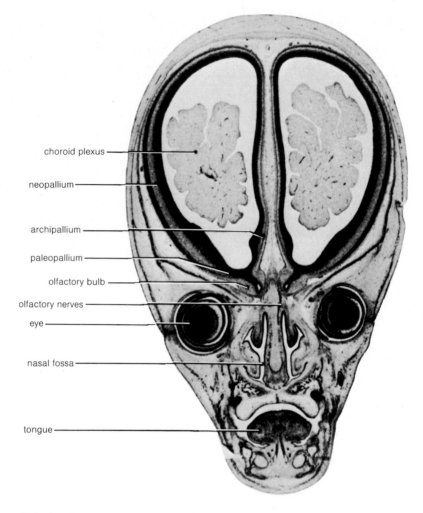

choroid plexus

neopallium

archipallium

paleopallium

olfactory bulb

olfactory nerves

eye

nasal fossa

tongue

Fig. 7.57. This frontal section of the head at 11 weeks illustrates the great volume occupied by the ventricles and choroid plexus in early gestation

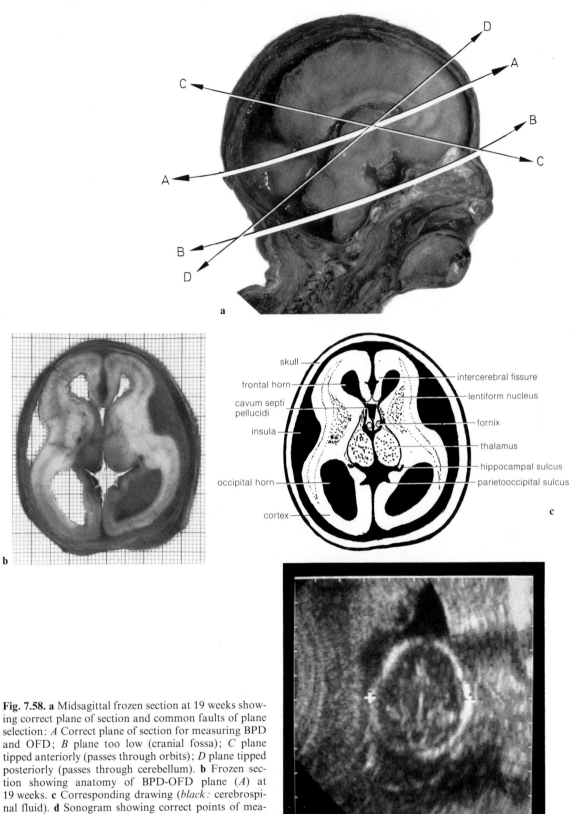

Fig. 7.58. a Midsagittal frozen section at 19 weeks showing correct plane of section and common faults of plane selection: *A* Correct plane of section for measuring BPD and OFD; *B* plane too low (cranial fossa); *C* plane tipped anteriorly (passes through orbits); *D* plane tipped posteriorly (passes through cerebellum). **b** Frozen section showing anatomy of BPD-OFD plane (*A*) at 19 weeks. **c** Corresponding drawing (*black:* cerebrospinal fluid). **d** Sonogram showing correct points of measurement and structural anatomy of reference plane (cf. **c**)

Labels in **c**:
skull — frontal horn — cavum septi pellucidi — insula — occipital horn — cortex — intercerebral fissure — lentiform nucleus — fornix — thalamus — hippocampal sulcus — parietooccipital sulcus

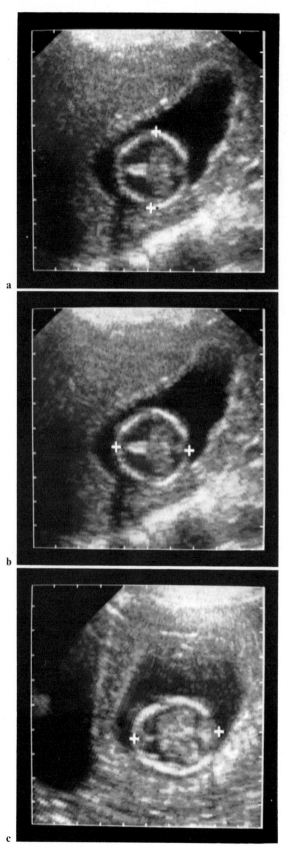

tronic caliper. With the latter technique, two electronic markers are positioned at the leading edge of the parietal bone echoes, and a digital readout gives the distance between the markers in millimeters. It is also possible to measure the BPD directly from the B-scan image (Fig. 7.64).

Hofmann and Holländer published their first report on B-scan cephalometry in 1967. Holländer (1972) later described the method in detail and reported the results of extensive studies, which correspond closely to our own with the B-scan technique. The main drawback of taking measurements directly from the B-scan is the poor resolution compared with the A-scan, particularly when real-time instruments are used. Nevertheless, one should not exaggerate the effect of inferior resolution, because what counts in practice is the net result of all factors which influence the accuracy of the measurement. Thus, considering the ability of real-time systems to provide images even in moving objects, and the practical difficulties of measuring the fetal skull in the early second trimester, even an examiner who is skilled in compound scanning will choose real time for fetal cephalometry, despite the attendant loss of resolution. Today, most measurements from sonograms are performed with the use of electronic caliper systems. Most of these systems are designed to operate only in the freeze-frame or stored-image mode. It is best to select a plane that will enable both BPD and OFD to be measured from a single image. Of course, this requires an image field of adequate width (approximately 12 cm in the late third trimester). Unfortunately, the quest for higher scanning rates to improve image quality has led to a progressive narrowing of the image field, with the result that many instruments today are unsuited for the important task of fetal biometry in the third trimester (Fig. 7.62).

Accuracy of Measurement. It is obvious that a measuring process is useful only if its accuracy

Fig. 7.59. a Measurement of BPD (30 mm): choroid plexuses visible on reference plane. **b** Incorrect points for measuring OFD: plane of section too high, giving a measurement of only 27 mm. **c** Extent of choroid plexus into occipital horns confirms correct selection of OFD plane (36 mm)

is known. Considering this problem in the context of ultrasonic biometry, we find that a basic distinction must be made between the reliability with which an indirectly determined quantity, such as fetal age, can be estimated, and the accuracy with which a correlating anatomic parameter, such as BPD, can be measured. While only the former is of interest to the clinician, it is the latter that concerns the ultrasonographer, for a precise measurement generally will ensure a better correlation. Nevertheless, one should always keep in mind the magnitude of error that is inherent in the measurement. Like other physical dimensions in the fetus, the accuracy of BPD measurements lies in the millimeter range, and values for the BPD should be stated accordingly (recommendation of European Study Group, Dubrovnik 1975).

Factors which compromise the accuracy of the result may be either random or systematic in nature and may occur anywhere in the triad of operator-equipment-structure. Whereas random errors such as faulty plane selection (Fig. 7.61 a, b) or reading errors can be minimized by obtaining multiple readings, errors of a systematic nature, such as faulty calibration or errors of scale, cannot be mitigated by repeating the examination. They are extremely difficult for the examiner to control, for generally he is unaware that they exist. For this reason, we repeat our appeal to equipment manufacturers to install simple test programs that will enable operators to check the functional status of their equipment. It is recommended that the equipment be tested with an approved test object on a regular basis.

It must be remembered that measurements with pulsed ultrasound are measurements of time, which are converted to distance on the basis of the assumed velocity of sound through the tissues. When the BPD is measured, the characteristic high-amplitude echoes returned

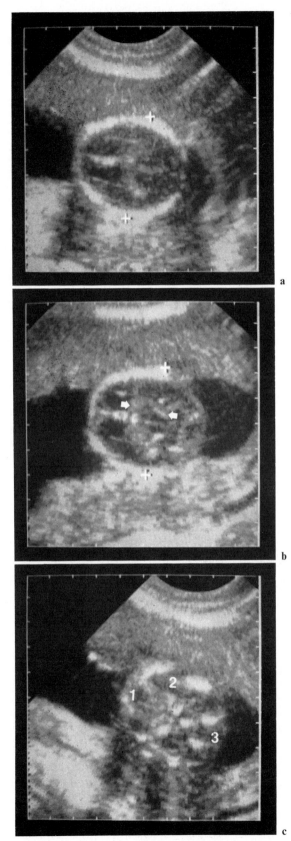

Fig. 7.60 a–c. Fetal cephalometry at various levels, 17 weeks. a The lateral ventricles and choroid plexuses are clearly visible in this section. b This section correctly demonstrates the choroid plexus, but the plane is angled too far posteriorly to measure the OFD, as indicated by the cerebellar echoes. The BPD can still be measured with reasonable accuracy. c Section through the base of the skull. The three cranial fossae are clearly delineated. Neither the BPD nor the OFD is measurable

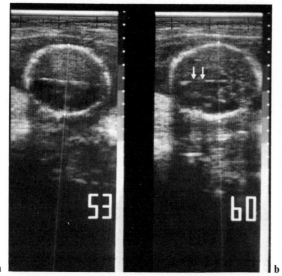

a   b

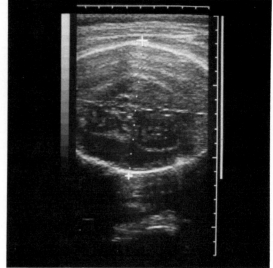

Fig. 7.61. a Faulty selection of BPD plane. The plane of section is too high; a midline echo is present, but the brain structure that identifies the reference plane is not visible (BPD 53 mm). **b** The same head imaged in the correct plane for measuring the BPD. In this scan the thalamus and frontal horns are visualized, and the cavum septi pellucidi (*arrows*) interrupts the midline echo (BPD 60 mm)

Fig. 7.62. Cephalometry in late pregnancy using an image field of insufficient width. This scan allows measurement of the BPD (95 mm), but the sound field is too small to measure the OFD

from the fetal skull (which are also used to generate a B-mode image) are reflected from the outer table of the proximal skull and the inner table of the distal skull. Thus, the distance measured with equipment calibrated to the usual velocity of 1,540 m/s (the average velocity of sound through human tissue at 37° C) will not directly represent the external BPD. One can either accept this discrepancy or attempt to correct it. Willocks et al. (1964) measured the skulls of dead fetuses weighing more than 2,000 g and found an average parietal bone thickness of 1.33 mm and average scalp thickness of 1.2 mm. This led some authors (Kratochwil 1968; Boog et al. 1969) to recommend that 2 mm be added to the measurement before the 36th week, and that 3 mm be added thereafter. To avoid this correction, Hansmann and Hoven (1971; Fig. 7.65) introduced a "biological calibration" based on an experimentally determined sound velocity of 1,582 m/s. This calibration provides an internal correction which correlates the distance between the leading edges of the wall echoes in the third trimester (to the degree of accuracy that is technically attainable) with the "true" BPD (Fig. 7.65). With real-time systems, the method described

by Holländer (1972) for measuring the distance from the outer margin of the near skull line to the outer margin of the far one ("outer-to-outer" BPD) leads to the same result, i.e., agreement of prenatal ultrasound measurements with postpartum caliper measurements. Since in North America the velocity calibration of compound as well as real-time scanners is the same (1,540 m/s) the leading edge method is commonly used for measurements with both types of equipment [see Jeanty (1984) and relevant growth curves in Appendix II]. We criticize the practice of some authors who publish "growth curves" or "normal values" without stating the velocity calibration used for the study (Aantaa and Forss 1974; Queenan et al. 1976; Varma 1973). To illustrate this problem, let us assume that the wall echoes in a skull scan are separated by a time interval of 60 µs. If the instrument is calibrated to 1,500 m/s, a value of 90 mm will be obtained for the BPD; if to 1,540 m/s, 92 mm; if to 1,582 m/s, 95 mm; and if to 1,600 m/s, 96 mm. If we assume that the examiner is using a calibration velocity of 1,500 m/s (perhaps without even knowing it) and attempts to use a correlation formula or chart that is based on a velocity of 1,600 m/s, it is not surprising if the examiner's results do not correlate with the clinical findings. Similar discrepancies can arise if the calibration is ther-

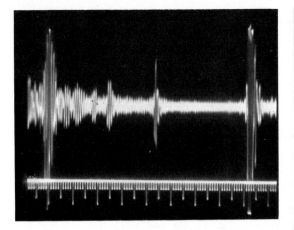

Fig. 7.63. Nondemodulated amplitude-mode image

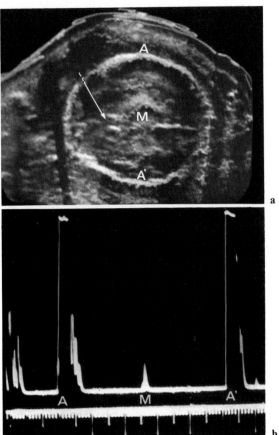

Fig. 7.64a, b. Measurement of BPD using a compound scan and A-scan. **a** Transverse scan demonstrating an oval cross-section of head: plane of section is anatomically correct (*arrow:* cavum septi pellucidi). **b** A-scan with electronic markers positioned at leading edge of skull echoes: BPD is read directly from a linear scale

molabile and "wanders" as the instrument heats up – a not uncommon occurrence in our experience.

Wladimiroff et al. (1975) have shown that the velocity of sound through fetal brain tissue can be highly variable and is also dependent on gestational age. This observation provides further evidence that there is probably no "ideal" calibration constant for BPD measurements that will satisfy all criteria. In an effort to standardize examination technique and improve the comparability of published data, the members of the European Study Group for Ultrasonography in Obstetrics and Gynecology, under the direction of Kratochwil, agreed at a 1975 meeting in Dubrovnik to recommend that A-mode systems be calibrated to a standard velocity of 1,600 m/s for BPD measurements.

In a final comment on the problem of accuracy in fetal cephalometry, we repeat that our own investigations in this area and those of most other authors (in which antenatal measurements were compared with caliper measurements in newborns) are of only limited value. In the final analysis they do not demonstrate the error of the ultrasound method, but only the discrepancies between values measured by two different methods, each of which is subject to error. Of greater interest to the operator are data on reproducibility, which affect only the ultrasound measurement. Davison et al. (1973) compared the variability of BPD measurements made (1) on a single occasion, (2) 24 h later, and (3) 4 weeks later under "blind" conditions; i.e., the examiner was not shown the results until the whole study was completed. When a set of three measurements was performed on a single occasion, the standard deviation was 1.21 mm. When sets of three measurements were performed 24 h apart, the standard deviation for the difference of the mean values was 2.74 mm. This error did not change when the interval was increased to 4 weeks. While this error is reasonably small, it nevertheless means that when a BPD of, say, 80 mm is measured, readings from 75 to 85 mm may be obtained when the measurement is repeated, for a confidence level of 96%. Pooling of these data yielded a standard deviation of 2.54 mm for the measured growth. The authors present the following formula for calculating the growth rate (GR):

$$GR = \frac{BPD_2 - BPD_1}{n} + \frac{SEM}{n} \; mm$$

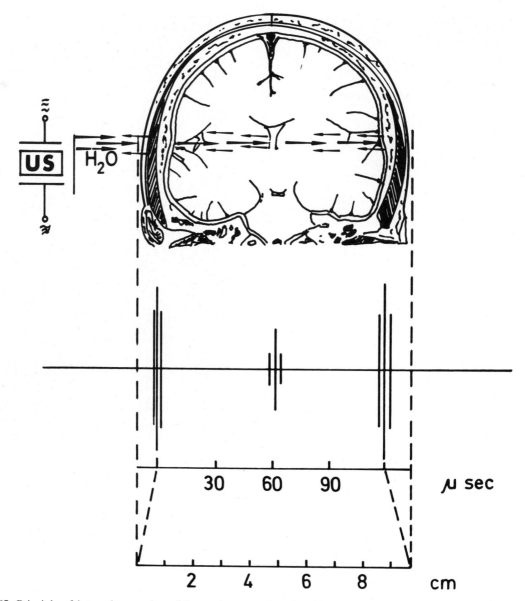

Fig. 7.65. Principle of internal correction of improving accuracy of BPD measurements. (After Hansmann and Hoven 1969; cf. text)

where *n* is the number of weeks elapsed between the two readings, and SEM is the standard error of mean of the difference between these readings. It follows that as the number of weeks between two observations increases, the effect of the total error on the growth rate declines. For example, if we assume that a BPD of 80 mm is measured initially and that a reading of 82 mm is obtained 1 week later, we find that the growth rate is 2 ± 2.54 mm; i.e., the BPD may have increased to 4.54 mm or it may have remained unchanged, if we exclude the possibil-

ity that it has decreased in size. Consequently, this time interval is of no use clinically. But if the same skull is measured 3 weeks later and the BPD is 86 mm, then the weekly growth rate would be $(6/3) + (2.54/3) = 2 \pm 0.84$ mm, with an obvious improvement in accuracy and reliability. Of course, the figures cited here are relevant only for the two experienced operators from Newcastle who participated in the study. From the data of Campbell (1970), an SEM of 1.68 mm was estimated for that author's measurements on the assumption that he always found the correct plane of section. In reality, no one can escape the sources of error that are inherent in the measuring system, such as those associated with wave interference or phase changes. In other words, even the most experienced examiner must recognize the magnitude of inherent errors and take that into account when evaluating his results.

Our Bonn study on intrauterine growth was based on a total of 4,858 ultrasound examinations performed in 2,014 pregnant women. All findings in the study, including history and information on the measurements, were recorded in computer-compatible fashion and stored and processed on the IBM 360-25 computer of the Institute for Medical Statistics, Documentation, and Data Processing of the Bonn University Clinics (Voigt and Hansmann 1975) using SEQAS, a programming language specially developed for that purpose (Voigt 1971).

To establish normal ranges for the different parameters, the program was designed to exclude data from multiple pregnancies and from pregnancies in which the gestational age was uncertain. Additional criteria for exclusion were maternal latent or overt diabetes, Rh incompatibility, fetal anomalies, and a transverse lie after 34 weeks. For each parameter, the arithmetic mean and standard deviation were calculated for the individual values and summarized on a weekly basis. Justification for stating the standard deviation was provided by a positive Lillie-Fors test.

For the BPD, 3,174 measurements in 1,348 pregnancies met the criteria established for the normal population. The period of observation extended from 9 to 42 weeks gestation, though only the interval from 13 to 42 weeks was statistically validated. All measurements were calibrated to a velocity of 1,600 m/s.

Besides the BPD and its rate of growth, the OFD and HC can be determined (Kratochwil 1971; Hansmann et al. 1972; Levi 1972; Stoger and Kratochwil 1974; Levi and Erbsmann 1975; Schillinger et al. 1975). With modern instruments, devices are available which allow measurement of the area or circumference of a structure directly from the ultrasound image.

A faster and easier way to calculate the HC is by using a modification of the formula for an ellipse:

$$HC = 2.325 \cdot \sqrt{BPD^2 + OFD^2}.$$

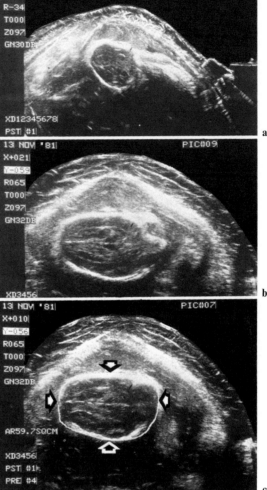

Fig. 7.66a–c. Typical fetal head configuration in a breech presentation with oligohydramnios. **a** Longitudinal scan showing head, back, and anterior placenta. **b** Occipitofrontal section showing typical dolichocephaly: measurement of BPD alone falsely implies growth retardation. **c** Measurement of HC indicates development appropriate for gestation

We use a table established from this formula for various BPD and OFD values so that the HC can be quickly found (see Appendix).

The combined measurement of BPD and OFD and the determination of HC is indicated in the following situations:

1. Unknown gestational age
2. BPD too small for a known gestational age
3. Transverse lie or breech presentation (Fig. 7.66)

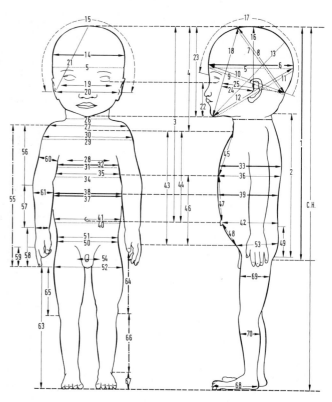

Fig. 7.67. Frontal and lateral views of a fetus with a 25-cm crown-heel length. The *arrows* indicate distances that may be relevant to ultrasound diagnosis. (Modified from Scammon and Calkins 1929)

4. Twin pregnancy
5. Suspected intrauterine growth retardation

7.2.3 Fetal Trunk Measurements

If one recognizes that the shape of the fetus is more cylindrical than spherical, and that this "cylinder" is composed of three main segments (head, trunk, extremities), each of which is subject to large variations independent of the others, it becomes clear that the measurement of only one linear dimension in one segment cannot be representative of the whole (Fig. 7.67). It is apparent that the key to better results in the assessment of fetal growth retardation lies not so much in the refinement of techniques for the measurement of BPD as in the inclusion of additional parameters from the fetal trunk and extremities.

Thompson et al. (1965) were the first to report on intrauterine measurement of fetal chest circumference. They did not measure the circumference directly, but calculated it from two transverse diameters. Despite the small number

of cases in the study (24) they found that fetal weight could be estimated more accurately from chest circumference than from BPD. This report prompted us to develop a technique for trunk measurements at our center. We were able to confirm the observation of Thompson et al. (1965), and published the first report on methodology and normal values (Hansmann et al. 1971, 1972). The most notable result of these efforts to improve fetal weight estimation was a significant improvement in the diagnosis of intrauterine growth abnormalities, especially in cases of maternal diabetes or suspected placental insufficiency. In that context we introduced the head-to-trunk ratio (H/T ratio) as an additional parameter for the assessment of fetal growth (Hansmann and Voigt 1973; Hansmann et al. 1973). It is defined as the ratio of the BPD to a trunk dimension [generally the transverse trunk diameter (TTD)] and thus provides a quantitative measure of the relationship between head and body.

Later a number of authors reported independently on fetal trunk measurements (Garrett and Robinson 1971; Bayer et al. 1972; Hollander 1972; Levi 1972; Levi and Erbsmann 1975; Prenzlau and Issel 1973; Schlensker 1973; Schlensker and Decker 1973; Issel and Prenzlau 1974; Stoger and Kratochwil 1974; Campbell 1974; Campbell and Wilkin 1975; Higginbottom et al. 1975; Schillinger et al. 1975). There is general agreement that prenatal trunk measurements improve the accuracy of fetal weight estimation and aid in the diagnosis of intrauterine growth retardation. There has been far less agreement on the technique of measurement, particularly with regard to the selection of standard planes. Although further studies in this area are needed, it is already clear that fetal trunk measurements have become an integral part of ultrasound diagnosis and should be routinely performed. In this section we shall describe and discuss our measurement technique, its problems, and the results that have been achieved, taking into account the principal modifications by other authors.

The main problem of ultrasound trunk measurements lies in the selection of a well-defined reference plane that avoids oblique sections. For simplicity, we propose that the trunk of the fetus be regarded as consisting of two truncated cones turned base-to-base, between which is interposed a cylindrical segment of variable thickness (Fig. 7.68).

In this simplified model the cranial truncated cone represents the chest with the heart, thymus, lungs, and upper portion of the liver. The middle segment represents the upper abdomen with the liver, spleen, pancreas, and stomach. The caudal truncated cone includes the mid and lower abdomen containing the bowel and urinary bladder. If we accept this model, it follows that the middle, cylindrical segment is the most advantageous site for fetal trunk measurements, for there the diameter and circumference are maximal and show the least variation in a craniocaudal direction. Thus, the anatomic target area is the liver, which is partly intrathoracic owing to the unexpanded state of the fetal lungs (Fig. 7.69a).

To locate this plane, we recommend that the following procedure be followed:

1. Locate the long axis of the fetus.

2. Rotate the transducer 90° and locate the lower thorax and liver.

3. Find the insertion of the umbilical cord in the transverse scan and move the transducer

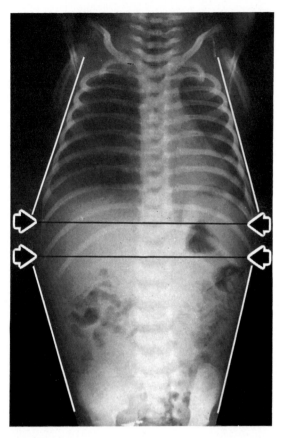

Fig. 7.68. Simplified geometric model of fetal trunk with radiograph. *Arrows* indicate target region for fetal trunk measurements

cranially, maintaining a transverse plane, until the umbilical vein disappears.

4. Avoid excessive pressure with the probe.

Particular attention should be given to the venous system of the fetal liver, including the umbilical vein, which presents on ultrasound as a nonpulsating double band coursing in an anteroposterior direction (Holländer 1972; Kossoff and Garrett 1972; Hansmann and Voigt 1973; Campbell 1974). Campbell and Wilkin (1975), using this method of fetal trunk measurement, find the umbilical vein in 95% of cases and consider it an important landmark for identifying the correct transverse plane. Kugener and Hansmann (1976) have investigated the topographic anatomy of the hepatic venous system (Fig. 7.69a, b) and have made the following observations:

1. The course of the umbilical vein does not define a specific plane, since the vein runs diagonally upward from the umbilicus at an angle

Fig. 7.69. a Midsagittal section through a male fetus with CRL of 140 mm: *1* Entry of umbilical vein into liver; *2* intrahepatic section of umbilical vein; ★, origin of ductus venosus; *upper arrow,* opening of ductus venosus into left hepatic vein; *lower arrow,* umbilical ring (an imaginary line connecting the arrows shows that the umbilical vein runs at about a 40° angle to the fetal longitudinal axis). **b** Corrosion preparation of a fetal liver, posterocaudal aspect: *1* Umbilical vein; *2* intrahepatic section of umbilical vein; *3* ductus venosus; *4* left hepatic vein; *5* inferior vena cava; ⊙ portal vein (left and right branch); ★origin of ductus venosus.(From Kugener and Hansmann 1976)

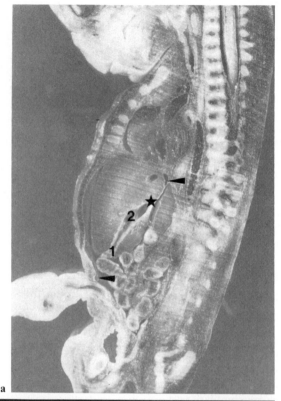

a

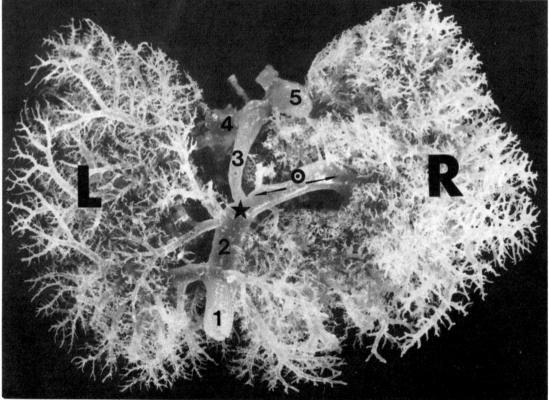

b

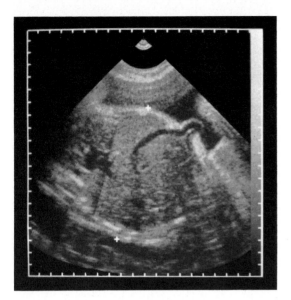

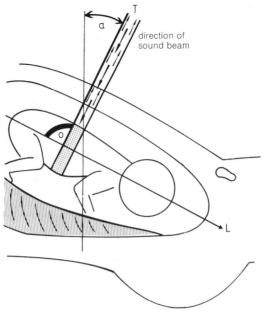

Fig. 7.70. Anterior sagittal scan showing site of entry of umbilical cord into abdomen and segment of umbilical vein ascending to liver

Fig. 7.71. Schematic diagram of correct level and plane for fetal trunk measurements. The plane of section is at right angles to the fetal long axis (*L*). When the plane is tilted about this axis, the scan becomes oblique. *T*, transducer

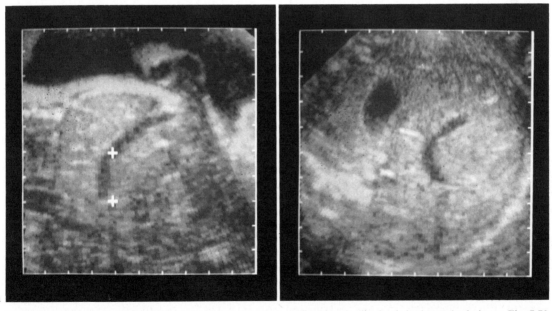

a   b

Fig. 7.72. a Course of umbilical vein in 3rd trimester: angle to fetal longitudinal axis is changed relative to Fig. 7.70 and reaches almost 90° posteriorly. **b** Corresponding transverse scan shows a long posterior segment of umbilical vein at level of junction with portal vein

of about 40° to the fetal long axis (Figs. 7.69a, 7.70). This angle becomes much greater as pregnancy progresses, and the course of the umbilical vein becomes highly variable (Fig. 7.72a, b).

2. A plane of measurement that is perpendicular to the fetal long axis (Fig. 7.71) will generally intersect the vascular band only over a relatively short segment (Fig. 7.73).

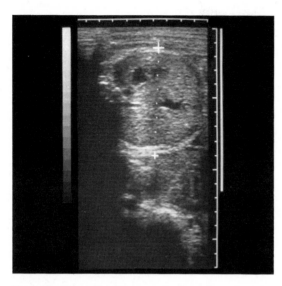

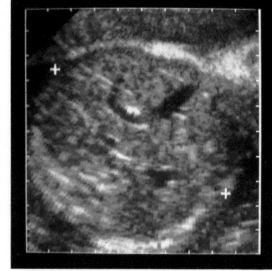

Fig. 7.73. Scan showing correct plane for measuring TTD: trunk profile circular; umbilical vein sectioned over only a short segment (oval), and intrahepatic; rib-profiles symmetric anteriorly and posteriorly

Fig. 7.74. Incorrect plane for measuring TTD: trunk elliptical rather than circular; long segment of umbilical vein depicted; ribs show asymmetric distribution

3. If a long segment of the vein is visualized (Fig. 7.74), it is likely that the plane is tilted frontally. This phenomenon, known as the "salami effect," does not alter the transverse abdominal diameter, but the anteroposterior diameter will increase as the plane is tilted, thus interfering with the circumference measurement. A plane tilted laterally will distort the TTD (Fig. 7.75a–c). In these cases the trunk will appear oval-shaped.

4. Transverse scans which demonstrate the site of entry of the umbilical vein into the abdominal wall are generally placed too low (Fig. 7.76).

5. The cranial end of the vascular band always marks the entry of the umbilical vein into the portal sinus and the origin of the ductus venosus. Because this junction lies in the lower thorax, it is a useful reference point (Fig. 7.77). Figure 7.78 A shows the plane of measurement in the frontal section.

For trunk measurements, then, it is necessary to locate the umbilical vein in transverse section and move the scan plane along the fetal axis until a short segment of the vein is imaged as far posteriorly as possible from the anterior abdominal wall. The presence of a long segment of vein probably indicates a tilted plane, in which case the AP diameter will appear too large.

If the plane of section is correct, it will also be possible to calculate area and circumference.

Reading errors can be minimized by measuring the circumference of the transverse section three times, adding the results and dividing the sum by three. For routine studies we measure diameters only, as this is easier and saves time. As a rule, we are not strong advocates of circumference measurement, because their theoretical advantage over diameter measurement is easily lost in practice due to unrecognized obliquity of the scanning plane (the salami effect).

To our knowledge, there is a paucity of research on the errors associated with fetal trunk measurements. The reason for this is that it is extremely difficult to verify the accuracy of ultrasound measurements because expansion of the fetal lungs at birth radically alters trunk dimensions compared with the antenatal state. In a study of 80 liveborn infants, Schlensker (1973) found that the chest circumference was an average of 31 mm greater than the value measured prenatally. Similar differences were reported by Stoger and Kratochwil (1974). On the other hand, Holländer (1972, 1975) observed that the chest circumferences measured with ultrasound were frequently too large (mean value of discrepancies 17.1 mm). This was probably due to unrecognized oblique

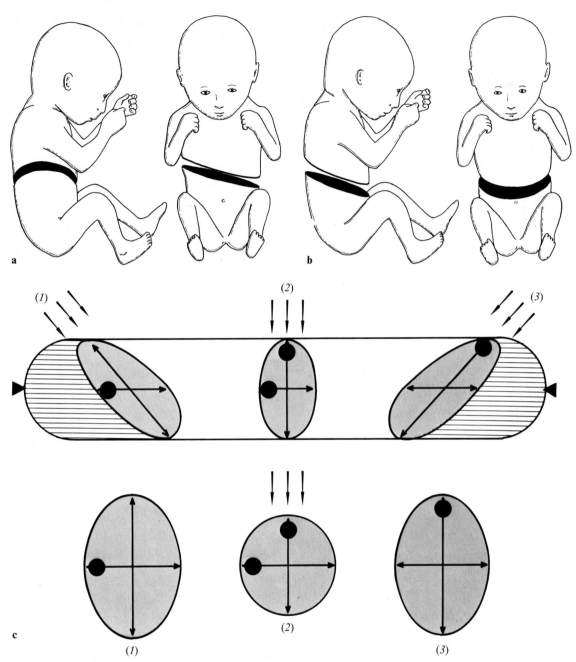

Fig. 7.75a–c. Schematic drawing of incorrect planes of section for fetal trunk measurements. **a** Lateral oblique; **b** frontal oblique; **c** salami effect

scans or to deformation of the fetal trunk from transducer pressure on the maternal abdomen. Holländer has shown that distorting a spherical trunk into an oval shape leads to an increase in the measured circumference.

Among our own patients, the discrepancies for the TTD are distributed symmetrically around a peak of ±5 mm, and around a peak of ±3 mm for the AP trunk diameter. After making suitable corrections, we found that 81.3% of all discrepancies between prenatal ultrasound measurements and postnatal caliper measurements fell within the range of ±7 mm. For the reproducibility of ultrasound measurements in a double-blind study, we calculated an mean error of ±2.8 mm with a standard

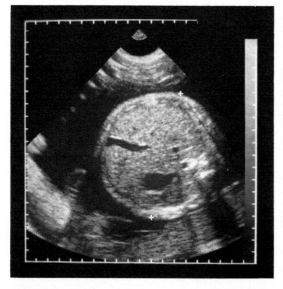 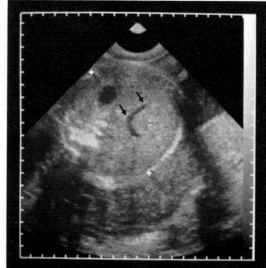

Fig. 7.76. In this scan the trunk profile appears symmetric and circular, but the level of the scan is too low. A long segment of umbilical vein is seen arising from the insertion of the umbilical cord into the abdomen

Fig. 7.77. Correct scanning plane. This scan is at a slightly higher level; the portal vein (*arrows*) is visualized

deviation of 2.1 mm (Hansmann 1975). On the whole, it appears that trunk measurements do not provide the same degree of accuracy as BPD measurements. But because the variability of trunk dimensions encompasses a far greater range of absolute values than that of the BPD, the relative magnitude of the error is reduced.

7.2.4 Measurement of the Fetal Extremities

It has been well established that fetal length correlates closely with gestational age. However, it is very difficult to measure the overall length of a fetus accurately by ultrasound.

One reason for this is the generally flexed posture of the fetus, which seldom if ever has enough room to extend to its full axial length, and seems reluctant to do so even when the opportunity presents itself (hydramnios). Another reason is that the imaging area of conventional ultrasound equipment is seldom large enough to depict the entire fetus after 20 weeks gestation.

An obvious alternative to the measurement of overall fetal length is the measurement of parts of the fetal body. It has been well documented in the literature that CRL when cor-

rectly measured, is an accurate parameter for assessing gestational age; however, its use is restricted to the relatively short interval between 7 and 14 weeks gestation. Other parts of the body, such as the arms and legs, are difficult to measure in their entirety because of their flexed position. On the other hand, the diaphyses of the long bones of the extremities are relatively easy to identify and measure by ultrasound. These facts were noted by Schlensker (1982), who, given sufficient time, was able to measure all the diaphyses between 13 and 27 weeks. The average time required to delineate all bones was 10 min, with a range of 5–20 min. The least amount of time was required between 16 and 20 weeks. Comparison with measurements of extremity bones from aborted fetuses indicated a maximum error of 4%.

Based on the degree of difficulty experienced in the imaging of different diaphyses, an obvious gradation was noted in favor of the proximal bones. In other words: The humerus and femur are more easily imaged than the distal diaphyseal bones (ulna, radius, tibia, and fibula). Also, the lower extremity is more accessible to measurement than the upper extremity, which is frequently in the acoustic shadow of the trunk and head and shows a greater mobi-

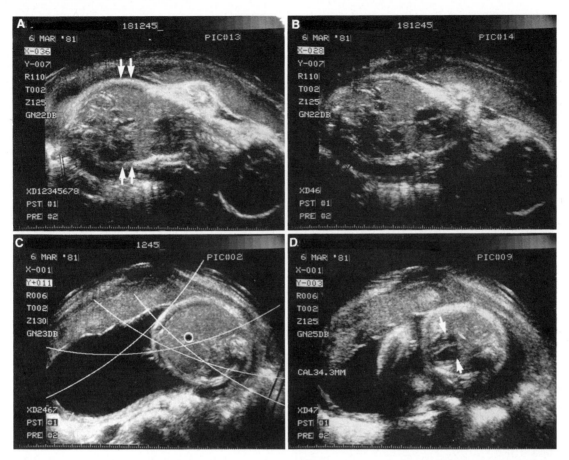

Fig. 7.78. Demonstration of planes of measurement with a compound scanner. **A** Frontal scan: level of measurement marked with *arrows*. **B** Paramedian sagittal scan depicting stomach. **C** Correct plane of measurement in transverse scan. **D** Cardiac structures (*arrows*) indicate that this plane is too high

lity than the leg. For these reasons, the majority of authors use the length of the femur, the longest extremity bone, as their favored parameter. The technique for measuring the femur was described in detail by Jeanty and Romero (1984).

Femur Length: Points of Measurement. After the femur has been visualized at the caudal end of the trunk, the transducer is rotated to depict its longest axis. It is recommended that the femur located within the focal zone of and closest to the transducer be used. The length of the diaphysis only should be measured; the femoral head is excluded. In many cases the femur will show a pronounced degree of curvature (especially when imaged in the frontal plane). Except in extreme cases, this curvature should not affect the accuracy of the measurement. The appearance of the ends of the diaphysis is a critical factor in identifying the longest axis

of the femur. Either the proximal or the distal end of the femur may appear curved or blunted (Fig. 7.82a). As shown by Lessoway and Wittmann (1985) in a water bath experiment (Fig. 7.82b), this is not due to reflection of soundwaves from the femoral head or the condyle, but represents the metaphyseal surface of the diaphysis. Oblique sectioning of the femur can be prevented if care is taken that the echo intensity and acoustic shadowing of the femur are uniform over its entire length. It is important in this regard that both ends of the diaphysis cast a well-defined acoustic shadow (Figs. 7.79 and 7.80). If the femurs of both extremities are oriented parallel to the transducer, the shadow from the diaphysis nearer the transducer may prevent accurate measurement of the other diaphysis. This underscores the importance of measuring the near femur. If the scanning plane traverses the femur at too great an

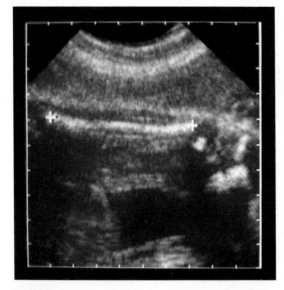

Fig. 7.79. Correct points for measurement of femur length. The femur closer to the transducer was selected for the measurement; the ends of the diaphysis are well defined, and the bone shows a uniform contour

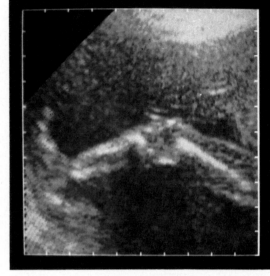

Fig. 7.81. This scan is unsatisfactory for femur length measurement. The proximal part of the femur is sectioned tangentially, and the end-point cannot be identified

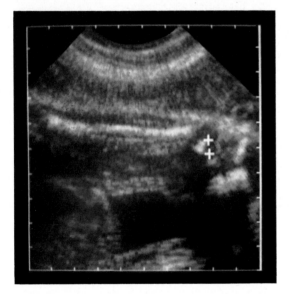

Fig. 7.80. Correct visualization of femur. The scan also shows the distal ossification center with corresponding points of measurement (same fetus as in Fig. 7.79: femur length is 59 mm, corresponding to 31 weeks)

angle, the proximal end of the diaphysis may be shadowed by the pelvic bone, and a false-short measurement may thus be obtained (Fig. 7.81). Apparent gaps in the bone are usually caused by structures overlying the diaphysis and should not be mistaken for "fractures."

These principles of femur length measurement can be applied with equal validity to the measurement of other diaphyses.

We have performed ultrasound measurements of the humerus, ulna, femur, and tibia in a series of 467 patients with accurate dates. From these values we were able to plot growth curves from 13 weeks to term (see Appendix).

For the exclusion of malformations or confirmation of gestational age in doubtful cases, only the measurement of femur length is thought to be of value (Farrant and Meire 1981; Hadlock et al. 1982; Hohler and Quetal 1982; Jeanty and Romero 1984; Jeanty et al. 1982; Jeanty et al. 1981).

Jeanty and Romero (1984) consider the measurement of femur length between 14 and 28 weeks as important as the determination of BPD. O'Brien and Queenan (1982) showed that by including femur length in the biometric evaluation of fetuses with suspected intrauterine growth retardation, it was possible in all cases to identify the pattern of growth retardation as being symmetric or asymmetric and to improve significantly the overall success rate in the detection of retarded growth.

On these grounds, and from the standpoint of recognizing limb malformations in the offspring of patients who are not at obvious risk, the measurement of femur length should be per-

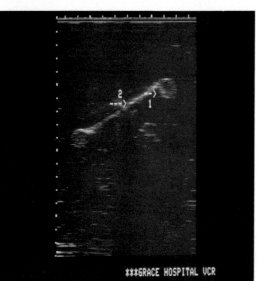

Fig. 7.82a, b. Femur measurement. **a** Femur from term infant immersed in waterbath. Line indicated by *1* represents metaphyseal surface of diaphysis, *not* femoral head. *2*, diaphysis. **b** Fetal femur at similar angle to **a**, displaying corresponding reflection of soundwaves from metaphyseal surface

center of the femur became increasingly well defined after 32 weeks and could always be demonstrated from 35 weeks onward. The proximal tibial center was visible in most cases by 36 weeks. Besides demonstrating these ossification centers, the author measured their diameters and found a marked increase in size as term approached. McLeary et al. (1983), in their study of 220 fetuses, had variable success in identifying the distal femoral epiphysis after 28 weeks. A 100% detection rate was not achieved until 37 weeks.

In the final analysis, these parameters are important only as additional criteria in cases where gestational age was not assessed sonographically before the third trimester and there is general doubt as to the age of the pregnancy.

formed in all patients. At the very least, this will furnish "practice" that will help the examiner to perform accurate measurements in more critical situations.

Ossification Centers. Bernaschek (1982) has investigated the sonographic visualization and measurement of fetal ossification centers (Figs. 7.79 and 7.80) in the region of the knee joint. He found that the distal ossification

References

Aantaa K, Forss M (1974) Determination of biparietal diameter by the ultrasonic B-scan technique. Acta Obstet Gynecol Scand 53:121

Bayer H, Issel EP, Schulte R (1972) Neue Meßgrößen bei der Erkennung einer intrauterinen Retardierung der Frucht mittels Ultraschalldiagnostik. Zentralbl Gynäkol 94:1169

Bernaschek G (1982) Die Besonderheiten einer neuartigen echographischen Bestimmung der Kniegelenkskerne des Feten. Geburtshilfe Frauenheilkd 42:94

Boog G, Irrmann M, Mot E de, Gandar R (1969) Céphalometrie foetale par ultrasons. I.-Technique, principe et précision de la méthode. Rev Fr Gynécol 64:303

Campbell S (1968) An improved method of fetal cephalometry by ultrasound. Br J Obstet Gynaecol 75:568

Campbell S (1969) The prediction of fetal maturity by ultrasonic measurement of the biparietal diameter. Br J Obstet Gynaecol 76:603

Campbell S (1970) Ultrasonic fetal cephalometry during the second trimester of pregnancy. Br J Obstet Gynaecol 77:1057

Campbell S (1974) The assessment of fetal development by diagnostic ultrasound. In: Milunsky A (ed) The pregnancy at risk. Saunders, Philadelphia (Clinics in perinatology, vol 1/2, p 507

Campbell S, Newman GB (1971) Growth of the fetal biparietal diameter during normal pregnancy. Br J Obstet Gynaecol 78:513

Campbell S, Wilkin D (1975) Ultrasonic measurement of fetal abdomen circumference in the estimation of fetal weight. Br J Obstet Gynaecol 82:689

Davison KM, Lind T, Farr V, Whittingham TA (1973) The limitations of ultrasonic fetal cephalometry. Br J Obstet Gynaecol 80:769

Donald I, Brown TG (1961) Demonstration of tissue interfaces within the body by ultrasonic echosounding. Br J Radiol 34:539

Durkan JP, Russo GL (1966) Ultrasonic fetal cephalometry. Accuracy, limitation and application. Obstet Gynaecol 27:399

Farrant B, Meire HB (1981) Ultrasound measurement of fetal limb length. Br J Radiol 54:660

Garrett WJ, Robinson DE (1971) Assessment of fetal size and growth rate by ultrasonic echoscopy. Obstet Gynaecol 38:525

Hadlock FP, Harrist RB, Deter RL (1982) Fetal femur length as a predictor of menstrual age: Sonographically measured. Am J Roentgenol 138:875

Hansmann M (1975) Ultraschallkephalo- und Thorakometrie zur Kontrolle des fetalen Wachstums unter besonderer Berücksichtigung der praepartalen Gewichtsschätzung. Habilitationsschrift, Med Fakultät Bonn

Hansmann M, Hoven R (1971) Eine abgewandelte Methodik zur Bestimmung des biparietalen Durchmessers mittels Ultraschall. In: Böck J, Ossoining (eds) Ultrasonographic Medica, Bd III. Verlag der Wiener Med Akademie, Wien, S 219

Hansmann M, Voigt U (1973a) Ultrasonic fetal thoracometry: an additional parameter for determining fetal growth. Excerpta Medica (Abstr), 2nd World Congress on Ultrasonics in Medicine, Rotterdam

Hansmann M, Voigt U (1973b) Ultraschall-Biometrie des Feten unter besonderer Berücksichtigung der Gewichtsschätzung bei intrauteriner Malnutrition. In: Saling E, Dudenhausen JW (eds) Perinatale Medizin, Bd IV. Thieme, Stuttgart

Hansmann M, Bäker H, Fabula S, Müller-Scholtes H, Nellen HJ, Voigt U (1972) Biometrische Daten des Feten. Ergebnisse einer modifizierten Methodik der Ultraschalldiagnostik. In: Saling E, Dudenhausen JW (eds) Perinatale Medizin, Bd III. Thieme, Stuttgart, S 136

Hansmann M, Voigt U, Lang N (1973) Ultraschallmeßdaten als Parameter zur Erkennung einer intrauterinen Wachstumsretardierung. Arch Gynecol 214:194

Hellmann LM, Kobayashi M, Fillisti L, Lavenhar M (1967) Sources for error in sonographic fetal mensuration and estimation of growth. Am J Obstet Gynecol 99:662

Higginbottom J, Slater J, Porter G (1975) Estimation of fetal weight from ultrasonic measurement of trunk circumference. Br J Obstet Gynaecol 82:698

Hinselmann M (1969) Ultraschalldiagnostik in der Geburtshilfe. Gynäkologe 2:45

Hofmann D, Holländer HJ (1968) Über den Nachweis fetalen Lebens und die Messung des kindlichen Schädels mittels des zweidimensionalen Ultraschallechoverfahrens. Gynaecologia 165:60

Hofmann D, Holländer HJ, Weiser P (1967) Über die geburtshilfliche Bedeutung der Ultraschalldiagnostik. Gynaecologia (Basel) 164:24

Hohler CW, Quetal TA (1982) Fetal femur length: Equations for computer calculation of gestational age from ultrasound measurement. Am J Obstet Gynecol 143:479

Holländer HJ (1972, ^{2}1975, ^{3}1984) Die Ultraschalldiagnostik in der Schwangerschaft. Urban & Schwarzenberg, München Berlin Wien

Issel EP, Prenzlau P (1974) Eine neue Methode zur Berechnung des fetalen Gewichtes mittels Ultraschall-B-Bild-Technik. Zentralbl Gynäkol 96:417

Jeanty P, Romero R (1984) Obstetrical ultrasound. Mc Graw-Hill, New York

Jeanty P, Kirkpatrick C, Dramaix-Wilmet M (1981) Fetal limb growth. Radiology 140:165

Jeanty P, Dramaix-Wilmet M, Kerkem J van (1982) Fetal limb growth, Part II. Radiology 143:751

Kohorn EI (1967) An evaluation of ultrasonic fetal cephalometry. Am J Obstet Gynecol 97:553

Kossoff G, Garrett WJ (1972) Ultrasonic film echography in gynecology and obstetrics. Obstet Gynecol 40:299

Kratochwil A (1966) Die diagnostische Anwendung des Ultraschalls in der Geburtshilfe und Gynäkologie. Zentralbl Gynäkol 88:1032

Kratochwil A (1968) Ultraschalldiagnostik in Geburtshilfe und Gynäkologie, 1. Aufl. Thieme, Stuttgart

Kratochwil A (1971) Biometrie des Feten mit Ultraschall. In: Saling E, Schulte EJ (eds) Perinatale Medizin, Bd II. Thieme, Stuttgart, S 247

Kugener H, Hansmann M (1976) Zur Topographie einer Referenzebene für die Ultraschallthorakometrie. Z Geburtshilfe Perinatol 180

Lessoway VA, Wittmann BK (1985) Femur – what do we actually see? Proceedings, 30th Annual Convention of the AIUM, Dallas, USA

Levi S (1972) Le diagnostic par les ultrasons en gynécologie et en obstétrique. Masson, Paris

Levi S (1973) Intra-uterine fetal growth studied by ultrasonic biparietal measurement – The percentiles of biparietal distribution. Acta Obstet Gynecol Scand 52:193

Levi S, Erbsmann F (1975) Antenatal fetal growth from the nineteenth week (Ultrasonic study of 12 head and chest dimensions). Am J Obstet Gynecol 121:262

Mc Leary, Lawrence RD, Kuhns R (1983) Sonographic evaluation of the distal femoral epiphyseal ossification center. J Ultrasound Med 2:437

O'Brien GD, Queenan JT (1982) Ultrasound fetal femur length in relation to intrauterine growth retardation. Am J Obstet Gynecol 144:35

Prenzlau P, Issel EP (1973) Die praktische Bedeutung der Messung der Schulter-Steißlänge (Trunkometrie) beim Fetus mittels Ultraschall. Zentralbl Gynäkol 95:1421

Queenan JT, Kubarych SF, Cook LN, Anderson GD, Griffin LP (1976) Diagnostic ultrasound for detection of intrauterine growth retardation. Am J Obstet Gynecol 124:865

Schillinger H, Müller R, Kretzschmar M, Wode J (1975) Gewichtsbestimmung des Feten durch Ultraschall. Geburtshilfe Frauenheilkd 35:866

Schlensker KH (1972) Reifegraddiagnostik mit Ultraschall. 155. Tagung der Niederrhein.-Westf. Gesellschaft für Gynäkologie u. Geburtshilfe, Düsseldorf

Schlensker KH (1973) Eine Ultraschallmethodik zur Thorakometrie beim Feten. Geburtshilfe Frauenheilkd 33:440

Schlensker KH (1975) Atlas of ultrasonic diagnosis in obstetrics and gynecology. Thieme, Stuttgart

Schlensker KH (1982) Biometrie der fetalen Extremitäten. Swiss Med 6.0:140

Schlensker KH, Decker I (1973) Voraussage des kindlichen Geburtsgewichtes aufgrund der Ultraschallkephalometrie und Thorakometrie am Feten. Geburtshilfe Frauenheilkd 33:859

Stöger H, Kratochwil A (1974) Ultraschallbiometrie des fetalen Wachstums. Geburtshilfe Frauenheilkd 34:611

Thompson HE, Holmes JH, Gottesfeld KR, Taylor ES (1965) Fetal development as determined by ultrasonic pulse echo techniques. Am J Obstet Gynecol 92:44

Varma TR (1973) Prediction of delivery date by ultrasound cephalometry. Br J Obstet Gynecol 80:316

Voigt U (1971) SEQUAS – eine Programmiersprache zur Sequentialdatenauswertung auf digitalen elektronischen Datenverarbeitungsanlagen. Dissertation, Med. Fakultät Bonn

Voigt U, Hansmann M (1975) Dokumentation und elektronische Datenverarbeitung von Ultraschallbefunden in der Geburtshilfe. Z Geburtshilfe Perinatol 179:450

Willocks J (1963) Fetal cephalometry by ultrasound. Thesis, Glasgow

Willocks J, Donald I, Duggan TC, Day N (1964) Foetal cephalometry ultrasound. Br J Obstet Gynecol 71:11

Wladimiroff JW, Craft IL, Talbert DG (1975) In vitro measurements of sound velocity in human fetal brain tissue. In: Ultrasound in medicine and biology, vol I. Excerpta Medica, Amsterdam, p 377

7.3 Diagnosis of Intrauterine Growth Retardation

Fetuses who suffer intrauterine growth retardation are small for gestational age (SGA) at birth, meaning that their birth weight is below the 10th percentile for the period of gestation (Bard 1970; Fedrick and Adelstein 1978; Frigoletto and Rothchild 1977). Gallbright et al. (1979) reported that the average incidence of intrauterine growth retardation in their population was approximately 5%.

Two-thirds of all growth-retarded infants come from "high-risk" pregnancies in which one or more risk factors are known to be present [hypertension, preexisting maternal heart or kidney disease, bleeding during pregnancy, multiple pregnancy (Fig. 7.83), or prior delivery of a growth-retarded infant] (Gallbright et al. 1979). The remaining one-third come from pregnancies that have no apparent risk factors (incidence 2.3%).

Growth-retarded infants have a four to eight times higher rate of perinatal mortality and morbidity than infants in the normal weight range (Low and Gallbright 1974; Scott and Usher 1966). Lang et al. (1977) recorded a mortality rate as high as 11%.

Children with growth retardation are at increased risk for abnormal physical and neu-

rologic development (Fitzhardinger and Steven 1972). However, Vohr et al. (1979) showed that with early diagnosis – the most important factor here – growth-retarded infants delivered between 32 and 36 weeks gestation can catch up to normal growth by the 8th month of life and show normal neurologic development after 2 years.

Before discussing the sonographic criteria for the diagnosis of intrauterine growth retardation, it is important to consider the different patterns of growth retardation that can occur. These have been described by Campbell (1974), Hansmann (1976), Wladimiroff et al. (1977), and De Vore and Hobbins (1979).

The observations made by ultrasound can be related to the pioneering studies of Gruenwald (1963), who showed that growth-retarded fetuses have a significantly higher brain-to-body weight ratio than premature infants, but have smaller intrathoracic and intraabdominal organs (most severely affected: thymus, lung, liver, spleen, adrenals). Accordingly, sonographic measurements yield considerably lower values for the trunk than for the head (Fig. 7.84). Myers et al. (1971) made similar observations in animal models. Naeye (1965, 1966, 1973) noted that a distinction can be made between growth-retarded infants whose weight is low by virtue of a decreased cell size and those whose weight is low as a result of

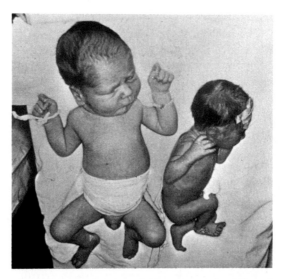

Fig. 7.83. Discordant growth in newborn twins delivered at 37 weeks. Twin on *left* is appropriate for gestational age, with a birth weight of 3,600 g. Twin on *right* is severely growth-retarded weighing only 1,600 g at birth

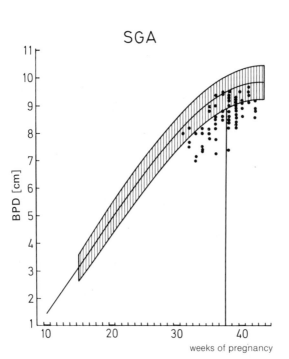

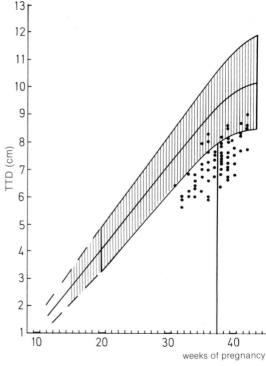

Fig. 7.84. Scattergrams of biometric data for intrauterine growth retardation (*SGA*). *Left:* last prenatal measure-ment of BPD; *right:* last measurement of TTD. (Explanation in text)

a reduced number of cells. Winick (1973) points out that there has been much evidence in recent years to show that antenatal cell growth follows definite time schedules in different organs. Three main phases of cell growth can be identi-fied:

1. Phase of pure proliferation (hyperplasia)
2. Phase of proliferation and hypertrophy
3. Hypertrophy with no increase in number of cells

Malnutrition during the proliferative phase can decrease the rate of cell division without altering the timing of the phase. The result is a small organ with a decreased number of cells – an irreversible condition. On the other hand, the same malnutrition in the hypertrophic phase will inhibit only the increase in cell size. These changes are reversible. Winick (1973) as-sumes that the conditions surrounding intrau-terine growth retardation in man are similar to those observed in animal models. According-ly, there are two basic forms of growth retarda-tion – the first causes a uniform reduction in the weight of all organs (including the brain) and in their protein, DNA, and RNA content,

while in the second these changes are less pro-nounced. The specific form that occurs ob-viously depends on the timing of the growth-retarding stimulus and on its duration, nature, and severity. The first form of growth retarda-tion, type 1 (Rosso and Winick 1974), can be

Fig. 7.85a–c. Examples of different types of intrauterine growth retardation: *left*, BPD; *right*, TTD. **a** Individual growth curve with early retardation of head and trunk growth (type 1: "low profile") in trisomy E (spontane-ous delivery at 39 weeks, male, weight 1,820 g, length 42 cm). **b** Individual growth curve with late retardation of head and trunk growth (type 2: "late flattening") secondary to chronic placental insufficiency with fall of HPL and pathologic NST (cesarean birth at 37 weeks, male, weight 1,730 g, length 47 cm). Growth retardation is earlier and more marked in the TTD curve. The H/T ratio is abnormally high (1.29) at 31 weeks, expressing a disproportion that persists until delivery (BPD 87 mm, TTD 68 mm). **c** Individual growth curve in a breech presentation with a fundal placenta. The BPD conforms to the late-flattening pattern, but trunk growth is undis-turbed. Endocrine parameters are within normal limits, NST is normal, BPD 87 mm (spontaneous delivery at 39 weeks, male weight 3,440 g, length 51 cm). (From Hansmann 1976)

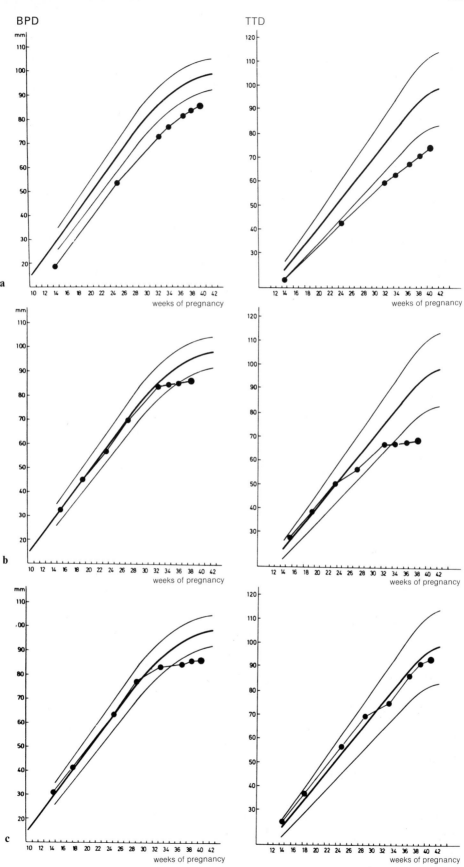

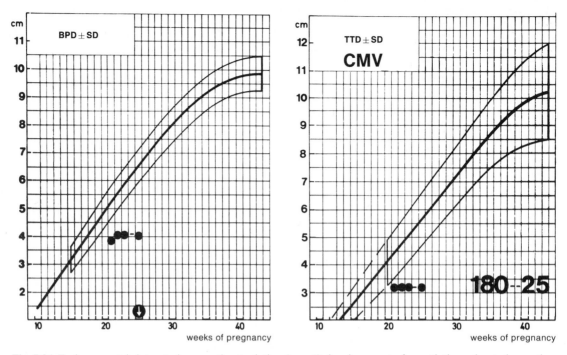

Fig. 7.86. Early symmetric intrauterine growth retardation (type 1) showing arrest of growth throughout observation period (20–24 weeks) secondary to a cytomegalovirus (CMV) infection. Stillborn fetus weighed 180 g and was approximately 25 cm long

produced in laboratory animals by a chronic maternal protein deficit during pregnancy. Type 2 growth retardation can be produced by ligating the uterine artery in rats (Wigglesworth 1964) or by causing partial separation of the placenta in rhesus monkeys (Myers et al. 1971). Sonographically, a variety of intrauterine growth patterns can be observed in accordance with the etiologic heterogeneity of the SGA syndrome. There are many patterns, which can never be exhaustively analyzed, because the onset, duration, and severity of the retarding stimulus and its specific site of action (mother/placenta/fetus) are rarely known and frequently cannot be identified. Nevertheless, the two basic types of fetal growth retardation can be described (Fig. 7.85):

Type 1: These fetuses exhibit growth retardation which begins in the second trimester and affects all parts of the body more or less uniformly. Affected fetuses are at much greater risk for congenital malformations than the general population (Ramzin et al. 1973). This group also includes babies that are genetically small but otherwise healthy. Campbell (1974) describes this growth pattern as "low profile"

and considers it a manifestation of reduced growth potential. In our experience, this group also includes a significant number of fetuses that suffered intrauterine infections (e.g., rubella or cytomegalovirus; Fig. 7.86).

According to Campbell (1976), type 1 growth retardation can also be classified as hypoplastic, since cell numbers are reduced. Approximately 20%–30% of all growth-retarded infants are assigned to this group. The possible causes of this retardation and its criteria are summarized below:

Time of onset: Second trimester
Form: Symmetric, the whole body being affected equally
Possible causes:
1. Genetic (small parents)
2. Chromosome abnormalities
3. Malformations (Fig. 7.87)
4. Intrauterine diseases
5. Exogenous substances (alcohol, drugs, nicotine)

Type 2: These fetuses experience normal head and trunk growth through the second trimester, followed by a relatively abrupt retardation of

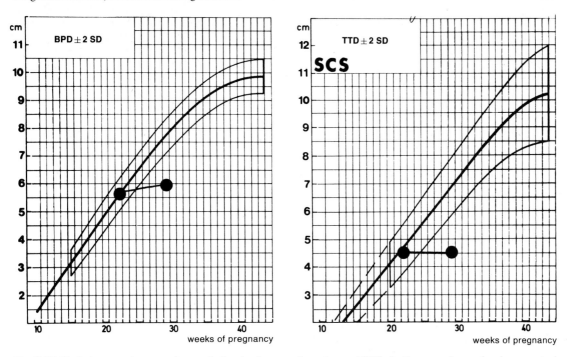

Fig. 7.87. Early intrauterine growth retardation in short-cord syndrome (*SCS*). In the case observed, a large central retroplacental hematoma apparently resulted from traction on the extremely short umbilical cord

growth in the third trimester. Generally, the trunk is affected earlier and more severely; head size may be normal or only slightly reduced. Hence a common feature of this condition is disproportion, which is present in over 66% of cases. Campbell (1974) calls this the "late flattening" type of growth retardation. This refers exclusively to the BPD, for which the term "late" is highly appropriate.

The main diagnostic feature of this disorder is an asymmetric retardation that affects weight more than length. It may be characterized as hypotrophic, since the cells are normal in number but decreased in size. As in every case of hunger, there is a primary reduction of fat with secondary compromise of the organs. In addition, the special circumstances of fetal circulation cause the head and brain to be supplied preferentially over the trunk. Fancourt et al. (1976) found that the prognosis of this type of growth retardation is closely related to the time of exposure to the growth-retarding stimulus. They found a retardation of brain growth only in cases where the BPD growth rate had decreased prior to 27 weeks.

To summarize the features of type 2 fetal growth retardation:

Time of onset: Third trimester
Form: Asymmetric, the trunk being affected earlier and more severely than the head
Possible causes:
1. Hypertension
2. Maternal renal or vascular disease
3. Placental insufficiency (partial separation)
4. Impairment of placental maturation
5. Idiopathic placental insufficiency

Basically this form of retardation is due to factors which compromise nutrition in an otherwise healthy fetus. Most of these factors relate to placental problems. This is by far the more common form of intrauterine growth retardation, accounting for 70%–80% of all cases.

7.3.1 Diagnostic Criteria, Possible Screening Methods

Investigators have used a variety of parameters in an effort to diagnose fetal growth retardation. All are based on the premise that the gestational age must be known before fetal growth retardation can be assessed. It would be pointless to try to differentiate an "error in dates"

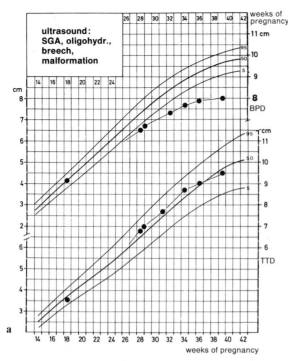
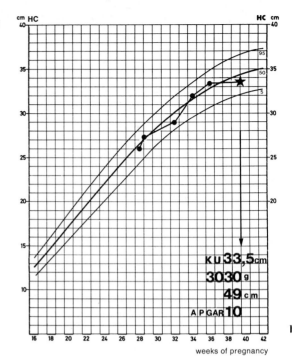

Fig. 7.88a, b. Fetal growth curves. Based on low BPD values in a breech presentation (**a**), the patient was referred at 27 weeks with suspected fetal growth retardation and/or fetal anomaly. Serial observations confirmed the measurements of the first examiner. It was found that the TTD was normal, while the head was dolichoce-phalic (as a result of the breech presentation with oligo-hydramnios). Further measurements of the HC (**b**) confirmed a normal development for brain volume, excluding microcephaly. A healthy infant was delivered at 39 weeks

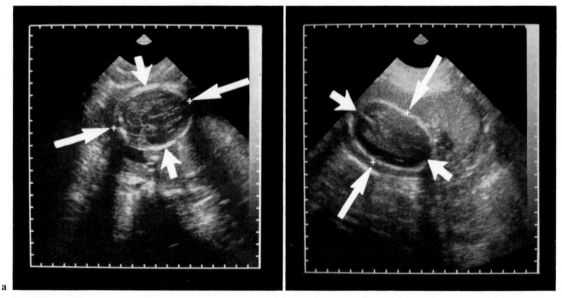

Fig. 7.89a, b. Example of measurements simulating early intrauterine growth retardation. **a** Transverse scan of fetal skull at 21 weeks. The head configuration is normal: BPD 5.4 cm (*short arrows*), OFD 6.8 cm (*long arrows*), HC 19.9 cm. All dimensions are properly proportioned and appropriate for dates. **b** Transverse scan at 21 weeks. The BPD (4.6 cm, *long arrows*) conforms to only 18 weeks, while the OFD (7.2 cm, *short arrows*) conforms to the mean for 23 weeks. The HC is 19.9 cm, "appropriate for dates." The dolichocephalic head configuration is the result of oligohydramnios in association with a breech presentation. The infant was healthy and of normal weight at birth

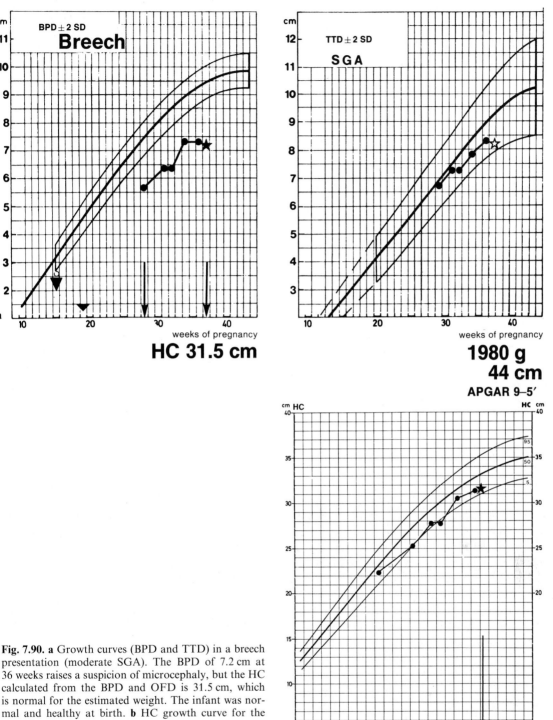

Fig. 7.90. a Growth curves (BPD and TTD) in a breech presentation (moderate SGA). The BPD of 7.2 cm at 36 weeks raises a suspicion of microcephaly, but the HC calculated from the BPD and OFD is 31.5 cm, which is normal for the estimated weight. The infant was normal and healthy at birth. **b** HC growth curve for the same fetus

from growth retardation at 30 weeks, or to identify a particular pattern of growth retardation without knowing the gestational age. Other clinical parameters, such as the height of the fundus, are inadequate as a basis for screening. Maternal obesity, variations in bladder fullness, changes in fetal position and lie, and the possible coexistence of a fetal anomaly with hydram-

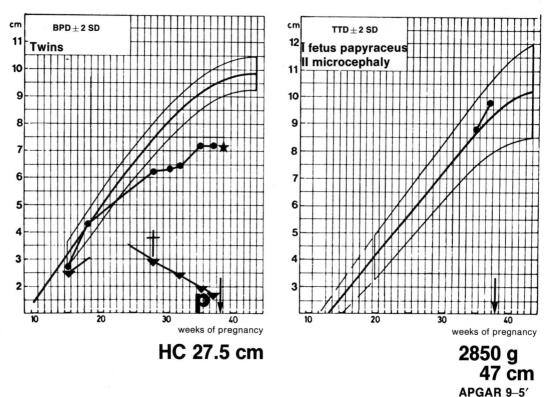

HC 27.5 cm

2850 g
47 cm
APGAR 9–5′

Fig. 7.91. Growth curves in a twin pregnancy. Fetus I (▲——▲) suffered severe growth retardation and died. Fetus II (●——●) likewise showed a significant retardation of BPD growth. Calculation of HC from BPD and OFD confirmed microcephaly; trunk dimensions were normal. The infant, delivered at 37 weeks, survived but was handicapped. HC at delivery was 27.5 cm

nios in the presence of growth retardation are only a few examples illustrating the unsuitability of clinical methods as a basis for accurate diagnosis. Establishment of the gestational age early in pregnancy is the only rational basis for screening. This is one reason why we have advocated routine baseline ultrasound scans during the second trimester, and why this recommendation has been generally adopted in the Federal Republic of Germany.

Once gestational age is accurately known, it is desirable to have more than one fetal growth parameter on which to base the diagnosis. It should be stressed from the outset that in evaluation for growth retardation, as in all ultrasound examinations (see Sect. 7.1), a general survey should be carried out before turning to specific details. The uterus, placenta, amniotic fluid volume, and general appearance and position of the fetus should be assessed before any measurements are performed. Thus, for example, an isolated measurement of the BPD without determining the OFD may be misleading in a breech presentation. It is common in breech presentations for the fetal head in the fundus to be molded into an elongated shape that will give a false result if only one measure (BPD) is employed (Fig. 7.88).

7.3.2 Technique and Accuracy of Measurement

Lang et al. (1977) state that fetal growth retardation can be diagnosed from a single, isolated measurement of the BPD in only about 60% of cases. Accuracy improves considerably when serial measurements are performed. Under these conditions Campbell (1974) and Campbell et al. (1979) found correlation in 72% of growth-retarded fetuses below the 10th percentile for BPD and in 82% below the 5th percentile.

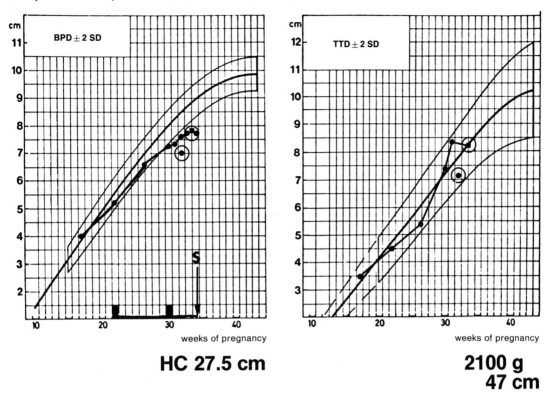

HC 27.5 cm

2100 g
47 cm

Fig. 7.92. Growth curves of the fetus "Jir." (see text). There had been chronic bleeding since 19 weeks due to a placenta previa, and markedly low BPD values (7.7 cm at 33 week) raised the suspicion of microcephaly. The pregnancy was terminated by Cesarean birth at 34 weeks. The HC at that time was 27.5 cm (medical examiner's report) and thus was below the 3rd percentile for gestational age (Largo and Duc 1977; Brandt 1979).

This value was close to the 50th percentile for 28 weeks, but the body length of 47 cm corresponded to 36 weeks. The small HC and body malproportion were classic signs of microcephaly, but the anomaly could not be definitively diagnosed from BPD measurements alone. Apparently the general impression of a "round" fetal head contributed to the suspicion of microcephaly

Our own research indicates that the "failure rate" of cephalometry based on the distribution of last measured value around the lower limit of the normal range (2 SD) is between 25% and 30%. This is consistent with the results of Campbell and Dewhurst (1971), who found a 21% incidence of normal BPD growth rates in fetuses with confirmed growth retardation.

Campbell and Wilkin (1975) used a computer model to show that when gestational age is known, a single abdominal circumference measurement at 33 weeks can detect fetal growth retardation in 81% of cases. If this measurement is done at 37 weeks, the success rate falls to 63.2%. Wladimiroff et al. (1981) used BPD and trunk area as their screening parameters. In fetuses with values below the 10th percentile, the BPD was a useful indicator in only 43% of cases, and the trunk area in 75%. In fetuses with values below the 5th percentile, these figures increased to 51% and 86% respectively. Hoffbauer et al. (1978) correctly diagnosed intrauterine growth retardation in only 80% of cases despite the use of seven or eight growth parameters.

Since we began using fetal trunk measurements (Hansmann et al. 1972a, b), our failure rate in the detection of growth-retarded fetuses has fallen to 10%. It should be noted that before the introduction of mass screening most patients were not evaluated for fetal growth retardation until the third trimester, at which time the assessment of gestational age introduced a significant error. Today such cases are rare, and generally one can rely on baseline ultrasound examinations made during the first half of the pregnancy for an accurate evaluation of fetal growth. It cannot be stated too strongly how

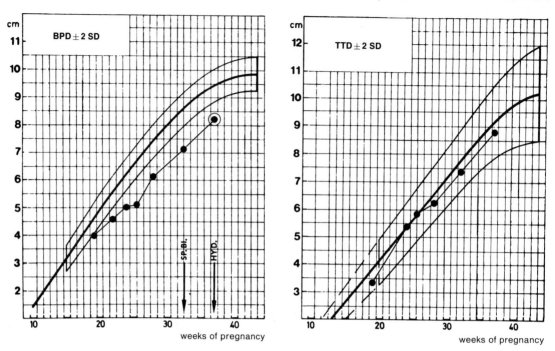

Fig. 7.93. Growth curves (BPD and TTD) for a fetus with spina bifida and hydrocephalus. Despite the development of hydrocephalus internus, we see the low BPD values that are characteristic of neural tube defects

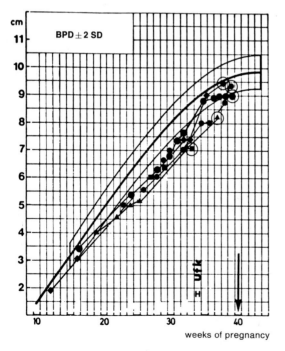

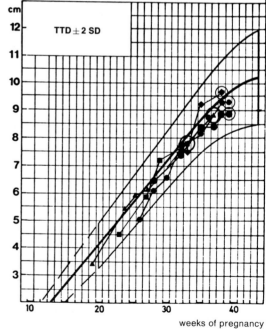

Fig. 7.94. Growth curves of five fetuses with spina bifida. Low BPD values up to 33 weeks led elsewhere to a presumptive diagnosis of intrauterine growth retardation. Normal trunk dimensions tended to refute this suspi- cion. The late catch-up growth results from the develop- ment of hydrocephalus, which is a consistent feature of this defect (cf. text). A correct diagnosis was made in all cases. (From Hansmann 1981)

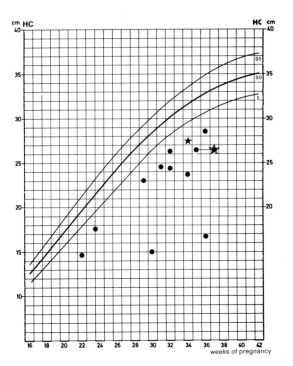

Fig. 7.95. Final HC measurements of 11 microcephalic fetuses that conformed to the definition (HC at 5th percentile with disproportion of brain and face; incidence 1 in 8,000). The Munich infant Jir. is shown by the *black star*, and the only surviving infant from the Bonn series by the *white star*

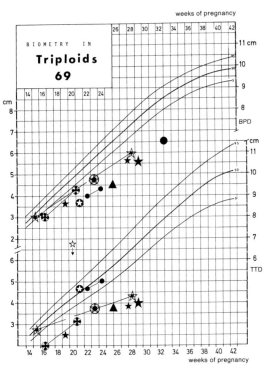

Fig. 7.96. Early and in some cases extreme intrauterine growth retardation in ten cases of triploidy (69 XXX, XXY)

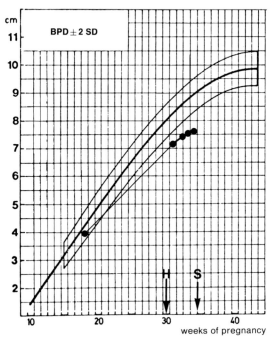

Fig. 7.97. Growth curves of a fetus with trisomy 21. When hospitalized (*H*) at 29 weeks, the mother (of a previous mentally retarded child) refused preterm delivery. NST showed no evidence of fetal distress. With bed

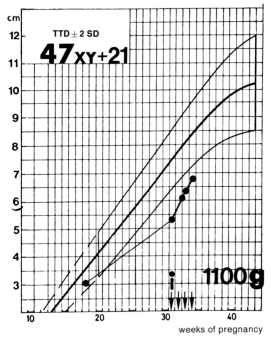

rest and the intraamniotic instillation (*i*) of amino acid solutions, fetal growth rates improved. Unfortunately, karyotyping was not performed prenatally. *S*: Cesarean birth

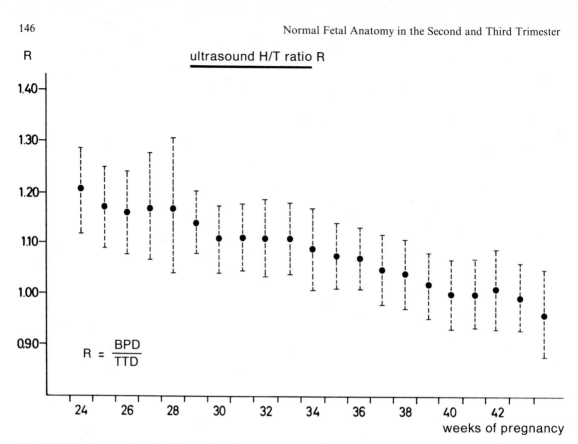

Fig. 7.98. Head-to-trunk ratio (*R*) as a function of gestational age (*n*=1,927; cf. text). (From Hansmann et al. 1973)

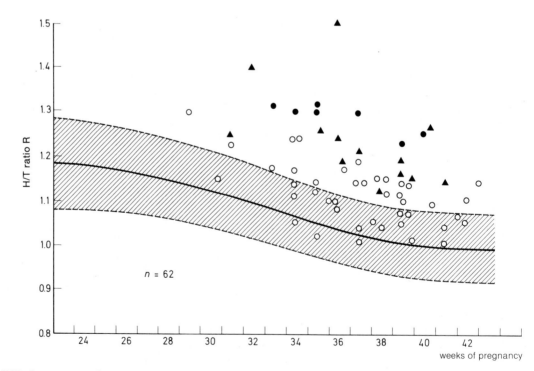

Fig. 7.99. Scattergram of H/T ratios in growth-retarded fetuses (*n*=62), ● perinatal section; ▲ coincidence with malformations; ○ survivals

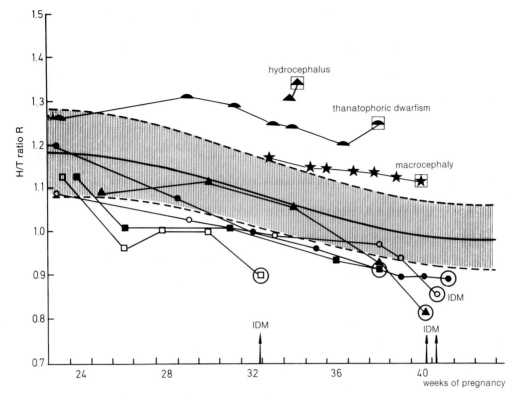

Fig. 7.100. Graphic representation of H/T ratios; The cases from Fig. 7.102 are shown in the *lower half* of the graph, using the same symbols. Three additional cases are shown in the upper half of the graph: 32-year-old G_1P_0: BPD always above 2 SD range from 31 weeks, TTD normal, spontaneous delivery at 39 weeks, female 3,690 g/52 cm, HC 38 cm, BPD 10.7 cm, TTD 9.5 cm, R 1.13, infant mature and healthy. 35-year-old G_2P_0, BPD above 2 SD range from 28 weeks, TTD below average, hydramnios, Cesarean birth at 37 weeks, female 2,810 g/40 cm, diagnosis: *thanatophoric dwarfism*. 36-year-old G_3P_2, BPD 11.2 cm, TTD 8.1 cm, R 1.36, Cesarean birth at 33 weeks, female 2,140 g/45 cm, diagnosis: *hydrocephalus* with multiple anomalies, infant of diabetic mother

much this early documentation of gestational age facilitates the interpretation of "late" ultrasound findings. When the classic one-dimensional parameters of BPD and TTD are used to screen for growth problems, it must be remembered that a small BPD does not necessarily imply a reduced brain volume. Frequently, a small BPD is the result of a dolichocephalic head shape related to the presentation of the fetus (Fig. 7.89) and possibly further aggravated by oligohydramnios. The latter, in turn, is an associated feature of many growth-retarded pregnancies and is almost always present in type 2 growth retardation ("late flattening"), being less common in type 1 "low profile".

A normal amount of amniotic fluid in the presence of type 2 fetal growth retardation is evidence that something more than "simple" growth retardation is involved. A very useful parameter for evaluating the significance of a low BPD reading is the HC. Some modern digital instruments permit the HC and head area to be measured by tracing around the sonographic image with a light pen or joystick. However, it is easier to calculate the HC by using the modified ellipse formula

$$HC = 2.325 \cdot \sqrt{BPD^2 + OFD^2}$$

This calculation requires that both the BPD and the OFD (at approximately the level of the cavum septi pellucidi) be known. We find it convenient to use a chart which shows a digital printout of the formula for various BPD and OFD values (see Appendix). The approximate brain weight can also be calculated by using a formula published by Dobbing and Sands (1978):

$$g = \frac{x^3}{100} - \frac{3,000}{2x},$$

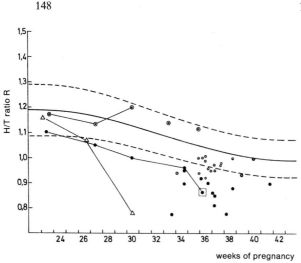

Fig. 7.101. H/T ratios (*R*) in fetuses of diabetic mothers (*n* = 31). Scattergram of last ratios determined prenatally: normal phenotype (*n* = 16), macrosomic phenotype (IDM) (*n* = 11), intrauterine growth retardation (*n* = 3) in the presence of hepatosplenomegaly, tracheoesophageal fistula, and abnormally developed genitalia. (For clarity, only three serial observations are shown)

where *g* is the brain weight in grams and *x* is the HC in centimeters. This formula is valid from 27 weeks gestation through the 2nd year of life (Brandt 1981). It has been shown that from 27 weeks to the 7th postnatal day, the human brain experiences a tremendous growth spurt that is not obvious from the growth curve of the one-dimensional BPD. Thus, for example, the brain weight normally doubles between 31 weeks and term from 183 g (SD 31 g) to 365 g (SD 40 g), but the BPD only increases by about 1 cm during this time, while the HC increases by 5 cm. Clearly, classification of the fetal head as "normal," "large," or "small" is more accurately accomplished by referral to the HC than the BPD, which we feel is suitable only for screening purposes, and even then is frequently misleading (Fig. 7.90). As the data illustrate, a plainly "abnormal" BPD growth curve with relatively low values (7.2 cm at 31 weeks) may represent a molding effect accompanied by moderate growth retardation, or

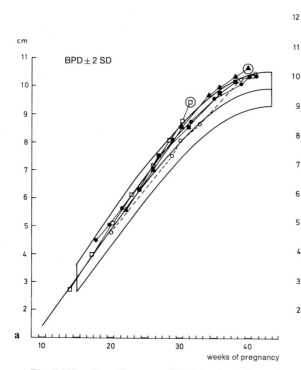

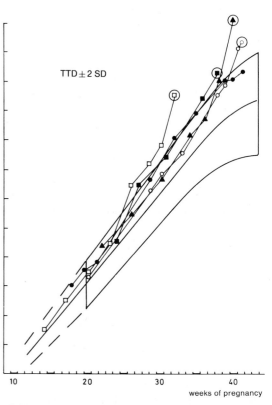

Fig. 7.102. a Growth curves of BPD for five infants classified as large for gestational age at birth. **b** Corresponding growth curves of TTD. 41-year-old G_6P_0; i.v. GTT abnormal; spontaneous delivery at 31 weeks, female

2,400 g/46 cm, macrosomia. 33-year-old G_3P_0; i.v. GTT suspicious; spontaneous delivery at 39 weeks, 4,470 g/ 54 cm, healthy. 34-year-old G_2P_0; i.v. GTT abnormal (cf. Fig. 7.100)

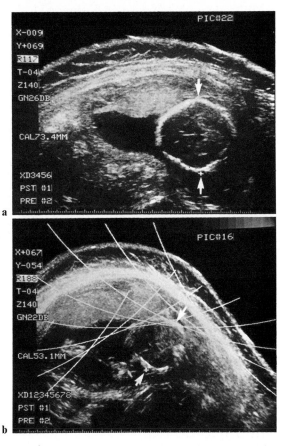

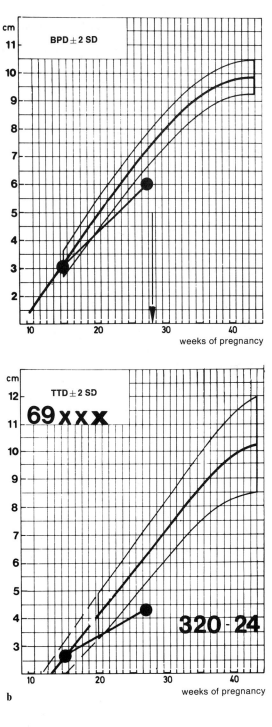

Fig. 7.103a, b. Severe growth retardation at 30 weeks. **a** BPD 7.3 cm, OFD 8.4 cm, HC 26.4 cm ($\hat{=}$ mean for 27 weeks). **b** TTD 5.1 cm, AC 17.5 cm ($\hat{=}$ mean for 23 weeks). The calculated H/T ratio is 1.38 (markedly abnormal); the three-parameter weight estimate is only 650 g

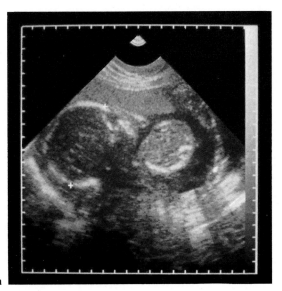

Fig. 7.104. a Extreme growth retardation at 26 weeks with obvious malproportion of head and trunk (H/T ratio = 1.5). **b** Growth curves of the same fetus. This case of triploidy (69 XXX) lacks the oversized, "moth-eaten" placenta that is a common feature of this chromosome abnormality

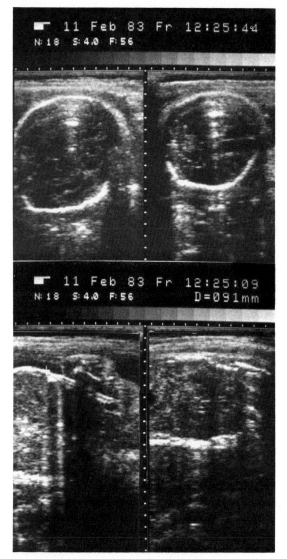

Fig. 7.105. Type 1 intrauterine growth retardation in a twin pregnancy at 35 weeks. Whereas the left twin is normal for gestational age, the right twin shows significant growth retardation affecting head and trunk equally (BPD 7.5 cm, TTD 7.0 cm)

ments is especially problematic in fetuses with neural tube defects (excluding anencephaly). The BPD values in our own series ($n = 20$) generally were below the 2 SD limit before 33 weeks. Accordingly, most were referred with suspected intrauterine growth retardation. In all cases, however, trunk measurements were normal (Fig. 7.93). The "late" catch-up growth of the BPD was the result of a progressive hydrocephalus, which is a consistent feature of these defects (Hansmann 1981). These cases offer convincing evidence that it is not enough to measure the BPD and HC without also evaluating the brain structure (Fig. 7.94). Finally, it should be recalled that "small" premature infants are at increased risk for malformations (Fig. 7.95) and genetic defects. As Ramzin et al. pointed out in 1973, these cases are subject to "early" and in some cases extreme retardation (Figs. 7.96, 7.97; see also Sect. 8.5, Potter's syndrome). Given these facts, it is reasonable to request that every case of a "small" fetus be investigated as intensively as possible before clinical treatment is initiated. We consider this to be one of the main applications of diagnostic ultrasound in clinical management of the future, especially in the case of the very small for gestational age fetus.

The head-to-trunk ratio (H/T ratio) is of particular interest in this context. It is defined as the ratio of the BPD to the TTD (Fig. 7.98) and is a measure of the relationship between the fetal head and trunk, which changes as gestation progresses. The curve of the H/T ratio demonstrates how the growth rates of the head and trunk differ during normal development. While the average daily growth rate of the BPD is 0.46 mm in the second trimester (14–27 weeks) and declines to 0.22 mm in the third trimester (28–42 weeks) (Hansmann 1975), the growth of the TTD maintains a more or less constant rate of 0.43 mm per day during this period. Accordingly, the smaller absolute trunk size in the second trimester catches up to the BPD in the third trimester, producing a final H/T ratio of about 1:1 at or shortly before term. If a disturbance in the growth of the head or trunk occurs during this period, the ratio will increase or decrease according to the nature of the disturbance (Fig. 7.99). For example, an abnormally high H/T ratio can result from an acceleration of head growth leading to absolute macrocephaly. The most striking example of

it may signify true microcephaly with a correspondingly poor prognosis (Fig. 7.91). While both fetuses had the same BPDs, their HCs differed by 4 cm; i.e., a brain volume of 265 g was calculated for the underweight, SGA fetus by the formula of Dobbing and Sands (1978), as opposed to only 153 g for the normal-weight microcephalic fetus. In the case of "Jir." (Fig. 7.92), the HC was again only 27.5 cm. The fetus was estimated to have a brain weight deficit of 43%. The significance of BPD measure-

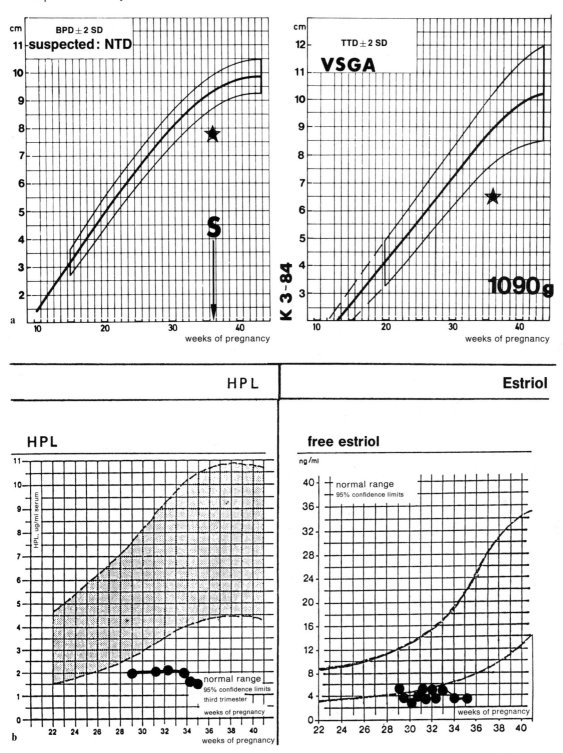

Fig. 7.106. a Asymmetric growth retardation diagnosed at 35 weeks. Sonograms raised the suspicion of lumbar meningocele associated with severe growth retardation; the latter was confirmed on referral, but no evidence of a neural tube defect was found. Fetal weight was estimated at 1,200–1,300 g on the basis of multiple parameters. **b** Pattern of hormonal parameters in the same case. **c** NST following confirmation of growth retardation (basal FHR 150/min, decreased variability, deceleration after every fetal movement and contraction); elective Cesarean birth of 1,090 g/43 cm infant, no complications

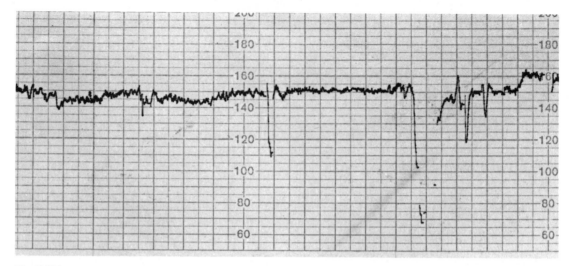

Fig. 7.106c

this is hydrocephalus (Fig. 7.100). In other instances, a high ratio can result from a retardation of trunk growth in the presence of normal head development. In this case the ratio expresses the malproportion resulting from the relative macrocephaly (Fig. 7.99). Conversely, a low ratio may result from an acceleration of trunk growth leading to absolute macrosomia, as in patients with diabetes (Fig. 7.101; Hansmann and Hinckers 1974), or from fetal microcephaly in the presence of normal somatic development (Hansmann et al. 1975). It is clear, then, that abnormally high or low H/T ratios are the result of accelerated growth in one body region or retarded growth in another and thus say nothing by themselves about the absolute size of the fetus.

Of particular clinical interest are the changes in the H/T ratio associated with intrauterine growth retardation. We have found that in the majority of cases the fetal trunk shows evidence of retarded growth earlier and to a more marked degree than the BPD (Hansmann et al. 1972; Hansmann and Voigt 1973; Hansmann et al. 1979; Hansmann and Bellmann 1974; Brandt and Hansmann 1974; Hansmann 1975). Thus, head growth, which reflects brain development, often progresses normally or with minimal disturbance in the growth-retarded fetus, whereas the trunk is almost always affected to a considerable degree. These changes always produce a high H/T ratio which reflects the degree of malproportion associated with the relative macrocephaly and may reach 1.5 or more in extreme cases (cf. Figs. 7.101 and 7.103).

It should be noted that the occurrence of an "early" malproportion does not preclude the presence of an abnormal karyotype. Even in the presence of chromosome defects, a classic type 2 growth retardation can develop as a result of secondary placental insufficiency (Fig. 7.104). Indeed, one must be careful about categorizing growth retardation as type 1 or 2, as a range of "mixed types" can occur, depending on the onset, severity and duration of the growth-retarding stimulus. This particularly applies to twin gestations (Fig. 7.105). In conclusion, we note that the ultrasound diagnosis of fetal growth retardation does not necessarily evaluate fetal well-being. In other words, ultrasound measurements will not identify a fetus that is subacutely or even acutely distressed. In every case of suspected intrauterine growth retardation, the operator is well advised to assess fetal well-being (Fig. 7.106) before scheduling a return visit.

References

Bard H (1970) Intrauterine growth retardation. Clin Obstet Gynecol 13:511

Brandt I, Hansmann M (1974) Postnatal catch-up growth in infants with prenatal ultrasound diagnosis of growth retardation. A combined longitudinal study. 4th European Congress of Perinatal Medicine, Prague

Campbell S (1974) The assessment of fetal development by diagnostic ultrasound. In: Milunsky A (ed) The pregnancy at risk. Saunders, Philadelphia (Clinics in perinatology, vol 1/2, p 507)

Campbell S (1976) Fetal growth. In: Beard RW, Nathanielsz PW (eds) Fetal physiology and medicine. Saunders, London

Campbell S, Dewhurst CJ (1971) Diagnosis of the small-for-dates fetus by serial ultrasonic cephalometry. Lancet II:1002

Campbell S, Wilkin D (1975) Ultrasonic measurement of fetal abdomen circumference in the estimation of fetal weight. Br J Obstet Gynecol 82:689

De Vore G, Hobbins JC (1979) Fetal growth and development: The diagnosis of intrauterine growth retardation. In: Hobbins JC (eds) Diagnostic ultrasound in obstretrics. Churchill Livingstone, New York Edinburgh London

Dobbing I, Sands J (1978) Head circumference, biparietal diameter and brain growth in fetal and postnatal life. Early Hum dev 2:81

Fedrick J, Adelstein P (1978) Factors associated with low birth weight of infants delivered at term. Br J Obstet Gynecol 85:1

Fitzhardinger FM, Steven EM (1972) The small for date infant. II. Neurological and intelectual sequence. Pediatrics 50:50

Frigoletto FD, Rothchild SB (1977) Altered fetal growth: an overview. Clin Obstet Gynecol 20:915

Gallbright RS, Karchmar EJ, Piercy WN, Low JA (1979) The clinical prediction of intrauterine growth redartation. Am J Obstet Gynecol 133:281

Gruenwald P (1963) Chronic fetal distress and placental insufficiency. Biol Neonate 5:215

Hansmann M (1975) Ultraschallkephalo- und Thorakometrie zur Kontrolle des fetalen Wachstums unter besonderer Berücksichtigung der präpartalen Gewichtsschätzung. Habilitationsschrift. Med Fakultät Bonn

Hansmann M (1976) Ultraschallbiometrie im II. und III. Trimester der Schwangerschaft. Gynäkologe 9:733

Hansmann M (1981) Nachweis und Ausschluß fetaler Entwicklungsstörungen mittels Ultraschallscreening und gezielter Untersuchung – ein Mehrstufenkonzept. Ultraschall Med 2:206

Hansmann M, Bellmann O (1974) Kombinierte Ultraschall- und HPL-Verlaufsstudien zur Erfassung der intrauterinen Wachstumsdynamik des Feten. In: Saling E, Dudenhausen JW (eds) Perinatale Medizin, Bd V. Thieme, Stuttgart

Hansmann M, Hinckers HJ (1974) Das große Kind. Gynäkologe 7:81

Hansmann M, Voigt U (1973) Ultrasonic fetal thoracometry: an additional parameter for determing fetal growth. Excerpta Medica. 2nd World Congress on Ultrasonics in Medicine, Rotterdam (Abstr)

Hansmann M, Bäker H, Fabula S, Müller-Scholtes H, Nellen HJ, Voigt U (1972) Biometrische Daten des Feten. Ergebnisse einer modifizierten Methodik der Ultraschalldiagnostik. In: Saling E, Dudenhausen JW (eds) Perinatale Medizin, Bd III. Thieme, Stuttgart, S 136

Hansmann M, Voigt U, Lang N (1973) Ultraschallmeßdaten als Parameter zur Erkennung einer intrauterinen Wachstumsretardierung. Arch Gynecol 214:194

Hofbauer H, Pachaly J, Arabin B (1978) Fetale Ultraschall-Somatometrie. In: Kratochwill A, Reinold E (eds) Ultraschalldiagnostik. Thieme, Stuttgart

Lang N, Bellmann O, Hansmann M, Nocke W, Niesen M (1977) Klinik und Diagnostik der intrauterinen Mangelentwicklung. Fortschr Med 95:482

Low JA, Gallbright RS (1974) Pregnancy characteristics of IUGR. Obstet Gynecol 44:122

Myers RE, Hill DE, Holt AB, Scott RE, Mellits ED, Cheek DB (1971) Fetal growth retardation produced by experimental placental insufficiency in the rhesus monkey. Biol Neonate 18:379

Naeye RL (1965) Lanutrion, probable cause of fetal growth retardation. Arch Pathol 79:284

Naeye RL (1966) Organ and cellular development in mice growing at simulated high altitude. Lab Invest 15:700

Naeye RL, Blanc W, Paul C (1973) Effects of maternal nutrition on the human fetus. Pediatrics 52:494

Ramzin US, Mendt OR, Hinselmann M (1973) Prognostic significance of abnormal ultrasonographic findings during the second trimester of gestation. J Perinat Med 1:60

Rosso P, Winick M (1974) Intrauterine growth retardation. A new systematic approach based on the clinical and biochemical characteristics of this condition. J Perinat Med 2:147

Scott KE, Usher R (1966) Fetal malnutrition: its incidence, causes and effects. Am J Obstet Gynecol 94:951

Vohr BR, Rosenfield AG, Cowett RM, Bernstein J (1979) The preterm small-for-gestational age infant: a two-year followup study. Am J Obstet Gynecol 133:425

Waldimiroff JW, Bloemsma CA, Wallenburg HCS (1978) Ultrasonic assessment of fetal head and body sizes in relation to normal and retarded fetal growth. Am J Obstet Gynecol 131:857

Winick M (1973) Fehlernährung und Nervensystem bei Tieren und Menschen. In: Dudenhausen JM, Saling E (eds) Perinatale Medizin, Bd IV. Thieme, Stuttgart, S 295

7.4 Estimation of Fetal Weight

During the first decade of clinical ultrasound, numerous attempts were made to estimate fetal weight (W) from measurements of the BPD. Most authors used linear regression formulae for this purpose. Willocks et al. (1964) devised the formula $W(oz) = 30 \cdot BPD - 177$. In a series of 152 cases, fetal weight could be estimated to an accuracy of ± 455 g in 66% of cases. Thompson et al. (1965) proposed the formula $W = 1.060\ BPD - 6.575$ with a standard deviation (SD) of ± 484 g. Kratochwil (1968) found a weight deviation of 400 g in 74% of cases using this formula. Kohorn (1967) devised the formula $W = 613 \cdot BPD - 2,569$ and with it achieved a mean deviation of 490 g in 68% of his series of 89 cases. Hellmann et al. (1967) used $W = 7,722.2 \cdot BPD - 3,973.8$ for their estimates and reported a mean error of 346 g. Levi (1970) found a weight deviation of ± 350 g in

90% of cases with the formula $W = (BPD - 60) \cdot 100$. Holländer (1972) published the formula $W = 95.08 \cdot BPD - 5,712$. The SD was 499 g in a series of 290 cases.

This survey shows that initial attempts at fetal weight estimation did not yield significantly better results than those obtained by conventional inspection and palpation (± 500 g in 75% of cases: Loeffler 1967; Ong and Sen 1972; Beazely and Kurjak 1973).

Given the poor degree of accuracy, investigators had to be content with stating the minimum weight for a particular BPD. Willocks et al. (1964) established the rule that a fetus with a BPD of 8.5 cm or more "probably" weighs over 1,816 g, and with 9.0 cm or more, over 2,270 g. The authors went on to say that these figures are "probable in more than 80% of cases." In a much-quoted publication on the same subject, Thompson et al. (1965) stated that when the BPD is 8.5 cm or more, fetal weight is greater than 2,500 g in 91% of cases. If we examine the data on which this statement is based, we find that the study population ($n = 100$) included only 11 fetuses below 2,500 g, and that 9 of these had a BPD greater than 8.5 cm. According to Holländer (1972), fetuses with a BPD over 9.2 cm will have a birth weight greater than 2,500 g in 98.5% of cases (179 out of 182). However, analysis of Holländer's data reveals that fetuses with a BPD in the range of $9.0 - 9.2$ cm still had a birth weight less than 2,500 g in 21.5% of cases (13 out of 60). The report of Schlensker and Decker (1973) seems to be more realistic. In their series of 2,166 newborns, these authors found that the BPD must be at least 9.4 cm before a minimum birth weight of 2,500 g can be predicted with confidence. In addition, a review of the literature indicates that, prior to 1974, no technical method was available for assessing the reliability of weight estimation for infants under 2,500 g or over 4,000 g.

To investigate the situation further, nonlinear regression formulae of sonographic values for the BPD, TTD, and the anteroposterior trunk diameter (APTD) were used (Hansmann 1975):

a) BPD

$$W = 0.933938 \cdot BPD + 0.109007 \cdot BPD^2 + 2.18744$$

b) TTD

$$W = 1.32545 \cdot TTD - 0.0423595 \cdot TTD^2 - 5.52699$$

c) APTD

$$W = 1.35655 \cdot APTD - 0.0432366 \cdot APTD^2 - 5.53386$$

It was found that the mean error of weight estimation of the three parameters was slightly less than ± 300 g with an SD of approximately 250 g and did not vary significantly. This result was already superior to the results of the authors cited above, all of whom used simple linear regression formulae with a higher mean error.

To improve the accuracy of the weight assessment, the number of independent parameters was increased by employing a multivariant statistical analysis (Hansmann and Voigt 1973). With this technique, polynomial approximations of fetal weight by BPD and TTD and by BPD and APTD were performed according to the method of least squares. Finally the effect of this technique on the accuracy of weight assessment was tested in the study population as a whole and in two subgroups of infants with birth weights under 2,500 g and over 4,000 g. A marked reduction of both the mean absolute error and the mean relative (percentage) error was found in all groups when two parameters were used for weight assessment. The accuracy of the weight estimate was best in the group of underweight infants, for whom prenatal weight estimation has the greatest clinical importance. Histograms of the percentage errors, which were plotted in increments of 5% for all groups, showed that the number of cases with large errors ($\pm 20\%$) was also decreased by more than half. The statistical significance of the improvement in accuracy effected by the change from one to two parameters was demonstrated by applying the McNemar test for significance of variance with the Yates continuity correction (Hansmann 1975).

For practical convenience, the formulae for the two-parameter estimations

$$W = -1.05775 \cdot BPD + 0.649145 \cdot TTD + 0.0930707 \cdot BPD^2 - 0.020562 \cdot TTD^2 + 0.515263;$$

$$W = 1.3345 \cdot BPD + 0.798429 \cdot APTD$$
$$+ 0.103458 \cdot BPD^2$$
$$- 0.0254788 \cdot APTD^2 + 1.3547$$

were tabulated in millimeter increments. Their graphic depiction in the form of a nomogram shows that small trunk diameters have a particularly marked effect on weight estimation (Fig. 7.107; see also Appendix). The mean error for the relation of BPD and APTD was ±7.4% (±223 g), and for the relation of BPD and TTD, ±7.9% (±240 g). With regard to reliability, it was found that 75% of the predicted birth weights were within ±10% of actual birth weight.

The effect of further increasing the number of independent parameters on the accuracy of the estimate was also investigated. Although further improvement was obtained, the degree was not sufficient to warrant the additional effort, and we still feel that determination of BPD and TTD is sufficient.

Our results were confirmed by Schlensker and Decker (1973), Boog et al. (1974), and Schillinger et al. (1975).

Based on their studies in 2,363 newborns, Schlensker and Decker first constructed a chart showing minimum and maximum weights as a function of BPD and chest circumference and then tested its validity on the basis of 216 cases using an appropriate correction (the addition of 31 mm to the sonographic chest circumference). They found that when both parameters were used, the mean weight deviation was ±238 g. Deviations greater than 500 g were found in only 6.8% of cases. When only the BPD was used, the mean deviation was ±300 g, and in 17.8% of cases the error was greater than 500 g. When chest circumference was used as the only predictive parameter, the mean deviation was ±285 g (with deviations over 500 g in 15% of cases). These results agreed very closely with our own.

Campbell and Wilkin published a study in 1975 in which abdominal circumference measurements were used to estimate fetal weight in a series of 140 cases. These authors found that 95% of the deviations in all weight ranges did not exceed 15%. Extrapolation of these results to the routine screening of an obstetric population showed that a single measurement between 32 and 38 weeks of pregnancy could

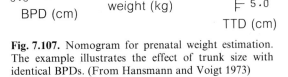

Fig. 7.107. Nomogram for prenatal weight estimation. The example illustrates the effect of trunk size with identical BPDs. (From Hansmann and Voigt 1973)

detect 87% of all fetuses with a weight below the 5th percentile for gestational age. The authors added, however, that this percentage falls to 63% from 37 weeks onward.

Schillinger et al. (1975) showed that measurements of the fetal abdomen provided only a slightly better accuracy of weight estimation than corresponding skull measurements (±423 g for BPD vs ±390 g for TTD). Again, only the combined use of head and abdominal parameters significantly improved the accuracy of the estimate. The best results in this study were obtained when planimetry was used to measure the areas of the skull and abdomen. This provided an accuracy of ±233 g in a small group of 108 normal and abnormal pregnancies, which is still less favorable than the result we achieved using two diameters in a larger population (±223 g with BPD and APTD). Following the basic principle that a simple technique is better than a more complex one as long as the results are the same it is reasonable to conclude that for routine evaluation, the measurement of two diameters is preferable to the more complicated and time-consuming measurement of area and circumference.

Dornan et al. recently (1982) confirmed the usefulness of our nomogram (under optimum conditions, 82% of predicted birth weights were

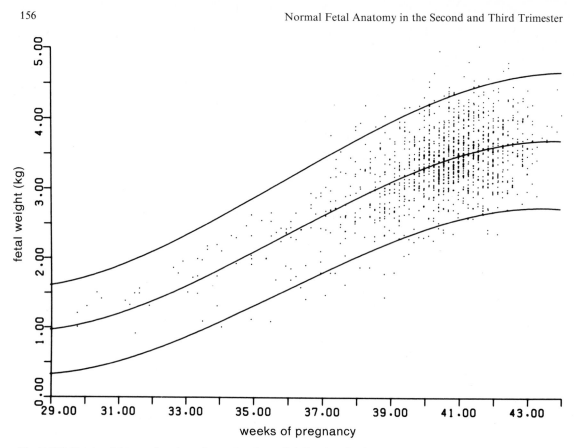

Fig. 7.108. Fetal weight as a function of gestational age (1,240 pairs of values and 3rd degree regression polynomial with 2 SD limits)

within 10% of actual birth weight, with a mean error of ±6% or ±150 g and a correlation coefficient of 0.98). To the authors' surprise, it was also found that prediction was most accurate in fetuses weighing less than 1,500 g. In the cases where measurements were obtainable (85%), the predictions provided useful information for clinical management (74% of estimates were within 10% of actual birth weight, with a mean error of ±7.2% or 165 g, $n = 100$).

Analyzing cases with large errors (±20%) in our study population, we find that growth-retarded fetuses tended to be underestimated at the conclusion of the pregnancy, while AGA premature infants were frequently overestimated. It would appear that gestational age has a positive influence on weight (W) that is not reflected in conventional fetal parameters (Figs. 7.108–7.111). We therefore performed a multiparametric, nonlinear assessment of weight (W) that included gestational age (GA) as a parameter and was based on 1,240 sets of values (Hansmann et al. 1977; Schuhmacher

1979). The regression formula calculated by Schuhmacher is as follows:

$$
\begin{aligned}
W(\text{g}) = \ & -0.001665958 \cdot \text{TTD}^3 + 0.4133629 \cdot \text{TTD}^2 \\
& -0.5580294 \cdot \text{TTD} - 0.01231535 \cdot \text{BPD}^3 \\
& +3.702 \cdot \text{BPD}^2 - 330.1811 \cdot \text{BPD} \\
& -0.4937199 \cdot \text{GA}^3 + 55.958061 \cdot \text{Ga}^2 \\
& -2{,}034.3901 \cdot \text{GA} + 32{,}768.19
\end{aligned}
$$

where

$$45 \leq \text{TTD} \leq 150 \ (\text{mm}),$$
$$66 \leq \text{BPD} \leq 110 \ (\text{mm}),$$
$$30 \leq \text{GA} \leq 44 \ (\text{weeks}).$$

To make it easier for the clinician to use this formula, we have put it in the form of a chart (Fig. 7.112; see also Appendix). A different chart is used for each week of gestation. The accuracy of this estimation is 9% for 68% of all cases and 18% in the 2 SD region. This applies to all weights between 1,000 and 4,500 g. The multiple correlation coefficient is 0.88. Be-

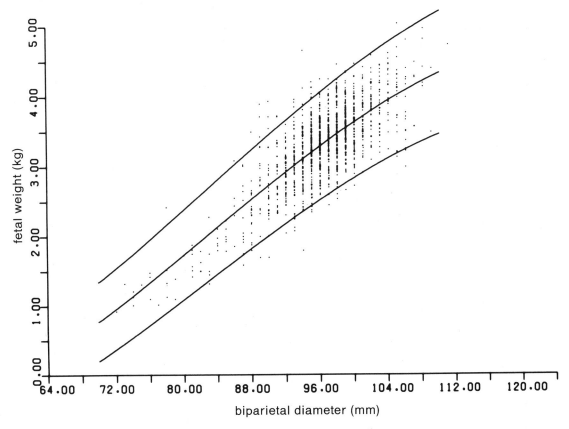

Fig. 7.109. Fetal weight as a function of BPD. (From Hansmann et al. 1978)

cause we usually know the age of a fetus at risk for growth problems with a fairly high degree of accuracy (as a result of early screening), we have been able to test this method. We have found that a knowledge of gestational age has vastly improved the accuracy of weight assessment for premature and growth-retarded infants (Fig. 7.112). The influence of time is illustrated by the following example:

A fetus with a BPD of 8.8 cm and an abdominal diameter of 8.4 cm is estimated at 2,416 g by the two-parameter method. If the fetus is in the 30th week of gestation, a weight of 1,988 g is calculated by the three-parameter formula. But if the fetus is already past term, the formula gives an estimate of 2,582 g. In the former case the fetus is classified as large for gestational age (LGA) and in the latter it is classified as small for gestational age (SGA), although the physical dimensions are identical! In conclusion, it should be noted that even the three-parameter method described above has not proved entirely satisfactory in practice.

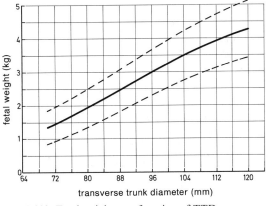

Fig. 7.110. Fetal weight as a function of TTD

Searching for the best method of fetal weight estimation, Bernaschek and Kratochwil (1981) compared the most popular current methods in a series of 123 cases. They concluded that with "normal" fetal development at term, a simple weight estimation from BPD and TTD yields the most accurate results. For LGA in-

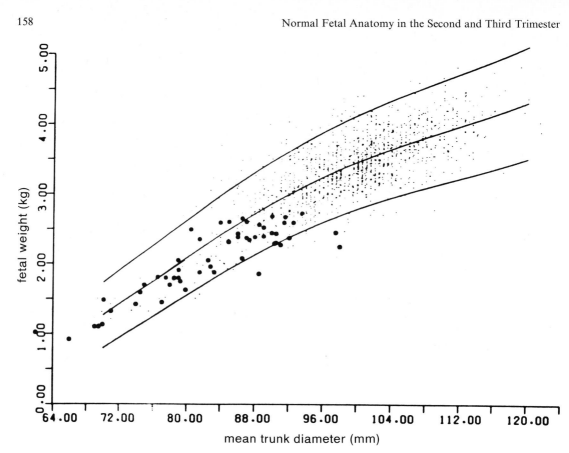

Fig. 7.111. Fetal weight as a function of the mean trunk diameter. Fetuses with intrauterine growth retardation ($n = 54$) are emphasized in the graph

fants, the head circumference and abdominal circumference were found to be more precise. For premature or SGA infants, on the other hand, the method of Campbell and Wilkin (1975), based entirely on the abdominal circumference, gave the most accurate estimate. Unfortunately, our three-parameter estimation was not compared with the other methods.

Eik-Ness (1980) published a weight estimation chart (Fig. 7.111) utilizing the following formula:

$$W = \text{BPD}^{1.856628} \cdot \text{TTD}^{1.34008} \cdot 1.43149 \cdot 10^{-3}$$

where weight is in grams and the BPD and TTD are in millimeters.

In the results of Eik-Ness, the relative error of the estimation was $\pm 12\%$ at weights of 2,000 g or less, and $\pm 7.3\%$ at weights of 2,001 g or more. Holländer (1984), having overestimated the weights of growth-retarded fetuses with our two-parameter method (Hans-

mann 1975, 1976), modified his 1972 formula

$$W = 7.344(\text{BPD}) + 17.525(\text{AC}) - 3,270$$

by replacing the abdominal circumference (AC) with the product $\pi \cdot \text{AC} = \text{AD}$ (mean abdominal diameter). This gave the equation

$$W = 7.344(\text{BPD}) + 55.056(\text{AD}) - 3,270$$

It is apparent that in this equation much more importance is given to the AD than to the BPD. Holländer (1984) obtained a SD of 384.3 g with this formula under clinical conditions. The relative error was no more than $\pm 10\%$ in 82% of estimates and no more than $\pm 20\%$ in 90.7% ($n = 323$). In Holländer's comparison of formulae, the formula of Warsoff et al. (1977) fared about as well as his own. The formula of Schillinger et al. (1975) proved the least accurate. Again, our three-parameter estimation, which we have been using for some years, was not tested. Probably every investigator ultimately seeks to prove that his method

weight estimation for 33 weeks (mean = 33 + 4 days = 235 th postmenstrual day)

BPD→ TTD↘	72*	74*	76*	78:	80:	82.	84.	86	88	90	92	94.	96.	98:	100:	102*	104*	106*	108*	↑
36*	171*	198*	232*	274*	322*	376*	436*	500*	569*	641*	717*	794*	874*	954*	1036*	1117*	1198*	1278*	1356*	36*
38*	217*	244*	279*	320*	369*	423*	482*	547*	615*	688*	763*	841*	920*	1001*	1082*	1164*	1245*	1324*	1402*	38*
40*	265*	292*	327*	368*	417*	471*	531*	595*	664*	736*	811*	889*	968*	1049*	1130*	1212*	1293*	1373*	1451*	40*
42*	315*	342*	377*	418*	467*	521*	580*	645*	713*	786*	861*	939*	1018*	1099*	1180*	1262*	1343*	1422*	1500*	42*
44*	367*	393*	428*	470*	518*	572*	632*	696*	765*	837*	912*	990*	1070*	1150*	1232*	1313*	1394*	1474*	1552*	44*
46*	420*	447*	481*	523*	571*	625*	685*	749*	818*	890*	965*	1043*	1123*	1203*	1285*	1366*	1447*	1527*	1605*	46*
48*	474*	501*	536*	577*	626*	680*	739*	804*	872*	945*	1020*	1098*	1177*	1258*	1339*	1421*	1502*	1581*	1659*	48*
50*	530*	557*	592*	633*	682*	736*	795*	860*	928*	1001*	1076*	1154*	1233*	1314*	1395*	1477*	1558*	1637*	1715*	50*
52*	587*	614*	649*	690*	739*	793*	853*	917*	986*	1058*	1133*	1211*	1290*	1371*	1452*	1534*	1615*	1695*	1773*	52*
54*	646*	673*	707*	749*	797*	851*	911*	975*	1044*	1116*	1192*	1269*	1349*	1429*	1511*	1592*	1673*	1753*	1831*	54*
56*	705*	732*	767*	808*	857*	911*	971*	1035*	1104*	1176*	1251*	1329*	1408*	1489*	1570*	1652*	1733*	1812*	1891*	56*
58*	766*	793*	827*	869*	917*	972*	1031*	1096*	1164*	1236*	1312*	1389*	1469*	1550*	1631*	1712*	1793*	1873*	1951*	58*
60:	828*	854*	889*	931*	979*	1033*	1093*	1157*	1226*	1298*	1373*	1451*	1531*	1611*	1693*	1774*	1855*	1935*	2013*	60:
62:	890*	917*	952*	993:	1042*	1096*	1155*	1220*	1288*	1361*	1436*	1514*	1593*	1674*	1755*	1837*	1918*	1997*	2075*	62:
64*	954*	980*	1015*	1057:	1105:	1159*	1219*	1283*	1352*	1424*	1499*	1577*	1656*	1737*	1819*	1900*	1981*	2061*	2139*	64*
66*	1018*	1044*	1079*	1121:	1169:	1223*	1283*	1347*	1416*	1488*	1563*	1641*	1721*	1801*	1883*	1964*	2045*	2125*	2203*	66*
68*	1082*	1109*	1144*	1185:	1234:	1288*	1348*	1412*	1481*	1553*	1628*	1706*	1785*	1866*	1947*	2029*	2110*	2190*	2268*	68*
70.	1148*	1175*	1209*	1251:	1299:	1353.	1413.	1477.	1546.	1618*	1694*	1771*	1851*	1931*	2013*	2094*	2175*	2255*	2333*	70.
72.	1214*	1241*	1275*	1317:	1365:	1419.	1479.	1543.	1612.	1684*	1759*	1837*	1917*	1997*	2079*	2160*	2241*	2321*	2399*	72.
74.	1280*	1307*	1341*	1383:	1431:	1486.	1545.	1610.	1678.	1751.	1826:	1903*	1983*	2064*	2145*	2227*	2307*	2387*	2465*	74.
76.	1347*	1373*	1408*	1450:	1498:	1552.	1612.	1676.	1745.	1817.	1892:	1970.	2050:	2130*	2212*	2293*	2374*	2454*	2532*	76.
78	1414*	1440*	1475*	1517:	1565:	1619.	1679.	1743	1812	1884.	1959.	2037.	2116:	2197:	2279*	2360*	2441*	2521*	2599*	78
80	1481*	1508*	1542*	1584:	1632.	1686.	1746.	1810	1879	1951	2027.	2104.	2184:	2264:	2346.	2427*	2508*	2588*	2666*	80
82	1548*	1575*	1609*	1651:	1699:	1754.	1813.	1878	1946	2019	2094	2171.	2251.	2332:	2413:	2494*	2575*	2655*	2733*	82
84	1615*	1642*	1677*	1718:	1767:	1821.	1880.	1945	2013	2086	2161	2239.	2318.	2399:	2480:	2562*	2643*	2722*	2800*	84
86	1682*	1709*	1744*	1785:	1834:	1888.	1948.	2012.	2081	2153	2228	2306.	2385.	2466:	2547.	2629*	2710*	2790*	2868*	86
88	1749*	1776*	1811*	1853:	1901:	1955.	2015.	2079.	2148.	2220	2295	2373.	2452.	2533:	2615:	2696*	2777*	2857*	2935*	88
90	1816*	1843*	1878*	1919:	1968:	2022.	2082.	2146.	2215.	2287.	2362	2440.	2519.	2600:	2681:	2763*	2844*	2924*	3002*	90
92	1883*	1910*	1944*	1986:	2034:	2089.	2148.	2213.	2281.	2353.	2429.	2506.	2586.	2667:	2748:	2829*	2910*	2990*	3068*	92
94.	1949*	1976*	2010*	2052:	2101:	2155.	2214.	2279.	2347.	2420.	2495.	2573.	2652.	2733:	2814:	2896*	2977*	3056*	3134*	94.
96.	2015*	2042*	2076*	2118:	2166:	2220.	2280.	2345.	2413.	2485.	2561.	2638.	2718.	2798:	2880:	2961*	3042*	3122*	3200*	96.
98:	2080*	2107*	2141*	2183:	2231:	2286.	2345.	2410.	2478.	2551.	2626.	2703.	2783.	2864:	2945:	3027*	3107*	3187*	3265*	98:
100:	2145*	2172*	2206*	2248:	2296:	2350.	2410.	2474.	2543.	2615.	2690.	2768.	2848.	2928:	3010:	3091*	3172*	3252*	3330*	100:
102:	2209*	2235*	2270*	2312:	2360:	2414.	2474.	2538.	2607.	2679.	2754.	2832.	2912.	2992:	3074:	3155*	3236*	3316*	3394*	102:
104:	2272*	2299*	2333*	2375:	2423:	2477.	2537.	2601.	2670.	2742.	2818.	2895.	2975.	3055:	3137:	3218*	3299*	3379*	3457*	104:
106:	2334*	2361*	2395*	2437:	2485:	2540.	2599.	2664.	2732.	2805.	2880.	2957.	3037.	3118:	3199:	3281*	3361*	3441*	3519*	106:
108:	2395*	2422*	2457*	2498:	2547:	2601.	2661.	2725.	2794.	2866.	2941.	3019.	3098.	3179:	3260:	3342*	3423*	3503*	3581*	108:
110*	2456*	2483*	2517*	2559:	2607:	2661.	2721.	2785.	2854.	2926.	3002.	3079.	3159.	3239:	3321:	3402*	3483*	3563*	3641*	110*
112*	2515*	2542*	2576*	2618:	2666:	2721.	2780.	2845.	2913.	2986.	3061.	3138.	3218.	3299:	3380:	3462*	3542*	3622*	3700*	112*
114*	2573*	2600*	2634*	2676:	2724:	2779.	2838.	2903.	2971.	3044.	3119.	3196.	3276.	3357:	3438:	3520*	3600*	3680*	3758*	114*
116*	2630*	2657*	2691*	2733:	2781:	2836.	2895.	2960.	3028.	3100.	3176.	3253.	3333.	3414:	3495:	3576*	3657*	3737*	3815*	116*
118*	2685*	2712*	2747*	2788:	2837:	2891.	2951.	3015.	3084.	3156.	3231.	3309.	3388.	3469:	3550:	3632*	3713*	3793*	3871*	118*
120*	2740*	2766*	2801*	2843:	2891:	2945.	3005.	3069.	3138.	3210.	3285.	3363.	3442.	3523:	3605:	3686*	3767*	3847*	3925*	120*
122*	2792*	2819*	2853*	2895:	2944:	2998.	3057.	3122.	3190.	3263.	3338.	3416.	3495.	3576:	3657:	3739*	3820*	3809*	3977*	122*
124*	2843*	2870*	2905*	2946:	2995:	3049.	3108.	3173.	3241.	3314.	3389.	3467.	3546.	3627:	3708:	3790*	3871*	3950*	4028*	124*
126*	2893*	2919*	2954*	2996:	3044:	3098.	3158.	3222.	3291.	3363.	3438.	3516.	3595.	3676:	3758:	3839*	3920*	4000*	4078*	126*
128*	2940*	2967*	3002*	3043:	3092:	3146.	3205.	3270.	3338.	3411.	3486.	3564.	3643.	3724:	3805:	3887*	3968*	4047*	4125*	128*
130*	2986*	3013*	3047*	3089:	3137:	3192.	3251.	3316.	3384.	3457.	3532.	3609.	3689.	3770:	3851:	3933*	4013*	4093*	4171*	130*
132*	3030*	3057*	3091*	3133:	3181:	3236.	3295.	3360.	3428.	3500.	3576.	3653.	3733.	3814:	3895:	3976*	4057*	4137*	4215*	132*

explanation of symbols ./:/* = at least one ultrasound parameter outside the 1st/2nd/3rd standard deviation (Schuhmacher 1977)

ultrasound parameters at 33 weeks

normal range percentile	−3STD* 0.13%	−2STD: 2.28%	−1STD. 15.87%	AM 50.00%	1STD. 84.13%	2STD: 97.72%	3STD* 99.87%
biparietal diameter = BPD (mm)	77.5*	81.5:	85.5.	89.5	93.5.	97.5:	101.5*
transverse trunk diameter = TTD (mm)	59.7*	68.0:	76.2.	84.5	92.7.	101.0:	109.2*
head-to-trunk ratio = BPD/TTD	0.8717*	0.9370:	1.0022.	1.0675	1.1328.	1.1980:	1.2633*
fetal weight = W (g)	760*	1180:	1600.	2020	2440.	2860:	3280*

Fig. 7.112. Tabulation of the three-parameter formula for estimating fetal weight. (From Hansmann and Schuhmacher 1977; see also tables in Appendix)

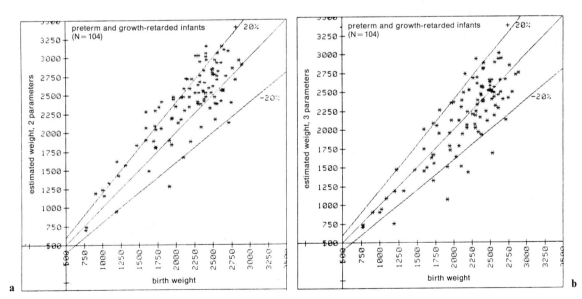

Fig. 7.113. **a** Correlation of the estimated weights of 104 preterm and growth-retarded infants with birth weight for the two-parameter estimation method (Hansmann and Voigt 1973; Hansmann 1975). **b** Correlation of estimated weight with birth weight for the three-parameter method (Hansmann and Schuhmacher 1977; Schuhmacher 1979). The number of overestimates is reduced (same population as in **a**)

is the best. In any event, differences in study populations and methods of data evaluation would seem to preclude a meaningful objective comparison.

We do not wish to describe our method as "unsurpassed," because we know that it does not eliminate the troublesome problem of erroneous estimates in clinical practice. In the future, attention should be focused on weight estimation in the VSGA (very small for gestational age) infant (birth weight $\leq 1,500$ g), whose prognosis depends heavily on accurate assessment. Birth weights over 2,000 g are less critical owing to the progress made in neonatology.

In summary, the following conclusions may be drawn:

1. Ultrasound is the method of choice for the assessment of fetal age and weight.
2. Clinical satisfactory estimates can be obtained only if fetal age and weight are considered separately.
3. Gestational age should be confirmed by ultrasound in the first half of pregnancy.
4. The analysis of growth abnormalities requires "expanded" ultrasound biometry and detailed evaluation of the fetus in serial examinations.
5. A satisfactory weight estimation must include consideration of fetal trunk dimensions. This is particularly important in preterm and growth-retarded infants.

References

Beazley JM, Kurjak A (1973) Prediction of foetal maturity and birthweight by abdominal palpation. Nurs Times, June 14

Bernaschek G, Kratochwil A (1981) Vergleich von Gewichtsschätzungsmethoden aus Kephalo- und Abdominometrie. Geburtshilfe Frauenheilkd 41:114

Boog G, Lierde M van, Schuhmacher JC, Kirstetter L, Gandar R (1974) Céphalométrie et thoracométrie foetales au cours des grossesses pathologiques. Rev Fr Gynécol 69:19

Campbell S, Wilkin D (1975) Ultrasonic measurement of fetal abdomen circumference in the estimation of fetal weight. Br J Obstet Gynaecol 82:689

Dornan KJ, Hansmann M, Redford DHA, Wittmann BK (1982) Fetal weight estimation by real-time ultrasound measurement of biparietal and transverse trunk diameter. Am J Obstet Gynecol 142:652

Eik Nes SH (1980) Ultrasonic assessment of human fetal weight, growth and blood flow. Habilitationsschrift

Eik Nes SH, Gröttum P (1982) Estimation of fetal weight by ultrasound measurement I. Development of a new formula. Acta Obstet Gynecol Scand 61:299

Eik Nes SH, Gröttum P, Andersson NJ (1981) Clinical evaluation of two formulas for ultrasonic estimation of fetal weight. Acta Obstet Gynecol Scand 60:567

Eik Nes SH, Gröttum P, Andersson NJ (1982) Estimation of fetal weight by ultrasound measurement II. Clinical application of a new formula. Acta Obstet Gynecol Scand 61:307

Hansmann M (1975) Ultraschallkephalo- und Thorakometrie zur Kontrolle des fetalen Wachstums unter besonderer Berücksichtigung der praepartalen Gewichtsschätzung. Habilitationsschrift, Med Fakultät Bonn

Hansmann M (1976) Ultraschallbiometrie im II. und III. Trimester der Schwangerschaft. Gynäkologe 9:133

Hansmann M (1982) Thorakoabdominometrie als Grundlage für die Gewichtsschätzung. Swiss Med 4:110

Hansmann M, Voigt U (1973) Ultrasonic fetal thoracometry. An additional parameter for determining fetal growth. (Abstr) Excerpta Medica, 2nd World Congress of Ultrasonics in Medicine, Rotterdam

Hansmann M, Schuhmacher H, Voigt U (1978) Mehrparametrische nicht lineare Gewichtsschätzung mittels Ultraschall unter Berücksichtigung des Gestationsalters. In: A Kratochwil, E Reinold, Ultraschalldiagnostik pp 69. Stuttgart: Georg Thieme Verlag

Hellmann LM, Kobayashi M, Fillisti L, Lavenhar M (1967) Sources for error in sonographic fetal mensuration and estimation of growth. Am J Obstet Gynecol 99:662

Holländer HJ (1972) Die Ultraschalldiagnostik in der Schwangerschaft, 1. Aufl. Urban & Schwarzenberg, München Berlin Wien

Holländer HJ (1984) Die Ultraschalldiagnostik in der Schwangerschaft, 3. Aufl. Urban & Schwarzenberg, München Berlin Wien

Kohorn EI (1967) An evaluation of ultrasonic fetal cephalometry. Am J Obstet Gynecol 97:553

Kratochwil A (1968) Ultraschalldiagnostik in Geburtshilfe und Gynäkologie. Thieme, Stuttgart New York

Levi S (1970) Ultrasonodiagnostic en obstétrique: Intérêt clinique de la mesure du diamètre bipariétal du foetus. Gynécol Ostét (Paris) 69:227

Loeffler FE (1967) Clinical foetal weight prediction. Br J Obstet Gynaecol 74:675

Ong HC, Sen DK (1972) Clinical estimation of fetal weight. Am J Obstet Gynecol 112:877

Schillinger H, Müller R, Kretzschmar M, Wade J (1975) Gewichtsbestimmung des Feten durch Ultraschall. Geburtshilfe Frauenheilkd 35:866

Schlensker KH, Decker I (1973) Voraussagen des kindlichen Geburtsgewichtes aufgrund der Ultraschallkephalometrie und – Thorakometrie am Feten. Geburtshilfe Frauenheilkd 33:859

Schumacher H (1979) Mehrparametrische nichtlineare fetale Gewichtsschätzung aus Ultraschallmeßwerten unter Berücksichtigung des Gestationsalters. Inaugural Dissertation, Med Fakultät Bonn

Thompson HE, Holmes JH, Gottesfeld KR, Taylor ES (1965) Fetal development as determined by ultrasonic pulse echo techniques. Am J Obstet Gynecol 92:44

Warsof SL, Gohari P, Berkowitz RL, Hobbins JC (1977) The estimation of fetal weight by computer-assisted analysis. Am J Obstet Gynecol 128:881

Willocks J, Donald I, Duggan TC, Day N (1964) Foetal cephalometry by ultrasound. Br J Obstet Gynaecol 71:11

7.5 Critical Reading of the Biometry Literature

P. Jeanty and R. Romero

7.5.1 Importance of a Critical Approach

The literature contains many tables and nomograms that describe the normal growth of various fetal parameters, such as the biparietal diameter, abdominal diameters, femur, and orbits. Some of these tables were established with great care, and respect basic mathematical principles. Others, however, were prepared in a less careful manner. Deciding which table to use and knowing its limitations is important in everyday practice. For instance, using a table whose "confidence limits" were graphically drawn, instead of mathematically computed, or worse, a table that does not provide confidence limits, would be difficult to justify should a legal problem arise. The basic principles involved are well established, and the software required for the analysis is currently available for most microcomputers. Finally, the knowledge of just a few basic concepts will permit you to understand the seemingly complicated and esoteric language used in the sonographic literature, and allow you to judge whether a study was performed correctly.

7.5.2 Why Fetal Biometry?

Before the development of ultrasound, fetal dimensions were measured using radiological techniques. The development of ultrasound made it possible to measure the bones and soft tissue structures of the fetus faster and more reliably than with X-rays. Fetal growth is so rapid that parameters such as the fetal biparietal diameter (BPD) and femur length change significantly within 1 to 2 weeks. The use of these measurements answers the following questions:

1. What is the age of the fetus?
2. Is the fetus of appropriate size for its age?
3. Are there any malformations?

Question 1 is crucial in the modern practice of obstetrics, and is one of the most frequent reasons for referral in countries where routine scanning is not the practice.

The evaluation of fetal growth and the detection of intrauterine growth retardation (IUGR) are also major concerns, since the growth retarded fetus is at a higher risk of morbidity and mortality.

Finally, with the decrease of the traditional causes of perinatal mortality, the detection of congenital malformations has become more important.

7.5.3 How Are Normal Values Derived?

The normal values (mean, lower, and upper limits of normal) of a given parameter at different gestational ages are defined by measuring that parameter in fetuses of normal patients with well-established gestational age. Data collection for this purpose can be either cross-sectional or longitudinal. The difference between the two is explained below.

7.5.4 Selection of the Patients

Gestational age is established with certainty if a record of the basal body temperature has been kept for the conceptional cycle or the date of conception is known. Since this information is rarely available, the combination of a regular menstrual history, a well-defined last menstrual period (LMP), and confirmation with early ultrasound is appropriate for purposes of dating the pregnancy. The precision of gestational age assessment of the patients included in the study is crucial for the accuracy of the study. Patients with doubtful dates should not be included in a study of fetal biometry.

Beside having a well-established menstrual history, patients should not have a history of medical, surgical, or obstetrical complications. Although it is obvious, let us emphasize that the infant should be delivered between 38 and 42 weeks with no evidence of growth retardation or congenital anomalies.

7.5.5 Type of Studies: Cross-Sectional or Longitudinal?

Fetal growth can be analyzed by two different kinds of studies: cross-sectional or longitudinal. In a cross-sectional study, many fetuses are examined only once during gestation. In a longitudinal study, a small number of fetuses are investigated serially.

Cross-sectional studies offer some important advantages: 1) they can be performed in a relatively short period of time; 2) the data are easier to collect because the patients are scanned only once; 3) statistical analysis is easier. On the other hand, they have important drawbacks: 1) they fail to characterize *individual* growth (they describe "population" growth); 2) the stability of the statistical analysis that can be performed on cross-sectional data is not always as good as that from longitudinal studies; 3) they are extremely susceptible to inclusion of fetuses with abnormal growth patterns and/or poorly established gestational age; 4) the follow-up of the newborns is complicated by the large number of cases; and 5) because of sampling artifacts, they often misrepresent the extreme values of the curve: the early and late gestation.

A very common error in the literature is failure to respect the principle that each fetus should contribute only one data point to the study. Otherwise, difficult variance assumptions are violated and the accuracy of the confidence limits is questionable. Yet, one can find in many articles statements such as: "150 patients were scanned for a total of 215 examinations."

Longitudinal studies have several advantages: 1) the gestational age has to be defined in fewer patients, 2) age is established only in early pregnancy, 3) abnormal growth curves are easily recognized, 4) the statistical analysis allows stronger curve fitting and computation of velocity curves, etc. Unfortunately, by their very design these studies necessitate that the same fetus be scanned throughout gestation, which considerably increases the time needed to collect the data and calls for a high motivation from the mother. There are many mathematical, biological, and epidemiological arguments to favor results obtained via longitudinal studies.

7.5.6 Sample Size

The optimal sample size depends on the variability of the parameter in question. In fetal biometry, samples of less than 100 cases (for cross-sectional studies) rarely permit polynomial regression to be calculated and are therefore less ideal. On the other hand, samples in excess of 500 are not necessary since the equation is well described and the standard deviation does not decrease significantly with larger samples. It must also be noted that increasing the sample (1,000 or in some case even 2,000 cases) makes it more and more difficult to obtain follow-up data and the probability of including data from abnormal population subgroups increases. It is more critical to have a well-distributed sample with the same number of observations throughout gestation. Should this condition not be fulfilled, there may well be a lack of precision at both ends of the curve.

7.5.7 Study Design

The three questions mentioned above are answered by two types of nomograms. One uses a parameter such as BPD to ascertain the gestational age. The other provides the gestational age, and attempts to determine the size of the BPD. This section will describe the underlying principles used to prepare those tables.

The data collected during a study concerning a certain parameter can be represented in graph form. The size of the parameter (one variable) is plotted on the y (vertical)-axis of the graph, and the gestational age at which this measurement was obtained (the other variable) is represented on the x (horizontal)-axis. The same procedure is repeated for all data that have been collected. The resulting graph is called a scattergram (Fig. 7.114).

The scattergram allows a visual analysis of the data. If all the data are grouped and aligned along a line, the data are said to correlate (Fig. 7.114). If the data are spread all over the graph without clear order (Fig. 7.115), they are said to have poor, or no, correlation.

When data that are correlated are represented in a scattergram, one can obtain an impression of the results of the study. To derive any prediction for clinical use, however, the correlation between the two variables must be described mathematically. The simplest form of mathematical analysis is to produce a series of means and standard deviations for each increment of the parameter for which data have been collected. This is a preliminary step for further analysis, but again, predictions based on this type of report are difficult and sample variability is not taken into account. The procedure that is commonly used consists of fitting a curve to the data.

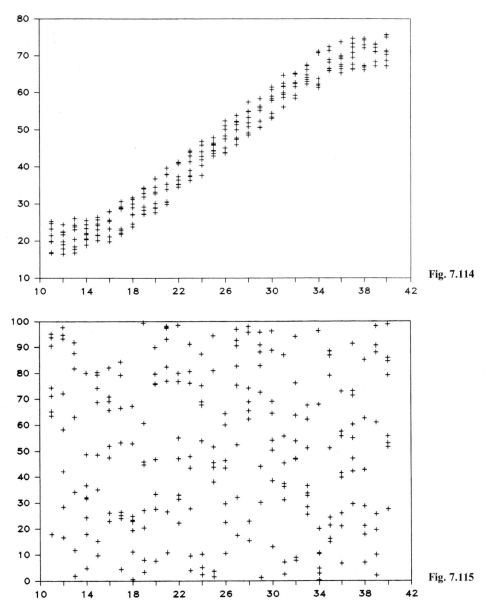

Fig. 7.114

Fig. 7.115

7.5.8 Curve Fitting

A simple technique to summarize the data of the scattergram is to draw a curve that passes through the mean of the data and compute the variability around this curve. Curve fitting is done by regression analysis, which is a statistical tool for evaluating the relationship between two variables. When this relationship is known, it is possible to predict values for one variable from the other (e.g., prediction of gestational age from BPD).

When two variables are used, one is called the independent or observed variable, the other the dependent or predicted variable. The independent variable is represented on the *x*-axis and the dependent variable is represented on the *y*-axis.

7.5.9 What is the Basic Idea of Regression Analysis?

The basic principle of regression analysis is to calculate a curve that best describes the relationship between two variables (hence the term "best curve fit"). Although details of the mathematical calculations are beyond the scope of

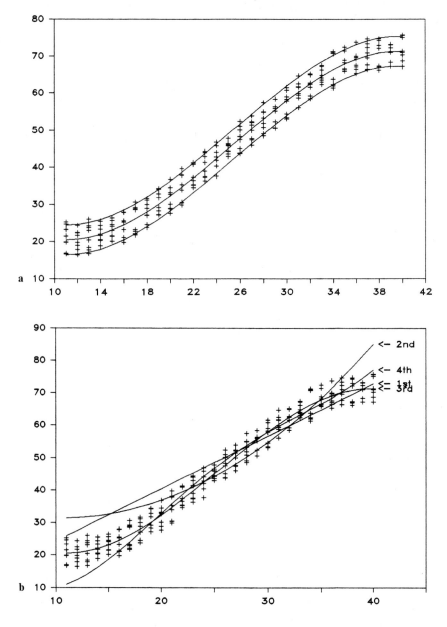

Fig. 7.116

this chapter, it is important to know that the usual procedure to fit a curve is called the "least squares technique". In simple words, a curve is proposed and the vertical distance between each individual data point and the curve is measured (Fig. 7.116). The sum of these distances is then added. Since some data will be above the curve and some below, taking the simple distances would not be sufficient. The sum of the distances from the "data above" would end up cancelling out the sum of the distances from the "data below." This is the reason why the sum of the square of the distances is taken:

by squaring these distances their signs are removed.

Either a straight or a curved line can be used; accordingly, the regression analysis is called linear or curvilinear polynomial (Fig. 7.116).

7.5.10 Linear Regression Analysis

In linear regression analysis, the best straight line that fits the relationship between the two variables is plotted. Since the straight line has a mathematical description, it is possible to use its formula for the prediction of the unknown variable. The formula of the straight line is

$$y = a + xb$$

where a is the value of y at the point of intersection with the x-axis and b is the slope of the line. This curve has one major advantage over all the others: it is so simple to calculate that even some wristwatch calculators can compute a linear regression from a sample of data. Linear regression is appropriate in the following situations: (i) for small samples; (ii) when the variability of the parameter is large; and (iii) when the accuracy of the prediction is not crucial, either because it is a preliminary study or because the variations from normal are considerably larger than the imprecision of the measurement. Conversely, linear regression analysis is not very powerful for accurate prediction because of the tendency to average the raw data.

Although linear regression lines are frequently used in the sonographic literature, most biological phenomena (e.g., fetal growth) are better described by curvilinear equations.

7.5.11 Polynomial Regression Analysis

When the sample is large, (i.e., more than 150 data points obtained over 20 weeks or more), it is possible to fit a curvilinear line that better describes the original evolution of the data. This technique is called polynomial regression analysis.

Polynomial regressions are described by mathematical formulas called polynomial equations, which have different orders according to the highest power to which the independent variable is raised.

For example:

First order: $y = a + bx$
Second order: $y = a + bx + cx^2$
Third order: $y = a + bx + cx^2 + dx^3$

The higher the order of the polynomial equation, the better it describes the data. The limit to such an approach would be to fit a curve that passes through each point. It can be demonstrated mathematically that such a curve would have an order that is equivalent to the number of points of the sample minus one. Obviously, such a high-order equation would make computation impractical and would no longer summarize the data.

In practice, the lowest order polynomial equation that summarizes the data is selected. The selection is made by comparing the coefficients of correlation of the different order polynomial equations for the same data.

7.5.12 The Coefficients of Correlation and of Determination

The quality of the fit of the equation is measured by the coefficient of multiple correlation, R, or by the square of this value: the coefficient of determination R^2. The better the correlation, the closer these coefficients will be to 1. If there is a perfect correlation between the two variables, all the points in the scattergram will be on the regression line. However, this rarely occurs, and it is more likely that some points will be outside the regression line. An R value of 0 indicates that there is no relationship between the two variables. Parameters that correlate very well have some R^2 values in the 0.90–0.99 range. After the second or third order, the curves will usually demonstrate R^2 values which are close to each other. Among the curves with a high R value, the most appropriate one is the curve with the lowest order. To discriminate these curves another test is needed: The F test.

7.5.13 The F Test

With an increase in the order of polynomial equations, the coefficients (b, c, d in the above equations) that multiply the independent variable (x in the above equations) become smaller. At high orders, the power by which the independent variable is raised results in values that become very large (40 weeks raised to the third power is 64,000). To compensate for this, the coefficient must become very small; otherwise the parameter would become immense. The coefficients may become so small that they are no longer different from 0. In this case the term does not add precision to the equation and should be eliminated. The F test is a variant of the T test designed to test the hypothesis that the coefficients (b, c, d, ... n) of the equations are different from zero. This test allows one to ascertain whether going to a higher order equation adds coefficients that are significant without unnecessarily complicating the equation.

7.5.14 Prediction from Equations

The purpose of fetal biometry is to predict information concerning a fetus and then verify how closely that fetus conforms to the predictions. The reference parameter which is represented on the *x*-axis of graphs, or at the extreme left column of nomograms (e.g., the gestational age) is called the *observed value*; and the *y*-axis value is called the *predicted value*. A common mistake consists in using the predicted value to obtain the observed value. For example, the BPD is measured and read from right to left to the gestational age column to obtain the age. This "two-directional" reading is mathematically incorrect. Among other reasons for this, the confidence limits will be expressed in the wrong scale or impossible to find. It appears a bit confusing that when data are collected, the relationship between the observed variable and the predicted variable is different from that between the predicted variable and the observed variable! One tends to assume that if a BPD of 45 mm corresponds to a gestational age of 19 weeks, then for 19 weeks the mean BPD would be 45 mm. You will note, however, in the following tables (Tables 7.2, 7.8) that the prediction is in fact 46 mm. This is due to the sum of squares technique described above. If you look at Fig. 7.117 you will see that the distance from the data to the curve are different when measured horizontally or vertically.

7.5.15 How to Compute the Confidence Limits

Besides being able to describe the mean growth, one must be able to answer the question: How far from the mean can an individual be and still be considered normal? In other words, what is the dispersion around the mean? The statistical parameter that measures this dispersion is the standard deviation. The smaller the standard deviation, the less the variability of the sample around the mean. The standard deviation is also used to define the statistical limits of "normality." These intervals are called confidence limits. Traditionally, the confidence limits are set at the 5th and 95th percentile (+ or − 1.66 standard deviations) or at the 1st and 99th percentiles (+ or − 2.38 standard deviations). Two standard deviations correspond to 95% of the population, 2.5% being below the normal limits, and 2.5% being above. Outside the lowest and highest percentiles, the parameter is considered abnormal. With the common 5th and 95th percentile, it is important to remember that 10 percent of patients tested with this nomsqrom will be outside "normal" limits. This does not mean, however, that the patient is abnormal. The predictive value of a given equation is greater if the standard deviation does not change significantly with variations of the observed value. The absence of variation of the standard deviation can be investigated by the Bartlett or Levene test.

7.5.16 Summary

When selecting an equation for your practice, use one derived from a study based on a large sample of data which covers a wide range of values for the independent variable and adequately represents the extremes of the curve. If there are many equations that fulfill these criteria, select the curve based on longitudinal rather than cross-sectional studies. Be careful to check that the study spans the range of gestational age that you want to cover. For instance, some studies describe the growth of the femur from 12 to 22 weeks: using these studies outside their limits is inaccurate. Finally, do not use the same table both to determine gestational age from a parameter, and to test the normality of this parameter against the gestational age.

The equations that follow (Sects. 7.6, 7.7) are always those of Jeanty and coworkers, except when specified. The rationale for the selection of the curve is expressed in the above conclusions. It is beyond the scope of this work to discuss all the curves that have been published. The guidelines expressed above should help the reader to decide which curves are correct. "Composite" curves which average several excellent curves with less optimal ones should be avoided.

In all nomograms presented, the observed value is listed in the left column and the predicted value in the right columns. A special effort towards standardization has been made. All measurements have been expressed in the same units: millimeters, weeks plus days from the *first* day of the LMP, and grams.

References

(Adapted from: Jeanty P, Romero R (1984) Obstetrical Ultrasound. McGraw-Hill, New York)

Colton T (1974) Statistics in medicine. Little Brown, Boston

Forsythe GE (1957) Generation and use of orthogonal polynomials for data fitting with digital computers. J Soc Indust Appl Math 5:2–17

Goldfarb N (1960) Longitudinal statistical analysis. Free Press, Glencoe, Illinois, pp 31–37

Goldstein H (1979) The design and analysis of longitudinal studies. Academic, New York, pp 1–47

Huff D (1954) How to lie with statistics. Norton, New York

Kleinbaum DG, Kupper LL (1978) Applied regression analysis and other multivariable methods. Duxbury, Boston

Preece MA (1978) Analysis of the human growth curve. In: Barltrop D (ed) Paediatrics and growth. Fellowship of Postgraduate Medicine, London, pp 77–86

Ralston A (1965) A first course in numerical analysis. McGraw-Hill, New York

Riegelman R (1981) Studying a study and testing a test: how to read the medical literature. Little Brown, Boston

Schulsinger F, Mednick SA, Knop J (1981) Longitudinal research. Nijhoff, Boston, pp 3–19

7.6 Estimation of Gestational Age

7.6.1 Definitions

Various estimates of the duration of pregnancy can be used. The conceptual age is calculated from ovulation. The menstrual age is calculated from the first day of the last menstrual period (LMP).

We use the gestational age, which is calculated from theoretical ovulation plus 2 weeks. This has the advantage over menstrual age of eliminating the problems associated with oligomenorrhea and delayed ovulation.

The weeks are always counted a completed weeks, not current weeks. A patient whose LMP started on January 1st will therefore be in her 4th week on February 1st.

7.6.2 Parameters Proposed for Estimation of Gestational Age

In all the tables in this section we have expressed gestational age in weeks and days from the (theoretical) onset of the normal menstrual period. We do not use tenths of weeks to avoid

difficulties in mental conversion into days. We have also expressed all measurements in millimeters instead of centimeters. This is consistent with the international system of units, in which the secondary units are related to the primary unit by ten raised to the power of three (thousand, million, billion, thousandth, micro, pico ...), and in which the use of centimeters is not recommended (Lippert and Lehman 1978).

The parameters that have been proposed to establish gestational age include:

Crown-Rump Length. The CRL (Table 7.1) is the longest demonstrable length of the embryo or fetus, excluding the limbs (Robinson and Fleming 1975). The reason for the high accuracy of the CRL is the excellent correlation between length and age in early pregnancy, when growth is rapid and minimally affected by pathological disorders, and even if differences do occur, they are too small to be detected by ultrasound. Although originally described with static scanners, CRL measurement is much faster and just as reliable when obtained with real time. In a scan that demonstrates a longitudinal section of the fetus, the calipers should be placed at the outer edge of the cephalic pole and the outer edge of the fetal rump. The average of three measurements should be used, and is predictive of menstrual age with an error of 3 days (90% confidence limits) from 7 to 10 weeks.

As growth progresses, however, the curvature of the fetus changes and the linear measurements that can be obtained with the calipers

Table 7.1. Estimation of gestational age (weeks and days) from the CRL (mm)

CRL	Age	CRL	Age	CRL	Age	CRL	Age
5	6+2	18	8+4	31	10+0	44	11+1
6	6+4	19	8+4	32	10+1	45	11+2
7	6+5	20	8+6	33	10+1	46	11+3
8	6+6	21	8+6	34	10+2	47	11+4
9	7+1	22	9+0	35	10+3	48	11+4
10	7+2	23	9+1	36	10+4	49	11+5
11	7+3	24	9+1	37	10+4	50	11+6
12	7+4	25	9+3	38	10+5	51	11+6
13	7+6	26	9+4	39	10+6	52	11+6
14	7+6	27	9+4	40	10+6	53	12+0
15	8+1	28	9+5	41	11+0	54	12+1
16	8+1	29	9+6	42	11+1		
17	8+3	30	9+6	43	11+1		

Table 7.2. Estimation of gestational age from the BPD

BPD (mm)	Percentile					BPD (mm)	Percentile				
	Jeanty			Hadlock	Shepard		Jeanty			Hadlock	Shepard
	5th	50th	95th	50th	50th		5th	50th	95th	50th	50th
10	6+4	9+1	11+6	9+4		54	18+6	21+4	24+1	22+4	20+2
11	6+6	9+4	12+1	9+6		55	19+1	21+6	24+4	22+6	20+5
12	7	9+5	12+3	10+1		56	19+4	22+1	24+6	23+1	21
13	7+2	10	12+5	10+2		57	19+6	22+4	25+1	23+4	21+3
14	7+4	10+2	12+6	10+4		58	20+1	22+6	25+4	23+6	21+5
15	7+6	10+4	13+1	10+6		59	20+4	23+1	25+6	24+1	22+1
16	8+1	10+6	13+3	11+1		60	20+6	23+4	26+1	24+4	22+3
17	8+3	11+1	13+5	11+3		61	21+1	23+6	26+4	25	22+6
18	8+4	11+2	14	11+5		62	21+4	24+1	26+6	25+2	23+1
19	8+6	11+4	14+1	12		63	21+6	24+4	27+1	25+5	23+4
20	9+1	11+6	14+4	12+1		64	22+1	24+6	27+4	26+1	23+6
21	9+3	12+1	14+6	12+4		65	22+4	25+2	27+6	26+3	24+2
22	9+5	12+3	15	12+6		66	22+6	25+4	28+2	26+6	24+4
23	9+6	12+4	15+2	13+1		67	23+2	26	28+4	27+1	25
24	10+1	12+6	15+4	13+2		68	23+5	26+3	29	27+4	25+3
25	10+4	13+1	15+6	13+4		69	24	26+5	29+3	28	25+6
26	10+5	13+3	16+1	13+6		70	24+3	27+1	29+6	28+2	26+1
27	11	13+5	16+3	14+1		71	24+6	27+4	30+1	28+5	26+4
28	11+2	14	16+4	14+4	11+6	72	25+1	27+6	30+4	29+1	26+6
29	11+4	14+1	16+6	14+5	12+1	73	25+4	28+2	30+6	29+4	27+2
30	11+6	14+4	17+1	15	12+4	74	26	28+5	31+2	29+6	27+5
31	12+1	14+6	17+3	15+2	12+6	75	26+3	29+1	31+5	30+3	28+1
32	12+2	15+1	17+5	15+4	13+1	76	26+6	29+4	32+1	30+6	28+3
33	12+4	15+2	18	15+6	13+3	77	27+1	29+6	32+4	31+1	28+6
34	12+6	15+4	18+2	16+1	13+5	78	27+4	30+2	33	31+4	29+1
35	13+1	15+6	18+4	16+4	14+1	79	28	30+5	33+3	32	29+4
36	13+4	16+1	18+6	16+6	14+3	80	28+4	31+1	33+6	32+4	30
37	13+5	16+3	19+1	17+1	14+5	81	28+6	31+4	34+2	32+6	30+3
38	14	16+5	19+3	17+3	15	82	29+2	32	34+5	33+2	30+6
39	14+2	17	19+5	17+5	15+2	83	29+6	32+4	35+1	33+6	31+1
40	14+4	17+2	19+6	18	15+4	84	30+1	32+6	35+4	34+1	31+4
41	14+6	17+4	20+1	18+2	16	85	30+5	33+3	36	34+5	32+1
42	15+1	17+6	20+4	18+4	16+2	86	31+1	33+6	36+4	35+1	32+4
43	15+3	18+1	20+6	18+6	16+4	87	31+4	34+2	37	35+4	32+6
44	15+5	18+3	21+1	19+1	16+6	88	32+1	34+6	37+3	36+1	33+2
45	16	18+5	21+3	19+4	17+2	89	32+4	35+2	37+6	36+4	33+5
46	16+2	19	21+5	19+6	17+4	90	33	35+5	38+3	37	34+1
47	16+4	19+2	22	20+1	17+6	91	33+4	36+1	38+6	37+4	34+4
48	16+6	19+4	22+2	20+4	18+2	92	34	36+5	39+3	38	35
49	17+1	19+6	22+4	20+6	18+4	93	34+4	37+1	39+6	38+4	35+3
50	17+4	20+2	22+6	21+1	18+6	94	35	37+5	40+3	38+6	35+6
51	17+6	20+4	23+1	21+4	19+2	95	35+4	38+2	40+6	39+3	36+2
52	18+1	20+6	23+4	21+6	19+4						
53	18+4	21+1	23+6	22+1	20						

are less accurate, the error increasing to 5 days between 10 and 14 weeks gestation.

Biparietal Diameter. Historically, BPD (Table 7.2) was the first parameter used to assess the gestational age. Its accuracy is maximal between 12 and 20 weeks.

The consensus that has been reached is to measure the BPD at the level of the thalami. Measurement rostral to the thalami (below the cerebral penduncles) may result in underestimation of the BPD and consequently of the gestational age. BPD charts are based on measurement from the outer table of the proximal skull

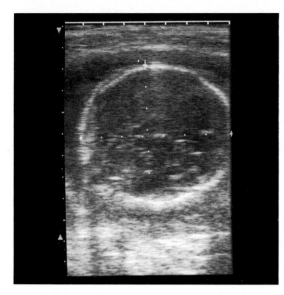

Fig. 7.117. Typical BPD plane: the landmarks are: interhemispheric fissure-septum pellucidum, thalami, insula and smooth symetrical shape. The BPD is obtained from the outer table of the proximal parietal to the inner table of the distal parietal. The occipito-frontal diameter (OFD) is obtained from mid echo to mid echo in the same plane. The cephalic index (CI) is the ratio of the BPD by the OFD

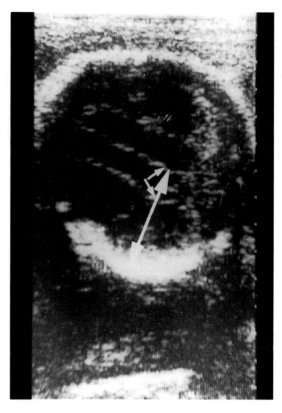

Fig. 7.118. The lateral ventricles appear as two linear echoes roughly parallel to the midline echo. The ventricle width is the distance between the midline to the first echoes of the lateral ventricles. The hemispheric width is the largest distance between the midline and the inner edge of the skull, measured perpendicularly to the midline. Both mearurements are taken on the same line. The binocular distance is measured from the lateral edge of one globe to the lateral edge of the other globe

to the inner table of the distal skull (Fig. 7.117) (Shepard and Filly 1982; Hadlock et al. 1982a), corresponding to the "leading edge to leading edge" measurement of the A-mode technique. Although the plane of largest BPD may vary with the gestational age (and move slightly rostrally), we prefer to use the same landmark throughout the pregnancy, to avoid unnecessary confusion. It is indeed ill-advised to change the plane in late pregnancy, since the reference charts were established with the fixed plane described above.

The fetal head can occasionally be flattened and elongated (dolichocephaly) and the BPD thereby artificially decreased. To check for this, the cephalic index (CI) should be obtained (Fig. 7.118). The CI is the ratio of the BPD divided by occipitofrontal diameter (OFD). (normal range: 0.75–0.85) (Jeanty and Romero 1984). When the CI is close to either end of the confidence limits, the BPD should *not* be used to assess gestational age.

Since shape, growth disturbances and individual variation affect the size of the head to an increasing degree after 20 weeks gestation, the BPD should not be used after this point.

The values derived from Shepard and Filly (1982) and Hadlock et al. (1982a) are included in Table 7.2, as well as those derived from our experience.

Femur Length. Femur length (Table 7.3) was originally measured to diagnose limb dwarfism. It was subsequently observed that femur length was an excellent parameter to determine fetal age (Jeanty et al. 1984a; Hohler and Quetel 1982; Hadlock et al. 1982b). The femur can be measured from 10 weeks onward.

The values derived from Hohler and Quetel (1982) and Hadlock et al. (1982b) are included in Table 7.3, as well as those derived from our experience.

Other Parameters. Femur length, CRL, and BPD are by no means the only parameters use-

Table 7.3. Estimation of gestational age from femur length

Femur length (mm)	Percentile					Femur length (mm)	Percentile				
	Jeanty			Hohler	Hadlock		Jeanty			Hohler	Hadlock
	5th	50th	95th	50th	50th		5th	50th	95th	50th	50th
10	10+3	12+4	14+6	12	12+6	50	24+6	27	29+1	26+4	26+4
11	10+5	12+6	15+1	12+2	13+1	51	25+1	27+3	29+4	27	27
12	11+1	13+2	15+4	12+4	13+3	52	25+4	27+6	30	27+3	27+3
13	11+3	13+4	15+6	12+6	13+4	53	26	28+1	30+3	27+6	27+6
14	11+5	13+6	16+1	13+1	13+6	54	26+3	28+4	30+6	28+2	28+1
15	12	14+1	16+3	13+4	14+1	55	26+6	29+1	31+2	28+5	28+5
16	12+3	14+4	16+6	13+6	14+4	56	27+2	29+4	31+5	29+1	29+1
17	12+5	14+6	17+1	14+1	14+6	57	27+5	29+6	32+1	29+4	29+4
18	13	15+1	17+3	14+4	15+1	58	28+1	30+2	32+4	30+1	30
19	13+3	15+4	17+6	14+6	15+3	59	28+4	30+5	32+6	30+4	30+4
20	13+5	15+6	18+1	15+1	15+5	60	28+6	31+1	33+2	31	30+6
21	14+1	16+2	18+4	15+4	16	61	29+3	31+4	33+6	31+4	31+3
22	14+3	16+4	18+6	15+6	16+2	62	29+6	32	34+1	31+6	31+6
23	14+5	16+6	19+1	16+1	16+4	63	30+1	32+3	34+4	32+3	32+2
24	15+1	17+2	19+4	16+4	16+6	64	30+5	32+6	35+1	32+6	32+6
25	15+3	17+4	19+6	16+6	17+1	65	31+1	33+2	35+4	33+2	33+2
26	15+6	18	20+1	17+1	17+4	66	31+4	33+5	35+6	33+6	33+6
27	16+1	18+2	20+4	17+4	17+6	67	32	34+1	36+3	34+2	34+1
28	16+4	18+5	20+6	17+6	18+1	68	32+3	34+4	36+6	34+6	34+5
29	16+6	19	21+1	18+2	18+4	69	32+6	35	37+1	35+2	35+1
30	17+1	19+3	21+4	18+4	18+6	70	33+2	35+4	37+5	35+6	35+5
31	17+4	19+6	22	19	19+1	71	33+5	35+6	38+1	36+2	36+1
32	17+6	20+1	22+2	19+3	19+4	72	34+1	36+3	38+4	36+6	36+5
33	18+2	20+4	22+5	19+5	19+6	73	34+4	36+6	39	37+2	37+1
34	18+5	20+6	23+1	20+1	20+2	74	35+1	37+2	39+4	37+6	37+5
35	19	21+1	23+3	20+4	20+5	75	35+4	37+5	39+6	38+2	38+2
36	19+3	21+4	23+6	20+6	21	76	36	38+1	40+3	38+6	38+6
37	19+6	22	24+1	21+2	21+3	77	36+3	38+4	40+6	39+2	39+2
38	20+1	22+3	24+4	21+5	21+6	78	36+6	39+1	41+2	39+6	39+6
39	20+4	22+5	24+6	22	22+1	79	37+2	39+4	41+5	40+2	40+3
40	20+6	23+1	25+2	22+3	22+4	80	37+6	40	42+1	40+6	40+6
41	21+2	23+4	25+5	22+6	22+6						
42	21+5	23+6	26+1	23+1	23+2						
43	22+1	24+2	26+4	23+4	23+5						
44	22+4	24+5	26+6	24	24+1						
45	22+6	25	27+1	24+4	24+4						
46	23+1	25+3	27+4	24+6	24+6						
47	23+4	25+6	28	25+2	25+2						
48	24	26+1	28+3	25+5	25+5						
49	24+3	26+4	28+6	26+1	26+1						

ful in estimating gestational age. Among the others that have been proposed are other fetal long bones (Jeanty et al. 1984a), binocular distance (Jeanty et al. 1984b) (Fig. 7.119), head perimeter (Deter et al. 1982; Hadlock et al. 1982c), the abdominal perimeter (Deter et al. 1982), and the size and shape of the fetal ears (Birnholz 1983). The abdominal perimeter has rapidly been abandoned because it is too sensitive to variations of fetal growth.

Among the other long bones, measurement of the humerus is surely the easiest to obtain and the most reproducible (Fig. 7.120). The tibia comes next, and the radius and ulna should be used only when confusing results are obtained from the other methods. In practice, we

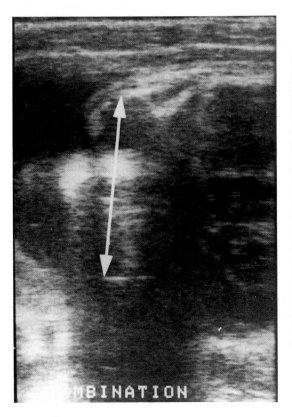

Fig. 7.119

Fig. 7.120. The femur is measured from the proximal portion of the shaft of the femur to its distal portion. The femoral head and the distal epiphysis are not included

average the bone-derived gestational ages and compare them with the BPD-derived gestational age. If the differences is greater than 1 week and 4 days, we prefer to use the bone-derived gestational age. Table 7.4 may be used to determine the gestational age from the long bones of the fetus.

The binocular distance is a recently introduced parameter that has proved useful in our practice. To obtain the right plane, one should start from the conventional section of the BPD and move the transducer caudally until the orbits are visualized (Fig. 7.121). In the correct plane: 1) both eyes should have the same diameter, 2) the largest diameter of the eye should be used, 3) the interocular distance should be the smallest, and 4) the image should be symmetrical. Table 7.5 may be used to derive the gestational age from the binocular distance.

The head perimeter is influenced by growth disorders but to a lesser extent than the BPD. The head perimeter is either measured with electronic calipers or computed using the formula (Jeanty and Romero 1984):

$$\text{head perimeter} = (\text{BPD} + \text{OFD}) \times 1.62$$

A nomogram that allows calculation of gestational age from the head perimeter is provided in Table 7.6.

7.6.3 Selection of Appropriate Table

In view of the large number of different parameters, it is important to know which one to measure and when. Different parameters have different reliability and ease of measurement at different gestational ages. In the list below, the parameters are given in decreasing order of preference. This order is established from reliability, confidence limits, and ease of measure-

Table 7.4. Estimation of gestational age from humerus, tibia, and ulna lengths

Bone length (mm)	Humerus Percentile			Ulna Percentile			Tibia Percentile		
	5th	50th	95th	5th	50th	95th	5th	50th	95th
10	9+6	12+4	15+2	10+1	13+1	16+1	10+4	13+3	16+2
11	10+1	12+6	15+4	10+4	13+4	16+4	10+6	13+5	16+4
12	10+3	13+1	15+6	10+6	13+6	16+6	11+1	14+1	17
13	10+6	13+4	16+1	11+1	14+1	17+2	11+4	14+3	17+2
14	11+1	13+6	16+4	11+4	14+4	17+5	11+6	14+6	17+5
15	11+3	14+1	16+6	11+6	15	18	12+1	15+1	18
16	11+6	14+4	17+2	12+2	15+3	18+3	12+4	15+4	18+3
17	12+1	14+6	17+4	12+5	15+5	18+6	13	15+6	18+6
18	12+4	15+1	18	13+1	16+1	19+1	13+2	16+1	19+1
19	12+6	15+4	18+2	13+4	16+4	19+4	13+5	16+4	19+4
20	13+1	15+6	18+5	13+6	16+6	20	14+1	17	19+6
21	13+4	16+2	19+1	14+2	17+2	20+3	14+4	17+3	20+2
22	13+6	16+5	19+3	14+5	17+5	20+6	14+6	17+6	20+5
23	14+2	17+1	19+6	15+1	18+1	21+1	15+1	18+1	21+1
24	14+5	17+3	20+1	15+4	18+4	21+4	15+4	18+4	21+3
25	15+1	17+6	20+4	16	19	22+1	16	18+6	21+6
26	15+4	18+1	21	16+3	19+3	22+4	16+3	19+2	22+1
27	15+6	18+4	21+3	16+6	19+6	22+6	16+6	19+5	22+4
28	16+2	19	21+6	17+2	20+2	23+3	17+1	20+1	23
29	16+5	19+3	22+1	17+5	20+6	23+6	17+4	20+4	23+4
30	17+1	19+6	22+4	18+1	21+1	24+2	18+1	21	23+6
31	17+4	20+2	23	18+4	21+5	24+6	18+4	21+3	24+2
32	18	20+5	23+4	19+1	22+1	25+1	18+6	21+6	24+5
33	18+3	21+1	23+6	19+4	22+5	25+5	19+2	22+1	25+1
34	18+6	21+4	24+2	20+1	23+1	26+1	19+5	22+4	25+4
35	19+2	22	24+6	20+4	23+4	26+5	20+1	23+1	26
36	19+5	22+4	25+1	21+1	24+1	27+1	20+4	23+4	26+3
37	20+1	22+6	25+5	21+4	24+4	27+5	21	23+6	26+6
38	20+4	23+3	26+1	22+1	25+1	28+1	21+4	24+3	27+2
39	21+1	23+6	26+4	22+4	25+4	28+5	21+6	24+6	27+5
40	21+4	24+2	27+1	23+1	26+1	29+1	22+3	25+2	28+1
41	22	24+6	27+4	23+4	26+5	29+5	22+6	25+5	28+4
42	22+4	25+2	28	24+1	27+1	30+2	23+2	26+1	29+1
43	23	25+5	28+4	24+5	27+5	30+6	23+5	26+4	29+4
44	23+4	26+1	29	25+1	28+2	31+2	24+1	27+1	30
45	24	26+5	29+4	25+6	28+6	31+6	24+4	27+4	30+4
46	24+4	27+1	30	26+2	29+3	32+3	25+1	28	30+6
47	25	27+5	30+4	26+6	29+6	33	25+4	28+4	31+3
48	25+4	28+1	31	27+3	30+4	33+4	26+1	29	31+6
49	26	28+6	31+4	28	31+1	34+1	26+4	29+3	32+2
50	26+4	29+2	32	28+4	31+4	34+5	27	29+6	32+6
51	27+1	29+6	32+4	29+1	32+1	35+2	27+4	30+3	33+2
52	27+4	30+2	33+1	29+5	32+6	35+6	28	30+6	33+6
53	28+1	30+6	33+4	30+2	33+3	36+3	28+4	31+3	34+2
54	28+5	31+3	34+1	30+6	34	37	29	31+6	34+6
55	29+1	32	34+5	31+4	34+4	37+5	29+4	32+3	35+2
56	29+6	32+4	35+2	32+1	35+1	38+2	30	32+6	35+6
57	30+2	33+1	35+6	32+6	35+6	38+6	30+4	33+3	36+2
58	30+6	33+4	36+3	33+3	36+3	39+4	31	33+6	36+6
59	31+3	34+1	36+6	34	37+1	40+1	31+4	34+3	37+2
60	32	34+6	37+4	34+4	37+5	40+6	32	34+6	37+6
61	32+4	35+2	38+1	35+2	38+2	41+3	32+4	35+3	38+2
62	33+1	35+6	38+5	35+6	39	42	33	35+6	38+6
63	33+6	36+4	39+2	36+4	39+4	42+5	33+4	36+4	39+3
64	34+3	37+1	39+6	37+1	40+2	43+2	34+1	37	39+6
65	35	37+5	40+4				34+4	37+4	40+3
66	35+4	38+2	41+1				35+1	38	41
67	36+1	38+6	41+5				35+5	38+4	41+4
68	36+6	39+4	42+2				36+1	39+1	42
69	37+3	40+1	42+6				36+6	39+5	42+4

Fig. 7.121. Both eyes should have the same diameter, the largest diameter of the eye should be used, and the image should be symmetrical. The binocular distance is measured from the lateral edge of one globe to the lateral edge of the other globe. The inter ocular distance is measured between the two eyes, and the ocular diameter is obtained along a transverse diameter in the same plane. All three measurements are obtained in the same plane

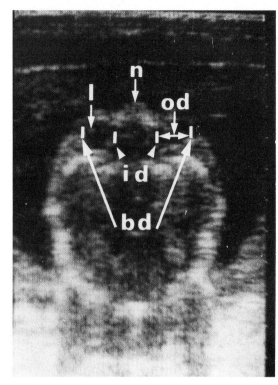

ment. It should not be regarded as definitive, and can be adapted to the particular circumstances.

From 7 to 10 weeks:
    CRL (Table 7.1)
From 10 to 14 weeks:
    CRL (Table 7.1)
    BPD (Table 7.2)
    femur length (Table 7.3)
    humerus length (Table 7.4)
From 15 to 28 weeks:
    BPD (Table 7.2)
    femur length (Table 7.3)
    humerus length (Table 7.4)

Table 7.5. Estimation of gestational age from binocular distance

Binocular distance (mm)	Percentile			Binocular distance (mm)	Percentile		
	5th	50th	95th		5th	50th	95th
15	7+1	10+3	13+6	40	22+0	25+2	28+4
16	7+5	11+0	14+3	41	22+4	25+6	29+1
17	8+2	11+4	15+0	42	23+1	26+4	29+6
18	8+6	12+1	15+4	43	23+6	27+1	30+3
19	9+4	12+6	16+1	44	24+3	27+5	31+0
				45	25+0	28+2	31+4
20	10+1	13+3	16+5	46	25+4	28+6	32+1
21	10+5	14+0	17+2	47	26+1	29+4	32+6
22	11+2	14+4	17+6	48	26+6	30+1	33+3
23	11+6	15+1	18+4	49	27+2	30+5	34+0
24	12+4	15+6	19+1				
25	13+1	16+3	19+5	50	27+6	31+2	34+4
26	13+5	17+0	20+2	51	28+4	31+6	35+1
27	14+2	17+4	20+6	52	29+1	32+4	35+6
28	14+6	18+1	21+4	53	29+5	33+0	36+3
29	15+4	18+6	22+1	54	30+2	33+4	37+0
				55	30+6	34+1	37+4
30	16+1	19+3	22+5	56	31+4	34+6	38+1
31	16+4	20+0	23+2	57	32+1	35+3	38+5
32	17+1	20+4	23+6	58	32+5	36+0	39+2
33	17+6	21+1	24+4	59	33+2	36+4	39+6
34	18+3	21+5	25+1				
35	19+0	22+2	25+5	60	33+6	37+1	40+4
36	19+4	22+6	26+2	61	34+4	37+6	41+1
37	20+1	23+4	26+6	62	35+1	38+3	41+5
38	20+6	24+1	27+3	63	35+5	30+0	42+2
39	21+3	24+5	28+0	64	36+2	39+4	42+6
				65	36+6	40+1	43+4

Table 7.6. Estimation of gestational age from head perimeter

Head perimeter (mm)	Percentile 10th	Percentile 50th	Percentile 90th	Head perimeter (mm)	Percentile 10th	Percentile 50th	Percentile 90th
80	11+3	13+2	15+2	220	21+6	23+6	25+6
85	11+5	13+5	15+4	225	22+3	24+3	26+2
90	12	14	15+6	230	22+6	24+6	26+6
95	12+2	14+2	16+2	235	23+3	25+3	27+2
100	12+4	14+4	16+4	240	23+6	25+6	27+6
105	13	14+6	16+6	245	24+3	26+3	28+2
110	13+2	15+2	17+1	250	25	26+6	28+6
115	13+4	15+4	17+4	255	25+4	27+3	29+3
120	13+6	15+6	17+6	260	26+0	28+0	30
125	14+2	16+2	18+1	265	26+4	28+4	30+4
130	14+4	16+4	18+4	270	27+1	29+1	31+1
135	15	16+6	18+6	275	27+6	29+5	31+5
140	15+2	17+2	19+2	280	28+3	30+2	32+2
145	15+5	17+4	19+4	285	29	31	32+6
150	16+0	18	20	290	29+4	31+4	33+4
155	16+3	18+3	20+2	295	30+2	32+1	34+1
160	16+6	18+5	20+5	300	30+6	32+6	34+6
165	17+1	19+1	21+1	305	31+4	33+4	35+3
170	17+4	19+4	21+3	310	32+2	34+1	36+1
175	18	19+6	21+6	315	32+6	34+6	36+6
180	18+3	20+2	22+2	320	33+4	35+4	37+4
185	18+6	20+5	22+5	325	34+2	36+2	38+2
190	19+1	21+1	23+1	330	35+0	37+0	39
195	19+4	21+4	23+4	335	35+6	37+5	39+5
200	20+1	22+0	24	340	36+4	38+4	40+3
205	20+4	22+3	24+3	345	37+2	39+2	41+2
210	21	23	24+6	350	38+1	40+0	42+0
215	21+3	23+3	25+3	355	38+6	40+6	42+6
220	21+6	23+6	25+6	360	39+5	41+5	43+4

head perimeter (Table 7.6)
binocular distance (Table 7.5)
other long bone lengths (Table 7.4)
After 28 weeks (inaccurate for dating):
  femur length (Table 7.3)
  humerus length (Table 7.4)
  binocular distance (Table 7.5)
  BPD (Table 7.2; check that the BPD is correct by evaluating the CI)
  other long bone lengths (Table 7.4)
  head perimeter (Table 7.6)

7.6.4 What to do when Different Parameters Provide Different Estimates

The general rule is that the earlier the estimation of the age, the more accurate it is. If estimation of the fetal age has been made at 15 weeks and a control scan at 27 weeks yields a different estimate, do not change the original estimate: it is more accurate. We consider that ages are equivalent when they are within 1 week and 4 days of each other (this is an arbitrary limit). Before 20 weeks, we only remeasure parameters when the difference exceeds 1 week.

During a given examination, when two similar parameters agree (e.g., two different bones) you can average the gestational age derived from them. When a few parameters provide estimates that are in the same range and only one is discordant, recheck the last one. If it is still abnormal, do not include it in the final estimate.

7.6.5 How to Report the Results

We are strongly in favor of reporting the lower 5th and the upper 95th confidence limits on the prediction for each measurement. This is especially important in late gestation, and may have legal implications.

7.6.6 The Use of Computers for the Reporting of Obstetrical Examinations

As any one knows who has reported a number of examinations, referring to charts is a tedious process. With the explosion of microcomputer systems, it was inevitable that the microcomputer would eventually be used to report ultrasound examinations. We have developed a low-cost reporting system (Jeanty 1985). It runs on an IBM PC, XT, or AT or 100% compatible computer, equipped with 384 K of RAM, and Lotus 1–2–3. This is a "user-supported" software, and a copy can be obtained from the author.

References

Birnholz J cited In: Ear scans reveal gestational age of abnormal fetuses. Diagn Imaging, Sept 1983, p 15

Deter RL, Harrist RB, Hadlock FP et al. (1982) Fetal head and abdominal circumferences. 2. A critical reevaluation of the relationship to menstrual age. J Clin Ultrasound 10:365–372

Hadlock FP, Deter RL, Harrist RB et al. (1982a) Fetal biparietal diameter: a critical reevaluation of the relation to menstrual age by means of realtime ultrasound. J Ultrasound Med 1:97–104

Hadlock FP, Harrist RB, Deter RL et al. (1982b) Fetal femur length as a predictor of menstrual age: sonographically measured. AJR 138:875

Hadlock FP, Deter RL, Harrist RB (1982c) Fetal head circumference: relation to menstrual age. AJR 138:649–653

Hohler CW, Quetel TA (1982) Fetal femur length: equations for computer calculation of gestational age from ultrasound measurements. Am J Obstet Gynecol 143:479–481

Jeanty P, Romero R (1984) Obstetrical ultrasound. McGraw-Hill, New York

Jeanty P, Rodesch F, Delbeke D (1984a) Estimation of fetal age by long bone measurements. J Ultrasound Med 3:75–79

Jeanty P, Cantraine F, Cousaert E et al. (1984b) The binocular distance: a new parameter to estimate fetal age. J Ultrasound 3:241–244

Jeanty P (1985) A simple reporting system for obstetrical ultrasound examination. J Ultrasound Med (in press)

Lippert H, Lehman HP (1978) SI units in medicine. An introduction to the international system of units with conversion tables and normal ranges. Urban & Schwarzenberg, Baltimore

Robinson HP, Fleming JEE (1975) A critical evaluation of sonar crown-rump length measurements. Br J Obstet Gynaecol 82:702–710

Shepard M, Filly RA (1982) A standardized plane for biparietal diameter measurement. J Ultrasound Med 1:145–150

7.7 Normal Growth of Fetal Parameters

This section will describe the normal values obtained for various fetal parameters. Since the techniques of measurement have already been exhaustively described, only a brief reminder of the preferred techniques will be included here.

7.7.1 Crown-Rump Length

Table 7.7. Normal mean CRL (mm) at each gestational age (weeks + days)

Age	CRL	Age	CRL	Age	CRL
6+0	4	8+0	15	10+0	31
6+1	5	8+1	16	10+1	32
6+2	6	8+2	17	10+2	33
6+3	6	8+3	18	10+3	35
6+4	7	8+4	19	10+4	36
6+5	8	8+5	20	10+5	38
6+6	8	8+6	21	10+6	39
7+0	9	9+0	22	11+0	40
7+1	10	9+1	23	11+1	41
7+2	10	9+2	24	11+2	43
7+3	11	9+3	26	11+3	44
7+4	12	9+4	27	11+4	46
7+5	13	9+5	28	11+5	47
7+6	14	9+6	29	11+6	49

7.7.2 Cranial Parameters

Biparietal Diameter

Although the BPD (Table 7.8) can be obtained in an infinity of planes, the most frequently used are the transverse and the coronal planes. The transverse plane is used when the head is in an occipitotransverse position, and the coronal sections when the head is in an occipitoanterior or occipitoposterior position. Transverse sections are preferred because they rely on the axial resolution of the ultrasound beam and because the appropriate plane can be identified by reference to the intracranial anatomy. Coronal sections, on the other hand, use lateral resolution and the intracranial anatomy is more difficult to display.

The plane of section for the BPD should meet the following criteria: (1) the section should be perpendicular to the midline; (2) the image should be recorded at medium/low gain to avoid artifactual thickness of the skull tables; (3) the image should be symmetrical, e.g., the distance between the midline and the skull tables should be the same on both sides; (4) the head shape should be ovoid (this can be verified with the cephalic index: if the cephalic index is greater than 85 or less than 75, do not use the BPD); (5) in the correct plane, the thalamus or the cerebral penduncles, the cavum septi pellucidi, part of the interhemispheric fissure, and the insula with the middle cerebral artery can be observed. The measurement is obtained from the outer edge of the proximal skull table to the inner edge of the distal skull table. The calipers are placed perpendicular to the midline echo.

Occipitofrontal Diameter. The OFD (Table 7.8) is measured in the BPD plane described above. These landmarks ensure that the longest anteroposterior cranial dimension is being measured. The measurement is obtained from mid-echo to mid-echo to render the measurement independent from variations due to increase in the TGC curve. The investigators that use outer-to-outer measurements have to adjust the TGC settings so that they are exactly the same from one patient to the other, otherwise the echoes could be larger and the OFD increased.

Head Perimeter. See Table 7.8.

Ocular Biometry. See Table 7.9.

Lateral Ventricle and Hemispheric Width. The lateral ventricles are measured in a section parallel to the BPD plane, although more cephalic. In such a section, the lateral ventricles appear as two linear echoes roughly parallel to the midline echo. The ventricle width is the distance between the midline and the first echoes of the lateral ventricles. The measurement is therefore slightly greater than the actual lateral ventricle. The hemispheric width is the largest distance between the midline and the inner edge of the skull, measured perpendicularly to the midline. Both measurements are taken on the same line. To avoid tilting errors, the lateral ventricles and the hemispheric width should be of the same size on each side. Frequently, the proximal hemisphere is obscured by artifactual echoes so that only the distal ratio can be obtained (Table 7.10).

Nomograms:

Table 7.8. Cranial parameters

Week	Biparietal diameter (mm)			Occipitofrontal diameter (mm)			Head perimeter (mm)		
	Percentile			Percentile			Percentile		
	5th	50th	95th	5th	50th	95th	5th	50th	95th
10	9	14	18	7	14	21	26	50	74
11	13	17	22	11	18	25	38	63	87
12	16	21	25	16	23	30	51	75	100
13	20	24	29	20	27	34	64	88	112
14	23	28	32	24	31	38	76	101	125
15	27	31	36	29	36	43	89	113	138
16	30	35	39	33	40	47	101	126	150
17	34	38	43	37	44	51	114	138	163
18	37	42	46	41	48	55	126	151	175
19	40	45	49	46	53	60	138	163	187
20	44	48	53	50	57	64	150	175	199
21	47	51	56	54	61	68	162	187	211
22	50	55	59	58	65	72	174	198	223
23	53	58	62	62	69	76	185	210	234
24	56	61	65	65	72	79	196	221	245
25	59	64	68	69	76	83	207	232	256
26	62	67	71	73	80	87	218	242	266
27	65	70	74	76	83	90	228	252	277
28	68	72	77	80	87	94	238	262	286
29	70	75	79	83	90	97	247	271	296

Table 7.8. Cranial parameters (continued)

Week	Biparietal diameter (mm)			Occipitofrontal diameter (mm)			Head perimeter (mm)		
	Percentile			Percentile			Percentile		
	5th	50th	95th	5th	50th	95th	5th	50th	95th
30	73	77	82	86	93	100	256	281	305
31	75	79	84	89	96	103	265	289	313
32	77	82	86	92	99	106	273	297	322
33	79	84	88	95	102	108	281	305	329
34	81	86	90	97	104	111	288	312	336
35	83	87	92	99	106	113	294	319	343
36	84	89	93	102	109	116	300	325	349
37	86	90	95	104	111	118	306	330	355
38	87	91	96	105	112	119	311	335	359
39	88	93	97	107	114	121	315	339	364
40	89	93	98	108	115	122	319	343	367

Table 7.9. Ocular biometry

Week	Ocular diameter (mm)			Binocular distance (mm)			Interocular distance (mm)		
	Percentile			Percentile			Percentile		
	5th	50th	95th	5th	50th	95th	5th	50th	95th
12	2	4	6	11	16	20	4	8	11
13	3	5	6	14	18	23	5	8	11
14	4	5	7	16	20	25	6	9	12
15	4	6	8	18	23	27	6	10	13
16	5	7	9	20	25	29	7	10	13
17	6	8	10	22	27	31	8	11	14
18	7	9	10	24	29	33	8	11	15
19	8	9	11	26	31	35	9	12	15
20	8	10	12	28	33	37	10	13	16
21	9	11	13	30	35	39	10	13	16
22	10	11	13	32	36	41	11	14	17
23	10	12	14	34	38	43	11	14	17
24	11	13	15	35	40	44	12	15	18
25	12	13	15	37	42	46	12	15	19
26	12	14	16	39	43	47	13	16	19
27	13	15	16	40	45	49	13	16	19
28	13	15	17	42	46	51	14	17	20
29	14	16	17	43	48	52	14	17	20
30	14	16	18	45	49	53	15	18	21
31	15	17	18	46	50	55	15	18	21
32	15	17	19	47	52	56	15	19	22
33	16	17	19	49	53	57	16	19	22
34	16	18	20	50	54	58	16	19	22
35	16	18	20	51	55	60	16	20	23
36	17	19	20	52	56	61	17	20	23
37	17	19	21	53	57	62	17	20	23
38	17	19	21	54	58	63	17	21	24
39	18	20	21	55	59	64	18	21	24
40	18	20	22	56	60	64	18	21	24

Table 7.10. The lateral ventricle: hemispheric width ratio

Week	Percentile			Week	Percentile		
	10th	50th	90th		10th	50th	90th
12	77	85	94	27	26	31	37
13	69	78	86	28	25	31	37
14	62	71	79	29	25	31	36
15	54	64	74	30	25	31	36
16	47	59	70	31	25	31	36
17	42	54	65	32	25	31	36
18	38	49	61	33	25	31	37
19	35	46	56	34	25	31	37
20	32	42	52	35	25	31	36
21	29	40	51	36	26	31	36
22	26	37	49	37	26	31	36
23	26	36	45	38	25	30	35
24	26	34	42	39	25	30	35
25	27	33	39	40	24	29	34
26	27	32	37				

Table 7.11. Cardiac diameters (mm)

Week	Transverse			Longitudinal		
	Percentile			Percentile		
	5th	50th	95th	5th	50th	95th
12	4	5	6	5	6	7
13	5	6	7	6	7	9
14	6	7	8	8	9	10
15	7	8	10	9	10	12
16	8	10	11	10	12	14
17	9	11	13	12	14	16
18	10	12	15	13	15	18
19	11	14	16	14	17	20
20	13	15	18	16	19	22
21	14	17	20	18	21	24
22	15	18	21	19	23	26
23	16	20	23	21	24	28
24	18	21	25	22	26	30
25	19	23	27	24	28	32
26	20	24	28	25	30	34
27	22	26	30	27	32	36
28	23	27	32	28	33	38
29	24	29	34	30	35	40
30	25	30	35	31	37	42
31	26	32	37	32	38	44
32	28	33	38	33	40	46
33	29	34	40	34	41	47
34	30	35	41	35	42	49
35	30	37	43	36	43	50
36	31	38	44	37	44	51
37	32	39	45	37	45	52
38	33	39	46	38	46	53
39	33	40	47	38	46	54
40	33	41	48	38	46	55

Table 7.12. Cardiac volume (cm^3)

Week	Percentile		
	5th	50th	95th
10	0.011	0.021	0.038
11	0.018	0.033	0.059
12	0.038	0.067	0.119
13	0.072	0.127	0.224
14	0.128	0.225	0.395
15	0.213	0.374	0.655
16	0.336	0.588	1.031
17	0.504	0.883	1.546
18	0.726	1.271	2.224
19	1.008	1.764	3.086
20	1.356	2.373	4.150
21	1.776	3.106	5.433
22	2.273	3.975	6.951
23	2.851	4.987	8.722
24	3.519	6.155	10.765
25	4.282	7.490	13.103
26	5.150	9.008	15.758
27	6.130	10.723	18.757
28	7.232	12.649	22.123
29	8.458	14.795	25.877
30	9.812	17.163	30.023
31	11.284	19.743	34.545
32	12.857	22.505	39.392
33	14.498	25.388	44.459
34	16.155	28.301	49.579
35	17.750	31.107	54.512
36	19.180	33.626	58.952
37	20.308	35.642	62.554
38	20.966	36.913	64.989
39	20.903	37.156	66.046
40	19.478	35.580	64.993

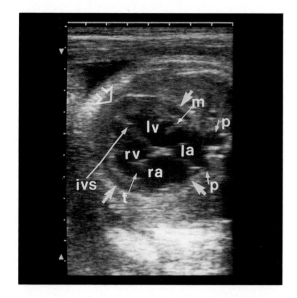

Fig. 7.122. The longitudinal diameter of the heart is measured from the apex to the highest part of the interauricular septum. The transverse diameter is obtained perpendicularly to the longitudinal diameter and is the largest possible diameter (approximately at the level of the atrio-ventricular groove). Both measurements are obtained from outside the myocardium

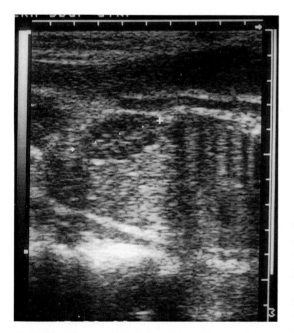

Fig. 7.123. The renal length is measured from the upper pole to the lower pole of the kidney in a longitudinal section of the fetus

Table 7.13. Abdominal perimeter (mm)

Week	Percentile			
	Computed (Jeanty)			Measured (Deter)
	5th	50th	95th	50th
12	35	57	80	63
13	45	67	90	74
14	55	77	100	84
15	65	88	110	95
16	76	98	120	106
17	86	109	131	117
18	97	119	142	128
19	108	130	152	139
20	119	141	163	150
21	129	152	174	161
22	140	163	185	172
23	151	173	196	183
24	162	184	206	194
25	172	195	217	205
26	183	205	227	216
27	193	215	238	227
28	203	225	248	238
29	213	235	257	249
30	222	244	267	260
31	231	254	276	271
32	240	262	285	282
33	248	271	293	293
34	256	279	301	304
35	264	286	309	315
36	271	293	316	326
37	278	300	322	337
38	283	306	328	348
39	289	311	333	359
40	294	316	338	370

7.7.3 Thoracic and Abdominal Organs

Cardiac Dimensions (Fig. 7.122)

The size of the two ventricles, and the thickness of the myocardial walls, are equal, since both are submitted to the same workload. Both sides of the heart indeed work in parallel, since they communicate at the level of the foramen ovale and the ductus. The normal dimensions of the transverse and longitudinal diameters are expressed in Tables 7.11 and 7.12.

The longitudinal diameter of the heart is measured from the apex to the highest part of the interauricular septum. The transverse diameter is obtained perpendicular to the longitudinal diameter and is the largest possible diameter. Both measurements are obtained from out-

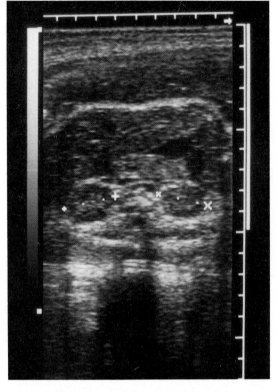

side the myocardium. The heart volume is estimated from the formula of the ellipsoid:

$$\text{heart volume} = (\text{transverse diameter})^2 \times \text{longitudinal diameter} \times 0.5233$$

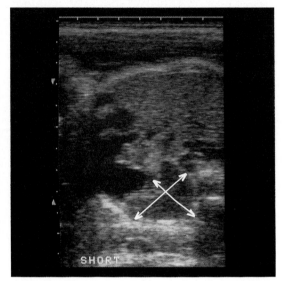

Fig. 7.124. The thickness, the width, and the kidney perimeter are measured in a transverse section of the fetal abdomen rather than a transverse section of the kidney, which would be more difficult to reproduce

Fig. 7.125. The longitudinal diameter of the spleen is measured from the extremity lateral to the spine to the extremity close to the anterior abdominal wall. The transverse diameter is the largest possible perpendicular to the longitudinal diameter

Table 7.14. Kidney biometry

Week	Volume (cm³)			Length (mm)			Width (mm)			Thickness (mm)		
	Percentile			Percentile			Percentile			Percentile		
	5th	50th	95th	5th	50th	95th	5th	50th	95th	5th	50th	95th
20	–	2	5.6	21	28	36	10	14	18	11	15	19
21	–	3	6	22	29	36	10	14	18	11	15	19
22	–	3	6.4	22	30	37	10	14	18	12	16	20
23	–	3	6.8	23	30	37	11	15	19	12	16	20
24	–	4	7.2	24	31	38	11	15	19	13	17	21
25	0.6	4	7.6	24	31	39	11	15	19	13	17	21
26	1	4	7.9	25	32	39	12	16	20	14	18	22
27	1.4	5	8.3	26	33	40	12	16	20	14	18	22
28	1.8	5	8.7	26	33	40	12	16	20	14	18	22
29	2.1	6	9.1	27	34	41	13	17	21	15	19	23
30	2.5	6	9.5	27	34	42	13	17	21	15	19	23
31	2.9	6	9.9	28	35	42	13	17	21	16	20	24
32	3.3	7	10.3	29	36	43	14	18	22	16	20	24
33	3.6	7	10.7	29	36	43	14	18	22	17	21	25
34	4	8	11.1	30	37	44	14	18	22	17	21	25
35	4.4	8	11.5	30	38	45	15	19	23	17	21	25
36	4.8	8	11.9	31	38	45	15	19	23	18	22	26
37	5.2	9	12.3	32	39	46	15	19	23	18	22	26
38	5.5	9	12.6	32	39	47	16	20	24	19	23	27
39	5.9	9	13	33	40	47	16	20	24	19	23	27
40	6.3	10	13.4	33	41	48	16	20	24	19	23	27

The transverse diameter is used to the second power because the perpendicular diameter (on the cephalocaudal axis) to both the longitudinal and transverse diameter is difficult to reproduce. Anatomical sections of abortuses have demonstrated that this dimension is very similar to the transverse diameter. The measurements are obtained at any time in the cardiac cycle, to avoid problems in the interpretation of the scans. The transverse diameter of the heart is equal to 45%–55% of the transverse thoracic diameter of the chest in the four-chamber-view plane.

Week	Length		
	Percentile		
	5th	50th	95th
20	6	9	12
21	6	10	13
22	7	10	13
23	8	11	14
24	8	11	14
25	9	12	15
26	9	12	16
27	10	13	16
28	10	14	17
29	11	14	17
30	12	15	18
31	12	15	18
32	13	16	19
33	13	16	20
34	14	17	20
35	14	18	21
36	15	18	21
37	16	19	22
38	16	19	23
39	17	20	23
40	17	21	24

Table 7.15. Adrenal gland thickness and length

Thickness (mm)	Weeks			
	<25	26–30	31–35	36–40
Mean	3	5	5	6
Range	2–5	2–8	3–7	4–9

Table 7.16. Spleen biometry

Age (weeks)	Length (mm)			Sagittal diameter (mm)			Transverse diameter (mm)			Volume (cm^3)			Perimeter (mm)		
	Percentile			Percentile			Percentile			Percentile			Percentile		
	5th	50th	95th	5th	50th	95th	5th	50th	95th	5th	50th	95th	5th	50th	95th
18	7	14	21	3	7	11	4	9	13		0.07	0.73	23	35	47
19	7	14	21	3	7	11	4	9	13		0.07	0.73	23	35	47
20	7	14	21	3	7	11	4	9	13		0.07	0.73	23	35	47
21	11	18	26	5	8	12	5	10	15	0.49	1.01	1.54	33	45	57
22	11	18	26	5	8	12	5	10	15	0.49	1.01	1.54	33	45	57
23	11	18	26	5	8	12	5	10	15	0.49	1.01	1.54	33	45	57
24	11	18	26	5	8	12	5	10	15	0.49	1.01	1.54	33	45	57
25	11	18	26	5	8	12	5	10	15	0.49	1.01	1.54	33	45	57
26	15	22	29	6	10	13	7	12	16	1.17	1.68	2.19	41	53	65
27	15	22	29	6	10	13	7	12	16	1.17	1.68	2.19	41	53	65
28	16	23	31	7	10	14	8	12	17	1.40	1.96	2.51	45	57	69
29	16	23	31	7	10	14	8	12	17	1.40	1.96	2.51	45	57	69
30	16	23	31	7	10	14	8	12	17	1.40	1.96	2.51	45	57	69
31	16	23	31	7	10	14	8	12	17	1.40	1.96	2.51	45	57	69
32	18	25	32	7	11	15	8	13	18	1.58	2.21	2.84	49	61	72
33	18	25	32	7	11	15	8	13	18	1.58	2.21	2.84	49	61	72
34	22	29	37	9	13	17	10	15	20	2.00	3.05	4.09	59	71	83
35	22	29	37	9	13	17	10	15	20	2.00	3.05	4.09	59	71	83
36	22	29	37	9	13	17	10	15	20	2.00	3.05	4.09	59	71	83
37	22	29	37	9	13	17	10	15	20	2.00	3.05	4.09	59	71	83
38	22	29	37	9	13	17	10	15	20	2.00	3.05	4.09	59	71	83
39	24	31	38	10	13	17	11	16	21	2.16	3.40	4.65	62	74	86
40	25	33	40	10	14	18	12	17	21	2.35	3.83	5.30	65	77	89

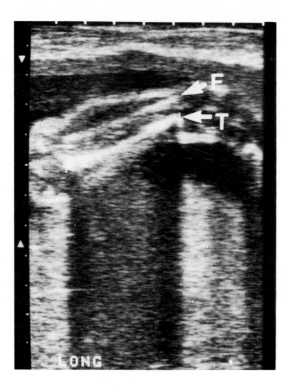

Fig. 7.126. The tibia is the thicker of the two leg bones and lies medial to the fibula

Abdominal Perimeter. It is important to obtain a section that is as "round" as possible. This will avoid the "salami" effect, in which an oblique section is obtained, resulting in a considerably increased anteroposterior diameter. The perimeter is computed from two diameters, using the formula:

abdominal perimeter = (transverse diameter + anteroposterior diameter) × 1.57

The anteroposterior diameter is measured from the abdominal wall facing the lowest part of the umbilical part of the left portal vein to the processus spinosus of the spine. The transverse diameter, instead of being the perpendicular diameter at the mid distance of the anteroposterior diameter, is the largest parallel to a virtual tangent to the processus spinosus. In the vast

Table 7.17. Long bones of leg (mm)

Week	Femur			Tibia			Fibula		
	Percentile			Percentile			Percentile		
	5th	50th	95th	5th	50th	95th	5th	50th	95th
12	4	8	13	–	7	–	–	6	–
13	6	11	16	–	10	–	–	9	–
14	9	14	18	7	12	17	6	12	19
15	12	17	21	9	15	20	9	15	21
16	15	20	24	12	17	22	13	18	23
17	18	23	27	15	20	25	13	21	28
18	21	25	30	17	22	27	15	23	31
19	24	28	33	20	25	30	19	26	33
20	26	31	36	22	27	33	21	28	36
21	29	34	38	25	30	35	24	31	37
22	32	36	41	27	32	38	27	33	39
23	35	39	44	30	35	40	28	35	42
24	37	42	46	32	37	42	29	37	45
25	40	44	49	34	40	45	34	40	45
26	42	47	51	37	42	47	36	42	47
27	45	49	54	39	44	49	37	44	50
28	47	52	56	41	46	51	38	45	53
29	50	54	59	43	48	53	41	47	54
30	52	56	61	45	50	55	43	49	56
31	54	59	63	47	52	57	42	51	59
32	56	61	65	48	54	59	42	52	63
33	58	63	67	50	55	60	46	54	62
34	60	65	69	52	57	62	46	55	65
35	62	67	71	53	58	64	51	57	62
36	64	68	73	55	60	65	54	58	63
37	65	70	74	56	61	67	54	59	65
38	67	71	76	58	63	68	56	61	65
39	68	73	77	59	64	69	56	62	67
40	70	74	79	61	66	71	59	63	67

majority of the cases, both techniques of obtaining the transverse diameter yield the same value, but when the fetal abdomen is deformed the two diameters are not strictly perpendicular and this technique provides a more meaningful measurement. Measurements should be obtained at medium gain from outer to outer edge (Table 7.13).

Kidney. The renal length is measured from the upper pole to the lower pole of the kidney in a longitudinal section of the fetus (Fig. 7.123). Usually, the easiest way is to image either the spine or the aorta and then move the transducer laterally until the entire length of the kidney is observed. Its thickness, width, and perimeter are measured in a transverse section of the fetal abdomen (Fig. 7.125) rather than a transverse section of the kidney, which would be more difficult to reproduce (Table 7.14). The trans-

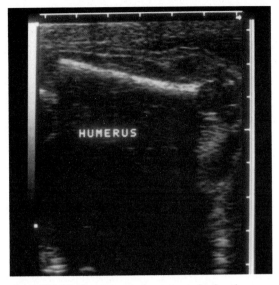

Fig. 7.127. The humerus can be measured using the same criteria as those used for the femur: i) complete acoustic shadow, ii) end-to-end shadow, iii) clear-cut margins

Table 7.18. Long bones of arm (mm)

Week	Humerus			Ulna			Radius		
	Percentile			Percentile			Percentile		
	5th	50th	95th	5th	50th	95th	5th	50th	95th
12	–	9	–	–	7	–	–	7	–
13	6	11	16	5	10	15	6	10	14
14	9	14	19	8	13	18	8	13	17
15	12	17	22	11	16	21	11	15	20
16	15	20	25	13	18	23	13	18	22
17	18	22	27	16	21	26	14	20	26
18	20	25	30	19	24	29	15	22	29
19	23	28	33	21	26	31	20	24	29
20	25	30	35	24	29	34	22	27	32
21	28	33	38	26	31	36	24	29	33
22	30	35	40	28	33	38	27	31	34
23	33	38	42	31	36	41	26	32	39
24	35	40	45	33	38	43	26	34	42
25	37	42	47	35	40	45	31	36	41
26	39	44	49	37	42	47	32	37	43
27	41	46	51	39	44	49	33	39	45
28	43	48	53	41	46	51	33	40	48
29	45	50	55	43	48	53	36	42	47
30	47	51	56	44	49	54	36	43	49
31	48	53	58	46	51	56	38	44	50
32	50	55	60	48	53	58	37	45	53
33	51	56	61	49	54	59	41	46	51
34	53	58	63	51	56	61	40	47	53
35	54	59	64	52	57	62	41	48	54
36	56	61	65	53	58	63	49	48	57
37	57	62	67	55	60	65	45	49	53
38	59	63	68	56	61	66	45	49	54
39	60	65	70	57	62	67	45	50	54
40	61	66	71	58	63	68	46	50	55

Table 7.19. Estimated fetal weights in "estimated grams," derived from the Shepard formula

Biparietal diameter (mm) — Abdominal perimeter (mm)

Biparietal diameter 30–39; Abdominal perimeter 40–150 mm

BPD	40	45	50	55	60	65	70	75	80	85	90	95	100	105	110	115	120	125	130	135	140	145	150
30	80	83	87	91	95	99	104	108	113	118	123	129	135	141	147	154	161						
31	83	86	90	94	98	103	107	112	117	122	128	133	139	145	152	159	166	173	181				
32			93	97	102	106	111	116	121	126	132	138	144	150	157	164	171	178	186				
33			97	101	105	110	115	120	125	130	136	142	148	155	162	169	176	184	192				
34			100	104	109	114	119	124	129	135	141	147	153	160	167	174	182	190	198	206	215		
35					113	118	123	128	134	139	145	152	158	165	172	180	187	195	204	213	222		
36					117	122	127	132	138	144	150	157	163	170	178	185	193	202	210	219	229		
37					121	126	131	137	143	149	155	162	169	176	183	191	199	208	217	226	235	245	256
38							136	142	148	154	160	167	174	182	189	197	206	214	223	233	243	253	263
39							141	146	153	159	166	173	180	187	195	203	212	221	230	240	250	260	271

Biparietal diameter 40–49; Abdominal perimeter 70–180 mm

BPD	70	75	80	85	90	95	100	105	110	115	120	125	130	135	140	145	150	155	160	165	170	175	180
40	145	152	158	164	171	178	186	193	202	210	219	228	237	247	257	268	279						
41			163	170	177	184	192	200	208	217	226	235	245	255	265	276	288	299	312				
42			169	176	183	190	198	206	215	223	233	242	252	262	273	284	296	308	321				
43			174	182	189	197	205	213	222	231	240	250	260	270	281	293	305	317	330				
44			180	188	195	203	211	220	229	238	247	257	268	279	290	302	314	326	340	353	368		
45					202	210	218	227	236	245	255	265	276	287	299	311	323	336	349	363	378		
46					208	217	225	234	244	253	263	274	285	296	308	320	333	346	359	374	389		
47					215	224	233	242	251	261	271	282	293	305	317	329	342	356	370	384	400	415	432
48							240	250	259	269	280	291	302	314	326	339	352	366	381	395	411	427	444
49							248	258	268	278	289	300	312	324	336	349	363	377	392	407	422	439	456

Biparietal diameter 50–62; Abdominal perimeter 100–230 mm

BPD	100	105	110	115	120	125	130	135	140	145	150	155	160	165	170	175	180	185	190	195	200	205	210	215	220	225	230
50	256	266	276	287	298	309	321	334	346	360	374	388	403	418	434	451	468	486	505								
51			285	296	307	319	331	344	357	370	385	399	414	430	447	464	481	500	519								
52			294	305	317	329	341	354	368	381	396	411	426	443	459	477	495	513	533								
53			304	315	327	339	352	365	379	393	408	423	439	455	472	490	508	527	547	568	589						
54					337	350	363	376	390	405	420	435	451	468	486	504	522	542	562	583	605						
55					348	360	374	388	402	417	432	448	464	482	499	518	537	557	577	598	620						
56					359	372	385	399	414	429	445	461	478	495	513	532	552	572	593	614	637	660	684				
57					372		397	412	426	442	458	474	492	509	528	547	567	587	609	631	654	677	702				
58							409	424	439	455	471	488	506	524	543	562	583	604	625	648	671	695	720				
59									453	469	485	503	520	539	558	578	599	620	642	665	689	713	739	765	792		
60									466	483	500	517	536	554	574	594	615	637	659	683	707	732	758	784	812		
61									480	497	514	532	551	570	590	611	632	654	677	701	725	751	777	804	832	883	
62											530	548	567	587	607	628	650	672	696	720	745	770	797	825	853	883	913

Rows 63–69

	170	175	180	185	190	195	200	205	210	215	220	225	230	235	240	245	250	255	260	265	270
63	545	564	583	603	624	645	668	691	714	739	764	790	818	846	875	905	936				
64	561	580	600	621	642	664	686	709	734	759	784	811	839	867	897	927	959				
65			617	638	660	682	705	729	753	779	805	832	860	889	919	950	982	1,015	1,050		
66			635	657	678	701	725	749	774	800	826	854	882	912	942	974	1,006	1,040	1,075		
67			654	675	698	721	745	769	795	821	848	876	905	935	966	998	1,031	1,065	1,100	1,137	1,174
68					717	741	765	790	816	843	870	899	928	959	990	1,023	1,056	1,091	1,127	1,164	1,202
69					738	762	786	812	838	865	893	922	952	983	1,015	1,048	1,082	1,117	1,154	1,191	1,230

Rows 70–79

	210	215	220	225	230	235	240	245	250	255	260	265	270	275	280	285	290	295	300	305	310	315	320	325	330
70	758	783	808	834	861	888	917	946	977	1,008	1,041	1,074	1,109	1,144	1,181	1,219	1,258	1,299	1,340						
71			830	857	884	912	941	971	1,002	1,034	1,067	1,101	1,136	1,172	1,209	1,248	1,287	1,328	1,371						
72			853	880	908	936	966	996	1,028	1,060	1,094	1,128	1,164	1,200	1,238	1,277	1,317	1,359	1,402						
73					932	961	991	1,022	1,054	1,087	1,121	1,156	1,192	1,229	1,268	1,307	1,348	1,390	1,433	1,478	1,524				
74					958	987	1,018	1,049	1,081	1,115	1,149	1,185	1,221	1,259	1,298	1,338	1,379	1,422	1,466	1,511	1,558				
75					983	1,013	1,044	1,076	1,109	1,143	1,178	1,214	1,251	1,290	1,329	1,370	1,411	1,455	1,499	1,545	1,592	1,641	1,691		
76							1,072	1,104	1,138	1,172	1,208	1,244	1,282	1,321	1,361	1,402	1,444	1,488	1,533	1,579	1,627	1,676	1,727		
77							1,100	1,133	1,167	1,202	1,238	1,275	1,313	1,353	1,393	1,435	1,478	1,522	1,568	1,615	1,663	1,713	1,764		
78							1,129	1,163	1,197	1,233	1,269	1,307	1,346	1,385	1,426	1,469	1,512	1,557	1,603	1,651	1,700	1,750	1,802	1,855	1,910
79									1,228	1,264	1,301	1,339	1,379	1,419	1,461	1,503	1,547	1,593	1,639	1,688	1,737	1,788	1,840	1,894	1,950

Rows 80–89

	250	255	260	265	270	275	280	285	290	295	300	305	310	315	320	325	330	335	340	345	350	355	360	365	370
80	1,260	1,296	1,334	1,373	1,412	1,453	1,495	1,539	1,583	1,629	1,677	1,725	1,775	1,827	1,880	1,934	1,990								
81			1,367	1,407	1,447	1,488	1,531	1,575	1,620	1,667	1,715	1,764	1,814	1,866	1,920	1,975	2,032	2,090	2,150						
82			1,402	1,441	1,482	1,524	1,568	1,612	1,658	1,705	1,753	1,803	1,854	1,907	1,961	2,017	2,074	2,133	2,193						
83			1,437	1,477	1,519	1,561	1,605	1,650	1,697	1,744	1,793	1,843	1,895	1,948	2,003	2,059	2,117	2,176	2,237	2,300	2,365				
84					1,556	1,599	1,643	1,689	1,736	1,784	1,834	1,885	1,937	1,991	2,046	2,103	2,161	2,221	2,282	2,346	2,411				
85					1,594	1,638	1,683	1,729	1,776	1,825	1,875	1,927	1,979	2,034	2,090	2,147	2,206	2,266	2,328	2,392	2,458				
86							1,723	1,770	1,818	1,867	1,918	1,970	2,023	2,078	2,134	2,192	2,252	2,313	2,375	2,440	2,506	2,574	2,644		
87							1,764	1,811	1,860	1,910	1,961	2,014	2,068	2,123	2,180	2,238	2,298	2,360	2,423	2,488	2,555	2,623	2,694		
88							1,806	1,854	1,903	1,954	2,005	2,059	2,113	2,169	2,227	2,286	2,346	2,408	2,472	2,538	2,605	2,674	2,745	2,817	2,892
89									1,947	1,998	2,051	2,104	2,160	2,216	2,274	2,334	2,395	2,457	2,522	2,588	2,656	2,725	2,797	2,870	2,945

Rows 90–100

	250	255	260	265	270	275	280	285	290	295	300	305	310	315	320	325	330	335	340	345	350	355	360	365	370
90	1,993	2,044	2,087	2,151	2,207	2,264	2,323	2,383	2,445	2,508	2,579	2,639	2,707	2,778	2,849	2,923	2,999								
91			2,145	2,199	2,256	2,313	2,372	2,433	2,495	2,559	2,624	2,692	2,760	2,831	2,903	2,977	3,054	3,132	3,212						
92			2,193	2,249	2,305	2,364	2,423	2,484	2,547	2,611	2,677	2,745	2,814	2,885	2,958	3,033	3,109	3,188	3,268						
93			2,243	2,299	2,356	2,415	2,475	2,537	2,600	2,665	2,731	2,799	2,869	2,941	3,014	3,089	3,166	3,245	3,326	3,409	3,494				
94					2,408	2,467	2,528	2,590	2,654	2,719	2,786	2,855	2,925	2,997	3,071	3,147	3,224	3,304	3,385	3,468	3,554				
95					2,461	2,521	2,582	2,645	2,709	2,775	2,842	2,912	2,982	3,055	3,129	3,205	3,283	3,363	3,445	3,528	3,614				
96							2,637	2,701	2,765	2,832	2,900	2,969	3,041	3,114	3,188	3,265	3,343	3,423	3,505	3,590	3,676	3,764	3,854		
97							2,694	2,757	2,823	2,890	2,958	3,028	3,100	3,173	3,248	3,325	3,404	3,485	3,567	3,652	3,738	3,827	3,918		
98									2,881	2,949	3,018	3,088	3,160	3,234	3,310	3,387	3,466	3,547	3,630	3,715	3,802	3,891	3,982	4,075	4,170
99									2,941	3,009	3,078	3,149	3,222	3,296	3,372	3,450	3,530	3,611	3,695	3,780	3,867	3,956	4,047	4,141	4,236
100									3,002	3,071	3,141	3,212	3,285	3,360	3,436	3,514	3,594	3,676	3,760	3,845	3,933	4,022	4,114	4,207	4,303

Normal Fetal Anatomy in the Second and Third Trimester

Table 7.20. Normal growth of the EFW (g)

Week	Number of standard deviations below the mean									Mean	Number of standard deviations above the mean								
	2.6	2.4	2.2	2	1.8	1.6	1.4	1.2	1		1	1.2	1.4	1.6	1.8	2	2.2	2.4	2.6
9	43	44	44	44	44	44	44	44	44	45	46	46	46	46	46	46	46	46	47
10	44	44	45	45	45	46	46	46	46	48	50	50	50	50	51	51	51	52	52
11	47	47	48	48	49	50	50	51	51	54	57	57	58	58	59	60	60	61	61
12	52	53	53	54	55	56	57	58	59	63	67	68	69	70	71	72	73	73	74
13	58	60	61	63	64	66	67	68	70	77	84	86	87	88	90	91	93	94	96
14	68	70	72	74	76	79	81	83	85	96	107	109	111	113	116	118	120	122	124
15	81	84	87	90	93	97	100	103	106	122	138	141	144	147	151	154	157	160	163
16	98	102	106	111	115	120	124	129	133	155	177	181	186	190	195	199	204	208	212
17	118	124	130	136	142	148	154	160	167	197	227	234	240	246	252	258	264	270	276
18	142	150	158	166	174	182	190	199	207	247	287	295	304	312	320	328	336	344	352
19	172	183	193	203	214	224	234	245	255	307	359	369	380	390	400	411	421	431	442
20	207	220	233	246	259	272	285	298	311	377	443	456	469	482	495	508	521	534	547
21	245	261	278	294	310	326	343	359	375	456	537	553	569	586	602	618	634	651	667
22	289	309	328	348	368	387	407	427	447	545	643	663	683	703	722	742	762	781	801
23	339	362	386	409	433	456	480	503	527	644	761	785	808	832	855	879	902	926	949
24	392	420	448	475	503	531	559	586	614	753	892	920	947	975	1,003	1,031	1,058	1,086	1,114
25	450	482	514	547	579	612	644	676	709	871	1,033	1,066	1,098	1,130	1,163	1,195	1,228	1,260	1,292
26	514	551	589	626	663	701	738	776	813	1,000	1,187	1,224	1,262	1,299	1,337	1,374	1,411	1,449	1,486
27	583	625	668	711	754	797	839	882	925	1,139	1,353	1,396	1,439	1,481	1,524	1,567	1,610	1,653	1,695
28	656	704	753	802	850	899	948	996	1,045	1,288	1,531	1,580	1,628	1,677	1,726	1,774	1,823	1,872	1,920
29	734	789	844	899	954	1,009	1,064	1,119	1,173	1,448	1,723	1,777	1,832	1,887	1,942	1,997	2,052	2,107	2,162
30	819	880	942	1,003	1,065	1,126	1,188	1,249	1,311	1,618	1,925	1,987	2,048	2,110	2,171	2,233	2,294	2,356	2,417
31	907	976	1,044	1,113	1,181	1,250	1,318	1,387	1,455	1,798	2,141	2,209	2,278	2,346	2,415	2,483	2,552	2,620	2,689
32	999	1,075	1,150	1,226	1,302	1,378	1,454	1,529	1,605	1,984	2,363	2,439	2,514	2,590	2,666	2,742	2,818	2,893	2,969
33	1,092	1,176	1,259	1,342	1,426	1,509	1,593	1,676	1,759	2,176	2,593	2,676	2,759	2,843	2,926	3,010	3,093	3,176	3,260
34	1,188	1,279	1,369	1,460	1,551	1,642	1,733	1,824	1,915	2,369	2,823	2,914	3,005	3,096	3,187	3,278	3,369	3,459	3,550
35	1,280	1,379	1,477	1,575	1,673	1,771	1,870	1,968	2,066	2,557	3,048	3,146	3,244	3,343	3,441	3,539	3,637	3,735	3,834
36	1,366	1,471	1,577	1,682	1,787	1,892	1,997	2,103	2,208	2,734	3,260	3,365	3,471	3,576	3,681	3,786	3,891	3,997	4,102
37	1,441	1,553	1,664	1,776	1,887	1,999	2,110	2,221	2,333	2,890	3,447	3,559	3,670	3,781	3,893	4,004	4,116	4,227	4,339
38	1,499	1,616	1,732	1,849	1,966	2,082	2,199	2,316	2,432	3,016	3,600	3,716	3,833	3,950	4,066	4,183	4,300	4,416	4,533
39	1,525	1,646	1,767	1,888	2,009	2,131	2,252	2,373	2,494	3,099	3,704	3,825	3,946	4,067	4,189	4,310	4,431	4,552	4,673
40	1,514	1,638	1,762	1,887	2,011	2,136	2,260	2,385	2,509	3,131	3,753	3,877	4,002	4,126	4,251	4,375	4,500	4,624	4,748

verse section is obtained at the level of the renal pelvis, if visible, otherwise at the level where the renal section is the largest as observed visually (Fig. 7.124).

Kidney Perimeter to Abdominal Perimeter Ratio

$$\frac{(\text{Kidney width} + \text{kidney thickness})}{(\text{Anteroposterior abdominal diameter} + \text{transverse abdominal diameter})} = 23\%$$

$+/-5\%$ for the 5th and 95th percentiles, normal range between 18% and 28%.

Adrenal Gland. The thickness of the adrenal gland is measured in a transverse section. A transverse scan of the kidney is obtained and the transducer is slowly moved cephalad until the right position is reached. The length and thickness of the adrenal can be measured in this section (Table 7.15).

The longitudinal section of the adrenal gland is of limited use, because acoustic shadowing from the ribs often conceals the interface between the kidney and the adrenal gland.

Spleen. On a transverse scan the spleen is lateral to the spine and posterior to the fluid-filled stomach. The longitudinal diameter of the spleen is measured from the posterior edge lateral to the spine to the anterior edge close to the anterior abdominal wall. The transverse diameter that can be obtained perpendicular to the longitudinal scan is the largest possible. The coronal diameter is measured in a coronal scan and is the largest obtained at the level of the stomach (Table 7.16).

The fetal spleen volume is estimated using the formula of the ellipsoid:

spleen volume = longitudinal × transverse × coronal diameter × 0.5233

The spleen perimeter is estimated using the formula of the ellipsoid:

spleen perimeter = longitudinal × transverse diameter × 0.5233

7.7.4 Long Bones

Femur, Tibia, and Fibula. A bright echo in close proximity to the bladder is the ilium. Once it is located, the next most external and caudal echo corresponds to the femur. Again, careful rotation of the transducer around the femoral section will display the femoral length. The tibia and fibula are slightly easier to demonstrate than the radius and ulna, because the latitude of movement permitted by the knee joint is smaller than that which occurs at the elbow. The tibia is the thicker of the two bones and lies medial to the fibula (Table 7.17, Fig. 7.126).

Humerus, Ulna, and Radius. The humerus can then be displayed by imaging the scapula and then rotating the transducer (Fig. 7.127).

The humerus is sometimes very close to the maternal anterior abdominal wall and therefore in the near field, where it can be difficult to delineate correctly.

Rotation of the transducer around the elbow then demonstrates a section with the ulna and radius, appearing as two bright dots. By further rotating the transducer, the whole length can be demonstrated. The ulna is distinguishable from the radius by virtue of its much deeper penetration into the elbow. The distal ends of the radius and ulna are sometimes fused, making individual identification difficult (Table 7.18).

7.7.5 Estimated Fetal Weight

The estimated fetal weight (EFW) is computed according to the formula proposed by Shepard. One uses the BPD and finds the intersection with the abdominal perimeter. The EFW can be read at this intersection.

References

Aubry JP, Aubry MC, Briard ML et al. (1981) Mesure prenatale de la croissance de la distance interorbitaire par echographie. Appoint dans le depistage des formes mineures d'holoprosencephalie. J Genet Hum 29:395–407

Birnholz JC (1980) Ultrasound characterization of fetal growth. Ultrasonic Imaging 2:135–149

Buttery B (1979) Occipito-frontal biparietal diameter ratio: an ultrasonic parameter for the antenatal evaluation of Down's syndrome. Med J Aust 2:662–664

Campbell S, Newman GB (1971) Growth of the fetal biparietal diameter during normal pregnancy. Br J Obstet Gynaecol 78:513–519

Campbell S, Thomas A (1982) Ultrasound measurement of the fetal head to abdomen circumference ratio in the assessment of growth retardation. Br J Obstet Gynaecol 89:165–174

Campbell S, Wilkin D (1975) Ultrasonic measurement of fetal abdomen circumference in the evaluation of fetal weight. Br J Obstet Gynaecol 82:689–697

Chervenak FA, Berkowitz RL, Romero R et al. The diagnosis of fetal hydrocephalus. Am J Obstet Gynecol (in press)

Denkhaus H, Winsberg F (1979) Ultrasonic measurement of the fetal ventricular system. Radiology 131:781–787

Deter RL, Harrist RB, Hadlock FP et al. (1982) Fetal head and abdominal circumferences. 1. Evaluation of measurement errors. J Clin Ultrasound 10:357–363

Deter RL, Harrist RB, Hadlock FP et al. (1982) Fetal head and abdominal circumferences. 2. A critical re-evaluation of the relationship to menstrual age. J Clin Ultrasound 10:365–372

Deter RL, Harrist RB, Hadlock FP et al. (1982c) Longitudinal studies of fetal growth with the use of dynamic image ultrasonography. Am J Obstet Gynecol 143:545

Farrant P, Meire HB (1981) Ultrasound measurement of fetal limb length. Br J Radiol 54:660–664

Filly R, Golbus MS, Carey JC et al. (1981) Short limb dwarfism: ultrasonographic diagnosis by measuration of fetal femoral length. Radiology 138:653

Gruenwald P (1966) Growth of the human fetus. I. Normal growth and its variation. Am J Obstet Gynecol 94:112

Hadlock FP, Deter RL, Harrist RB et al. (1982) Fetal biparietal diameter: rational choice of plane of section for sonographic measurement. AJR 138:871–874

Hadlock FP, Deter RL, Harrist RB et al. (1982) Fetal head circumference: relation to menstrual age. AJR 136:649–653

Hadlock FP, Deter RL, Harrist RB, Roecker E, Park SK (1983) A date-independent predictor of intrauterine growth retardation: femur length/abdominal circumference ratio. AJR 141:979

Hadlock FP, Harrist RB, Deter RL et al. (1982) Fetal femur length as a predictor of menstrual age: sonographically measured. AJR 138:875

Hohler CW, Quetel TA (1982) Fetal femur length: equations for computer calculation of gestational age from ultrasound measurements. Am J Obstet Gynecol 143:479–481

Jeanty P, Dramaix-Wilmet M, Delbeke D (1981) Ultrasonic evaluation of fetal ventricular growth. Neuroradiology 21:123–131

Jeanty P, Kirkpatrick C, Dramaix-Wilmet M et al. (1981) Ultrasonic evaluation of fetal limb growth. Radiology 140:165–169

Jeanty P, Dramaix-Wilmet M, Elkazen N (1982) Measurement of fetal kidney growth on ultrasound. Radiology 144:159–162

Jeanty P, Dramaix-Wilmet M, Gansbeke D van (1982) Fetal ocular biometry by ultrasound. Radiology 143:513–516

Jeanty P, Dramaix-Wilmet M, Kerkem van (1982) Ultrasonic evaluation of fetal limb growth, part II. Radiology 143:751–754

Jeanty P, Cantraine F, Romero R (1984) A longitudinal study of fetal weight growth. J Ultrasound Med 3:321–328

Jeanty P, Chervenak F, Grannum P (1984) Normal ultrasonic size and characteristics of the fetal adrenal glands. Prenat Diagn 4:21–28

Jeanty P, Cousaert E, Cantraine F (1984) Normal growth of the abdominal perimeter. Am J Perinatal 1:129–135

Jeanty P, Cousaert E, Cantraine F (1984) A longitudinal study of fetal limb growth. Am J Perinatal 1:136–144

Jeanty P, Cousaert E, Hobbins JC (1984) A longitudinal study of fetal head biometry. Am J Perinatal 1:118–128

Jeanty P, Romero R, Cantraine F (1984) Fetal cardiac dimensions: a potential tool for the diagnosis of congenital heart defects. J Ultrasound Med 3:359–364

Jeanty P, Romero R, Hobbins JC (1985) Fetal limb volume: a new parameter to assess fetal growth. J Ultrasound Med 4:273–282

Johnson ML, Dunne MG, Mack LA et al. (1980) Evaluation of fetal intracranial anatomy by static and real-time ultrasound. J Clin Ultrasound 8:311–318

Kurtz A, Wagner RJW, Kurtz RJ (1980) Analysis of biparietal diameter as an accurate indicator of gestational age. J Clin Ultrasound 8:319–326

Mayden K, Tortora M, Berkowitz RL et al. (1982) Orbital diameters: a new parameter for prenatal diagnosis and dating. Am J Obstet Gynecol 144:289–293

O'Brien GD, Queenan JT (1981) Growth of the ultrasound femur length during normal pregnancy. Am J Obstet Gynecol 141:833

Ott WJ, Doyle S (1982) Normal ultrasonic fetal weight curve. Obstet Gynecol 59:603

Pedersen JF (1982) Fetal crown-rump length measurement by ultrasound in normal pregnancy. Br J Obstet Gynaecol 89:926

Robinson HP (1973) Sonar measurement of fetal crown-rump length as means of assessing maturity in first trimester of pregnancy. Br Med J 4:28

Robinson HP, Fleming JEE (1975) A critical evaluation of sonar crown-rump length measurements. Br J Obstet Gynaecol 82:702–710

Robinson HP, Sweet EM, Adam AH (1979) The accuracy of radiological estimates of gestational age using early fetal crown-rump length measurements by ultrasound as a basis for comparison. Br J Obstet Gynaecol 86:525

Schmidt W, Yarkoni S, Jeanty P (1982) Fetal spleen measurement by ultrasound and its clinical implications. J Ultrasound Med (in press)

Shepard M, Filly RA (1982) A standardized plane for biparietal diameter measurement. J Ultrasound Med 1:145–150

Shepard MJ, Richards VA, Berkowitz RL et al. (1982) An evaluation of two equations for predicting fetal weight by ultrasound. Am J Obstet Gynecol 142:42–54

Yarkoni S, Schmidt W, Jeanty P Fetal clavicle measurements by ultrasound. J Ultrasound Med (in press)

8 Fetal Malformations

8.1 Signs Suggesting the Presence of a Malformation

Fetal biometry for the confirmation of gestational age and the monitoring of growth was the dominant theme of diagnostic ultrasound during the first decade of its use. But in the past 5 years (1979–1984), a great deal of interest has been focused on the use of ultrasound for the detection of fetal malformations. This was made possible by improvements in static and real-time imaging techniques and by the integration of ultrasound as a screening procedure into prenatal care.

The purpose of this chapter is to acquaint the reader with the capabilities of diagnostic ultrasound within the limits imposed by current technology so that the potential of ultrasound for the diagnosis of fetal anomalies can be better appreciated and utilized. A multistage approach to diagnosis is proposed. Main consideration is given to the timing of the diagnosis, its specificity, and the question of reliability. In addition, it will be shown that the prenatal diagnosis of a fetal malformation presents a range of management options that go well beyond elective termination.

The Federal Republic of Germany was the first country in the world to implement ultrasound screening as a routine part of prenatal care. For the first time, it became possible to screen *all* pregnancies for evidence of fetal malformation. While evaluation for fetal abnormalities is only one aspect of the diagnostic spectrum of obstetric sonography, the efficacy of the method and the absence of adverse effects represent important factors which will motivate the patient and her spouse to attend for ultrasound examination. In a scale published by Stauber, the fear of congenital malformations ranked first among the anxieties expressed by pregnant women.

This fear is not unfounded, considering that the incidence of major congenital anomalies is approximately 2 per 100 live births. Assuming 500,000 births annually in the Federal Republic of Germany, this means that 10,000 families are affected each year.

The responsibility of the operator, then, is to alleviate this fear by careful examination, or to draw the correct conclusions if a fetal malformation is confirmed. The key to the successful diagnosis of fetal abnormalities lies in the detailed visualization of the relevant part of the fetal anatomy, combined with a knowledge of "normal" fetal anatomy in all its variations and expertise in the conduct of special biometric studies. It is a general rule that every ultrasound examination of a gravid patient, whether it involves a basic scan or a detailed investigation, should begin with a careful inspection of the general anatomy of the fetus and its environment.

Experience has shown that the following easily recognized indirect signs are suggestive of a fetal malformation in a high percentage of cases:

1. Anhydramnios or oligohydramnios before 20 weeks
2. Polyhydramnios independent of gestational age
3. Early growth retardation when gestational age is confirmed (by BBT, pregnancy test, ultrasound, etc.)
4. Abnormal body shape (e.g., failure to demonstrate an oval head)
5. Structural fetal anomalies (e.g., echo-free areas: cysts and other fluid collections)
6. Discrepancies in size between different parts of the body
7. Large placenta
8. Absence of an umbilical artery
9. Abnormal pattern of fetal activity (e.g., inactivity, excessive activity)

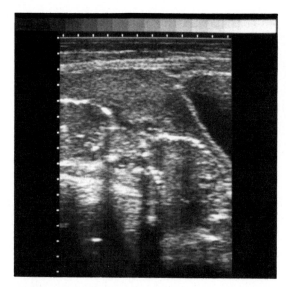

Fig. 8.1. Anhydramnios at 18 weeks

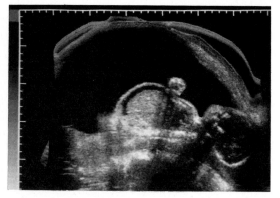

Fig. 8.2. Polyhydramnios at 24 weeks

Anhydramnios or Oligohydramnios Before 20 Weeks. The amount of amniotic fluid increases by an average of 50 ml/week between 15 and 20 weeks, attaining a volume of approximately 400 ml at 20 weeks (Queenan and Thompson 1972). Because quantitative determination of amniotic fluid volume is not yet practical, the examiner must rely on general appearance (and his own experience) in order to recognize deviations from the norm.

Generally, polyhydramnios is said to be present if the uterine cavity would be large enough to accommodate a second fetus comfortably (definition of Holländer 1972). Oligohydramnios may be diagnosed if no echo-free areas are seen between the fetus, placenta, and uterine wall that would permit movements of the fetal extremities. Moreover, the quality of the ultrasound image deteriorates as amniotic fluid volume decreases.

In our experience, the presence of oligohydramnios or anhydramnios before 20 weeks usually reflects a reduction or absence of fetal urine excretion, and thus is suggestive of a urogenital anomaly. Occasionally it may be associated with complex syndromes such as chromosome abnormalities. Only rarely can a prior rupture of the membranes be verified. In most cases it is difficult to make a definitive diagnosis due to the poor image definition and the difficulty of examining the internal organs (Fig. 8.1). Because oligohydramnios is always indicative of pathology, the patient must be

diagnosed as quickly as possible at a center with experience in this area.

Polyhydramnios. Polyhydramnios (Fig. 8.2) is associated with detectable fetal malformations in only about 30% of cases (Ramzin et al. 1973). Clinically relevant polyhydramnios practically always occurs in the second half of pregnancy. It has a much greater range of etiologies than oligohydramnios. Accordingly, it is no easier to establish a diagnosis, despite the usually excellent image quality afforded by the ideal acoustic conditions (large water-coupling path). With regard to etiology, polyhydramnios may be divided into two groups:

a) Cardiovascular decompensation (e.g., anemia secondary to Rh incompatibility, fetomaternal transfusion syndrome, fetofetal transfusion in multiple pregnancy, cardiac defects, premature closure of fetal vessels, arrhythmias; Figs. 8.7, 8.8)

b) Obstructive malformations of the gastrointestinal tract proximal to the ileum, particularly esophageal and duodenal atresia

It is not uncommon for the latter to occur in association with much more complex anomalies, including chromosome abnormalities.

Generally the diagnosis of polyhydramnios is easily made. However, it is important to confirm that the fluid collection is extrafetal. We have seen several cases in which fetal obstructive uropathy (prune-belly syndrome) was discovered in patients who had been referred for polyhydramnios (Fig. 8.3a, b).

Early Growth Retardation. As explained in the chapter on the first trimester, variations of fetal body size are minimal in early pregnancy and

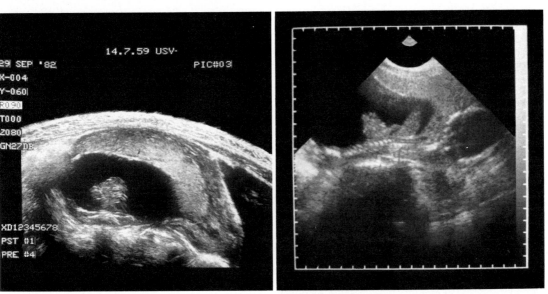

Fig. 8.3a, b. Referral for polyhydramnios at 19 weeks. The longitudinal scan (**a**) shows only the anterior placenta and a large fluid volume with fetal parts. Scan **b** shows that the fluid represents not hydramnios, but fetal ascites in association with anhydramnios (prune-belly syndrome with urinary ascites)

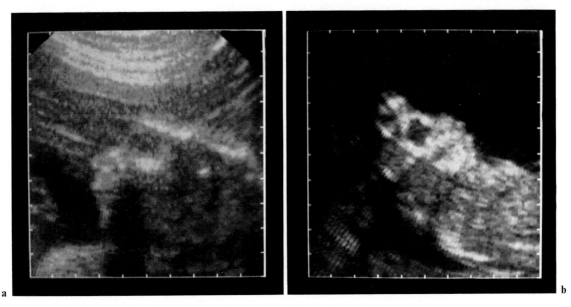

Fig. 8.4. a Abnormal profile: microcephaly. **b** Abnormal profile at 20 weeks: anencephaly

increase as gestation progresses. A body size that is small for a confirmed gestational age *before 20 weeks* should raise the suspicion of a severe fetal anomaly with a generally impaired growth potential. *Chromosome abnormalities* are of particular concern in this respect (see Chap. 10).

Abnormal Body Shape, Structural Anomalies. The recognition of abnormal body shape or intrafetal morphologic abnormalities (parenchymal defects, displacements, herniations, fluid collections in organs or body cavities) is of course suggestive of a fetal malformation (Figs. 8.3–8.10).

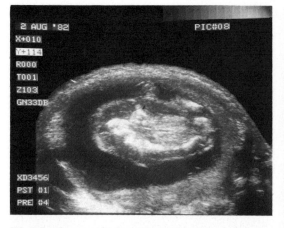

Fig. 8.5. Abnormal body outline at 23 weeks: acephalus with skin edema

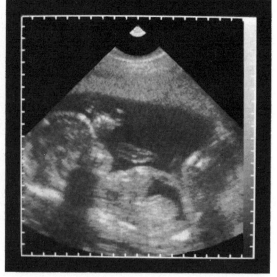

Fig. 8.7. Free fluid in fetal abdomen: ascites with complete AV block

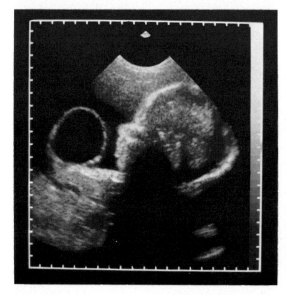

Fig. 8.6. Abnormal anterior trunk: omphalocele

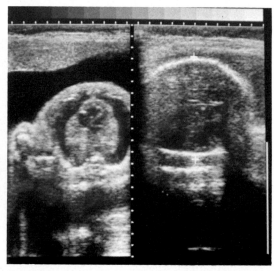

Fig. 8.8. Fluid in fetal thorax: pleural effusions with cardiac decompensation

Size Discrepancies Between Body Parts. Malproportions between individual body parts are most easily demonstrated by the use of multiple scanning planes. Even discrepancies between head and trunk size can yield valuable information. Inclusion of a third parameter in the analysis, such as the length of an extremity bone (femur), makes it easier to classify the malproportion.

Large Placenta, Absence of Umbilical Artery. The volume and structural features of the placenta can point toward fetal malformation. For example, a placental thickness greater than

6 cm (measured at the apex), increased echogenicity, and/or the presence of numerous sonolucent "holes" in the placental substance may be suggestive of an anomaly (Fig. 8.14). Finally, the absence of an umbilical artery should lead to more intensive investigation (Figs. 8.11–8.13).

Abnormal Fetal Activity. Since the introduction of real-time ultrasound, the observation of fetal movements has become an integral part of the

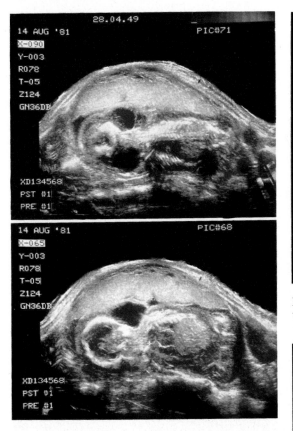

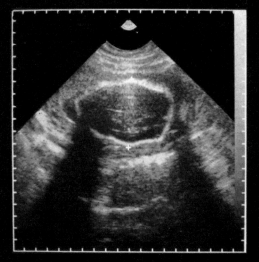

Fig. 8.10. Irregular outline of head associated with intrauterine death at 28 weeks (BPD: 22 weeks)

Fig. 8.9. Abnormal body outline, hyperechoic placenta, and fluid in fetal thorax with oligohydramnios: cystic hygroma, pleural effusions in Noonan syndrome

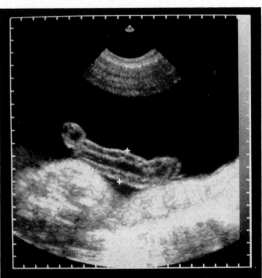

Fig. 8.11. Longitudinal scan of a normal umbilical cord demonstrating both arteries and umbilical vein

examination process. Investigators have attempted to derive diagnostic criteria from the quantitative assessment of fetal movements. However, these studies are still too time-consuming to have wide application at the clinical level. Based on our experience, we feel that a qualitative assessment of fetal movements is more worthwhile – e.g., harmonious movement of the hand to the head, thumb sucking, scratching movements, swallowing and stretching. Familiarity with normal patterns of fetal behavior will make it easy to recognize the abnormal nature of very rapid, spasmodic, uncoordinated movements of the extremities, particularly when there is a repeated alternation between excessive movements and immobility.

If only *one* of these suggestive signs is noted initially, the examiner should make an effort to search for additional signs, since they frequently occur in combination. As a general rule, it may be said that the likelihood of the presence of a fetal malformation increases with the number of suggestive signs that are observed.

If the first examiner is unable to make a definitive diagnosis, it is essential that he refer the patient to a facility with expertise in this area for more intensive evaluation.

Experience in recent years has proved that the problem of diagnosing fetal malformations can be solved only through a multistage approach that begins with an examination before

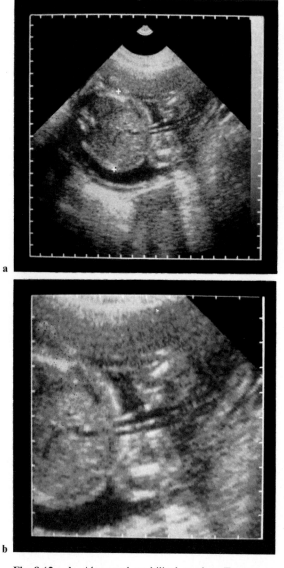

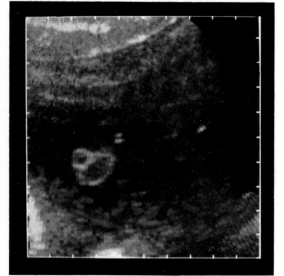

Fig. 8.13. Abnormal umbilical cord showing "signet ring" sign; only one artery and the vein

Fig. 8.12a, b. Abnormal umbilical cord. **a** Transverse scan of trunk showing insertion of umbilical cord between lower extremities. **b** Detail of **a** showing only two blood vessels in the cord (one vein and one artery)

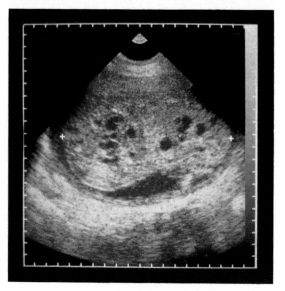

Fig. 8.14. Placental appearance in triploidy

20 weeks and, if findings are suspicious, proceeds to more specific examinations at specialized centers (Hansmann 1981). According to our records, 50% of cases that had been referred for investigation of a suspected fetal anomaly proved to be negative, while in the "positive" cases, the final diagnosis did not agree with the initial presumptive diagnosis in more than 50% of cases. There is no question that a specific diagnosis and the knowledge of its reliability are absolute prerequisites for prognosis and management planning.

References

Hansmann M (1981) Nachweis und Ausschluß fetaler Entwicklungsstörungen mittels Ultraschallscreening und gezielter Untersuchung – ein Mehrstufenkonzept. Ultraschall 2:206

Hepp H (1982) Schwangerschaftsabbruch aus kindlicher Indikation – anthropologisch – philosophische Aspekte des Arzt-Patienten-Konfliktes. In: Boland P, Krone HA, Pfeiffer RA (eds) Wissenschaftliche Informationen, Bamberger Symposium. Milupa, Friedrichsdorf

Holländer HJ (1972, ²1975, ³1984) Die Ultraschalldiagnostik in der Schwangerschaft. Urban & Schwarzenberg, München Wien Baltimore

Queenan JT, Thompson W (1972) Amniotic fluid vol-
    umes in normal pregnancies. Am J Obstet Gynecol
    114:34
Ramzin MS, Meudt RO, Hinselmann JJ (1973) Prognos-
    tic significance of abnormal ultrasonographic findings
    during the second trimester of gestation. J Perinat
    Med 1:60

8.2 Neural Tube Defects

Malformations of the central nervous system
based upon a failure of neural tube closure
(dysraphia) mainly include anencephaly, spina
bifida, and meningomyeloceles. Their incidence
in the Federal Republic of Germany (FRG) is
estimated to be 1 per 1,000 births (Warkany
1971). Weitzel (1983) found an incidence of
only 0.4 per 1,000 in his field study conducted
in the Hanover/Lower Saxony region of the
FRG, while the U.K. Collaborative Study
(1977) reported an incidence of 4.5 per 1,000.
The recurrence risk following the prior birth
of an affected fetus is approximately 5% in England (Brock 1979) and approximately 3% in
the FRG and rises to 10% after the birth of
a second affected fetus. Thus, neural tube defects are relatively common compared with
other fetal anomalies and have assumed a correspondingly high clinical significance.

8.2.1 Anencephaly

Anencephaly accounts for 50%–65% of all neural tube defects. Its hallmark sonographically
is the absence of the cerebral hemispheres (te-
lencephalon). This accounts for the absence of
an oval cranial vault. The term "anencephaly"
is not entirely correct, for the brain stem and
portions of the midbrain (mesencephalon) are
generally present. The defect which results from
a failure of closure of the neural tube at its
cranial end, develops "early," between 3 and
4 weeks menstrual age. The defect is covered
by a membrane of vascular stroma, but virtually never by bone or skin. Because the normal skull is visible sonographically as an oval
with a midline echo as early as 8–9 weeks menstrual age (Fig. 8.15), anencephaly is amenable
to early diagnosis. The main criteria are absence
of the cranial vault, inability to establish a reference plane for measuring the BPD, and large
"eyeglass-like" orbits (Figs. 8.16–8.22). Poly-

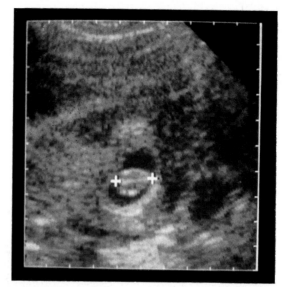

Fig. 8.15. Fetal head at 9 weeks day 6 (BBT). OFD
12 mm, BPD 10 mm (one fetus of a sextuplet pregnancy)

hydramnios is frequently present owing to increased secretion from the vasular membrane.
The anomaly may be somewhat more difficult
to diagnose if the head is low in the pelvis.
In these cases it is advisable to perform serial
examinations with progressive filling of the maternal bladder. This will either cause the shadowed portion of the fetal head to present
through the "window" of the bladder, or it
will stimulate strong fetal movements that place
the fetus in a more accessible position (this is
particularly common in anencephaly).

Once the diagnosis has been confirmed, it is
advisable (and instructive) to examine the fetus
for other malformations and observe the pattern of its movements. Up to 50% of anencephalic fetuses will have an associated spinal defect, which can be far more difficult to diagnose. The more experienced examiner should
also make an effort to confirm or exclude facial
midline defects, which are a commonly associated anomaly (Figs. 8.21 and 8.22).

Finally, omphalocele and complete eventration are more common in anencephalics than
in normocephalics. With regard to fetal movement, an abrupt alternation between episodes
of complete immobility and excessive activity
is characteristic. The latter can also be pro-
voked by percussing the maternal abdomen.
The spasmodic, jerky, uncoordinated "storms"
of movement differ dramatically from the har-

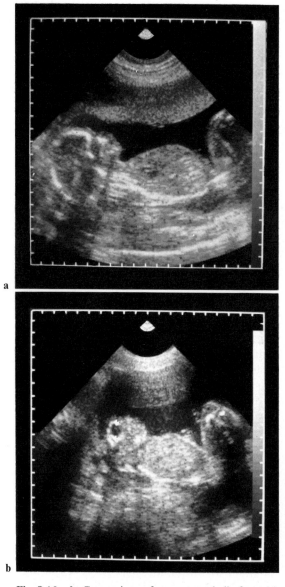

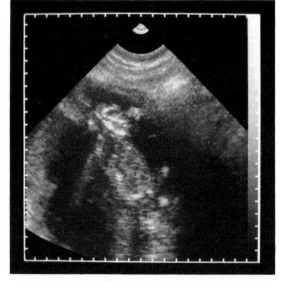

Fig. 8.17. Anencephaly at 17 weeks, the fetus here in a "sitting" breech position

Fig. 8.16a, b. Comparison of a normocephalic fetus (**a**) and an anencephalic fetus (**b**) at 18 weeks in longitudinal scans. In **b** note the absence of a calvarium over the orbits (diameter 12 mm)

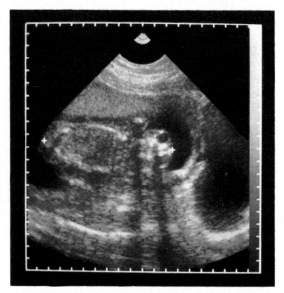

Fig. 8.18. Anencephaly at 19 weeks: head on *right* of sonogram. Crown-rump length only 107 mm

monious motor patterns of the healthy fetus, which by 14 weeks is already capable of coordinated movements (e.g., raising the hand to the mouth, assuming a comfortable position and posture). Twin pregnancies in which one fetus is anencephalic and the other is normal offer particularly striking evidence of behavioral differences. In one of three cases of this type that we have followed, we became concerned that constant punching and kicking by the an-

encephalus might cause a behavioral disorder in the normal twin.

Difficulties may be encountered in differentiating anencephaly from severe microcephaly. The flat cranial vault of microcephaly may be missed in frontal scans of the head, but it is easily appreciated in longitudinal scans (Fig. 8.4). In the case depicted the total brain weight was only 30 g, half of which was accounted for by the rudimentary cerebrum.

From a clinical standpoint, the prognosis for this case was extremely poor regardless of the specific diagnosis. This is not altered by the presence of "normal" alpha-fetoprotein values.

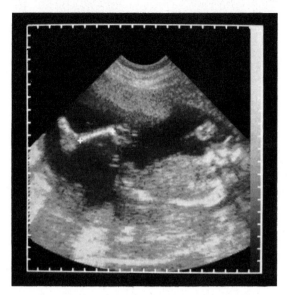

Fig. 8.19. Anencephaly at 20 weeks (*left:* tibia 27 mm)

The delay in arriving at the correct diagnosis in this case resulted in a 6-week ordeal for the couple involved. Amniotic band syndrome, a relatively rare anomaly, is typically distinguished from anencephaly by a marked asymmetry of the remaining portion of the calvarium. Finally, it is necessary to differentiate anencephaly from the acrania that is present in the acardius acephalus twin. The latter condition occurs exclusively in monozygotic twins, and in twins is even rarer than anencephaly. In one of the two cases we have seen to date (Fig. 8.5), the acardius twin led to significant cardiac decompensation in the healthy twin, acting similarly to a large, fast-growing tumor.

Today it should be possible to detect anencephaly routinely on early ultrasound examination between 16 and 20 weeks gestation. At the Gynecologic Center of Bonn University, not one case of anencephaly has been missed since 1968. Of the 50 cases diagnosed, 32 were detected prior to 24 weeks. A "late" diagnosis was invariably the result of a late referral. The earliest diagnosis of anencephaly was at

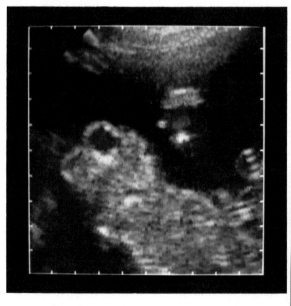

a

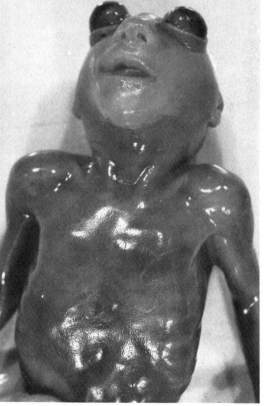

b

Fig. 8.20a, b. Anencephalic fetus at 20 weeks with extreme exophthalmos

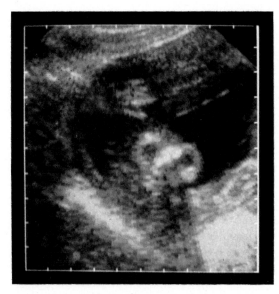

Fig. 8.21. Frontal view of face of an anencephalic fetus at 16 weeks, illustrating "eyeglass" phenomenon

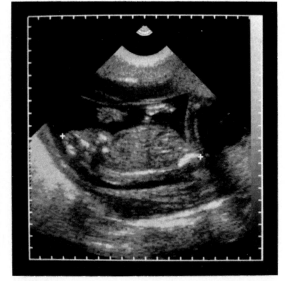

Fig. 8.23. Anencephaly in a twin pregnancy at 19 weeks. Anencephalic neonate was resuscitated to serve as kidney donor. (Dr. Scheel, personal communication 1984)

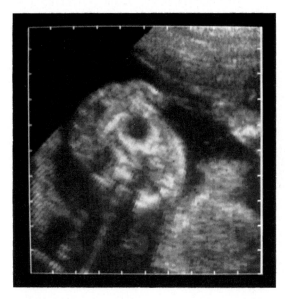

Fig. 8.22. Frontal view of face of an anencephalic fetus at 22 weeks, with facial cleft

12 weeks. We may regard the prenatal detection of anencephaly as a quality control criterion for ultrasound diagnosis. If an examiner records an anencephalus as "normal," this is an indication either that the equipment is faulty or (more likely) that the operator is not adequately trained. If the examiner notes that he is not getting a "normal" skull image and that the BPD cannot be measured, immediate referral to a specialized center is indicated. There is no excuse for an operator following the "do-it-yourself" principle, to examine a patient five or six times without making a definitive diagnosis. This not only wastes time and money, but imposes a needless psychological burden on the parents. In general, it may be said that no second form of investigation is needed to confirm the diagnosis of anencephaly. This pertains only to that anomaly, however. When considering the entire spectrum of neutral tube defects, the importance of the alpha-fetoprotein (AFP) assay as a screening method cannot be denied (U.K. Collaborative Study 1977). Kurjak (1980) reported on 37 cases of anencephaly without a single false-negative result. Robinson (1979) reported similar findings in a series of 321 high-risk cases that included 33 anencephalics. The amniocenteses for determining the amniotic fluid AFP were performed essentially for reasons of academic interest. In Campbell's series (1979) 17 anencephalics were detected in 409 high-risk pregnancies. Recently (1981) Campbell reported on 114 neural tube defects diagnosed prior to the 26th week. Only 14 of these were detected on routine ultrasound screening. All the others were high-risk patients, i.e., patients who either had a prior af-

fected fetus or were found to have a significant serum elevation of AFP during AFP screening, which is routinely practiced in parts of the U.K. (Ferguson-Smith et al. 1978).

When anencephaly is confirmed, the parents generally elect to have the pregnancy terminated. Since ultrasound screening enables the early recognition of an increasing number of fetal anomalies (18 of 21 cases before the 24th week at the Bonn University Gynecologic Center, 1982/83), it should generally be possible to terminate the pregnancy safely and within legal limits. When an anencephalic fetus is carried to term, it will probably become necessary to induce labor, because labor is often not initiated spontaneously due to the absence of a fetal neurohypophysis. This fact has to be considered in planning the obstetric management. A new rationale for electing the term delivery of an anencephalic fetus is offered by the possibility of using the fetus as an organ donor e.g. for kidneys (Fig. 8.23; Dr. Scheel, personal communication 1984).

8.2.2 Spina Bifida

Spina bifida is an abnormality of neural tube closure in which one or more vertebral arches fail to fuse (Figs. 8.24, 8.25). Between the extremes of rachischisis and spina bifida occulta, any number of intermediate forms may occur. Spina bifida cystica (aperta) is the most common and has the greatest clinical significance (Fig. 8.26). In this form the meninges (arachnoideae) herniate through the bony defect, forming an extracorporeal sac of variable size. This sac is termed a meningocele if it contains no nervous tissue, a meningomyelocele if it contains spinal cord. The latter carries a poorer prognosis. Approximately 90% of lesions are located in the lumber or lumbosacral region, with 6% affecting the thoracic spine and 3% the cervical spine (Fig. 8.30a, b). As a rule, the higher the level of the defect, the less favorable the prognosis in terms of neurologic function. This does not mean, however, that a "low" spina bifida implies a favorable prognosis. In the series of Ferguson-Smith et al. (1978), 70% of infants described as having "minor" neural tube defects were classified as severely handicapped. This means that in the cases that are most favorable in terms of the location and size

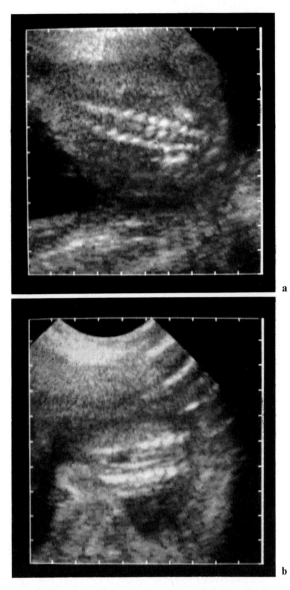

Fig. 8.24. a Longitudinal scan of lumbosacral spine in a healthy fetus. (Note segmentation of sacrum, caudal tapering.) Iliac wings flank spine. **b** A slightly more dorsal longitudinal scan in lumbar spina bifida. Note absence of spinous processes

of the lesion, it cannot be predicted with certainty whether the child will learn to walk or whether it will be continent. Moreover, the demonstration of intact leg function and bladder dynamics in utero does not necessarily imply a favorable prognosis in postnatal life (Campbell 1983, personal communication). Conversely, evidence of intrauterine cord paralysis in a fetus with a neural tube defect is always a poor prognostic sign. In our experience, the degree and rate of progression of the hydrocephalus that is generally associated with neural tube defects also have an important bearing on prognosis. Attention should also be given to the form and position of the feet. For example, we have found that when "early" clubfeet are discovered in association with a neural tube defect, a poorer prognosis is indicated.

With this in mind, one can appreciate the difficulties involved in the diagnosis of a neural tube defect by ultrasound. These difficulties result both from the varied presentations of the defect and from the challenging detailed examination which is required. It is not surprising that, in contrast to the positive record of sonography in anencephaly, it is quite common for spina bifida to be missed in initial examinations. It is unlikely that this situation will change significantly until a nationwide program of AFP screening is instituted. To date, convincing figures on the success rate of ultrasound in the detection of spina bifida have come only from England, where high-risk patients were examined by ultrasound experts. Campbell (1979) missed only 3 of 19 spina bifida cases in the second trimester. No false-positive diagnoses were made. However, eight of the fetuses in this series had associated hydrocephalus, and two had associated encephaloceles.

Both of these anomalies are easily recognized, and both are suggestive of a concomitant neural tube defect. Robinson (1979) had 15 cases of spina bifida in his series of 321 high-risk pregnancies. In 11 cases he was confident enough to make a diagnosis before amniocentesis was performed. In four cases he repeated the ultrasound examination after elevated AFP values were found, and in three of these cases the defect was recognized at that time. Only one small lumbosacral lesion was missed.

Our own experience (to the end of 1983) encompasses 35 spina bifida cases (Table 8.5). In 27 cases the lesion was correctly diagnosed pre-

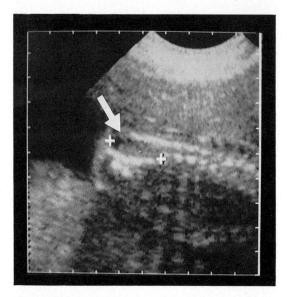

Fig. 8.25. Posterior coronal view of a large lumbar spina bifida at 22 weeks

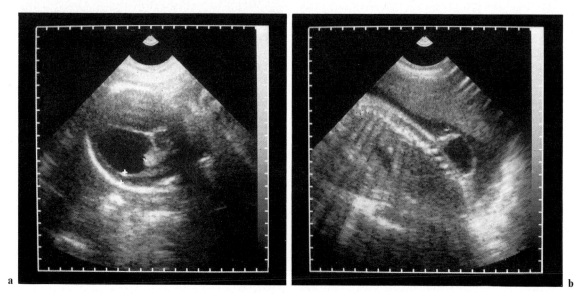

a   b

Fig. 8.26. Hydrocephalus (**a**) with concomitant lumbosacral meningomyelocele (**b**) at 32 weeks

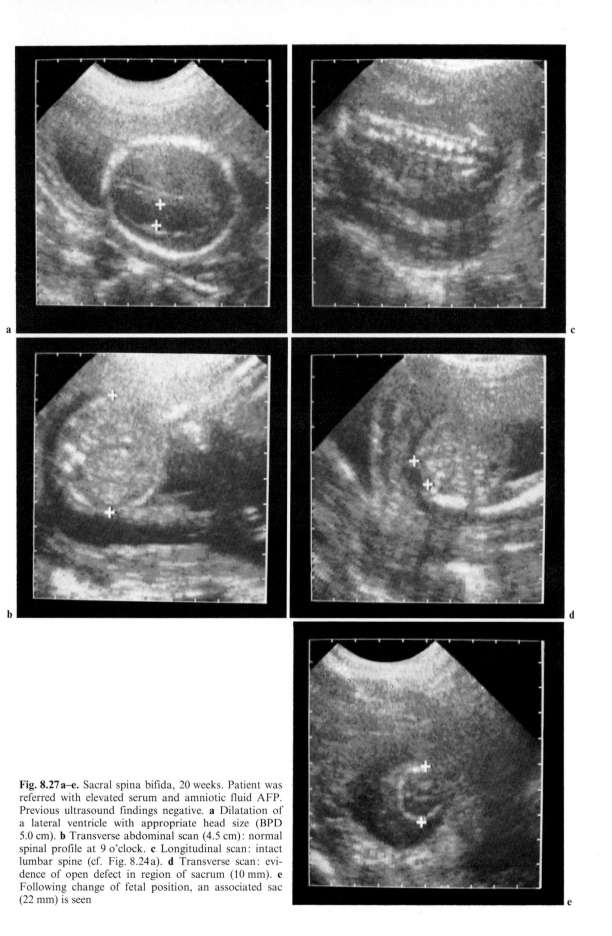

Fig. 8.27a–e. Sacral spina bifida, 20 weeks. Patient was referred with elevated serum and amniotic fluid AFP. Previous ultrasound findings negative. **a** Dilatation of a lateral ventricle with appropriate head size (BPD 5.0 cm). **b** Transverse abdominal scan (4.5 cm): normal spinal profile at 9 o'clock. **c** Longitudinal scan: intact lumbar spine (cf. Fig. 8.24a). **d** Transverse scan: evidence of open defect in region of sacrum (10 mm). **e** Following change of fetal position, an associated sac (22 mm) is seen

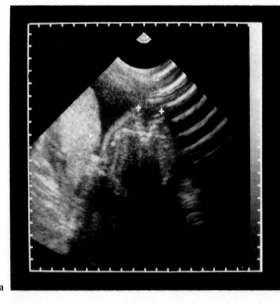

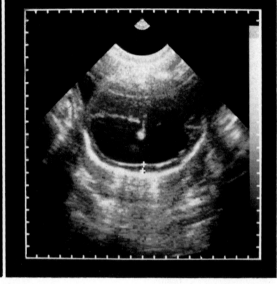

a

b

Fig. 8.28. a Spina bifida in transverse scan of trunk: open, V-shaped defect in vertebra is characteristic. b Fetal head shows marked hydrocephalus with a cortex only 5 mm thick

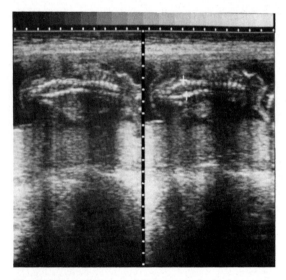

Fig. 8.29 Typical Y-shaped divergence of spinal contours in longitudinal scan of lumbar spina bifida

natally. Fourteen of the pregnancies were before 24 weeks; 8 were referred for an elevated AFP, 3 had a prior affected fetus, and the remainder were diagnosed on routine screening. One "early" case of lumbar spina bifida was not diagnosed until the 32nd week despite an intensive search prompted by an elevated amniotic fluid AFP at 18 weeks (1979). Serial observations of fetuses with spina bifida are summarized in Fig. 7.94. A typical pattern is demonstrated consisting of an initial microcephaly followed by a period of "catch-up" head growth. We attribute this late growth to the development of hydrocephalus. Nine of 19 "late" spina bifida cases that we have observed were referred for ultrasound evaluation with suspected intrauterine growth retardation. In each case we found that the BPD was small at the time of referral, but that the abdominal diameter was in the normal range. Growth patterns of this kind are suggestive of spina bifida.

By far the most important suggestive sign is dilatation of the cerebral ventricles, or hydrocephalus internus (Figs. 8.27 and 8.28). Whenever hydrocephalus is detected, the index of suspicion for associated anomalies is high, and the fetal spine should be carefully examined with all available means. In many cases this will mean referring the patient to a center specializing in the diagnosis of fetal anomalies.

During selective examination, the fetal spine is examined by segments on both longitudinal and transverse scans. As described above, a normal scan will demonstrate the parallel "double contour" of the lateral vertebral arches. A separation or Y-shaped divergence of the lateral margins is the classic feature of an open spinal defect on the longitudinal scan (Fig. 8.29). On transverse scans the affected segments will display a U- or V-shaped profile.

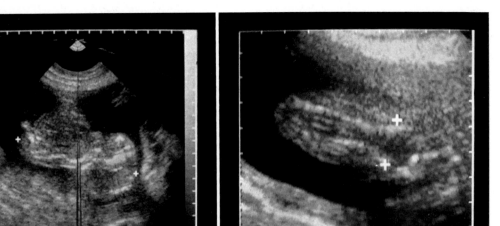

Fig. 8.30a, b. Cervical spina bifida in an iniencephalic fetus at 20 weeks (patient referred for early fetal growth retardation.) **a** Longitudinal scan of neckless fetus (*top*) with CRL of only 103 mm. **b** Cervical spina bifida in longitudinal zoom image

Unless the fetal spine is favorably positioned, it may be difficult or impossible to demonstrate the often subtle interruptions of vertebral contour that signify spina bifida (Fig. 8.27e). It is essential that the examiner proceed as patiently and carefully as possible. As in other situations, stimulation of the fetus with resultant changes in position (by percussing the maternal abdomen) and/or the scheduling of repeat examinations can be very helpful. If oligohydramnios is present, image definition can be enhanced by instilling an isotonic solution (e.g., 50–200 ml Normofundin) into the uterus. The benefits of this procedure should always be weighed against its risks (infection, induction of labor, rupture of fetal membranes, premature delivery), which should be discussed with the parents before a decision is made.

There is no question that even a "late" diagnosis of spina bifida is of value to the patient, as this will enable the timing and mode of the delivery to be selected. Emergency cesarean birth can be avoided, and the parents can be prepared psychologically for the birth of a malformed child. In our experience, spina bifida children who were diagnosed antenatally and delivered by elective cesarean birth have had remarkably good outcomes. Presumably the cesarean birth avoids the bacterial contamination and traumatization that may accompany a vaginal delivery.

The AFP screening program introduced in the U.K. has as its goal the "early" diagnosis of neural tube defects, with subsequent safe termination within the legal limits (in the U.K., before the end of the 26th week). Among our own patients, there have been three cases in which the parents elected to continue the pregnancy despite an early diagnosis of sacral or lumbosacral spina bifida. All three children have shown fair to good development following planned surgical correction of their defects. Admittedly, it is not possible to draw general conclusions on the basis of such a small sample. But it is clear that as experience is gained, our ability to assess the prognosis of fetal anomalies on a more individualized basis, and thus to calculate risks and benefits, will improve.

8.2.3 Encephalocele

Encephaloceles are less common. We have seen only 12 cases, 10 of which were found in screening examinations after 20 weeks. Almost all were associated with hydrocephalus (Figs. 8.31 and 8.32). Two of the fetuses were microcephalic, and there was one case of polyhydram-

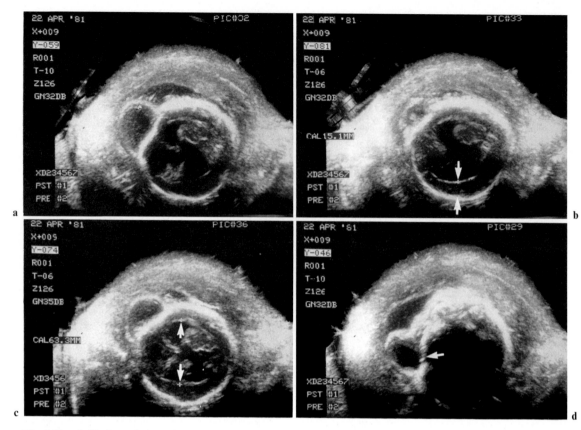

Fig. 8.31 a–d. Hydrocephalus with occipital infratentorial encephalocele at 34 weeks. **a** overview; **b** lateral brain mantle 15 mm; **c** dilatation of occipital horns; **d** defect in occiput (*arrow*)

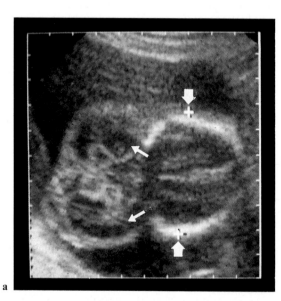
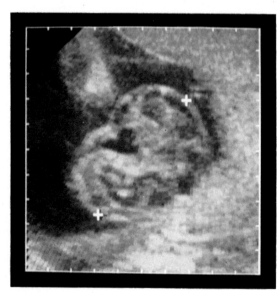

Fig. 8.32. a Exencephaly at 27 weeks: horizontal display. Greater part of cerebrum is prolapsed posteriorly (*small arrows*). In consequence, BPD is only 48 mm (marked microcephaly). **b** Exencephaly at 23 weeks: entire cerebrum presents as soft tissue mass outside skull

nios. Eleven of the 12 encephaloceles were occipital or dorsonuchal in location. To arrive at a prognosis in such cases, it is necessary to obtain the most complete sonographic "brain status" possible. It is particularly important to delineate the ventricles and the cerebellum and to check the symmetry of larger brain structures. It is also important to assess the topographic relations of the bony defect. If the defect is supratentorial, the sac most likely arises from the cerebrum; if the defect is infratentorial, the sac probably contains portions of the cerebellum. If this is the case, a poorer prognosis is indicated. In most cases, however, the sac contains no brain tissue at all, despite the presence of "soft tissue" echoes in the sonogram – usually these represent venous plexus. The absolute size of a purely "cystic" sac is of only secondary importance. Whenever an encephalomeningocele is detected, it is important to check for associated anomalies that might indicate a complex malformation syndrome (such as Meckel-Gruber syndrome, which has a gloomy prognosis). This means that a complete examination in the sense of exclusionary diagnosis should be performed (see Sect. 8.9). Differentiation from cervical cystic hygroma (frequent) or hemangioma (rare) can be difficult.

In our experience it is worthwhile to discuss the case with a neurosurgeon (using video documentation if possible) before obstetric decisions are made.

References

Brock DJH (1979) Prenatal diagnosis of neural tube defects. In: Weitzel HK, Schneider J (eds) Alpha-Fetoprotein in clinical medicine. Thieme, Stuttgart New York, p 1

Campbell S (1979) Early prenatal diagnosis of fetal abnormality by ultrasound B-scanning. In: Murken J-D, Stengel-Rutkowski S, Schwinger E (eds) *Prenatal Diagnosis*. Proceedings of the 3rd European Conference on Prenatal Diagnosis of Genetic Disorders, Enke, Stuttgart, p 183

Campbell S (1981) Ultrasonic diagnosis of cranial spinal defects. In: Kratochwil A, Kurjak A (eds) *Ultrasound in Medicine*. Proceedings of the 4th European Congress on Ultrasound in Medicine, Dubrovnik. Amsterdam, Excerpta Medica

Ferguson-Smith MA, May HM, Vince JD, Robinson HP, Rawlinson HA, Tait HA, Gibson AAM, Ratcliffe JG (1978) Avoidance of anencephalic and spina bifida births by maternal serum-alpha-fetoprotein screening. *Lancet* 1330

Kurjak A (1980) Fetal abnormalities in early and late pregnancy. In: Kurjak A (ed) Progress in Medical Ultrasound, Amsterdam, Excerpta Medica

Robinson HP (1979) The role of ultrasound in the prenatal diagnosis of neural tube defects. In: Murken J-D, Stengel-Rutkowski S, Schwinger W (eds) *Prenatal Diagnosis*. Stuttgart, Enke

U.K. Collaborative Study on Alpha-fetoprotein in: Amniotic-fluid alpha-fetoprotein measurement in antenatal diagnosis of anencephaly and open spina bifida in early pregnancy. Relation to neural tube defects. *Lancet*, 651–662, 1979

Warkany J (1971) *Congenital malformations. Notes and comments*. Chicago. Year Book Medical, pp 189–352

Weitzel H (1983) Alpha-Fetoprotein in der Geburtshilfe. Gynäkologe 16:148

8.3 Malformations of the Brain

8.3.1 Hydrocephalus

Congenital obstructive hydrocephalus unassociated with other neural tube defects has an incidence of about 1 in every 2,000 live births. The recurrence rate for communicating hydrocephalus is approximately 0.5%–1%. Obstructive hydrocephalus that is secondary to aqueductal stenosis is inherited as an X-linked trait and has a recurrence rate of 50% in male offspring. In the Dandy-Walker syndrome, the risk of recurrence is 25% or less based on the autosomal recessive transmission of the disorder.

Prior to 1975 hydrocephalus could be diagnosed with ultrasound only in cases where the fetal head was already enlarged. Hobbins et al. (1983) found in one case of obstructive hydrocephalus that ventricular dilatation was apparent by 23 weeks, but that the BPD did not show measurable enlargement until 27 weeks. This explains why all diagnoses prior to 1975 were made during the third trimester. With subsequent improvement in the resolution and graytone display of ultrasound equipment, it became possible to delineate intracranial structures with increasing clarity. Today, the recognition of ventricular dilatation forms the basis for the early diagnosis of hydrocephalus.

A number of authors have described the ventricle-to-hemisphere (V/H) ratio as a method for evaluating ventricular size (Garret 1979; Denkhaus and Winsberg 1979; Campbell et al.

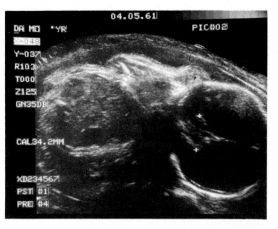

Fig. 8.33. Hydranencephaly at 34 weeks: longitudinal scan

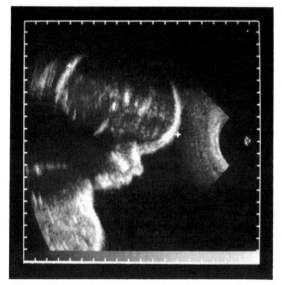

Fig. 8.34. Typical profile of hydrocephalic fetus (27 weeks), protruding forehead and depressed nasal root; OFD 104 mm

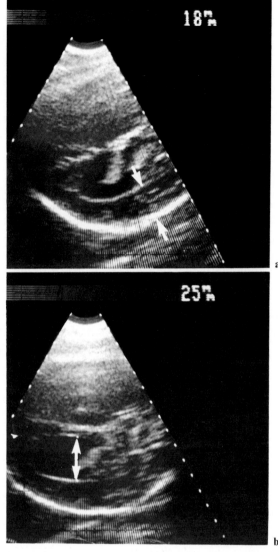

Fig. 8.35a, b. Moderate hydrocephalus internus. **a** Cortex 18 mm; **b** width of lateral ventricle 25 mm

1981). Garret (1979) states that a V/H ratio greater than 0.5 after 18 weeks gestation justifies a diagnosis of hydrocephalus. Jeanty and Romero (1984) and Hobbins (1981) point out that correct plane selection is all-important for obtaining an accurate measurement. The plane must traverse the lateral ventricles at the correct level and must be absolutely symmetrical in its orientation. It is illustrated in Fig. 7.17.

There are several factors which weaken the value of this method for the routine diagnosis of hydrocephalus: Only a slight deviation of the scanning plane will invalidate the measure-

ment. In addition the values reported to date show a large scatter. For example, Jeanty and Romero (1984) report that the normal ratio for 23 weeks is 0.34, with values ranging from 0.26 at the 10th percentile to 0.42 at the 90th percentile.

Hydrocephalus is a symptom, and can have various underlying causes. Accordingly, it is not surprising that it can manifest a variety of forms at different stages of pregnancy. Campbell (1979) reported on 14 cases in the second trimester. Ten of them had associated spina bifida. Campbell placed particular emphasis on his observation that fetal head circumference was not enlarged in any of his "early" cases. It follows that the diagnosis of hydrocephalus in the second trimester depends directly on the ability to visualize the cerebral ventricles with ultrasound. Extensive information on the intracranial anatomy of the fetus was published by Hadlock et al. (1981). They emphasized the advantages of real-time equipment, which can demonstrate vascular pulsations that are useful for orientation.

We have found that the earliest manifestation of hydrocephalus is a dilatation of the frontal and occipital horns (Figs. 8.35, 8.36, 8.37a, 8.40b). When hydrocephalus is advanced, profile views will show the characteristic bulging forehead (Fig. 8.34). However, it must be remembered that head enlargement is also present in thanatophoric dwarfs and in the cloverleaf skull syndrome. Other criteria are available for differentiating these conditions from hydrocephalus. Denkhaus and Winsberg (1979) consider the bifrontal horn width to be the most important parameter for assessing the development of hydrocephalus. They state that this width normally increases linearly from 11 mm at 12 weeks to approximately 25 mm at term.

Once hydrocephalus has been detected sonographically, a search should be made for associated malformations (meningomyelocele, spina bifida, omphalocele, etc.) so that an overall prognosis can be made. This should be done at an experienced ultrasound facility.

With regard to intrauterine therapy, Birnholz and Frigoletto (1981) have discussed the potential of repeated "atraumatic" cephalocentesis under ultrasound control. In their case report five successive cephalocenteses were performed

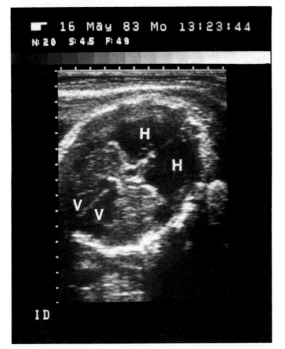

Fig. 8.36. Moderate hydrocephalus at 34 weeks: occipital horns (*H*) affected more severely than frontal horns (*V*)

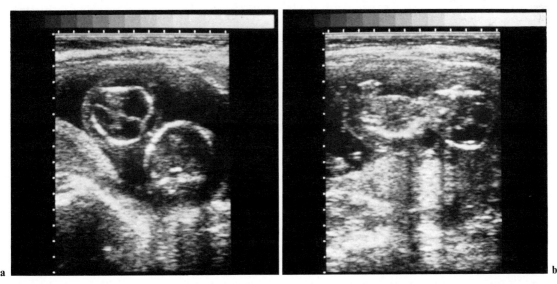

Fig. 8.37a, b. Twin pregnancy at 18 weeks. **a** Transverse scan of both heads, which are approximately equal in size, reveals hydrocephalus. **b** Longitudinal scan of affected fetus showing coexisting trunk edema

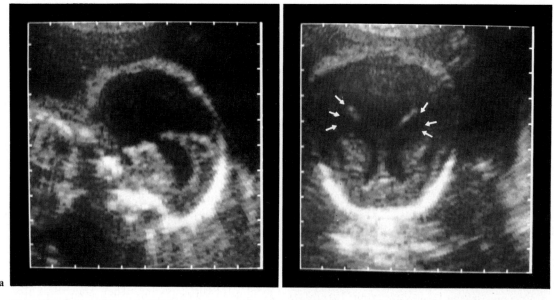

Fig. 8.38a, b. Special form of hydrocephalus at 24 weeks, with dilatation of fourth ventricle (Dandy-Walker syndrome). **a** Sagittal scan demonstrating echo-free occipital region. **b** Transverse scan showing normal-sized lateral ventricles (*arrows* indicate occipital horns)

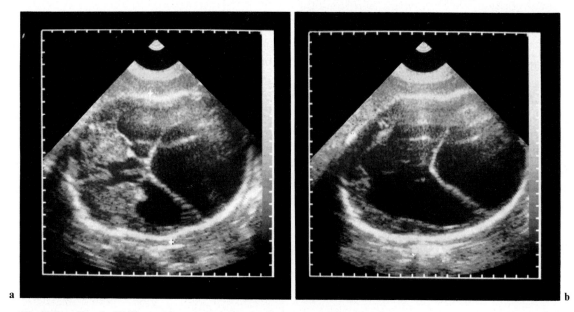

Fig. 8.39. a Dandy-Walker syndrome: tentorium well demarcated by dilated fourth ventricle, third ventricle also enlarged. **b** Slightly higher scan: dilatation of lateral ventricles secondary to obstruction

starting at 25 weeks. The fetus was delivered by cesarean birth at 35 weeks. According to the authors, no signs of injury were visible on the scalp after delivery. It is clear that only a few selected cases will derive benefit from such therapy. Jeanty and Rodesch (1981) introduced the prototype of a small shunt designed to provide continuous intrauterine drainage of cerebrospinal fluid into the amniotic cavity. The shunt consists of a 3- to 4-cm-long polyethylene catheter that is introduced into a ventricle under ultrasound guidance with the aid of a special needle. (When the needle is withdrawn, the ends of the catheter curl to keep it from slipping

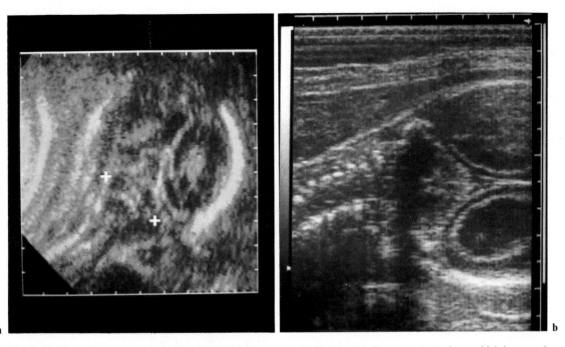

Fig. 8.40a Frontal scan through head at level of spine. *Crosses* indicate cerebellum over tentorium, which is normal for gestation. Choroid plexus echoes are seen in the ventricles. b Hydrocephalus: frontal scan at level of spine over normal cerebellum. Note marked dilatation of occipital horns (29 weeks)

into or out of the ventricle.) At the center of the catheter is a valve that permits flow in one direction only. Of the various intrauterine therapies for hydrocephalus that have been proposed to date, this method seems to us to be the most promising.

Other Intracranial Anomalies

There are several rare types of intracerebral pathology which vary in their prognosis and present typical ultrasound features. Their recognition is important in terms of prognosis and management.

Figure 8.33 shows the typical sonographic appearance of hydranencephaly. The cerebral hemispheres are absent, and in their place is a collection of fluid that fills the cranial vault up to the calvarium. Only the brain stem, tentorium, and cerebellum are intact. This malformation is believed to result from on occlusion of the internal carotid artery early in development (Lee and Warren 1977). The prognosis is grave.

Another anomaly that is easily recognized sonographically is the Dandy-Walker syndrome (Figs. 8.38 and 8.39). Neuropathologically, this syndrome involves a combination of hydrocephalus with a cystic dilatation of the fourth ventricle, maldevelopment of the cerebellum, and enlargement of the posterior fossa (Fischer 1973). It is important to distinguish this malformation from isolated cysts of the posterior fossa. Because these cysts do not cause significant disruption of brain anatomy, their prognosis is more favorable (Dempsey and Koch 1981).

A rare but easily recognized abnormality is unilateral ventricular dilatation (Hartung and Yiu-Chiu 1983). In our population we observed three cases (Fig. 8.41). Figure 8.41b, c shows a case of "late" detected papilloma of the choroid plexus with concomitant unilateral hydrocephalus and compression of the contralateral hemisphere. After extirpation of this tumor the baby is doing fine. Subarachnoid cysts may be misleading concerning hydrocephalus. In one case of ours (Fig. 8.42b–d), after postpartum drainage of the cyst the dilatation of the ventricular system decreased, and the baby is so far without any neurological handicap.

It should again be emphasized that a fetus with confirmed hydrocephalus should always be screened for associated malformations. The search should be an intensive one, for the detec-

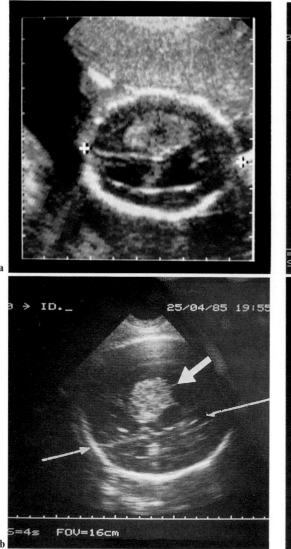

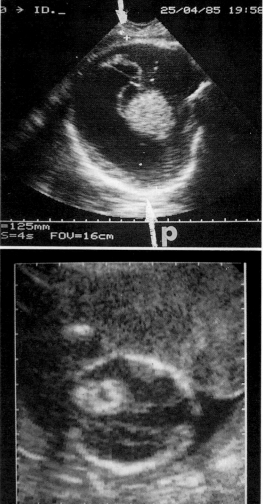

Fig. 8.41. a Unilateral ventricular dilatation: unusual structure of choroid plexus in region near transducer remained unexplained (autopsy was refused). **b** Frontal scan of papilloma of choroid plexus at 37 weeks: hyper-reflective mass (*arrow*) surrounded by dilated lateral ventricle, resulting in marked midline shift and compression of contralateral hemisphere. **c** Same case as **b,** sagittal scan: OFD 125 mm. *a,* anterior; *p,* posterior. **d** Intraventricular hemorrhage in a very small for gestational age fetus at 29 weeks: BPD 58 mm (proven on autopsy)

tion of coexisting anomalies will critically influence individual obstetric management.

The presence of cystic structures within the choroid plexus has no pathologic significance (Fig. 8.42a). Such defects should be differentiated from the lesions of macroporencephaly (Fig. 8.43). The latter is characterized by the presence of smooth-walled cavities in the hemispheres that occasionally communicate with the ventricles. They are believed to result from hypoxic injury, and their diagnosis has been well

described in the context of neonatal ultrasonography (Bliesener 1984).

There is evidence that it is possible to diagnose cerebral hemorrhages prenatally with ultrasound. Kim and Elyaderani (1982) described the intrauterine diagnosis of a ventricular hemorrhage culminating in fetal death at 28 weeks. Dann et al. (1983) and Chinn and Fill (1983) presented case reports of intracranial hemorrhages diagnosed soon after delivery which, based on their morphology and temporal set-

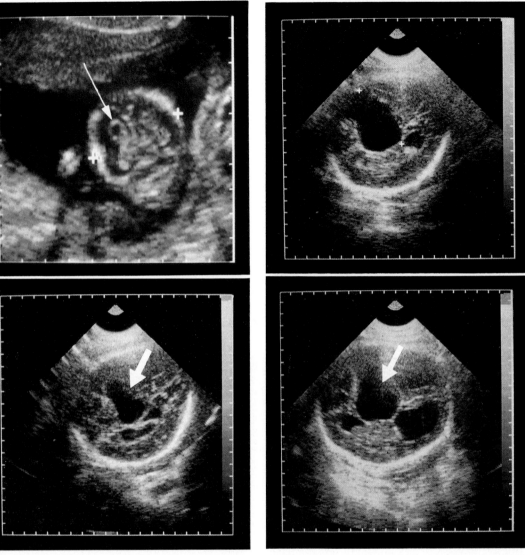

Fig. 8.42. a Cyst within choroid plexus at 17 weeks. **b** Subarachnoid cyst (*arrow*) originating inferior to sella and causing midline shift: detected at 35 weeks. **c** Inferi-or horizontal head scan: widest expansion of cyst at 35 weeks. **d** Same case at 38 weeks: cyst has not grown, but now there is progressive hydrocephalus

ting, had obviously developed antenatally. These reports suggest a broad range of new applications for obstetric ultrasonography and raise new possibilities for the elucidation of significant causal relationships in perinatology.

The improved resolution of modern equipment has made it possible to delineate intracerebral structures with increasing detail, permitting evaluations to go beyond a simple assessment of skull contour. But this can also lead to errors of diagnosis, especially in cases where the equipment is newly acquired. An examiner who is accustomed to seeing only the skull outline and midline echo on a sonogram must know how to interpret the details visible on a higher quality image, and also how the sizes of structures normally vary at different stages of gestation. Figure 8.44 shows a frozen section of a normal fetal brain at 20 weeks. The section passes through the region of the lateral ventricles. The ventricular cavities are still relatively large at this stage, and the lateral sulcus is not yet narrowed by the surrounding gyri. Particular physical characteristics, depending on the

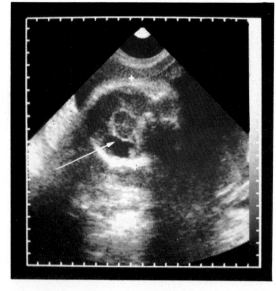

Fig. 8.43. Porencephaly: brain tissue is replaced by an isolated, well-defined cavity (*arrow*)

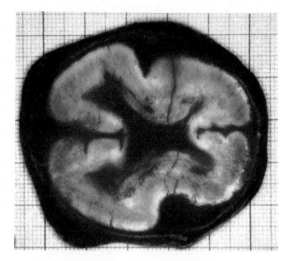

Fig. 8.44. Frozen section of normal brain at 20 weeks: section traverses lateral ventricles, which are still physiologically large; gyri have not yet narrowed insula

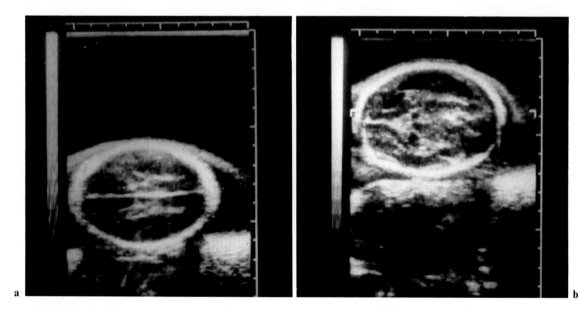

a   b

Fig. 8.45. a Pseudohydrocephalus in far ventricle. **b** Pseudohydrocephalus in near ventricle. These artifacts change as distance between head and transducer is reduced

type of instrument, can also lead to errors of diagnosis. In a biparietal transverse scan, the two halves of the brain may show differences in echodensity depending on their distance from the transducer, with fewer echoes occurring in the region farther from the acoustic source. If the head is brought closer to the transducer

than usual, the echogenic area will "migrate" from the near to the far hemisphere (Fig. 8.45). This artefact can be corrected to some extent by adjusting the gain control (Staudach and Lassmann 1984). In doubtful cases, however, referral for detailed expert evaluation is always preferable to a false-negative diagnosis.

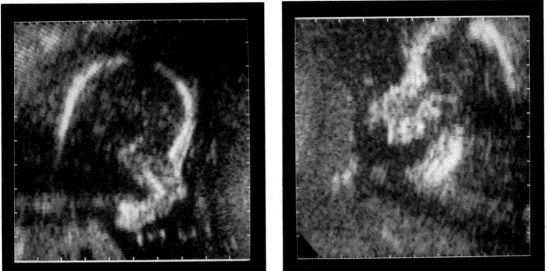

Fig. 8.46. a Microcephaly at 23 weeks: profile shows high forehead but shortened OFD. **b** Same case with opened mouth: disproportion of size of face to cranial skull is revealed. **c** Extreme case of microcephaly: weight of brain 15 g

8.3.2 Microcephaly

Microcephaly is defined as abnormal smallness of the head (Fig. 8.46). It may be the result of abnormal changes in bony structures with no significant disruption of brain anatomy (craniosynostosis), or it may occur in association with microencephaly, in which case mental retardation is inevitable.

Microcephaly is estimated to occur in 1 in every 6,200–8,000 births (Book et al. 1953; Koch 1959). Etiologically, it may be inherited as an autosomal recessive trait associated with Meckel-Gruber syndrome or parental consanguinity, or it may result from prenatal exposure to harmful agents. Not infrequently, it is associated with chromosome abnormalities, indicating that karyotyping may be of value in doubtful cases. Microcephaly should not be diagnosed biometrically unless the BPD is below the 2 SD limit, and many authors recommend that 3 SD be accepted as the criterion. As always, the basis for this evaluation is a well-established gestational age. Relatively few cases of prenatal diagnosis of microcephaly have been described in the literature, due to the rarity of the condition (Rose 1977; Garret et al. 1975).

The problems involved in the prenatal detection of microcephaly are reviewed by Kurtz et al. (1980). Initial biometry indicates that the BPD is definitely small for gestational age in the presence of normal trunk size. It is essential in these cases that the OFD and HC be determined. In doubtful cases, femur length should additionally be measured. If trunk size and femur length are found to be appropriate for age, and all head dimensions are below the 2 SD limit, a presumptive diagnosis of microcephaly may be made, and the patient should be referred for more intensive evaluation. As mentioned above, the possible association of microcephaly with chromosome abnormalities (trisomy 13, trisomy 18) is also an indication for genetic testing. During intensive examination all relevant biometric data are checked, and meticulous screening is carried out on intracerebral structures, the facial skeleton, and facial soft tissues. True microcephaly is almost always associated with a shift in the proportions of the cranium and facial skeleton. Frequent serial examinations are performed in which fetal profile, facial dynamics, orbital dimensions, etc. are evaluated. It is therefore obvious that microcephaly should not be diagnosed by a relatively inexperienced examiner alone, and even those with considerable experience should be extremely cautious in view of the legal problems involved.

References

Birnholz JC, Frigoletto FD (1981) Antenatal treatment of hydrocephalus. N Engl J Med 30:1021

Bliesener JA (1984) Sonographie der normalen und pathologischen Hirnanatomie bei Neugeborenen und Säugling. Habilitationsschrift, Köln

Book JA, Schult JW, Reed SC (1953) A clinical and genetical study of microcephaly. Am J Ment Defic 57:637

Campbell S (1979) Early prenatal diagnosis of fetal abnormality by ultrasound B-scanning. In: Murken JD, Stengel-Rutkowski S, Schwinger E (eds) Prenatal diagnosis. Enke, Stuttgart, S 183

Campbell S, Griffin D, Little D (1981) Ultrasonic diagnosis of cranial spinal defects. In: Kurjak A, Kratochwill A (eds) Recent advances in ultrasound diagnosis. 3. Excerpta Medica International Congress Series 553, Amsterdam

Chinn DH, Fill RA (1983) Extensive intracranial hemorrhage in utero. J Ultrasound Med 2:285

Dann StM, Di Pietro MA, Faix RG, Bowermann RA (1983) The sonographic appearance of old intraventricular hemorrhage present a birth. J Ultrasound Med 2:283

Dempsey PJ, Koch HJ (1981) In utero diagnosis of Dandy-Walker-Syndrome: Differentiation from extra-axial posterior fossa cyst. J Clin Ultrasound 9:403

Denkhaus H, Winsberg F (1979) Ultrasonic measurement of the fetal ventricular system. Radiology 131:781

Fischer EG (1973) Dandy-Walker-Syndrome: an evaluation of surgical tratment. J Neurosurg 39:615

Garret WJ (1979) Ultrasound in discerning normal fetal anatomy. In: Hobbins JC (ed) Diagnostic ultrasound in obstetrics. Churchill Livingstone, New York Edinburgh London

Garret WJ, Fisher CC, Kosoff G (1975) Hydrocephaly, microcephaly and anencephaly diagnosed in pregnancy by ultrasonic echography. Med J Aust 2:587

Hadlock FP, Deter RL, Park SK (1981) Real-time sonography: Ventricular and vascular anatomy of the fetal brain in utero. AJR 136:137

Hartung RW, Yiu-Chiu V (1983) Demonstration of unilateral hydrocephalus in utero. J Ultrasound Med 2:369

Hobbins JC, Winsberg F, Berkowitz RL (1983) Ultrasonography in obstetrics and gynecology. Wiliams & Wilkins, Baltimore London

Jeanty P, Rodesch F (1981) Is antenatal diagnosis enough? Free lecture: 4th European congress on ultrasonics in medicine, Dubrovnik

Jeanty P, Romero R (1984) Obstetrical ultrasound. McGraw-Hill, New York

Kim MS, Elyaderani MK (1982) Sonographic diagnosis of cerebro-ventricular hemorrhage in utero. Radiology 142:479

Koch G (1959) Genetics of microcephaly in man. Acta Genet Med Gemellol (Roma) 8:75

Kurtz AB, Wappner RJ, Rubin CS, Cole-Beuglet C, Ross RD, Goldberg BB (1980) Ultrasound criteria for in utero diagnosis of microcephaly. J Clin Ultrasound 8:11

Lee TG, Warren BH (1977) Antenatal diagnosis of hydranencephaly by ultrasound: Correlation with ventriculography and computed tomography. J Clin Ultrasound 5:271

Rose JS (1977) The ultrasound diagnosis of fetal neural tube abnormalities. Ann Radiol 1:19

Staudach A, Laßmann R (1984) Ultraschalldiagnostik von fetalen Mißbildungen. Oester Aerztetg 39/7:476

U.K. Collaborative Study (1977) On alpha-fetoprotein in relation to neural tube defects. Maternal serum-alpha-fetoprotein measurement in antenatal screening for anencephaly and spina bifida in early pregnancy. Lancet I:1323

Warkany J (1971) Congenital malformation. Year Book Medical Publishers, Chicago

8.4 Malformations Involving the Abdomen and Gastrointestinal Tract

From a pathologic standpoint it would seem reasonable to continue to review fetal anomalies by organ systems, but from the standpoint of diagnostic ultrasound, sonographic morphology is the most rational basis for diagnosis. In this regard it is appropriate to distinguish between abdominal wall defects and intrafetal structural abnormalities. Defects in the fetal abdominal wall have typical sonographic appearances both in anterior midsagittal scans and in transverse scans owing to the presence of extruded viscera. In the assessment of intrafetal anomalies, the relationship of cystic structures to the gastrointestinal tract or urogenital tract (Sect. 8.5) is fundamental. Generally we recommend that the urogenital tract be examined first.

8.4.1 Abdominal Wall Defects

The primary distinction to be made is between omphalocele and gastroschisis.

Omphaloceles range in reported frequency from 1 in 2,280 to 1 in 10,000. The pathogenesis involves an inhibitory malformation in which the small bowel fails to reenter the abdomen with rotation of the umbilical loop. Umbilical hernias of this type may contain liver, spleen, and pancreas in addition to bowel. Accordingly, a distinction is drawn between small omphaloceles (umbilical funicular hernia) and large omphaloceles (hepatomphalos). In all cases the hernial sac is covered by amniotic epithelium from the umbilical cord.

Gastroschisis, also called paraomphalocele or "omphalocele without a sac," differs from om-

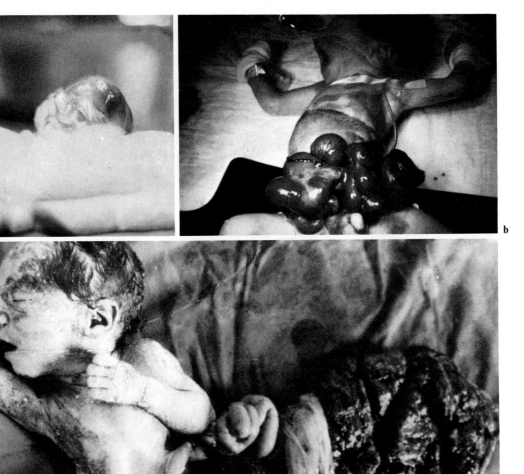

Fig. 8.47a–c. Phenotypes: **a** Omphalocele; **b** gastroschisis; **c** eventration

phalocele in the absence of a hernial sac and in its location, which is usually to the right of the umbilicus. The umbilical cord enters the abdomen separate from the hernial opening, and the extruded abdominal viscera float freely in the amniotic fluid.

A special form is *eventration,* in which the contents herniate through a large, central defect and are in direct contact with the chorion of the placenta, covered only by a short piece of umbilical cord. The morphology of the three different wall defects is shown in Fig. 8.47a–c.

Omphalocele. The ability to diagnose fetal omphalocele with ultrasound is well documented with case reports (Roberts 1978; Lomar et al. 1979; Zaleski et al. 1978; Meyenburg and Maasen 1979; Niesen and Hansmann 1979). The various forms were surveyed by Schaffer et al. (1983). Our own collective experience is summarized in Sect. 8.9. The earliest time at which omphalocele can be diagnosed is 12 weeks gestation (Fig. 8.48a, b; Schmidt et al. 1981; Hansmann 1983). The relationship between diagnosis and management options has been well

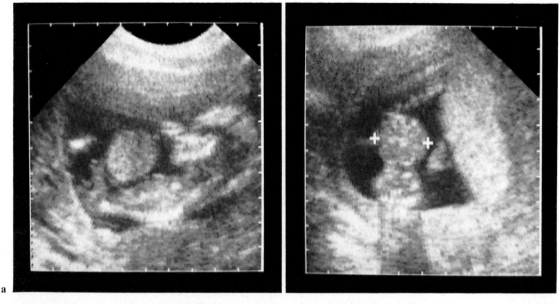

a   b

Fig. 8.48a, b. Omphalocele. **a** Longitudinal scan at 12 weeks: spherical, echo-dense structure anterior to abdomen. **b** Transverse scan at 12 weeks: mass (diameter 2 cm) is in front of fetal abdomen (spine at 6 o'clock)

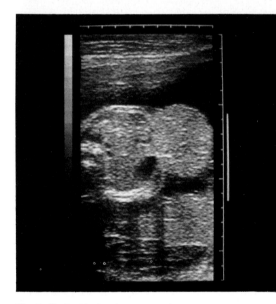

Fig. 8.50. Omphalocele at 25 weeks in trisomy 13: umbilical vein (*arrows*) coursing through omphalocele

Fig. 8.49. Omphalocele at 28 weeks: hernial sac contains liver tissue, stomach is intraabdominal

explored (Niesen and Hansmann 1979; Staudach et al. 1984). Our policies in this area remain essentially unchanged. For omphalocele diagnosed in early pregnancy, we feel that termination is the best option in view of the high incidence of associated malformations (30%–60%) and the diminished chance of infant survival. The not infrequent association of

omphalocele with chromosome abnormalities (Staudach et al. 1981) emphasizes the importance of genetic evaluation. When an omphalocele is detected at a later stage of pregnancy, decisions will have to be made with regard to the timing and mode of the delivery. Large omphaloceles (Figs. 8.49–8.51) may cause mechanical interference with delivery or may rupture at birth. The risk of infection by bacterial contamination and the potential need for prompt surgical intervention further worsen the prognosis. In these cases delivery by elective cesar-

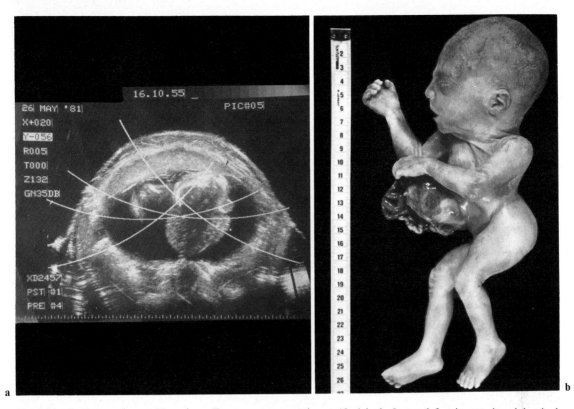

Fig. 8.51 a, b. Eventration at 28 weeks. **a** Transverse scan: spine at 12 o'clock. Large defect in anterior abdominal wall. **b** Phenotype

ean birth will eliminate the problem of dystocia and maximize the infant's chance of survival. Preparations should be made for primary care of the omphalocele in the delivery room and for subsequent management by a pediatric surgeon.

The risk of recurrence of this malformation is small, and only sporadic cases have been described. In cases of a prior affected fetus, the risk should be discussed with the parents, taking special care to mention that selective ultrasound examination in the first half of pregnancy can exclude omphalocele with certainty. The most favorable period for the examination is from 15 to 21 weeks.

Gastroschisis. Gastroschisis is less common and, if small, is not always easy to diagnose. Usually it is not the abdominal wall defect that is first noticed, but the floating loops of bowel, which present on certain planes as multiple circular echoes in the amniotic cavity (Fig. 8.52e). In many cases they appear as convoluted structures distant from the fetal trunk (Fig. 8.52a–

d). By tracing these structures to the abdominal wall, it is often possible to find the site of emergence of the bowel through the hernial defect (Fig. 8.52a).

Flexed position of the fetal extremities can prevent the direct visualization of small loops. In these cases the diagnosis should be confirmed by serial examinations once indirect warning signs have been noted. The main indirect sign is a change in the relative proportions of the chest and abdomen, with the latter appearing small. This is confirmed by thoracoabdominometry. Deviation of the abdominal aorta on sagittal and frontal scans (lateral or anterior bowing of a short segment) is another indirect warning sign. Extruded bowel loops almost always cause aortic deviation due to traction on the mesenteric vessels.

A late diagnosis of gastroschisis is likewise an indication for cesarean birth following the exclusion of associated anomalies. The opportunity to prepare postnatal care in cooperation with the pediatric surgeon is reason enough for this approach, quite apart from the increased

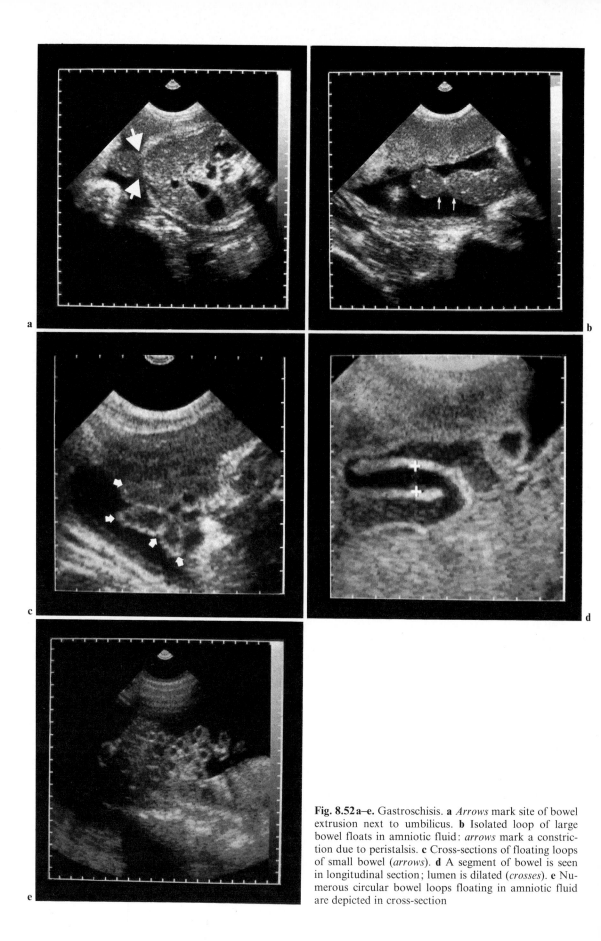

Fig. 8.52 a–e. Gastroschisis. **a** *Arrows* mark site of bowel extrusion next to umbilicus. **b** Isolated loop of large bowel floats in amniotic fluid: *arrows* mark a constriction due to peristalsis. **c** Cross-sections of floating loops of small bowel (*arrows*). **d** A segment of bowel is seen in longitudinal section; lumen is dilated (*crosses*). **e** Numerous circular bowel loops floating in amniotic fluid are depicted in cross-section

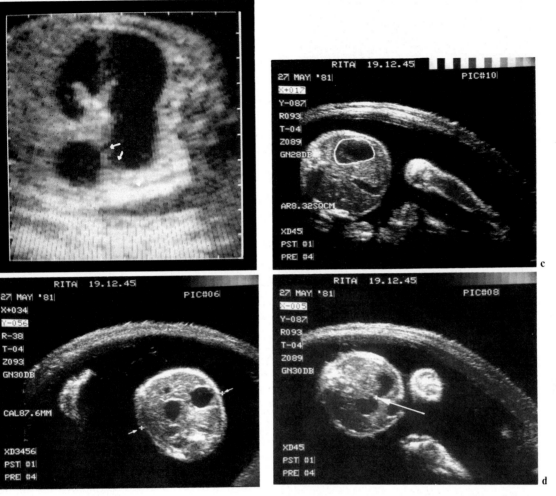

Fig. 8.53a–d. Duodenal atresia. **a** Double bubble sign at 30 weeks. **b** Transverse abdominal scan: pronounced double bubble sign in presence of hydramnios: spine at 5 o'clock. **c** Transverse scan of trunk. Region used to measure stomach area (32 cm^2) is outlined: spine at 10 o'clock. **d** *Arrow* marks junction of stomach and duodenum (pylorus)

risk of traumatization and infection that would accompany a vaginal delivery (Dunne and Johnson 1979; Giulian and Alvear 1978; Lomar et al. 1979). It is still unclear whether preterm delivery improves the prognosis of the affected fetus. However, it is noteworthy that as term approaches and the amniotic fluid volume decreases, the risk of intrauterine compression of the bowel loops increases.

8.4.2 Intraabdominal Structural Abnormalities

If sonograms reveal fluid-filled, "cystic" structures within the abdomen, and the urogenital tract appears normal, the following possibilities should be considered in making a differential diagnosis:

Proximal bowel atresia
Malrotation
Choledochal cyst
Mesenteric cyst
Meconium ileus
Microcolon
Anal atresia
Ovarian cyst

In contrast to severe urogenital malformations and anal atresia, obstructive lesions of the upper digestive tract are generally associated with polyhydramnios. Purely cystic lesions (choledo-

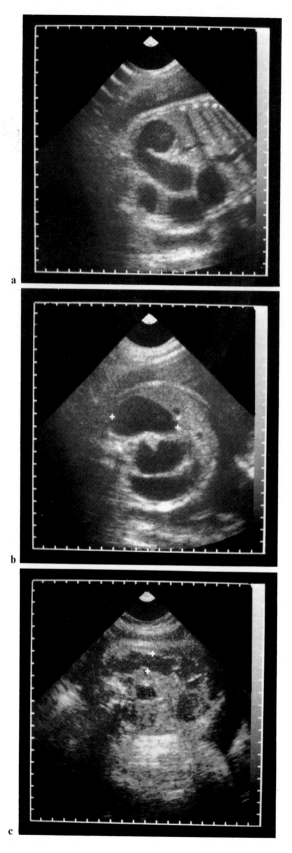

chal cyst, mesenteric cyst, ovarian cyst) are usually not associated with polyhydramnios. Duodenal atresia is recognized by the familiar "double bubble" sign (Fig. 8.53), one bubble representing the overdistended stomach and the other the fluid-filled segment of duodenum between the pylorus and the stenosis (Fig. 8.53d). This double structure may be seen in all planes of section, because a similar phenomenon can be simulated on a tangential scan of the stomach. Duodenal atresia may be associated with chromosome defects (trisomy 21), so karyotyping is indicated. The prenatal diagnosis of meconium ileus was described by Winter (1981). With anal atresia (Fig. 8.54), there may be massive engorgement of the bowel loops proximal to the obstruction (Fig. 8.54a, b). In the case of Fig. 8.54c, megacolon was also present. With a cloacal malformation, no division is apparent between the bladder and rectum in the lower abdomen – there is only a large, common, fluid-filled cavity.

Duplication of parts of the intestine may also create abnormal intraabdominal structures (Fig. 8.55). It is important in these cases to watch for hyperperistalsis and/or signs of perforation (ascites, fibrin flags etc.). Immediate surgery may save the baby's life.

Diaphragmatic Malformations. The primary communication between the thorax and abdominal cavity is closed secondarily during the course of development by the formation of two pleuroperitoneal membranes that are reinforced by ingrowth of muscular elements. If this development is anomalous, defects of varying size and location will result. The majority of these defects [80% according to Brandesky (1983)] occur on the left side. The incidence of diaphragmatic malformations is approximately 1 in 2,200 (Moore 1980). Large diaphragmatic defects are of perinatal interest because of the acute symptoms that occur postnatally, but even small defects can often produce vague symptoms over a period of days. A large defect may allow the stomach, bowel, spleen, and sometimes even portions of the liver to herniate

Fig. 8.54a–c. Anal atresia at 32 weeks: **a** Longitudinal scan: distended loops of large bowel. **b** Transverse scan of same fetus: overfilled stomach (*crosses*), greatly distended bowel loops. **c** Anal atresia and megacolon (*crosses:* distended colon)

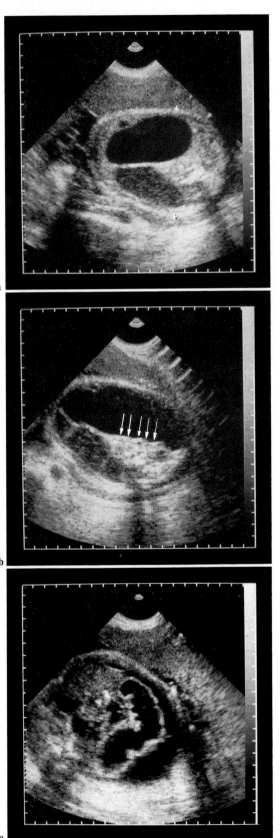

into the chest, causing displacement of the mediastinal organs and pulmonary compression and accounting for postnatal symptoms of respiratory distress. Cardiac displacement is usually toward the right side. Compression of the lung can cause severe pulmonary hypoplasia. This is why the anomaly has a 50%–90% mortality, despite the relative ease of surgical closure of the defect after birth (Harrison and Lorimier 1981).

It is possible to diagnose diaphragmatic defects prenatally using ultrasound (Jeanty and Romero 1984). To date we have made this diagnosis sonographically in ten cases. Figure 8.56 shows the typical appearance of a defect. The herniation of bowel into the chest almost always causes cardiac displacement.

The ability to diagnose such defects prenatally, together with the high postnatal mortality, have prompted investigators to use animal models to determine whether prenatal correction of the defect can prevent the occurrence of pulmonary hypoplasia by relieving lung compression. Harrison et al. (1980) succeeded in preventing hypoplasia by the intrauterine correction of experimentally produced diaphragmatic defects in fetal lambs. Harrison (1983) recommends that a confirmatory amniogram be obtained in cases where suspicion of the defect is raised by sonograms. The extent to which findings in laboratory animals can be applied to human medicine remains unclear.

But even a presumptive diagnosis can significantly improve the prognosis of affected fetuses by allowing preparation for primary care.

The prenatal diagnosis of all the abnormalities discussed above has as its main goal not termination of the pregnancy, but improvement of the prospects for specific, organized, adequate postnatal therapy. Particularly in cases

Fig. 8.55. a. Duplication of intestine with threatened perforation at 34 weeks: abdominal cross-section shows two dilated parts of intestine. Anterior part contains pure fluid and shows no peristalsis, while in posterior part, containing a soup-like mass (speckled cells), marked hyperperistalsis can be seen. Side-to-side anastomosis was performed on day of delivery, and baby is doing fine. **b** A more inferior oblique section in same case: part of "empty" distal small bowel (*arrows*). **c** Perforation of intestine in another case of duplication of small bowel due to inferior stenosis at 34 weeks. Oblique abdominal section shows widened loop of intestine with hyperperistalsis, surrounded by ascites

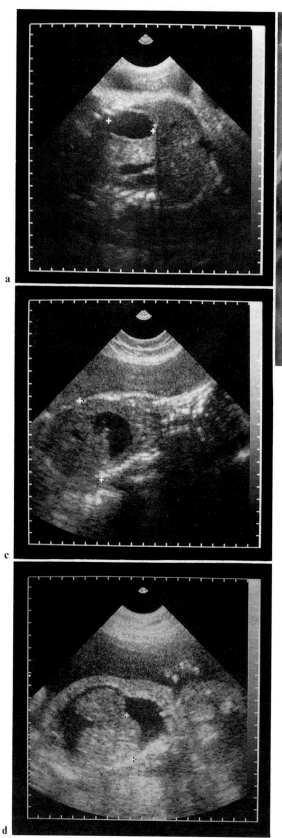
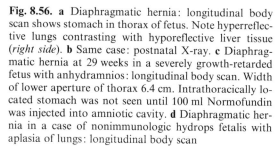

Fig. 8.56. a Diaphragmatic hernia: longitudinal body scan shows stomach in thorax of fetus. Note hyperreflective lungs contrasting with hyporeflective liver tissue (*right side*). **b** Same case: postnatal X-ray. **c** Diaphragmatic hernia at 29 weeks in a severely growth-retarded fetus with anhydramnios: longitudinal body scan. Width of lower aperture of thorax 6.4 cm. Intrathoracically located stomach was not seen until 100 ml Normofundin was injected into amniotic cavity. **d** Diaphragmatic hernia in a case of nonimmunologic hydrops fetalis with aplasia of lungs: longitudinal body scan

where the need for pediatric intervention is anticipated, the delivery should take place at a tertiary obstetric/neonatal facility.

Esophageal Atresia. Esophageal atresia, which has an incidence of 1 in 1,500 live births, is difficult to detect prenatally with ultrasound. Ninety percent of these fetuses have concomitant esophagotracheal fistulas which allow passage of fluid into the stomach (Scott and Wilson 1957). Thus, a filled stomach does not exclude esophageal atresia. However, if hydramnios is present and the stomach is difficult to identify even on serial examinations, and if no fetal swallowing movements are observed, one should suspect esophageal atresia and examine for it after delivery.

If a differential diagnosis of intraabdominal lesions is not obtainable during initial examination, particularly with regard to distinguishing between urogenital and intestinal anomalies, one should strive for urgent clarification of the findings in cooperation with a center specializing in diagnostic ultrasound.

References

Brandesky G (1973) Zwerchfell. In: Kunz H (ed) Operationen im Kindesalter. Thieme, Stuttgart

Dunne MG, Johnson ML (1979) The ultrasonic demonstration of fetal abnormalities in utero. J Reprod Med 23:195

Giulian BB, Alvear DT (1978) Prenatal ultrasonographic diagnosis of fetal gastroschisis. Radiology 129:473

Hansmann M (1984) Möglichkeiten und Grenzen sonographischer Diagnostik bei fetalen Erkrankungen und Mißbildungen. In: Kowalewski (ed) Pädiatrische Intensivmedizin VI. Thieme, Stuttgart New York

Harrison MR (1983) Perinatal management of the fetus with a curable defect. In: Callen PW (ed) Ultrasonography in obstetrics and gynecology. Sounders, Philadelphia London Toronto

Harrison MR, De Lorimier AA (1981) Congenital diaphragmatic hernia. Surg Clin North Am 61:1023

Harrison MR, Bressack MA, Churg AM (1980) Correction of congenital diaphragmatic hernia in utero. II. Simulated correction permits fetal lung growth with survival at birth. Surgery 88:260

Jeanty P, Romero R (1984) Obstetrical ultrasound. Mc Graw, New York

Lomar F, Stattford-Bell M, Tymms A (1979) Prenatal ultrasound in diagnosis and management of fetal exomphalos case reports. Br J Obstet Gynecol 86:581

Meyenburg M, Maaßen V (1979) Praepartale Erkennung einer Omphalocele. Geburtshilfe Frauenheilkd 39:1021

Moore KL (1980) Embryologie. Schattauer, Stuttgart New York

Niesen M, Hansmann M (1979) Omphalocele, praepartale Ultraschalldiagnostik und Konsequenzen. Gynäkologie 12:80

Roberts C (1978) Intrauterine diagnosis of omphalocele. Radiology 127:762

Schaffer RM, Barone C, Friedman A (1983) The ultrasonographic spectrum of fetal omphalocele. J Ultrasound Med 2:219

Schmidt W, Gabelmann J, Garoff L, Kubli F (1981) Ultrasonographische Diagnose einer Omphalocele im ersten Schwangerschaftsdrittel. Geburtshilfe Frauenheilkd 41:562

Scott JS, Wilson JK (1957) Hydramnions as an early sign of oesophageal atresia. Lancet II:569

Staudach A, Laßmann R, Menzel C (1982) Mißbildungsdiagnostik vor der 24. Woche. In: Kratochwill A, Reinold R (eds) Ultraschalldiagnostik 1981. Thieme, Stuttgart New York

Staudach A, Laßmann R, Rosenkranz W, Engels M, Joos H, Rücker J (1984) Praenatale Diagnose fetaler Entwicklungsstörungen, das Model eines interdisziplinären Teams. In: Kowalewski (ed) Pädiatrische Intensivmedizin VI. Thieme, Stuttgart New York

Warkany J (1971) Congenital malformation. Year Book Medical Publishers, Chicago

Winter R (1981) Die Diagnose angeborener Mißbildungen mittels Ultraschall. Ultraschall 2:235

Zaleski AM, Cooperberg PL, Kliman MR (1979) Ultrasonic diagnosis of extrafetal masses. J Can Assoc Radiol 30:55

8.5 Malformations of the Urogenital Tract

With high-resolution gray-scale ultrasound it is possible to demonstrate the fetal kidneys and bladder at 12 weeks gestation, given a normal amniotic fluid volume. This is also the reason why abnormalities of the fetal urogenital tract (polycystic kidneys, hydronephrosis, and other obstructive changes) are being recognized and reported with increasing frequency. However, detailed anatomic differentiation of urogenital tract lesions is usually made difficult by the concomitant presence of oligohydramnios.

The sonographic visualization of the fetal kidneys, the ability to distinguish pelvis from parenchyma, the significance of the presence or absence of a full bladder, and the assessment of amniotic fluid volume form the basis for the prenatal evaluation of the fetal genitourinary tract. The correct interpretation of sonographic findings demands a basic knowledge of renal development (McCrory 1972; Oliver 1968), of the normal sizes of urogenital structures at various stages of development (Grannum et al. 1980), of fetal urine production (Campbell et al.

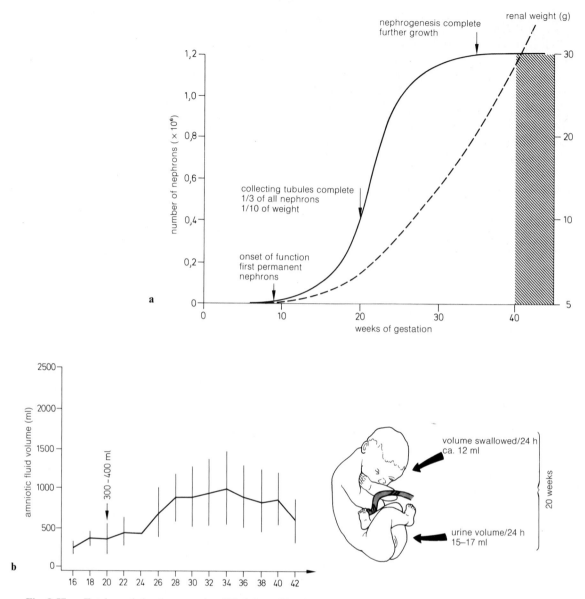

Fig. 8.57. a Fetal renal development (modified from Harrison 1983). **b** Amniotic fluid volume during pregnancy and fetal contribution (urination and swallowing) at 20th weeks

1973), and of the normal range of amniotic fluid volumes (Queenan and Thompson 1972).

The essential points are summarized in Fig. 8.57a, b, which clearly shows that development of the fetal kidneys continues beyond embryogenesis, and is most rapid between 20 and 30 weeks. Major congenital anomalies (bilateral renal agenesis, multicystic kidneys) invariably lead to early oligohydramnios or anhydramnios (21 weeks; Hansmann et al. 1979) due to a failure of urine excretion. With other anomalies, it often takes some time for urinary tract ob-

struction to produce obvious sonographic changes. Because the fate of the fetal kidneys may well depend on the time that elapses between diagnosis and treatment, and little time is required to perform the standard scans, evaluation of the fetal urogenital tract should be a routine part of every ultrasound examination. The basic procedure is as follows:

1. A transverse scan is performed through the upper abdomen (with the fetus prone or supine, if possible) to evaluate the renal pelvises.

2. Comparative left and right paravertebral

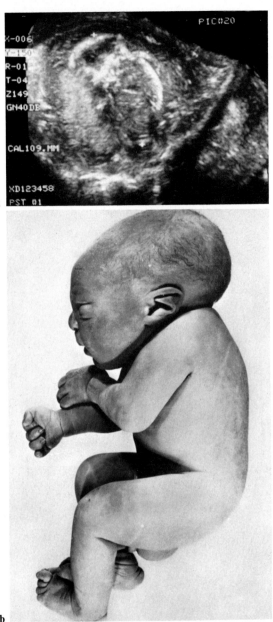

Fig. 8.58a, b. Potter's syndrome at 17 weeks: bilateral renal agenesis. **a** Fetus in breech presentation with posterior fundal placenta and anhydramnios (CRL 100 mm). **b** Typical phenotype

The recognition of pathology during routine baseline examinations is essential. A more thorough differentiation and evaluation of suspicious findings generally should be done in cooperation with a specialized center in view of the experience, equipment and time required. We caution against "experimentation" without sufficient prior experience.

For example, when ultrasound reveals a unilateral subpelvic stenosis producing moderate dilatation (no trunk distension) prior to 27 weeks, it may be tempting to try to decompress the fetal urinary tract by the introduction of a shunt catheter. However, it is not known for certain whether drainage is beneficial in such cases (usually the pressure causes only a saclike dilatation of the proximal ureter without visibly distending the renal pelvis). Moreover, there is a significant risk of premature rupture of the membranes, possibly resulting in loss of the fetus. When weighing the risks and benefits in such cases, it is important to consider that only one kidney is necessary for survival.

The experience of centers that deal with large numbers of fetal urinary tract abnormalities indicates that there is as yet no generally accepted scheme of management that offers specific options based on morphology, function, and gestational age (Harrison 1983). The prompt intrauterine diagnosis of correctible urologic defects can reduce the number of pediatric "problem cases" in which a diagnosis is delayed until symptoms of organ damage are apparent (Straub 1983).

The prenatal diagnosis before the 22nd week of urinary tract malformations that are incompatible with life lifts a heavy burden from perinatal medicine. To make it easier to survey the complex field of fetal urogenital tract pathology, we have listed the principal diagnoses in order of their functional importance:

scans are obtained to evaluate renal topography, size, and number.

3. A prevertebral frontal scan is performed just anterior to the spine (at the level of the aorta) to permit a direct comparison of both kidneys. Tilting the plane caudally will outline the fetal bladder; dilated ureters, if present, are most easily identified in this plane.

Diagnosable Lesion of the Fetal Urogenital Tract

Bilateral renal agenesis (classic Potter's syndrome)
Renal cystic diseases (Potter types I–IV)
Isolated renal cysts
Changes secondary to urinary tract obstruction:
  subpelvic
  prevesical
  urethral
Functional dilatation

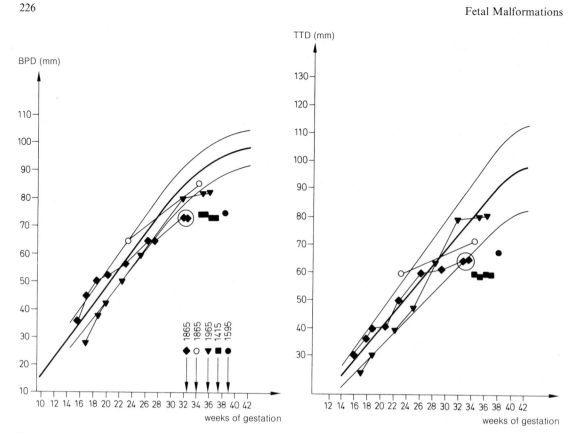

Fig. 8.59. Serial observations in five cases of Potter's syndrome: *left,* BPD; *right,* TTD. Common feature: growth retardation in third trimester. (From Hansmann et al. 1979)

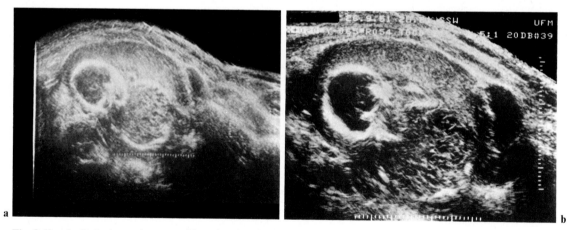

Fig. 8.60a, b. Potter's syndrome at 20 weeks: longitudinal scan. Anhydramnios, bilateral cystic kidneys (Potter type II)

8.5.1 Potter's Syndrome (Renal Agenesis)

Almost 40 years ago Edith Potter described in detail the congenital malformation syndrome of renofacial dysplasia which now bears her name (Potter 1946). She observed that newborn infants with a characteristic "senile" facies (widely spaced eyes, epicanthal folds, flattened nose, micrognathia, and large, low-set, floppy ears; Fig. 8.61 a, b) also tended to have bilateral renal agenesis. Other features of the syndrome

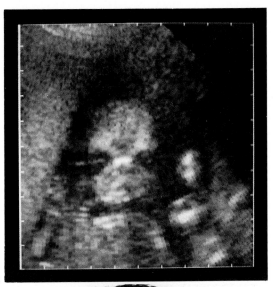

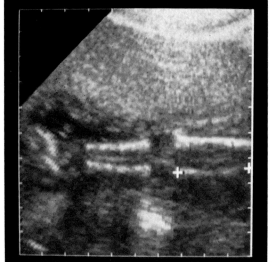

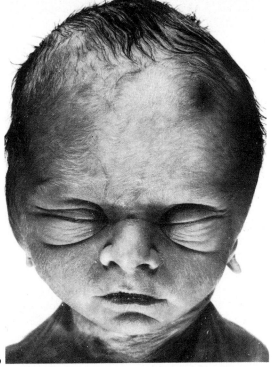

Fig. 8.61. **a** Ultrasound imaging of Potter facies after intraamniotic instillation of 100 ml Normofundin to improve visualization. **b** Phenotype (compare perioral region). **c** Sirenomelia in Potter's syndrome at 18 weeks. Points for left femur length measurement are indicated

are loose skin, spade hands, foot deformity, contractures of the major joints, and malformations of the genital tract, central nervous system, gastrointestinal tract, heart, and other internal organs. The prognosis of these infants, 70% of whom are male, is grave (Potter 1965; Ratten 1973). The majority of live-born infants develop signs of respiratory insufficiency within 4 h of birth as a result of pulmonary hypoplasia (Potter 1965; Warkany 1971; Harrison et al. 1979). No numerical or gross structural chromosome abnormalities have been observed.

The incidence of Potter's syndrome varies. Reported incidence is between 1 in 3,000 and 1 in 4,000 births (Bain 1960; Potter 1965). Six cases have been recorded at our center since 1969. The clinical impression in the initial cases was one of severe intrauterine growth retardation (Fig. 8.59).

Potter's syndrome (renofacial dysplasia) is not treatable. All cases lead to severe oligohydramnios or anhydramnios (Fig. 8.58a), which is apparent in the first half of pregnancy and thus is an important indicator of the disorder (Hansmann et al. 1979). Because severe oligohydramnios is recognizable during routine ultrasound examination it should be possible in the future to diagnose more of these cases before 23 weeks.

Generally, however, Potter's syndrome is not an easy condition to diagnose, and suspected cases should be confirmed at a specialized facility before clinical conclusions are drawn. The adrenals are frequently enlarged in Potter's syndrome and are apt to be mistaken for kidneys (Figs. 8.62, 8.63), and not every echo-free mass within the lower abdomen is the fetal bladder! A cystic mass may be identified as the bladder only if it manifests the functions of filling and

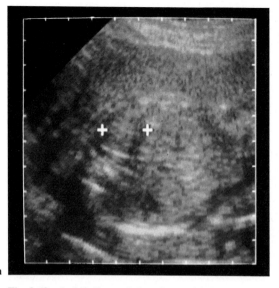

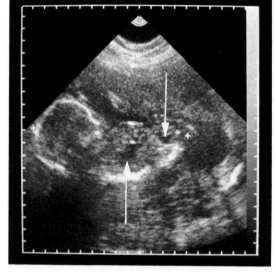

Fig. 8.62a, b. Misdiagnosis in a fetus with Potter's syndrome. **a** Hypoechoic areas (*crosses*) represent adrenals and were misinterpreted as kidneys (common in Potter's syndrome). **b** After instillation of Normofundin (180 ml at 18 weeks), improved visualization with demonstration of fetal stomach and bladder

emptying. This is confirmed or excluded by serial observations. The value of administering furosemide to the mother to provoke fetal diuresis remains to be proved. Among our own patients, we have made one false-positive diagnosis of Potter's syndrome in a case of triploidy (69 XXX) which exhibited anhydramnios and early growth retardation.

One notable feature of Potter's syndrome is that affected fetuses tend to show little body movement. Many of these fetuses have malformations of the extremities, or at least large, stiff joints. The latter has been interpreted as a secondary effect of the anhydramnios, which leads to prolonged immobilization of the fetus (Hansmann et al. 1979). The most conspicuous malformation of the lower extremities is sirenomelia, which, when present, may serve as a diagnostic criterion (Fig. 8.61c). Of course, the examiner must recognize that this anomaly can manifest a variety of forms and degrees. Genital anomalies are also not uncommon in fetuses with Potter's syndrome, and may be a useful diagnostic aid. Due to the poor acoustic transmission that results from the anhydramnios, we adopted the practice in 1983 of artificially filling the amniotic sac in doubtful cases. We initially instill 50–100 ml Normofundin SK over a period of 10 min, followed by up to 300 ml more depending on image quality, gestational age,

and uterine size. With the uterus thus filled, it is easier to evaluate the phenotype and recognize malformations. Usually fetal swallowing movements can be observed after the solution is instilled, followed by the appearance of fluid in the stomach. Shortly thereafter we have frequently observed a marked hyperperistalsis in the fluid-filled loops of bowel, and we have seen several instances of bladder filling in cases where one functioning kidney was present.

In other cases we have observed the filling of irregularly bordered cloacae. According to the literature, about 50% of fetuses with Potter's syndrome have associated anal and rectal atresia, with or without a cloacal malformation (Knöpfle et al. 1982). In coping with the diagnostic problems of this syndrome, it is important to recognize that bilateral renal agenesis, – the classic Potter's syndrome – is present in only a minority of cases. In a series of 32 of our own cases, bilateral renal agenesis was present in 10. The rest involved uni- or bilateral cystic dysplasias of Potter type IIA or IIB. Prognosis becomes very difficult in cases where both kidneys are hypoplastic but retain some function and produce definite urine after fluid is ingested. In one such case we observed that when an adequate intraamniotic fluid pool was maintained for 3 months by multiple instillations, the infant was phenotypically normal at

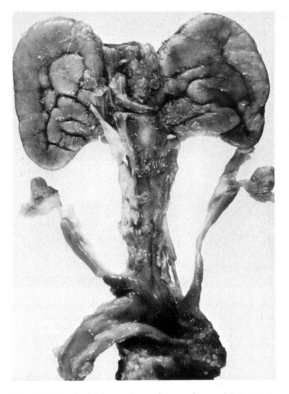

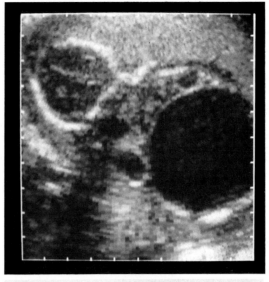

Fig. 8.63. Pathologic specimen from a fetus with Potter's syndrome. Failure of renal development allowed expansive growth of the adrenals. (Courtesy Dr. Foedisch Bonn)

birth and showed no pulmonary hypoplasia, which usually prevents effective postpartum ventilation. The infant in question could be ventilated without difficulty and survived for 8 weeks with its hypoplastic kidneys. This case clearly illustrates that Potter's syndrome is by no means a uniform entity, and that the term "renal nonfunction syndrome," proposed by Bain and Scott (1960), does better justice to the heterogeneity of its forms.

8.5.2 Cystic Kidneys (Potter Type I)

Synonym: Infantile polycystic kidneys.

The cystic lesions of this disease result from the secondary dilatation of normally formed collecting tubules. The nephrons are normal in number and morphology. There is no connective tissue proliferation.

The disease has an autosomal recessive inheritance. Its reported incidence varies between 1:6,000 and 1:14,000.

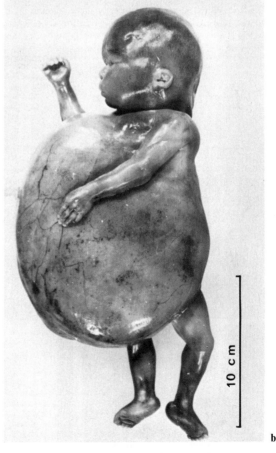

Fig. 8.64a, b. Prune-belly syndrome at 15 weeks. a Longitudinal scan: fetus in breech presentation with anterior fundal placenta, large cystic mass, anhydramnios. b Phenotype (different case)

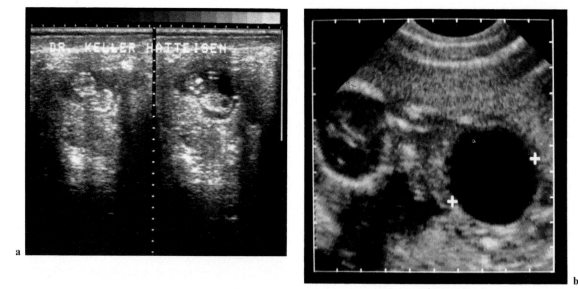

Fig. 8.65. a Fetus with abnormally large bladder at 12 weeks (Photo kindly provided by Dr. Keller-Hatteisen) **b** Same fetus at 18 weeks, with fully developed obstructive uropathy

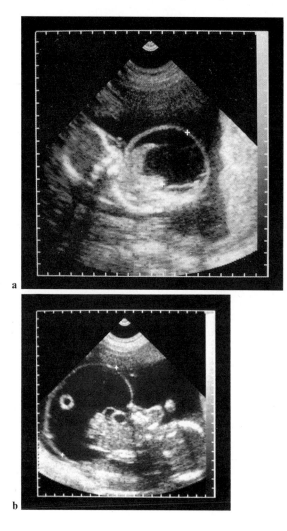

Both kidneys are affected symmetrically (Potter 1972). A fetal lobation of the kidneys is typical (Potter 1972) and can be seen in sonograms. The cystic lesions consist of dilated renal tubules and are only 1–2 mm in diameter – too small to be resolved by ultrasound as individual cysts (Fig. 8.71 b). Because the kidneys probably develop normally, at least in the first half of pregnancy (Zerres 1981), oligohydramnios need not be present. The typical sonographic appearance is that of a uniformly enlarged kidney that contains no visible cysts and presents a patchy, echogenic structure (Fig. 8.71 a–c). Type I cystic kidneys are rarely diagnosed in the first half of pregnancy, because urinary output is not yet affected, and the cardinal symptom of oligohydramnios has not yet developed. In cases where oligohydramnios does not occur, it may be possible to diagnose the disease later from the general enlargement of both kidneys in patients who have a history of a previously affected fetus. An association of elevated AFP values with cystic kidneys has not been established. Further studies are needed to determine whether the elevation of trehalase activity reported by Merin et al. (1981) is a useful indicator of infantile polycystic kidneys.

Fig. 8.66a, b. Longitudinal scans in obstructive uropathy after rupture of bladder. **a** At 24 weeks. **b** Same case showing contracted, almost empty bladder

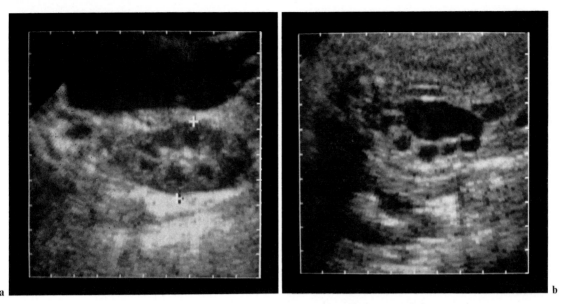

Fig. 8.67a, b. Sonograms of fetal kidney at 34 weeks. **a** Normal finding; **b** moderate hydronephrosis with caliceal dilatation

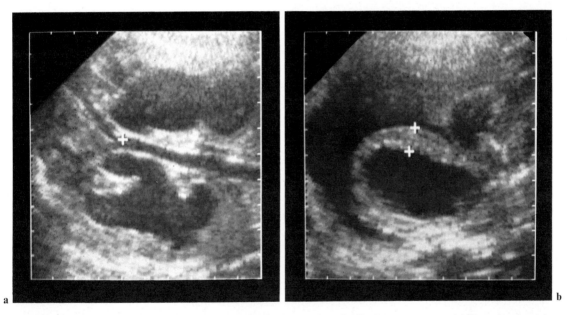

Fig. 8.68a, b. Advanced hydronephrosis with urethral valves. **a** Longitudinal scan: aorta and bifurcation (*cross*). **b** Bladder wall hypertrophy (*crosses*). There is urinary ascites from a bladder fistula

8.5.3 Cystic Kidneys (Potter Type II)

Synonym: Multicystic renal dysplasia.

In this rare disease all collecting tubules and nephrons in the affected region are abnormal, and there is a heavy proliferation of connective tissue.

The disease is characterized by the presence of multiple cystic lesions larger than 1 cm in diameter (Fig. 8.60a, b). One or both kidneys may be affected. Even after the administration of furosemide, the fetal bladder cannot be visualized. In type IIA there is enlargement of the affected kidney(s), whereas in type IIB the kidneys are smaller than normal. Thus, ultrasound diagnosis in these cases may be difficult or impossible if adequate urine is being produced.

Type IIA is more commonly diagnosed prenatally. This is possible in the second trimester, because the underlying abnormal embryonic development is present prior to 11 weeks.

In most cases only one kidney is affected (Fig. 8.70a, b). Contrary to prevailing opinion, function of the contralateral kidney is also impaired in a high percentage of cases (e.g., valve formation, hydronephrosis, ureterocele). A careful assessment of amniotic fluid volume and the contralateral kidney is indicated. Up to 50% of patients with multicystic kidneys have anomalies of other organ systems. When both kidneys are affected, the prognosis is grave.

8.5.4 Cystic Kidneys (Potter Type III)

Basically this is the adult form of polycystic renal disease. It is rare in infants and seldom diagnosed in utero. We have described only one case in which type III cystic kidneys were diagnosed prenatally in a patient who had a relevant family history (Weiss et al. 1981; Fig. 8.72a, b). The features of the disease are reviewed in detail by Zerres (1981).

8.5.5 Urinary Tract Obstruction

A detailed description of obstructive changes of the fetal urogenital tract that can be diagnosed prenatally was presented by Harrison (Callen 1983). The ultrasound appearance of ureteral and urethral stenoses was discussed by Staudach et al. (1983) on the basis of typical examples. The main pathological finding common to all these changes is a dilatation of the urinary tract proximal to the site of the obstruction (Fig. 8.73). Thus, with a subpelvic obstruction, only the renal pelvis on the affected side will be dilated. If the obstruction is prevesical, both the ureter (Fig. 8.66a, b) and the renal pelvis will be dilated. With obstruction of the

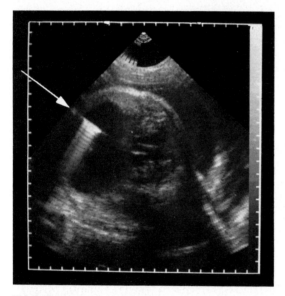

Fig. 8.69. Aspiration of bladder in megacystis: needle is in place (*arrow*)

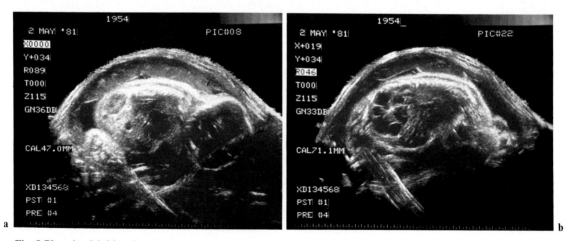

Fig. 8.70a, b. Multicystic dysplastic kidney (Potter type II). **a** Longitudinal scan of healthy kidney. **b** Contralateral cystic dysplasia with normal amniotic fluid volume

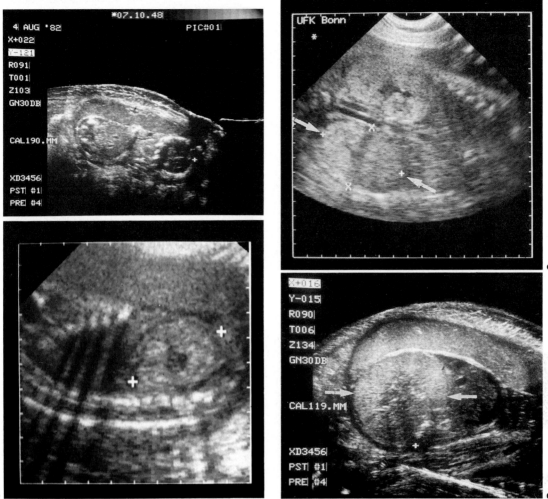

Fig. 8.71 a–d. Infantile polycystic kidneys (Potter type I): serial observations. **a** Findings normal up to 23 weeks: anhydramnios noted at 25 weeks. **b** Scan showed enlarged, hypoechoic kidneys: the small cystic lesions could not be demonstrated. **c** Same case 8 weeks later, now with massive enlargement of kidneys: longitudinal diameter 7.5 cm, transverse diameter 4 cm. Again, no cysts demonstrable (see text). **d** Longitudinal scan of cystic kidneys near term: total anhydramnios, kidney diameter increased to 11.9 cm. Note difference between lower echogenicity of liver (*right*) and highly reflective kidney (*arrows*). Cysts are hardly seen

urethra (regardless of etiology), there will be distension of the bladder, ureters, and renal pelvises. While a subpelvic or prevesical ureteral obstruction may be isolated and unilateral (Fig. 8.67 a, b), a constriction of the urethra necessarily affects both sides. However, the degree of dilatation can vary markedly, being severe on one side and mild on the other. The earlier the obstruction develops and becomes functionally significant, the more pronounced the changes (Figs. 8.64, 8.65, 8.68 a, b).

Dilatation that is secondary to urinary tract obstruction and accompanied by a rise in pressure cannot be distinguished sonographically from adynamic, pressure-free dilatations unless a supplementary invasive technique is used (Fig. 8.73 a, b). The hypertrophic wall of a bladder that is distended by obstruction (Figs. 8.68 b, 8.74 a) serves to distinguish that condition from a neurogenic disturbance of bladder emptying (Fig. 8.74 b). It should be noted that the renal collecting system is also subject to transient dilatation that may not be present on repeat examinations. In no case should a final evaluation be made at a center without experience in this area. As long as an

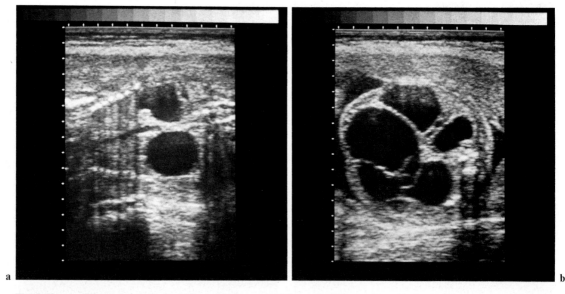

Fig. 8.72a, b. Bilateral dysplastic kidneys (Potter type III) at 21 weeks. **a** Longitudinal scan; **b** transverse scan: grossly distended abdomen

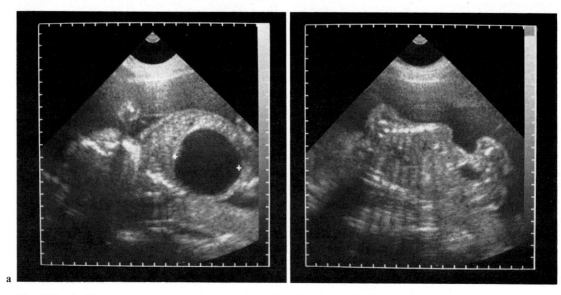

Fig. 8.73a, b. Hydronephrosis secondary to unilateral stenosis at ureteropelvic junction. **a** Longitudinal scan prior to aspiration. **b** Fetus after diagnostic aspiration (70 ml): the flank appears sunken, and there is a small amount of bladder urine. Body contour normalized within a few hours

adequate volume of amniotic fluid is present, the dilated collecting system is surrounded by a distinct mantle of renal parenchyma, and renal function appears to be intact on the basis of bladder dynamics, one should be wary about undertaking invasive procedures prematurely. On the other hand, one should not hesitate too long, as in some rare cases even organ rupture can be observed (Fig. 8.75). The survey article by Harrison (1983), which is based on a large number of cases, shows that beyond a certain degree of dilatation, even intrauterine decompression and preterm delivery may not be of significant benefit (Fig. 8.69).

The range of diagnosable fetal urogenital tract lesions is reviewed in Sect. 8.9.

For clarity of understanding, the key aspects of fetal urogenital tract anomalies, their ultra-

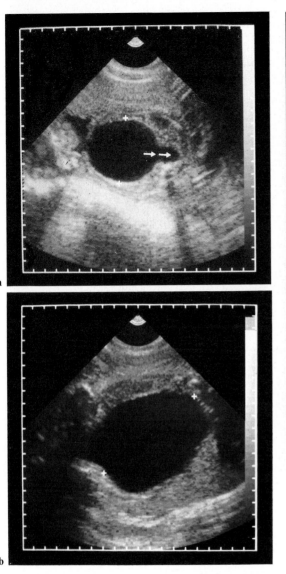

Fig. 8.74c–e. Urinoma at 39 weeks. **c** Kidney ruptured spontaneously, urine created large tumor in renal capsule. **d** Flattened kidney (*arrows*) on longitudinal scan. **e** Kidney after decompression. Surgery immediately after delivery saved child's life

Fig. 8.74a, b. Megalocystis. **a** In urethral obstruction at 21 weeks: proximal part of urethra is keyhole-like (*arrows*), bladder wall is thickened. **b** In late pregnancy secondary to a neurogenic voiding disturbance: bladder wall is not hypertrophic. There was spontaneous onset of micturition post partum, and surgical intervention was unnecessary

sound appearance, and the available diagnostic and therapeutic options are summarized in Tables 8.1 and 8.2. It should be remembered that a urogenital tract malformation often represents only one aspect of a more complex syndrome or one symptom of a chromosomal disorder. Table 8.3 shows the relationship between chromosome abnormalities and various urogenital malformations.

As mentioned in Sect. 8.4, the first step in the differential diagnosis of an intraabdominal cystic mass is to relate it to a particular organ system. Specifically in the region of the left kidney, a fluid-filled loop of colon may, without careful analysis, be mistaken for an abnormality. Doubts are resolved by maintaining the standardized scanning planes described previously.

Table 8.1. Ultrasound findings in urogenital malformations compatible with postnatal life

Kidney, renal pelvis	Bladder, ureters	Amniotic fluid	Diagnosis and implications
Kidney demonstrable, parenchyma visible, pelvis demonstrable in isolation and not dilated, calices not distended, isolated cyst, moon-shaped displacement of parenchyma	Normal	Normal	Renal cyst, postpartum urologic and radiologic evaluation *Caution:* Misdiagnosis from visualization of left descending colon
Kidney enlarged, parenchyma demonstrable, calices and pelvis distended	Bladder normal, ureters not obstructed	Normal	Subpelvic stenosis; serial observations at frequent intervals; preterm delivery if progression is noted; urologic evaluation and treatment
Kidney enlarged, parenchyma demonstrable, calices and pelvis distended	Bladder enlarged, ureters obstructed	Normal Reduced Reduced, with extremely thin abdominal wall, associated encephalocele and polydactyly	Infravesical obstruction Decompensating infravesical obstruction Prune-belly syndrome Meckel-Gruber syndrome

Table 8.2. Ultrasound findings in fetuses with urogenital malformations incompatible with postnatal life

Kidney, renal pelvis	Bladder	Amniotic fluid	Diagnosis	Occurrence
Not demonstrable on either side	Not demonstrable	Oligo- or anhydramnios	Bilateral agenesis, Potter's syndrome: 1:4,800 births, 4:1,000 stillbirths	Not hereditary; familial increased incidence
Both kidneys enlarged, parenchyma replaced by large cysts ($\varnothing$ 2 cm), pelvis not congested, not demonstrable	Not demonstrable	Oligo- or anhydramnios	Multicystic renal dysplasia (Potter type II) (very rare)	Not familial
Kidney replaced by "large cyst," no parenchyma	Not demonstrable	Oligo- or anhydramnios	Complete agenesis distal to kidneys	

Table 8.3. Developmental anomalies of urogenital tract and associated syndromes

Urogenital tract	Syndrome	Inheritance
Obstructive uropathy, cystic dysplasia, horseshoe kidney	Trisomy 18	
Obstructive uropathy, horseshoe kidney, duplications	Turner (XO)	Chromosomal
Obstructive uropathy, cystic dysplasia	Trisomy 21, 13	
Obstructive uropathy	Apert	
Renal dysplasia	Holt-Oram	Autosomal dominant
Obstructive uropathy, unilateral agenesis	Leopard	

Table 8.3. (continued)

Urogenital tract	Syndrome	Inheritance
Renal dysplasia	Beckwith-Wiedemann	
Obstructive uropathy, cystic renal dysplasia	Ectromelia with ichthyosis	
Obstructive uropathy, renal dysplasia	Laurence-Moon-Biedl	
Cystic renal dysplasia	Meckel-Gruber-Gruber	
Cystic renal dysplasia	Roberts	Autosomal recessive
Cystic renal dysplasia	Zellweger	
Obstructive uropathy	Johanson-Blizzard	
Bilateral agenesis	Potter	
Primary ectasia, adynamia	Prune-belly	

References

Bain AD, Scott JS (1960) Renal agenesis and severe urinary tract dysplasia. Br Med J 1:841

Campbell S, Wladimiroff JW, Dewhurst CJ (1973) The antenatal measurement of fetal urine production. Br J Obstet Gynecol 80:680

Grannum P, Bracken M, Silverman R, Hobbins JC (1980) Assessment of kidney size in normal gestation by comparison of ratio of kidney circumference to abdominal circumference. Am J Obstet Gynecol 136:249

Hansmann M, Niesen M, Födisch J (1979) Praenatale Ultraschalldiagnose des Potter-Syndroms. Gynäkologe 12:69

Harrison MR (1983) Perinatal management of the fetus with a correctable defect. In: Callen PW (Ed) Ultrasonography in obstetrics and gynecology. Sounders, Philadelphia

Knöpfle G, Födisch HJ, Hansmann M (1982) Das Potter-Syndrom. Prä- und postnatale Diagnostik. Verh Dtsch Ges Pathol 66:278

McCrory WW (1972) Developmental nephrology. Harvard University, Cambridge, p 40

Merin PR, Portter M, Dallaire L, Melancon SB, Boisuert I (1981) Prenatal detection of the autosomal recessive type of polycystic kidney disease by trehalase assay in amniotic fluid. Prenat Diagn 1:75

Oliver J (1968) Nephrons and kidneys. Harper & Row, New York, p 1

Potter EL (1946a) Bilateral renal agenesis. J Pediatr 29:68

Potter EL (1946b) Facial characteristics of infants with bilateral renal angenesis. Am J Obstet Gynecol 51:885

Potter EL (1965) Bilateral absence of ureters and kidneys. A report of 50 cases. Obstet Gynecol 25:3

Potter EL (1972) Normal and abnormal development of the kidney. Chicago

Queenan JT, Thompson W (1972) Amniotic fluid volumes in normal pregnancies. Am J Obstet Gynecol 114:34

Ratten GJ, Beischer NA, Fortune DW, Path MRC (1973) Obstetric complications when the fetus has Potter's syndrome. Am J Obstet Gynecol 115:890

Staudach A, Laßmann R, Rosenkranz W, Engels M, Joos H, Rücker J (1984) Pränatale Diagnose fetaler Entwicklungsstörungen, das Modell eines interdisziplinären Teams. In: Kowalewski (ed) Pädiatrische Intensivmedizin VI. Thieme, Stuttgart New York

Straub E (1983) Pädiatrisch-urologische Gesichtspunkte. In: Hohenfellner R, Zingg EJ (eds) Urologie in Klinik und Praxis. Thieme, Stuttgart New York

Warkany J (1971) Congenital malformations. Year Book Medical Publishers, Chicago, p 1036

Weiß H, Zerres K, Hansmann M (1981) Pränatale Diagnose zystischer Nierenveränderungen mit Hilfe der Ultraschalltechnik. Ultraschall 2:244

Zerres K (1981) Zystennieren, klinische, pathologisch anatomische und genetische Gesichtspunkte. Dissertation, Bonn

8.6 Skeletal Malformations

The ability to demonstrate bony structures with ultrasound has been discussed in Sects. 4.1 and 7.1. In connection with the diagnosis of skeletal malformations, it should again be emphasized that progressive ossification forms the basis of skeletal imaging in the fetus. This process varies substantially from one area of the skeleton to the next. For example, while the clavicle manifests an ossification center at 7 weeks gestation, the carpal bones do not develop ossification centers until after birth. Most relevant to the diagnosis of skeletal malformations are the ossification processes in the major long bones, the spine, the thorax (ribs), and the skull.

A discussion of the complete range of theoretically recognizable fetal skeletal abnormalities would exceed the scope of this book. Instead, we shall focus our attention on suggestive signs that can be identified during the routine examination of patients not considered to be at risk. The specific exclusion of malformations in high-risk patients is discussed in Sect. 8.9.

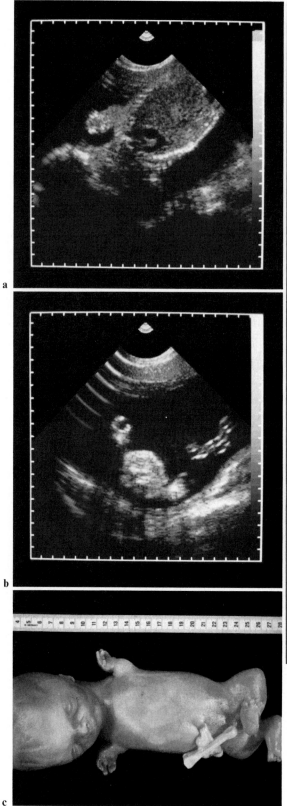

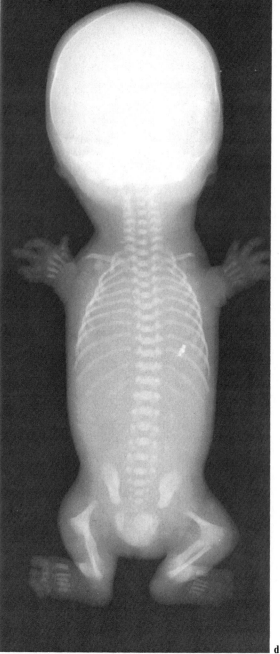

Fig. 8.75a–f. Limb malformations at 26 weeks: patient referred for polyhydramnios. **a** Thorax in longitudinal section: marked phocomelia evident in upper extremity. **b** Transverse scan through same fetus: hands arise directly from thorax. **c** Phenotype. **d** Radiograph of phocomelic fetus. **e** Sonogram of foot: femur length measurement indicates extreme shortening (16 mm). **f** Measured tibia length (29 mm) also short for gestational age

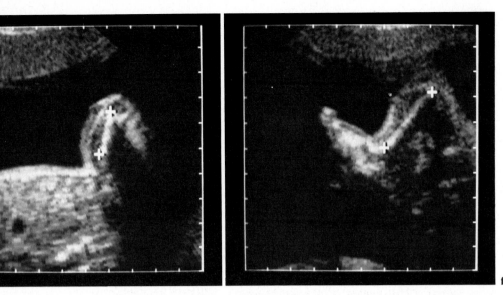

e   f

Fig. 8.75e, f

Three main groups of skeletal malformations are recognized:

1. Defects confined to certain segments of the limbs
2. Complex skeletal malformations that are compatible with postnatal viability
3. Skeletal malformations that are incompatible with postnatal viability

8.6.1 Radial Aplasia

Defects involving specific parts of the limbs are either one feature of a more complex syndrome (e.g., numerical anomalies of the digits or deformities), or the effect of an exogenous agent that may or may not be known. Every case of a partial skeletal malformation is an indication for karyotyping and detailed evaluation in cooperation with a specialized center.

An example of a partial skeletal malformation is shown in Fig. 8.75a–f. This case featured polyhydramnios and two stumplike hands attached directly to the thorax (Fig. 8.75a, b). In the lower extremities ultrasound confirmed the presence of a femur and tibia, but there was marked deformity with significant shortening of the diaphyses (Fig. 8.75e, f). The phenotype is shown in Fig. 8.75c. Another example of a partial but severe skeletal malformation is presented in Fig. 8.76. The humerus of this fetus was normal in length, but the distal portion of the limb could not be visualized in any plane (Fig. 8.76a). On further screening the same anomaly was noted in both lower extremities (Fig. 8.76b). In a lately observed case of bilateral lobster claws at 15 weeks the mother was suffering from the same symptoms (Fig. 8.76 c, d). In cases of this type it is extremely difficult to speculate about "quality of life," and ethical questions are raised that will not be addressed in the present context.

A close association exists between aplasia of the radius and complex syndromes. The typical sonographic appearance of radial aplasia is shown in Fig. 8.77. Radial aplasia occurs as the cardinal feature of approximately 25 syndromes. Hamburg et al. (1982) have classified these into four main etiologic groups:

1. Syndromes of genetic origin that are associated with radial aplasia: acheiropodia; Arias, Syndrome and Baller-Gerold syndrome; Fanconi panmyelopathy; Goldenhar's syndrome and Harris-Osborne syndrome; hemidysplasia with psoriasis; Holt-Oram syndrome and congenital thrombocytopenia syndrome; Ladd's syndrome and Nager-de Reynier syndrome; Robert's syndrome, SC syndrome and Thomson's syndrome

2. Quantitative and qualitative chromosome abnormalities associated with radial aplasia: trisomy 13, 18, and 22, and deletion of the long arm of chromosome 4 (4q or 4r)

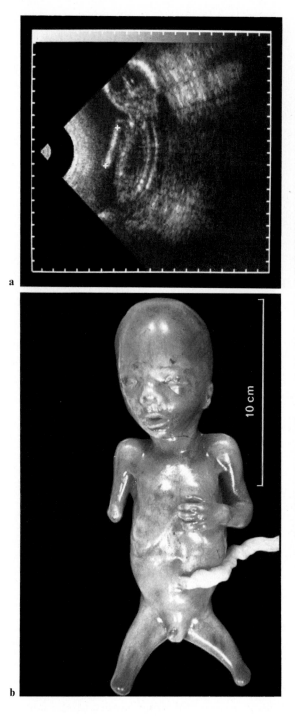

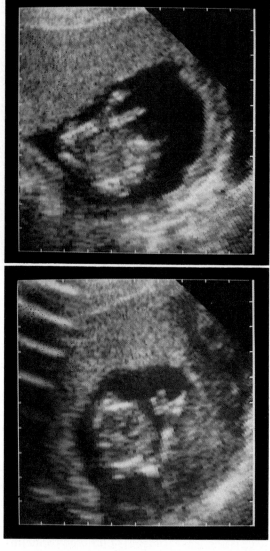

Fig. 8.76a, b. Limb malformations of hemimelic type at 20 weeks in a patient with family history of hemimelia. **a** Humerus measurement is normal, but bone tapers distally to a stump. **b** Phenotype: concomitant hemimelia of lower limbs. **c, d** Bilateral lobster claws at 15 weeks (pregnancy continued)

3. Radial aplasia of undetermined etiology: Adam's complex, anencephaly and spina bifida, in very rare cases unilateral pulmonary agenesis, various peromelia syndromes, ulnar duplication and VACTERL syndrome

4. Radial aplasia due to exogenous agents, e.g. thalidomide

Thus, radial aplasia is a classic example of the path from symptom to diagnosis that is so frequently followed by the sonographer. Of course, differential diagnosis in such cases is an extremely lengthy process that encompasses a range of diverse syndromes. Indeed, in the majority of cases a definitive diagnosis must

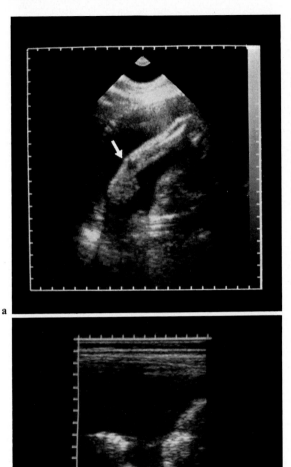

a

b

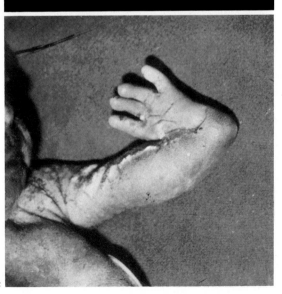

c

await examination after delivery and cytogenetic analysis.

8.6.2 Malformations Incompatible with Postnatal Viability

If initial examination demonstrates marked disproportion between the thorax and abdomen (small or narrow thorax, poorly defined ribs) in combination with markedly short femurs, this is usually a warning sign of skeletal anomalies that will seriously compromise viability. The term "nonviable" generally refers to the inability of the newborn to develop normal respiration. Usually this results from a skeletal anomaly in which the thorax is too small or too narrow to permit normal pulmonary excursions. The most important of these anomalies are:

Achondrogenesis type I (Saldino-Noonan), short rib-polydactyly syndrome
Achondrogenesis type II
Thanatophoric dwarfism
Congenital recessive form of osteogenesis imperfecta
Camptomelic dysplasia
Asphyxiating thoracic dysplasia
Congenital hypophosphatasia

Achondrogenesis Type I (Saldino-Noonan Dwarfism). Several cases have been reported to date in which achondrogenesis type I suspected on the basis of ultrasound findings was subsequently confirmed at delivery (Richardson et al. 1977; Smith et al. 1981). We have diagnosed one such case at 19 weeks gestation (Fig. 8.78). The criteria for a sonographic diagnosis are:

1. A narrow thorax with extremely short ribs (Fig. 8.78 b, c)
2. Marked shortening of the diaphyses (Fig. 8.78 a)
3. Polydactyly (Fig. 8.78 d)

Achondrogenesis Type II. Achondrogenesis type II is a rare, severe, and invariably lethal congen-

Fig. 8.77 a–c. Radial aplasia in VACTERL syndrome: a hand attaches directly to elbow (*arrow*). b Same case: fingers appear to arise directly from humerus. c Phenotype

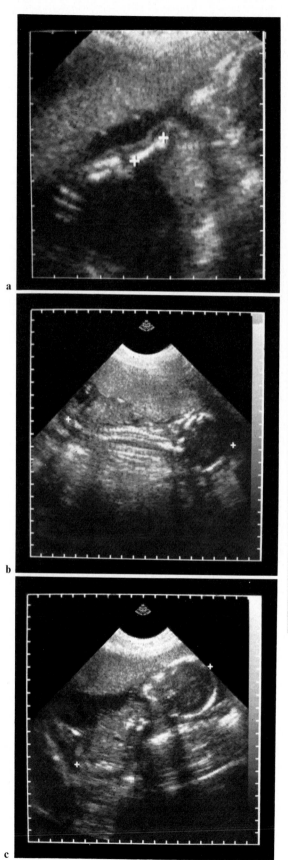

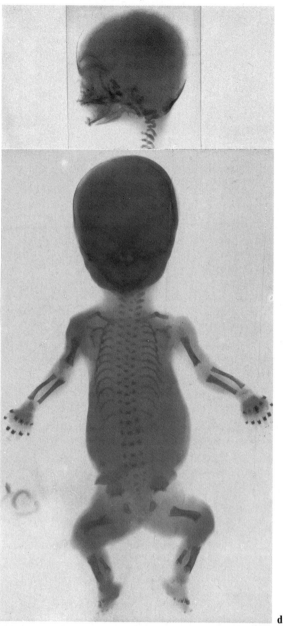

Fig. 8.78a–d. Achondrogenesis type I (Saldino-Noonan dwarfism) at 19 weeks. **a** Long bones of extremities (here, humerus) severely shortened (humerus 15 mm instead of 30 mm). **b** Sagittal scan: deformed ribs within thorax. **c** Bony structures of thorax are rudimentary. **d** Radiographic confirmation of short limbs and polydactyly of left hand

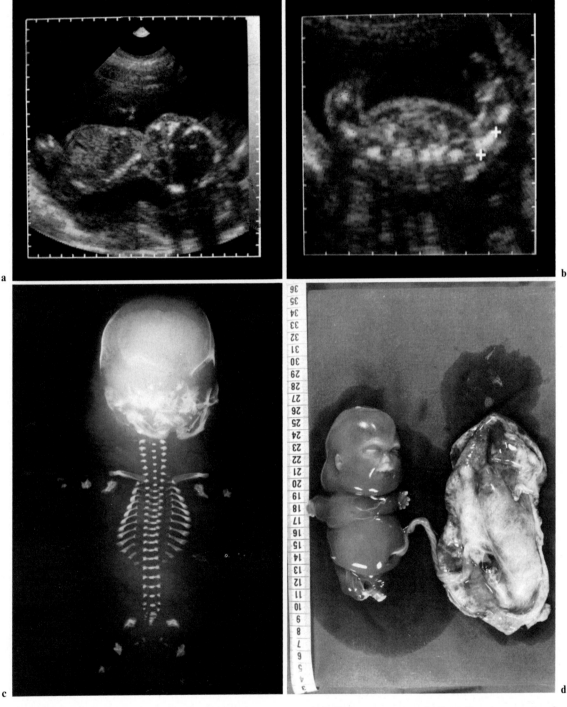

Fig. 8.79 a–d. Achondrogenesis type II. **a** Sagittal scan: short, deformed thorax and relative macrocephaly. **b** Transverse scan through pelvis and upper leg: *crosses* mark rudimentary, extremely short (1 cm) segments of femur. **c** Radiograph. **d** Phenotype

ital skeletal dysplasia. So far we have diagnosed two cases by ultrasound, both before 24 weeks (Fig. 8.79). The typical sonographic criteria are:

1. A short trunk with a protuberant abdomen (Fig. 8.79 a)
2. Macrocephaly (Fig. 8.79 a)
3. Extremely short limbs in which the dia-

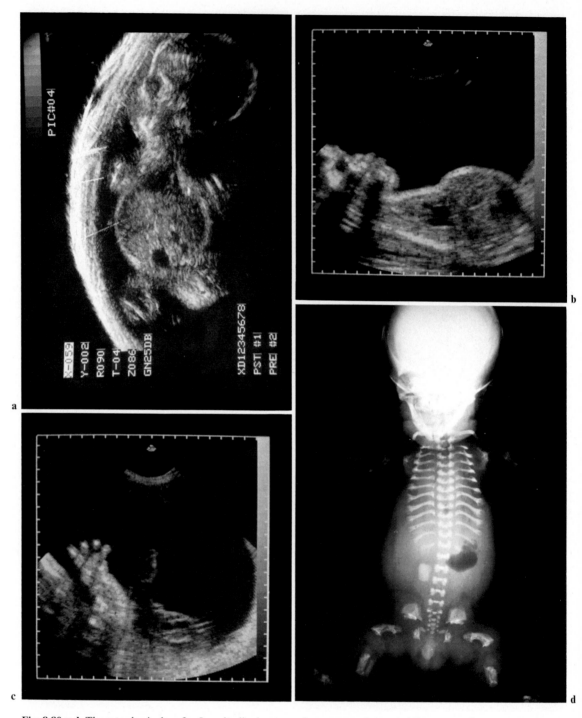

Fig. 8.80 a–d. Thanatophoric dwarf. **a** Longitudinal scan at 31 weeks showing typical "champagne cork" phenomenon: thorax narrow, abdomen distended, head markedly enlarged. **b** Sagittal scan at 28 weeks: small thorax, protuberant abdomen, sunken nasal bridge. **c** Extremely short arms with short, stubby fingers. **d** Radiograph

physes appear only as short, stubby vestiges (Fig. 8.79 b)

Not infrequently, hydrops is an associated finding (Fig. 8.79 d). A postpartum radiograph (Fig. 8.79 c) confirms the rudimentary diaphyses of the limbs.

Thanatophoric Dwarfism. Thanatophoric dwarfism is rare among the severe fetal malformation syndromes, with an estimated incidence of 1 in 100,000 births (Thompson and Parmley 1971). Because it can be diagnosed prenatally with great confidence when specifically sought, and because major risks, including serious maternal psychological stress, can be avoided with appropriate obstetric management, the inclusion of this anomaly in differential diagnosis is necessary during the prenatal investigation of a suspected anomaly. The main diagnostic criteria are:

1. A small, narrow thorax and protuberant abdomen ("champagne cork" phenomenon; Fig. 8.80 a, b, d)
2. Short diaphyses (Fig. 8.80 c)
3. Macrocephaly, depressed nasal bridge, possibly hydrocephalus (Fig. 8.80 a, b)

To date approximately 100 cases have been described. Hobbins and Mahoney (1980) have described one case diagnosed with ultrasound. We have observed seven fetuses with thanatophoric dwarfism, and all six after the first case in 1974 (published in 1979) were correctly diagnosed without difficulty. The main warning symptom in all cases was extreme hydramnios at the end of the second trimester. The earliest diagnosis was made at 25 weeks, and an earlier diagnosis might well have been possible if the patient had been referred sooner (see also Sect. 8.9).

Maroteaux et al. (1967) have differentiated thanatophoric dwarfism from other skeletal chondrodysplasias on the basis of clinical and radiographic findings. They found that thanatophoric dwarfs exhibit typical skeletal changes characterized by general shortening and bowing of the long bones with thickening of the endochondral ossification zones, especially in the ribs and long bones. Another feature is extreme flattening of the vertebral bodies with widening of the interspaces (Fig. 8.80 d). These changes produce such characteristic radiographic features that the condition can be readily diagnosed from X-rays alone. With sufficient technical expertise, the anomaly can even be recognized in utero, given an adequate degree of skeletal calcification (20–22 weeks).

Besides radiography, an important aid to differentiating thanatophoric dwarfism from achondroplasia (to which it was once assigned) is that with the former, the parents of the fetus are healthy and phenotypically normal. Finally, all thanatophoric dwarfs are characterized by an inability to survive after birth, with most dying within the first 48 h. The longest reported survival time was 25 days (Lander et al. 1969). The presumed cause of death is respiratory failure secondary to narrowness of the thorax and pulmonary hypoplasia.

If fetal trunk measurements are correctly performed, the extreme narrowing of the thorax that is typical of thanatophoric dwarfism can be recognized; it results in an increased head-to-trunk ratio. Prenatal diagnosis justifies elective abortion, because the anomaly is incompatible with life.

In summary, it may be said that thanatophoric dwarfism is a special form of micromelic dwarfism that usually leads to death within hours after birth as a result of pulmonary hypoplasia. It is readily diagnosed prenatally on the basis of its typical appearance.

Osteogenesis Imperfecta. Osteogenesis Imperfecta (Fig. 8.81) presents a great diversity of forms. The most severe form, osteogenesis imperfecta congenita, is inherited as an autosomal recessive trait. Affected fetuses are frequently stillborn and show multiple fractures, which produce a marked shortening of the limbs. We have observed three cases of this anomaly, one at 17 weeks (Staudach et al. 1982). The diagnostic signs were:

1. A bell-shaped thorax (Fig. 8.81 c)
2. Extremely short limbs in which the diaphyses appear fragmented (Fig. 8.81 d, e, g, i)
3. High acoustic transmission through the poorly mineralized, membrane-like skull (Fig. 8.81 a, b, f)
4. Cranial deformation and visible movement of the brain ("jello" phenomenon; Fig. 8.81 a, b) caused by the slightest compression of the fetal head (e.g. by percussing the material abdomen)

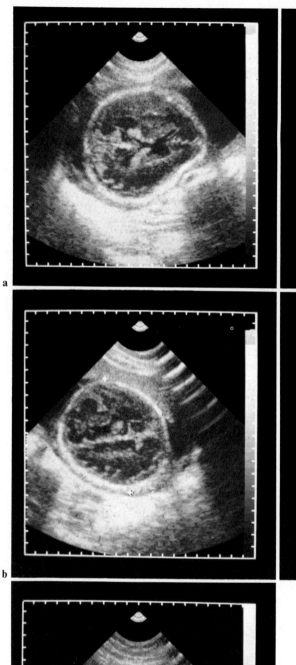

Fig. 8.81 a–i. Osteogenesis imperfecta (Vrolik type). **a** Hypoechoic skull allows an unusually clear depiction of intracranial structures. Slight pressure on maternal abdomen causes marked change in shape of skull. **b** Note detail of cerebral structures. **c** Longitudinal scan of trunk: deformity of ribs (bell-shaped thorax). **d** Extreme shortening of humerus. Gaps in diaphyses result from pathologic fractures. **e** Caudal end of body and extremely short fingers (*arrows*) are seen. **f** Longitudinal scan at 17 weeks: picture of pseudohydrocephalus results from sonolucency of membrane-like cranial bone. **g** Limbs are shortened and deformed, diaphyses have a "patchy" appearance (17 weeks). **h** Typical frontal view of face. **i** Radiograph at 17 weeks

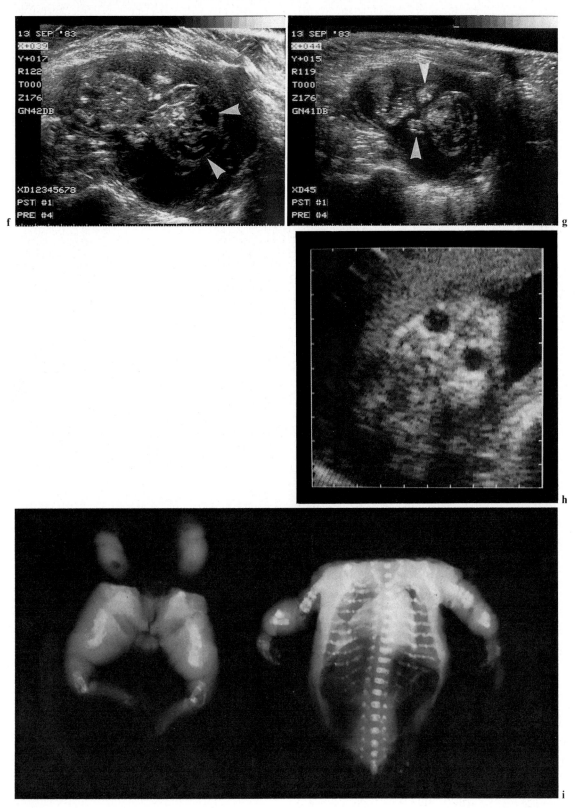

Fig. 8.81 f–i.

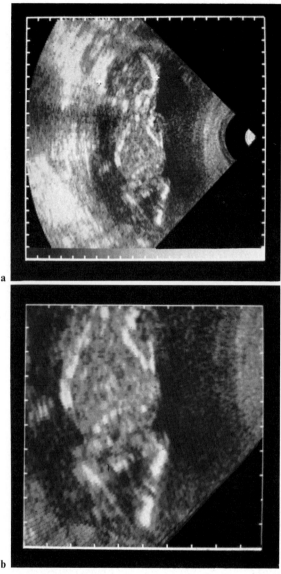

a

b

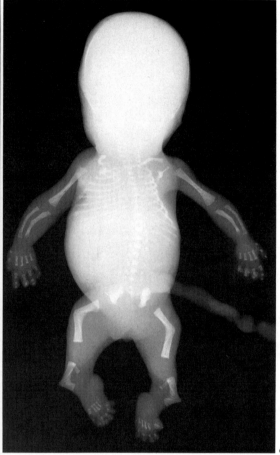

c

Fig. 8.82a–c. Camptomelic dysplasia. **a** Frontal scan at 18 weeks: shortened and deformed thorax, BPD 47 mm. **b** Lower extremity: diaphyses shortened and angulated. **c** Radiograph

Two of our cases were diagnosed at 28 weeks. In the third case, pathology was suspected as early as 14 weeks because of the unusual clarity with which brain structures were seen. The primary suspicion on subsequent examinations was hydrocephalus. In fact, it was only the thin membrane of the calvarium that permitted such a remarkably clear definition of intracranial structures (Fig. 8.81 f). Further screening revealed extremely short limbs with rudimentary diaphyses (Fig. 8.81 g). The findings were confirmed at autopsy following elective abortion at 17 weeks. The postpartum radiograph is shown in Fig. 8.81 i.

Camptomelic Dysplasia. Camptomelic dysplasia is a typical but rare syndrome (Fig. 8.82); only 50 cases were described prior to 1980. The prenatal diagnosis of this condition was described by Winter and Rosenkranz (1984). We have been able to diagnose one case sonographically at 18 weeks. The prognosis of this syndrome is grave, with death occurring in the first week of life. The criteria for sonographic diagnosis are:

1. A narrow, bell-shaped thorax (Fig. 8.82a)
2. Short and angulated bones of the lower limbs, clubbed feet (Fig. 8.82b, c)
3. Micrognathia and auricular dysplasia

Asphyxiating Thoracic Dysplasia. Figure 8.83 shows the typical sonographic appearance of asphyxiating thoracic dysplasia. The bony thorax is extremely narrow relative to the abdomen.

Congenital Hypophosphatasia. Congenital hypophosphatasia is a lethal autosomal recessive disorder. Wladimiroff et al. (1984) diagnosed it

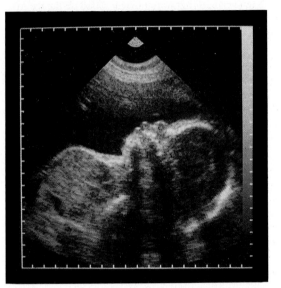

Fig. 8.83. Asphyxiating thoracic dysplasia: Longitudinal scan: Thorax appears extremely narrow in relation to abdomen + head

sonographically as early as 15 weeks. The main diagnostic criteria are:

1. Inability to demonstrate the calvarium clearly from 11 weeks onward
2. Bowing and shortening of the limbs

Figure 8.84 shows the limb shortening associated with chondrodystrophia punctata ossificans at 22 weeks gestation. This syndrome will be discussed further in connection with the ultrasound examination of high-risk pregnancies.

References

Hamburg K, Grossheim M, Födisch JH, Schwanitz G (1982) Leitsymptom: Radiusaplasie. Verh Dtsch Ges Pathol 66:475

Hobbins JC, Mahoney MJ (1980) The diagnosis of skeletal dysplasia with ultrasound. In: Sanders RC, James AE (eds) The principles and practice of ultrasonography in obstetrics and gynecology. 2nd edn. Appleton-Century-Crofts, New York, pp 191, 203

Lang M, Hansmann M, Bellmann O, Azubuike J (1979) Thanatophorer Zwergwuchs – pränatale Diagnostik und Geburtsleitung. Gynäkologe 12:84

Langer LO, Spranger JW, Greinacker I, Herdmann RC (1969) Thanatophoric dwarfism. Radiology 92:285

Maroteaux P, Lainy M, Robert JM (1967) Le nanisme thanatophore. Presse Med 75:2519

Richardson MM, Beaudet AL, Wagner ML, Malini S, Rosenberg HS, Lucci JA (1977) Prenatal diagnosis of reccurence of saldino-noonan dwarfism. J Pediat 91:467

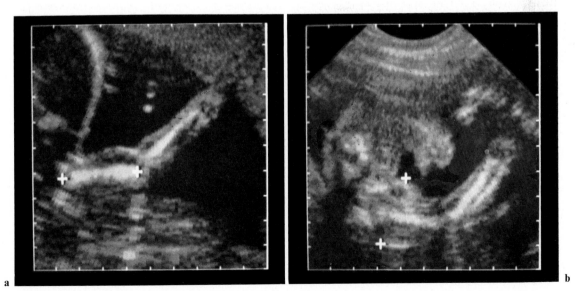

Fig. 8.84a, b. Chondrodystrophia punctata ossificans at 22 weeks. **a** Humerus length 28 mm, corresponding to only 18 weeks. **b** Scan through lower limb: marked shortening of femur. *Crosses* indicate malproportion

Smith WL, Breitweiser TD, Dinno N (1981) In utero diagnosis of achondrogenesis typ I. Clin Genet 19:51
Staudach A, Laßmann R, Menzel C (1982) Mißbildungsdiagnostik vor der 24. Woche. In: Kratochwill A, Reinold E (eds) Ultraschalldiagnostik 81. Thieme, Stuttgart New York

8.7 Tumors

A separate discussion of fetal tumors that can be diagnosed prenatally is presented purely for didactic reasons and is not based on any specific difference between these lesions and other types of fetal malformations. It may well happen that a fetal tumor is detected which does not conform to the features of a syndrome or disease. The goal of prenatal sonography in such cases is to arrive at a diagnosis on the basis of the structure of the tumor and the aspiration findings. In some cases the aspiration alone may be curative.

Congenital tumors are a rare finding but often can be diagnosed prenatally by their relationship to a particular organ. The importance of tumor diagnosis is illustrated by the following case reports:

Case 1: On routine examination at 36 weeks a mass was noted in the fetal heart, raising the suspicion of a cardiac tumor (rhabdomyoma; Fig. 8.85). Following interdisciplinary consultation, a cesarean birth was planned with the intent of surgically removing the tumor postpartum. On repeat examination immediately before the planned cesarean birth, a second mass was noted in the fetal head (Fig. 8.86). Neurosurgical consultation at this time led us to suspect a malignant intracranial tumor. The elective delivery was cancelled, and autopsy confirmed the diagnosis of rhabdomyoma while identifying the intracranial tumor as an astrocytoma. Both occurred in the setting of tuberous sclerosis.

Case 2: In a patient who did not have an ultrasound examination prior to admission (1974), non strep test (NST) showed highly pathologic fetal heart rate (FHR) patterns (silent oscillation type and decelerations) as soon as monitoring was initiated. Based on the reported association between this type of NST pattern (Fig. 8.87b) and anomalies of the central nervous system (Fischer 1982), a sonographic examination was performed, revealing the presence of intracranial partly cystic and partly solid masses consistent with a diagnosis of intracranial teratoma (Fig. 8.87b). Despite the pathologic FHR pattern, we decided against cesarean birth. Autopsy confirmed the prenatal diagnosis.

Case 3: A cystic intraabdominal mass was noted during screening at 16 weeks of pregnancy. The urogenital tract appeared structurally normal, and there was a normal amount of amniotic fluid. When aspirated, the mass diminished in size, and the fetus did not appear to be compromised. This prompted a second aspiration in which the entire content of the mass (serous fluid) was withdrawn. Subsequent observation showed no further evidence of pathology; the mass did not recur. As the fetus was a male, the possibility of an ovarian cyst was not considered. The infant was healthy at birth and developed normally. There was no reason for invasive procedures, and so the exact nature of the mass remained unknown (Fig. 8.88a–c).

These cases illustrate that accurate prenatal diagnosis, aided if necessary by invasive tech-

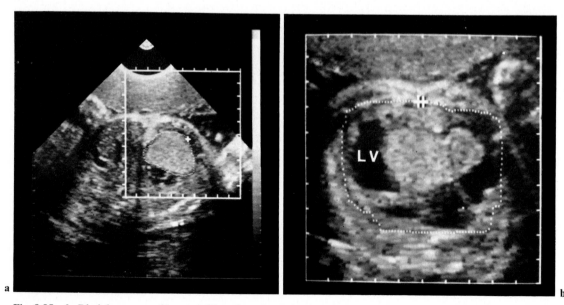

a   b

Fig. 8.85a, b. Rhabdomyoma of heart at 36 week. **a** Cardiac tumor noted during screening: circumference 112 mm. **b** Detail: tumor presents as highly echogenic, spherical mass at wall of left ventricle. Spine at 6 o'clock

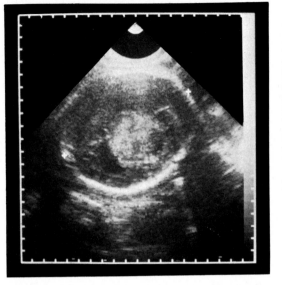

Fig. 8.86. Transverse scan through head, with a large, right-sided echogenic mass that was first discovered shortly before planned delivery

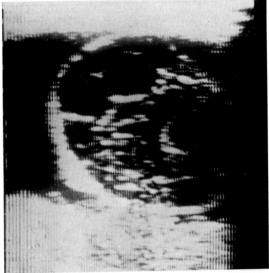

Fig. 8.87. a Intracranial teratoma: entire brain structure replaced by a mixture of cystic and solid masses. **b** Abnormal NST in immediate prepartal period (no variability, decelerations) ▽

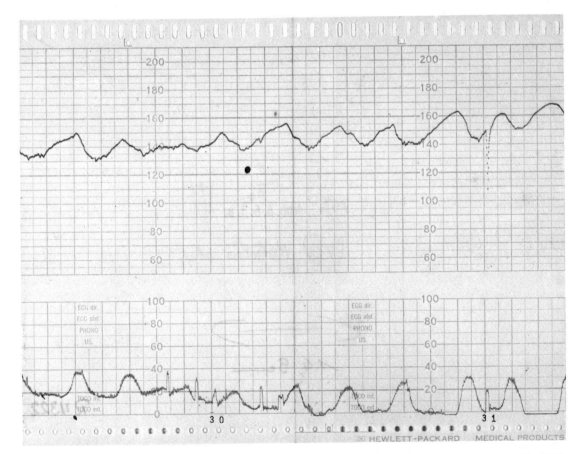

Fig. 8.87 b

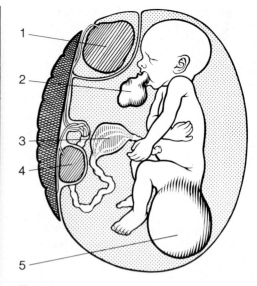

Fig. 8.89. Schematic drawing showing potential sites of occurrence of congenital teratomas: *2* epignathus, *3* teratoma of umbilical cord, *4* teratoma of placenta, *5* sacrococcygeal teratoma. Placental teratoma (*4*) must be differentiated from acardius acephalus with its own amnion and amniotic fluid (*1*). (From Schaller 1975)

niques, can have a decisive impact on prognosis and obstetric management.

8.7.1 Teratomas

Teratomas occur most frequently at the cranial and caudal poles of the fetus. Those that protrude from the oral cavity are called epignathi, and those attached to the sacral region are called sacrococcygeal teratomas (sacral parasites). According to Goerttler (1964), teratomas are a developmental anomaly based on an early rupture of the blastomere as a result of partial necrosis. These tumors can occur in various body regions (Fig. 8.89), and all contain derivatives of the three germinal layers. Thus, it is common to find tumors containing both solid and cystic elements on sonograms. A cranial teratoma was described by Callen (1983). Sac-

Fig. 8.88. a Cystic mass of unknown etiology in fetal upper abdomen. **b** Aspiration of 30 ml of fluid causes partial collapse of mass with no alteration of vital signs. **c** Two hours after a second aspiration, abdominal structure appears normal. Infant was healthy at birth and showed no subsequent evidence of disease

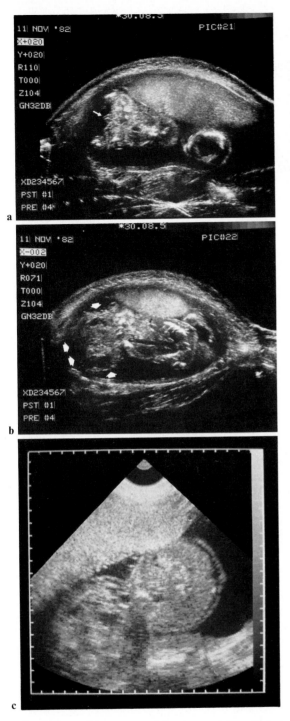

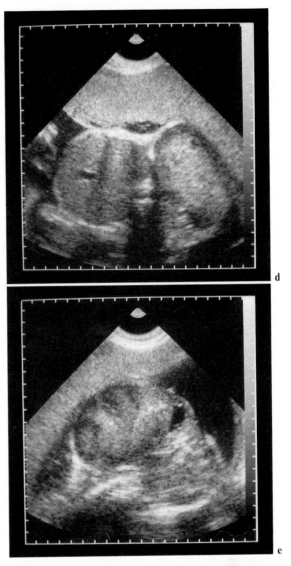

Fig. 8.91. a Sacrococcygeal teratoma in longitudinal section. Tumor arises from caudal pole of fetus and does not involve neural tube. **b** Same tumor in cross-section: cystic and solid structures fill the mass. **c** Gross appearance of sacrococcygeal teratoma in a newborn. **d** Appearance of region following surgical correction. **e** Minimal scarring is evident 1 year postoperatively. **c, d, e** see page 254

Fig. 8.90 a–c. Sacrococcygeal teratoma at 31 weeks. **a** Frontal scan: thighs are abducted in a "frogleg" posture, male genitalia are visible between them. **b** Frontal scan on a slightly more posterior plane: tumor (*arrows*) now clearly visible at caudal pole of fetus. **c** Transverse scan: tumor arising at 7–8 o'clock from coccygeal region

rococcygeal teratomas are relevant to obstetric management. Although they can obstruct delivery, even large teratomas may have a good prognosis. The often "dramatic" appearance of the lesion belies the good prognosis that is assured by prompt surgical correction. Figures 8.90 and 8.91 a, b show the typical sonographic appearance of a large sacrococcygeal teratoma. Figure 8.91 a–e illustrates the good

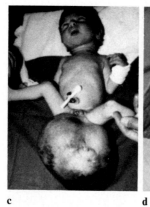

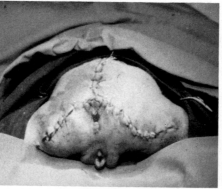

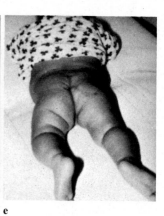

c   d   e

Fig. 8.91

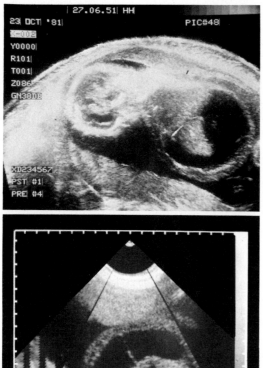

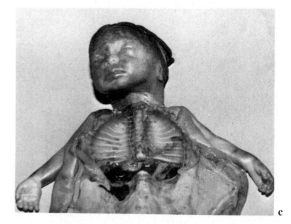

a

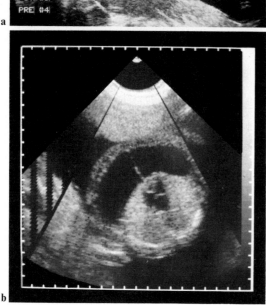

b

Fig. 8.92a–c. Cystic adenomatoid dysplasia of lungs with ascites. **a** Longitudinal scan. **b** Transverse scan: spine at 5 o'clock. Heart, surrounded by hyperechoic lung tissue, is seen in foreshortened four-chamber view. **c** Autopsy findings

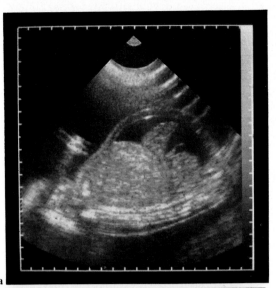

a

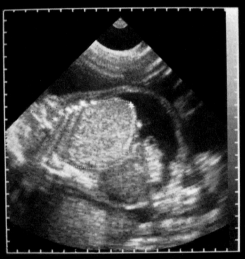

b

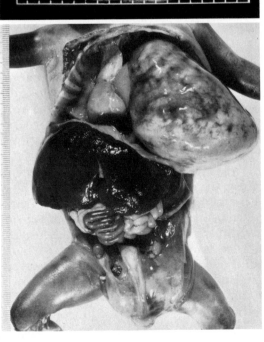

c

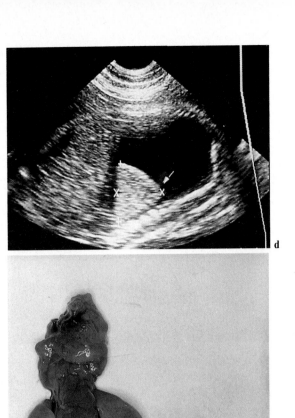

d

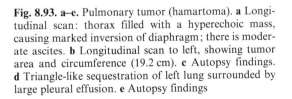

e

Fig. 8.93. a–e. Pulmonary tumor (hamartoma). a Longitudinal scan: thorax filled with a hyperechoic mass, causing marked inversion of diaphragm; there is moderate ascites. b Longitudinal scan to left, showing tumor area and circumference (19.2 cm). c Autopsy findings. d Triangle-like sequestration of left lung surrounded by large pleural effusion. e Autopsy findings

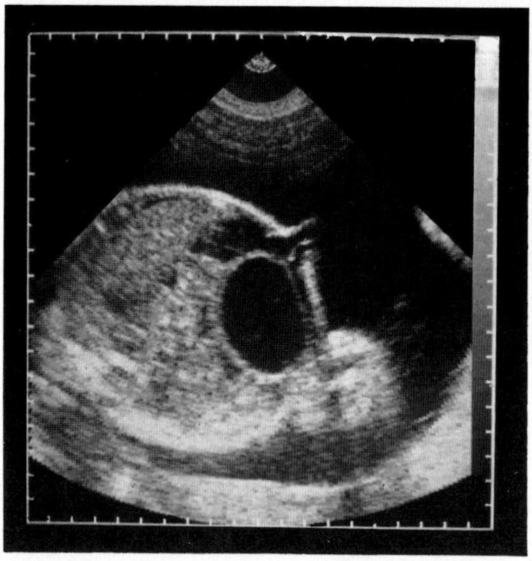

Fig. 8.94. Cystic mass of lower abdomen (ovarian cyst). Mass did not recur following diagnostic aspiration

cosmetic and functional results that can be achieved with surgery (Staudach 1982).

In all cases of this type it should be determined whether the caudal part of the neural tube is involved in the tumor, as this will influence the prognosis.

8.7.2 Pulmonary Tumors

Another tumor that is detectable prenatally occurs within the fetal thorax and affects the pulmonary tissues. Figure 8.92 shows the sonographic appearance of a cystic adenomatoid malformation of the lung. Vascular compression can result in a massive hydrothorax that hampers structural analysis. The prenatal diagnosis of this condition was described by Callen (1983), Don et al. (1981), and Garrett et al. (1975). Another pulmonary tumor is shown in Fig. 8.93a–c. This is a hamartoma of the fetal lung, characterized sonographically by pronounced ascites and an enlarged echogenic lung.

Figure 8.94 shows a cystic mass of the lower abdomen. In a fetus with female genitalia and no apparent urogenital anomalies, we felt that the most likely diagnosis was an ovarian cyst. We performed a diagnostic aspiration, and the mass did not recur.

Ehman et al. (1983) reported on the prenatal diagnosis of other less common types of tumor, including a congenital malignant mesoplastic nephroma. Nakamoto et al. (1983) diagnosed a hepatic hemangioma in utero by means of ultrasound.

In the future, selective aspiration and fetal tissue sampling could significantly aid further evaluation of these types of tumors.

References

Donn SM, Martin JN, White SJ (1981) Antenatal ultrasound findings in cystic adenomatoid malformation. Pediatr Radiol 10:180
Ehmann RL, Nicholson StF, Machin GA (1983) Prenatal sonographic detection of congenital mesoblastic nephrome in a monozygotic twin pregnancy. J Ultrasound Med 2:555
Garret WJ, Kossoff F, Lawrence R (1975) Gray scale echography in the diagnosis of hydrops due to fetal lung tumor. J Clin Ultrasound 3:45
Goerttler KI (1964) Kyematopathien. In: Becker PE (ed) Humangenetik, Bd II. Thieme, Stuttgart
Knochel JQ, Lee TG, Melendez MG, Henderson SC (1983) Fetal anomalies involving the thorax and abdomen. In: Callen PW (ed) Ultrasonography in obstetrics and gynecology. Sounders, Philadelphia London Toronto
Nakamoto StK, Dreilinger A, Dattel B, Mattrey RF, Key TC (1983) The sonographic appearance of hepatic hemangioma in utero. J Ultrasound Med 2:239
Schaller A (1975) Geburtsmedizinische Teratologie. Urban & Schwarzenberg, München Berlin Wien
Staudach A (1982) Möglichkeit und Grenzen der Mißbildungsdiagnostik. Swiss Med 4:67, 6a

8.8 Heart Defects and Cardiovascular Diseases

Congenital heart defects have an incidence of 0.7%–0.8%. The recurrence rate of these defects and their association with syndromes are discussed in Sect. 8.9. Conditional to the understanding of this section is a knowledge of the normal cardiovascular anatomy.

With patience and proper plane selection, cardiac dynamics can be studied even with a linear scanner (Fig. 8.95a–c). The state of arterial and chamber filling, the motion of the septum secundum, the tricuspid and mitral valves, and the myocardium and ventricular septum can be assessed. It is also possible to measure the transverse diameter of the heart at the level of the AV valves ("short axis"; Figs. 8.95–8.97).

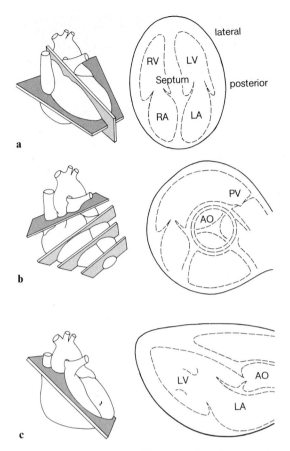

Fig. 8.95a–c. Schematic diagrams of **a** four-chamber view; **b** short-axis view; **c** long-axis view

Fig. 8.96. Four-chamber view of fetal heart: transverse cardiac diameter 38 mm. In this scan the foramen ovale is open, and the septum primum is visible (*arrow*)

In our experience, most severe congenital defects have a sonographic presentation that is at the very least "suspicious," and the great majority are readily identifiable. The obstetric examination is usually performed with conventional real-time B-mode instruments, while further evaluation by the pediatric cardiologist requires the use of instruments integrated with M-mode and Doppler flow analysis.

The sonographic features used in the qualitative and quantitative evaluation of the causes of fetal cardiac failure are presented below.

Fetal cardiovascular diseases that can lead to fetal cardiac failure and hydrops fetalis

1. *Dysrhythmias*
   a) Tachyarrhythmias: paroxysmal supraventricular tachycardia, atrial flutter, atrial fibrillation
   b) Bradyarrhythmias: complete AV block
   c) Complex dysrhythmias

2. *Premature closure of fetal blood passages* (Foramen ovale and ductus arteriosus)

3. *Impaired myocardial function*
   a) Endocardial fibroelastosis
   b) Cardiomyopathies (e.g., diabetic cardiomyopathy)
   c) Myocardial infarction from coronary artery thrombosis
   d) Intrauterine myocarditis (e.g., cytomegalovirus)

4. *Cardiac malformations*
   a) AV canal with mitral regurgitation
   b) Absence or insufficiency of pulmonary valve
   c) Tricuspid insufficiency
   d) Ebstein's anomaly
   e) Complex cardiac malformations

5. *Intracavitary space-occupying lesions* (e.g., tumor, thrombus)

6. *Idiopathic generalized arteriosclerosis*

7. *Any defect occuring in association with the causes listed above (1–6)*
   Especially common with dysrhythmias (e.g., AV canal, single ventricle, tetralogy of Fallot)

Examination of the Heart

1. The standard four-chamber view is obtained, noting the position, shape, and size of the heart.

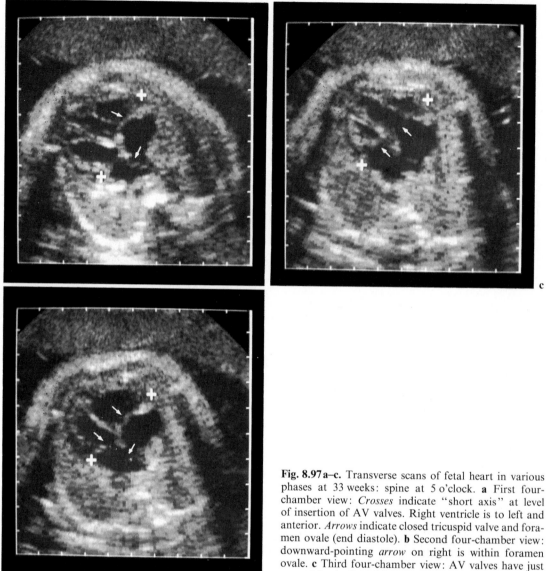

Fig. 8.97 a–c. Transverse scans of fetal heart in various phases at 33 weeks: spine at 5 o'clock. **a** First four-chamber view: *Crosses* indicate "short axis" at level of insertion of AV valves. Right ventricle is to left and anterior. *Arrows* indicate closed tricuspid valve and foramen ovale (end diastole). **b** Second four-chamber view: downward-pointing *arrow* on right is within foramen ovale. **c** Third four-chamber view: AV valves have just opened (early diastole)

2. The short axis is imaged and measured (transverse diameter at the level of the AV valve)

3. Special studies (where indicated): diameter of both ventricles in systole and diastole; diameter of the right atrium; diameters of the large vessels; thickness of septum and ventricular walls; quantitative evaluation of the function of both ventricles; measurement of systolic intervals of both ventricles (in conjunction with fetal ECG); etc.

Examination of Other Organs

1. Diameters of intra- and subhepatic veins
2. Diameter of umbilical vein
3. Qualitative and quantitative assessment of
 — pericardial effusion
 — ascites
 — pleural effusion
 — skin edema
 — hydramnios
 — placental edema or placental thickness
 — number of umbilical arteries

8.8.1 Cardiovascular Disease

The prenatal diagnosis of cardiovascular disease has been pursued intensively by several groups of investigators since 1980 (Allan et al. 1980; Kleinman et al. 1980; Hansmann and Redel 1982; Redel and Hansmann 1984; Sahn et al. 1980). This diagnosis relies essentially on the use of high-resolution real-time sector scanners which incorporate M-mode and pulsed Doppler blood flow analysis into the two-dimensional image. Increasingly, qualitative and quantitative echocardiography is enabling physicians to monitor the anatomy and function of the fetal heart, diagnose cardiac malformations in utero, and evaluate the efficacy of fetal cardiotherapeutic measures. In addition, ultrasound techniques are providing new sources of information on the physiology and pathophysiology of fetal hemodynamics.

Previous experience has shown that cardiovascular disease in the fetus has varying effects on fetal hemodynamics and on that basis can be divided into two broad groups:

The first includes all cardiac malformations that are compatible with normal fetal circulation and do not produce symptoms until the occurrence of circulatory changes after birth. The majority of congenital defects fall within this category, including the tetralogy of Fallot, truncus arteriosus, and transposition of the great arteries.

The second include fetal disease states that produce symptoms in utero ranging from mild cardiac failure to hydrops fetalis. These decompensating diseases include dysrhythmias, premature closure of fetal blood passages, and myocardial disease. Dysrhythmias and myocardial disease can also produce symptoms postnatally, whereas premature closure of the foramen ovale and ductus arteriosus become asymptomatic after birth owing to the physiologic closure of these structures.

The majority of patients with fetal heart disease are referred to our center for detailed sonographic evaluation after initial assessment has demonstrated dysrhythmias, polyhydramnios, hydrops fetalis, or any combination of these conditions (Hansmann 1981). A second, larger group is comprised of patients examined between 19 and 22 weeks gestation because their personal or family history places them at increased risk for fetal cardiac anomalies or disease (see Sect. 8.9).

To date, the following therapeutic measures have been used in the treatment of fetal cardiac failure:

1. Pharmacologic treatment with digoxin, propafenone, verapamil, or flecainide, administered (a) transplacentally through maternal administration or (b) directly to the fetus by intravascular (umbilical vein), intramuscular, or intracavitary injection under sonographic vision
2. Ultrasound-guided aspiration of pleural and pericardial effusions, ascites, and hydramnios
3. Elective preterm delivery (if possible after confirmation of lung maturation)

8.8.2 Heart Disease

Fetal heart disease that is symptomatic in utero commonly produces the complete picture of hydrops fetalis (ascites, pleural effusion, pericardial effusion (Fig. 8.98), skin edema, cardiomegaly, hepatomegaly, splenomegaly) with accompanying hydramnios and placental edema. They are the cause of nonimmunologic hydrops fetalis in approximately 50% of cases (Hansmann and Redel 1982; Kleinman et al. 1982). It is always necessary to consider and exclude a wide range of other fetal diseases that can cause nonimmunologic hydrops fetalis (e.g., chromosome abnormalities, especially when hydrops develops before 24 weeks). Anomalies of organ systems (e.g., urogenital tract, diaphragmatic hernia, tumors), infections, chorioangioma of the placenta, and various other conditions can also cause hydrops (Etches and Lemons 1979; Hansmann 1981; Maidman et al. 1980; Perlin et al. 1981; Davis 1982).

Fetal heart failure, whether of cardiac or extracardiac origin (AV fistula, fetal transfusion syndrome, chronic anemia), generally manifests itself as a right-sided failure due to the unique characteristics of the fetal circulation. With a high pulmonary vascular resistance, low pulmonary blood flow (only 5%–10% of the ejection volume of both ventricles), and shunting of blood by the ventricles (Rudolph 1974), pulmonary edema will not develop during intrauterine life, even in left-sided cardiac disease. The common mechanism of all diseases that produce fetal cardiac failure is increased pressure and

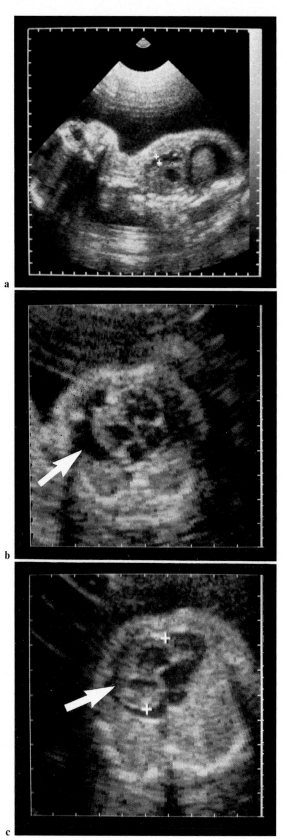

volume load on the right atrium. Besides actual cardiac diseases (obstruction of fetal blood passages, dysrhythmias, myocardial disease), various cardiac anomalies can lead to hydrops fetalis, such as an AV canal in the presence of left ventricular to right atrial shunting through mitral insufficiency. However, this does not account for the observation of fetal hydrops in association with hypoplastic left heart syndrome. Two of these cases were twin gestations in which fetofetal transfusion was the presumed cause of the hydrops (Hansmann and Redel 1982; Leake et al. 1979). Sahn et al. (1982) reported on one case of hypoplastic left heart syndrome and hydrops fetalis in which cardiac failure was attributed to a restriction of the foramen ovale and the presence of an organized thrombus filling approximately one-third of the left ventricle.

The compensatory mechanisms of the fetal heart in the face of pressure and volume overload appear to be less efficient than those in the adult (Rudolph 1974; Kleinman et al. 1982). This explains why even relatively minor disturbances of the fetal circulation, such as paroxysmal supraventricular tachycardia, can precipitate heart failure and even intrauterine death. The rapid development of symptoms of right-sided failure, including severe hydrops fetalis, within the space of a few days is just as characteristic of fetal pathophysiology as is the complete regression of congestive phenomena after removal of the cause, e.g., following the spontaneous or drug-induced cardioversion of fetal tachyarrhythmias. This also may occur over a period of days, or it may require weeks or even months if hydrops is advanced.

To illustrate this, we present the case of an hydropic fetus with massive ascites and skin edema and a heart rate of 200–300/min referred to us at 22 weeks for evaluation and therapy (Fig. 8.99a–e). Fetal echocardiography showed no significant cardiac anomaly. Pharmacologic cardioversion was achieved through maternal digitalization (loading dose of digoxin, then maintenance dose of 0.3 mg/day with monitor-

Fig. 8.98. a Longitudinal scan: pericardial effusion in a univentricular, decompensated heart. **b** Isolated pericardial effusion at 29 weeks: etiology unknown. **c** Same case 2 weeks later: regression of effusion, which disappeared altogether after a further couple of weeks. Spontaneously delivered child doing fine

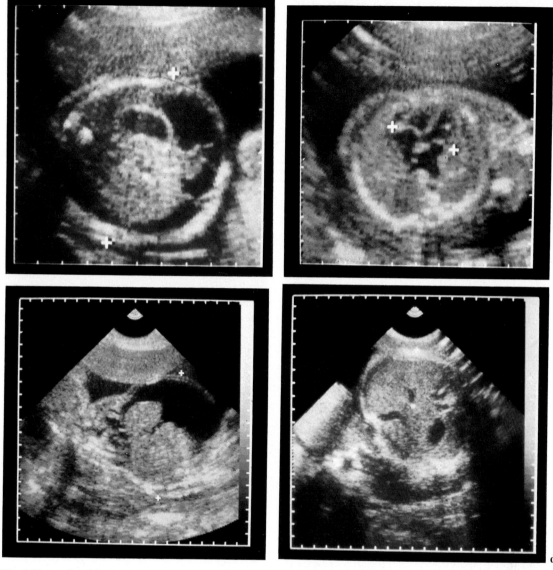

Fig. 8.99a–e. Fetal hydrops at 21 weeks, secondary to fetal tachyarrhythmia of 280–300/min. **a** Transverse abdominal scan: spine at 10 o'clock, diameter 6.8 cm. **b** Four-chamber view of fetal heart 14 days after start of therapy (23 weeks gestation). **c** Following conversion to sinus rhythm, ascites initially persits (26 weeks). **d** As therapy is continued (digitalis and antiarrhythmics), complete regression of ascites is achieved. Infant was delivered spontaneously at 37 weeks and was healthy. **e** see page 262

ing of maternal serum digoxin levels), followed by treatment with an antiarrhythmic drug (verapamil: 5 × 80 mg/day). An early attempt to treat the arrhythmia directly by the intravascular injection of propafenone during amniocentesis for chromosomal diagnosis had shown that cardioversion was possible, but the effect was only transitory. The transplacental regime of digoxin followed by verapamil finally resulted in cardioversion at 24 weeks. The initial highly unstable rhythm gradually gave way, via occasional bradyarrhythmias, to a sustained, normal sinus rhythm. With a sinus rhythm of about 140/min, fetal fluid accumulation began to diminish within a few weeks and then declined steadily, until skin edema had cleard by 26 weeks and ascites by 34 weeks (Fig. 8.99a–e). Antiarrhythmic medication was continued until 37 weeks, when a healthy female infant was spontaneously delivered.

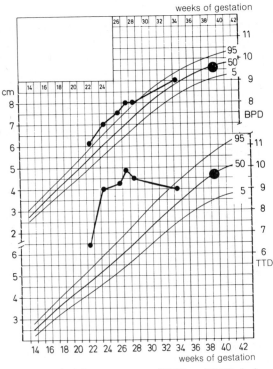

Fig. 8.99e. Serial measurement of BPD and TTD during therapy

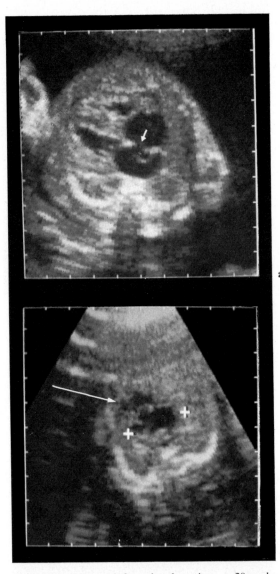

Fig. 8.100. a Normal four-chamber view at 28 weeks demonstrating foramen ovale (*arrow*): transverse thoracic scan, spine at 6 o'clock. **b** Complete AV canal at 22 weeks. *Crosses* indicate common atrium, *arrow* indicates ventricular portion: common AV valve is visible between them

Another characteristic of the fetal heart is the immaturity of the conduction system, which accounts for the high incidence of dysrhythmias, especially reentry tachycardias (Gembruch et al. 1982). In addition, the detection of any fetal arrhythmia, even if hemodynamically insignificant, should always prompt a search for associated cardiac malformations, particularly AV canal, single ventricle, tetralogy of Fallot, and Ebstein's anomaly (Hansmann and Redel 1984).

The main criteria for the sonographic diagnosis of fetal cardiac failure are summarized on p. 297, and are based essentially on changes associated with generalized fetal hydrops. Findings such as (a) the presence of skin edema or its absence in association with ascites and (b) the size of the liver and the caliber of its veins play an important role in this evaluation. For example, fluid accumulation confined to the upper body half (hydrothorax, skin edema) is strongly suggestive of premature closure of the foramen ovale (Hansmann et al. 1982; Redel and Hansmann 1981). Selective echocardiography can disclose further anatomic anomalies of the fetal heart and vessels, as well as functional disturbances (e.g., in brady- and tachyarrhythmias), which can be further differentiated (paroxysmal supraventricular tachycardia, atrial fibrillation or flutter) by means of M-mode recordings (DeVore et al. 1983).

Indications for fetal echocardiography

A. History

1. Family (genetic) history:
   a) cardiac defects
   b) other malformations associated with cardiac defects

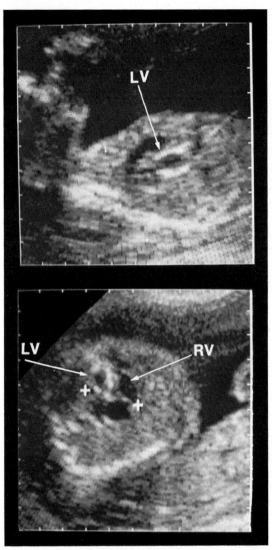

Fig. 8.101 a, b. Left ventricular endocardial fibroelastosis at 22 weeks. **a** Longitudinal scan with head to left: small, rigid left ventricle (*LV*). **b** Four-chamber view: endocardial fibroelastosis of left ventricle (*LV*). *Crosses* mark plane of AV valves

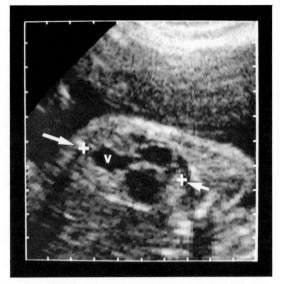

Fig. 8.102. Univentricular heart showing points for measuring long axis. *V,* ventricle

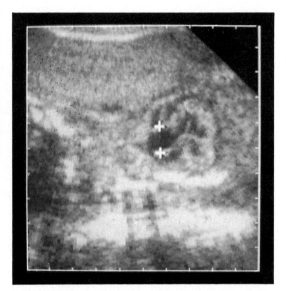

Fig. 8.103. Hypoplastic left heart with pseudotruncus arteriosus (*crosses,* 10 mm)

2. Exposure Insult during pregnancy:
   a) exogenous substances (alcohol, hydantoin, trimethadione, lithium, phenothiazines, amphetamines, etc.)
   b) large doses of ionizing radiation
   c) suspected infection (rubella, cytomegalovirus, coxsackie virus, etc.)
   d) other maternal disease (diabetes mellitus, phenylketonuria, systemic lupus erythematosus)

B. Detection of fetal abnormalities

1. Cardiovascular system:
   a) dysrhythmias
   b) nonimmunologic hydrops fetalis
2. Fetal malformations that may be associated with cardiac anomalies (chromosome aberrations, many syndromes, omphalocele, VACTERL)
3. Intrauterine growth retardation

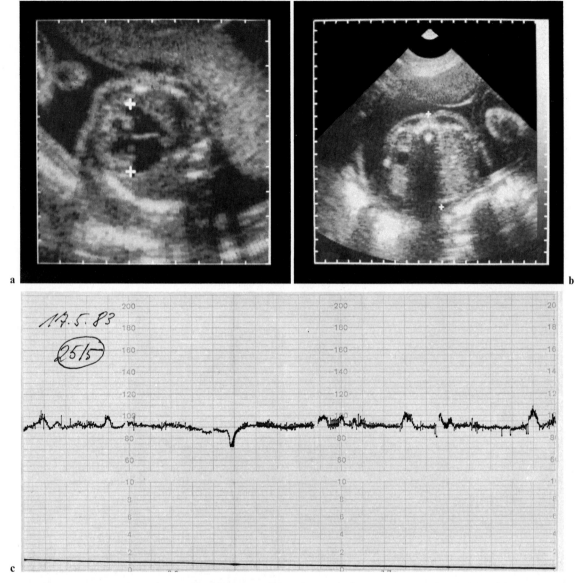

Fig. 8.104. a Transverse scan of trunk at 25 weeks: abnormal four-chamber view. Ventricle on right side (left ventricle with situs inversus) is abnormally small. Defect in ventricular septum, complete AV canal. **b** Transverse scan of trunk: stomach on right, situs inversus. **c** NST at 24 weeks

Only an accurate diagnosis of the underlying cardiovascular disorder can provide the prognosis and information needed to develop an individualized approach to management in general and intrauterine therapy in particular. The basic principles of such therapy may be summarized as follows:

1. The transplacental cardioversion of fetal tachyarrhythmias can be accomplished through maternal medication (Redel and Hansmann 1982, 1984; Kleinman et al. 1983). The direct administration of drugs to the fetus under sonographic guidance (combined if necessary with other measures such as aspiration for chromosome analysis, exclusion of anemia, or therapeutic decompression) is justified only if there is an immediate threat to the fetus. Digoxin is the primary drug of choice. If cardioversion is not obtained, additional antiarrhythmic drugs – propafenone, verapamil, flecainide – are administered. Procainamide may also be used (Dumesic et al. 1982). In view of the unde-

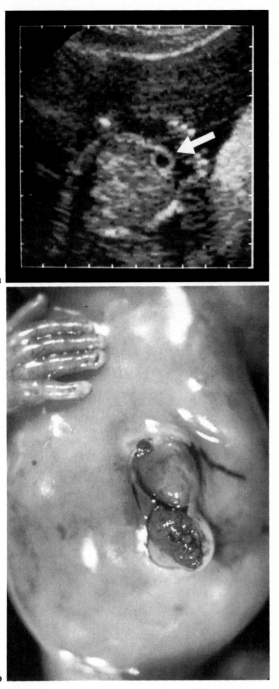

Fig. 8.105. a Transverse scan of trunk: spine at 7 o'clock. Partially ectopic univentricular heart (*arrow*). b Morphologic findings

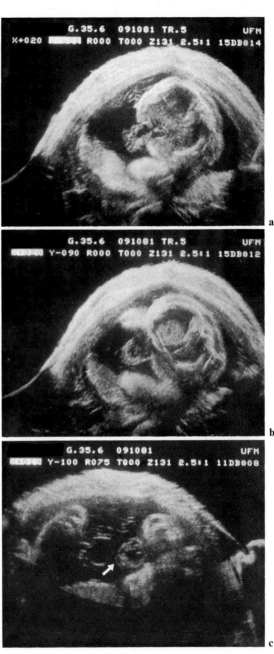

Fig. 8.106a–c. Ectopic heart at 34 weeks. Serial scans of trunk on caudal-to-cranial transverse planes: spine at 2 o'clock. a Thoracic wall defect; b exteriorized portion of aorta; c complete ectopia cordis (*arrow*)

sirable side effects of β-receptor blocking drugs (e.g., propranolol) in newborn infants (low Apgar score, hypoglycemia, and bradycardia in the first 72 h of life; Tamari et al. 1982), we refrain from using them if at all possible.

2. Even with complete AV block, digitaliza-tion of the fetus may cause cardiac stabilization with no change in heart rate and regression of the hydrops (Hansmann and Redel 1982).

3. Aspiration of abdominal, pleural, and pericardial effusions is of only temporary value and is recommended only if there is a response to

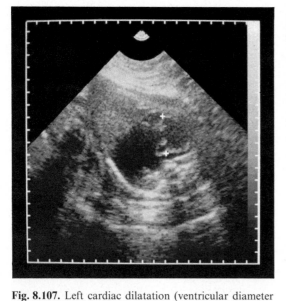

Fig. 8.107. Left cardiac dilatation (ventricular diameter 29 mm!). Right ventricle severely compressed, aneurysmatic dilatation of atrial region

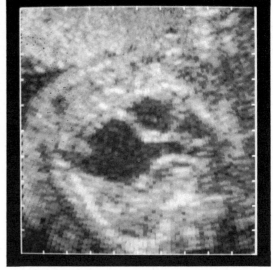

Fig. 8.109. Tricuspid atresia

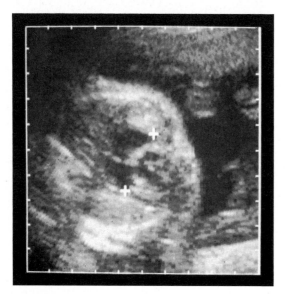

Fig. 8.108. Severely distended left ventricle in myogenic dilatation

pharmacologic therapy, or in the immediate prepartal period to improve the chance of successful postpartum resuscitation (pulmonary expansion; Hansmann et al. 1982).

4. Elective preterm delivery is considered the therapy of choice for the premature closure of fetal blood passages (Hansmann et al. 1982). It may also be indicated in cases of hydrops fetalis and growth retardation based on dys-

rhythmias that are unresponsive to drugs. In these cases, the options offered should be intensive postnatal therapy with intravenous drugs, cardioversion, or the implantation of a temporary or permanent pacemaker (Kleinman et al. 1982; DeVore et al. 1983).

To date, we have not had to terminate a pregnancy due to hydrops fetalis of cardiac origin. Generally, this option is not available, since this condition rarely manifests itself before 23 weeks gestation, unlike the hydrops associated with chromosome abnormalities (Hansmann and Redel 1982).

In contrast, we have terminated two pregnancies because of fetal cardiac malformations following an interdisciplinary review that included a cardiac surgeon and pediatric pathologist. The examinations, which were performed in selected, high-risk patients at 22 weeks gestation, resulted in the diagnosis of severe, untreatable cardiac anomalies. (*Case 1:* complete AV canal with common atrium, single AV valve, and rudimentary ventricular septum; Fig. 8.100. *Case 2:* marked left ventricular endocardial fibroelastosis with mitral and aortic hypoplasia; Fig. 8.101.) Both pregnancies had been asymptomatic prior to examination; the patients were selected solely on the basis of their increased risk for cardiac malformations as indicated by their family and obstetric history.

The prenatal diagnosis of cardiac defects will only be possible in centers where there is close collaboration between specially trained obstetric sonographers and pediatric cardiologists familiar with intrauterine echocardiography. It should be stressed, however, that the recognition of suspicious or abnormal findings during the initial examination is a necessary preliminary to more detailed evaluation (Figs. 8.102–8.109).

References

Allan LD, Tynan MJ, Campbell S, Wilkinson JL, Anderson RH (1980) Echocardiographic and anatomical correlates in the fetus. Br Heart 44:444

Davis CL (1982) Diagnosis and management of nonimmune hydrops fetalis. J Reprod Med 27:594

DeVore GR, Siassi B, Platt LD (1983) Fetal echocardiography. III. The diagnosis of cardiac arrhythmias using real-time-directed M-Mode ultrasound. Am J Obstet Gynecol 146:792

Dumesic DA, Silverman NH, Tobias S, Golbus MS (1982) Transplacental cardioversion of fetal supraventricular tachycardia with procainamide. N Engl J Med 307:1128

Etches PC, Lemons JA (1979) Nonimmune hydrops fetalis: Report of 22 cases including three siblings. Pediatrics 64:326

Gembruch U, Venn HJ, Redel DA, Hansmann M (1982) Wolff-Parkinson-White-Syndrom mit paroxysmalen supraventrikulären Tachykardien des Feten und des Neugeborenen – Fallbeschreibung. Klin Pädiat 194:320

Hansmann M (1981) Nachweis und Ausschluß fetaler Entwicklungsstörungen mittels Ultraschallscreening und gezielter Untersuchung – ein Mehrstufenkonzept. Ultraschall 2:206

Hansmann M, Gembruch U (1984) Gezielte sonographische Ausschlußdiagnostik fetaler Fehlbildungen in Risikogruppen. Gynäkologe 17:19

Hansmann M, Redel DA (1982) Prenatal symptoms and clinical management of heart disease. In: 1er symposium international d'echocardiologie foetale, Strasbourg 1982, p 137

Hansmann M, Redel DA, Födisch HJ (1982) Premature obstruction of the foramen ovale detected, treated and reconfirmed by help of ultrasound. In: Burruto F, Hansmann M, Wladimiroff JW (eds) Fetal ultrasonography: The secret prenatal life. Wiley, Chichester New York, p 151

Kleinman CS, Hobbins JC, Jaffe CC, Lynch DC, Talner NS (1980) Echocardiographic studies of the human fetus: prenatal diagnosis of congenital heart disease and cardiac dysrhythmias. Pediatrics 65:1059

Kleinman CS, Donnerstein RL, DeVore GR, Jaffe CC, Lynch DC, Berkowitz RL, Talner NS, Hobbins JC (1982) Fetal echocardiography for evaluation of in utero congestive heart failure. N Engl J Med 306:568

Kleinman CS, Donnerstein RL, Jaffe CC, DeVore GR, Weinstein EM, Lynch DC, Talner NS, Berkowitz RL,

Hobbins JC (1983) Fetal echocardiography. A tool for evaluation of in utero cardiac arrhythmias and monitoring of in utero therapy: Analysis of 71 patients. Am J Cardiol 51:237

Leake RD, Strimling B, Emmanouilides GC (1973) Intrauterine cardiac failure with hydrops fetalis. Case report in a twin with the hypoplastic left heart syndrome and review of the literature. Clin Pediatr 12:649

Maidman JE, Yeager C, Anderson V, Makabali G, O'Grady P, Arce J, Tishler DM (1980) Prenatal diagnosis and management of nonimmunologic hydrops fetalis. Obstet Gynecol 56:571

Nora JJ, Nora AH (1978) The evolution of specific genetic and environment counseling in congenital heart diseases. Circulation 57:205

Perlin BM, Pomerance JJ, Schifrin BS (1981) Nonimmunologic hydrops fetalis. Obstet Gynecol 57:584

Redel DA, Hansman M (1981) Fetal obstruction of the foramen ovale detected by two-dimensional doppler echocardiography. In: Rijsterborgh H (ed) Echocardiology. Nijhoff, The Hague Boston London, p 425

Redel DA, Hansmann M (1984) Fetale Echokardiographie – ihre Anwendung in Diagnostik und Therapie. Gynäkologe 17:41

Rudolph A (1974) Congenital diseases of the heart. Year Book Medical Publishers, Chicago

Sahn DJ, Lange LW, Allen HD, Goldberg SJ, Anderson C, Giles H, Haber K (1980) Quantitative real-time cross-sectional echocardiography in the developing normal human fetus and newborn. Circulation 62:588

Sahn DJ, Shenker L, Reed KL, Valdes-Cruz LM, Sobonya R, Anderson C (1982) Prenatal ultrasound diagnosis of hypoplastic left heart syndrome in utero associated with hydrops fetalis. Am Heart J 104:1368

Tamari I, Eldar M, Rabinowitz B, Neufeld HN (1982) Medical treatment of cardiovascular disorders during pregnancy. Am Heart J 104:1357

8.9 Ultrasound Evaluation of Patients at Risk of Fetal Anomalies

Up to this point we have dealt primarily with the diagnosis of fetal malformations during the general screening of patients not considered to be at risk. Now we shall examine the problem as it relates to the evaluation of selected patients who are at risk of delivering a malformed fetus. Of course, one cannot draw a strict dividing line between general and high-risk screening. However, we consider this approach to be useful didactically, particularly since sonographers at all levels of experience increasingly have occasion to examine high-risk patients and therefore must be familiar with the capabilities and limitations of ultrasound diagnosis in this population.

Today, pregnant patients who are at high risk of bearing a child with malformations may be

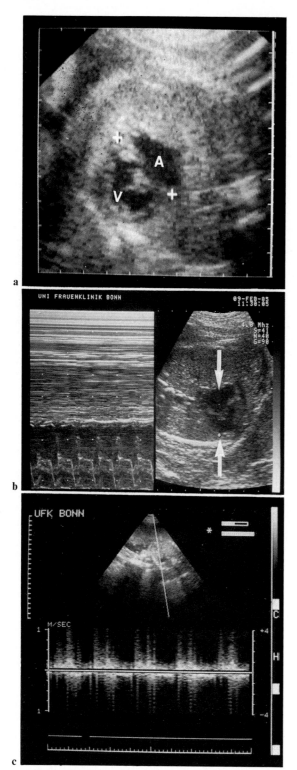

Fig. 8.110. a Cor biloculare: complete AV channel at 32 weeks. *A,* atrium; *V,* ventricle. Short axis (+——+) 30 mm. **b** Time-motion display in same case: registration time 10 s, frequency 60 beats/min. **c** Pulsed Doppler display in third-degree AV block: registration time 10 s, frequency 50 beats/min, atria 100 beats/min

offered an "early" prenatal sonographic evaluation that can exclude or establish an increasing number of fetal defects with a high degree of confidence (Hansmann and Gembruch 1984). If this evaluation is done in time, the parents will have the option of terminating the pregnancy if severe malformations are found. Thus, this diagnosis offers a chance of healthy offspring to families that previously would have been counseled against further pregnancies due to excessive risk of recurrence of a severe anomaly. Finally, the diagnosis of fetal malformations and diseases offers the opportunity to develop specific, individualized approaches to intrauterine therapy (Golbus et al. 1984). In other cases, the ability to choose the timing and mode of delivery and provide immediate neonatal care by specialists (e.g., neonatologists, neurosurgeons, pediatric surgeons, pediatric cardiologists) is an important advantage. It is anticipated that early diagnosis will significantly reduce mortality and morbidity in these infants (Kowalewski 1984).

Frequent problems of differential diagnosis in the assignment of symptoms, variations in the expressivity of symptoms in syndromes, and unresolved questions of prognosis underscore the need for close teamwork among disciplines. In many cases extensive genetic evaluation and counseling are necessary to define a given familial risk. This in turn relies on an accurate assessment of the risk factors (e.g., malformations in previous pregnancies) present in the family (Födisch 1982; Rehder 1982). Frequently this assessment is inadequate due to an obscure family history, sketchy postmortem records, or undiagnosed living relatives (Födisch and Knöpfle 1984). Drawing on the results of our previous investigations, we shall describe the current capabilities and limitations of sonography in the evaluation of high-risk pregnancies and present a range of indications that may be helpful in genetic counseling and in the planning and care of these pregnancies.

The instrumentation required for detailed evaluations is more sophisticated than for a basic examination. A sufficient quantity of instruments should be available to permit uninterrupted operation in the event of a malfunction. Both sector and linear systems should be available and should have a minimum image width of 10 cm at a depth of 6 cm. In addition to the photodocumentation required for a basic examination the facility should be equipped for video documentation, preferably using $^3/_4$-in. tape owing to its superior image quality.

Staffing of the facility should also be commensurate with the need for continuous screening. If a department is rendered inoperative by the absence of one staff member, it cannot be properly called a referral facility.

The optimum time for establishing or excluding a fetal anomaly is between 17 and 21 weeks gestation. By that time the fetal organs have formed, and their growth has progressed sufficiently for anatomic details and abnormalities to be verified sonographically. Also, this allows sufficient time for further investigation of suspicious findings prior to the legal limit of elective abortion for a fetal indication. These may consist of serial examinations, organ function tests, special sonographic studies using other types of instruments (e.g., two-dimensional pulsed Doppler echocardiography), or the use of supplemental diagnostic procedures such as fetoscopy or amniocentesis for chromosomal and biochemical amniotic fluid analysis. Interdisciplinary consultations (e.g., with neonatologists, pediatric surgeons, neurosurgeons, pediatric cardiologists, urologists, and pediatric radiologists) are also helpful in many cases.

Basically, the sonographic evaluation of high-risk patients is not limited to the confirmation or exclusion of organ anomalies for which the pregnancy is judged to be at risk, but also requires an assessment of overall fetal development including positive or negative findings relating to other organ systems. This demands that a systematic procedure be followed during the examination:

1. Survey of the uterus with assessment of amniotic fluid volume and the location, size, and appearance of the placenta

2. Measurement of all pertinent fetal parameters (BPD and OFD, head circumference, abdominal diameters and circumference, length of long bones, intraorbital distance, etc.)

3. Evaluation of skull and brain structure, noting brain symmetry and ventricular size

4. Inspection of the face in frontal and profile views, delineating the eyes, nose, mouth, ears, and jaws

5. Examination of the spine in longitudinal scans and of individual segments in transverse scans

6. Visualization of the heart in the four-chamber view and measurement of the transverse diameter at the level of the AV valves (short axis)

7. Exclusion of abnormal structures in the chest (fluid, cyst, stomach, bowel)

8. Evaluation of the outline of the diaphragm, liver, and stomach (with serial scans if the stomach is "empty")

9. Visualization of the kidneys and bladder (with assessment of urinary dynamics if oligohydramnios is present)

10. Examination of all four extremities with delineation of the hands and feet

11. Evaluation of fetal behavior (e.g., coordinated motion of hand to head, thumb sucking, swallowing, yawning, stretching)

An examination of this type requires an average of 30–60 min to complete. If special studies are needed, the examination may take several hours over a period of days.

Since 1978 we have used ultrasound to search for fetal malformations prior to 24 weeks in selected patients belonging to high-risk groups, i.e., considered to have an increased risk of bearing an abnormal child [see Gembruch et al. (1983) for earlier results]. To date, more than 1,500 high-risk patients have been evaluated under this protocol. As of October 1983, information on pregnancy outcome was available for 878 cases from four different high-risk groups:

1. Six hundred sixteen patients (70.2%) with a family history of malformations of various organ systems (Table 8.4). 96% of these had affected first-degree relatives, mostly offspring of previous pregnancies.

2. Two hundred five patients (23.3%) exposed in early pregnancy to toxic or teratogenic agents: 165 (80.5%) to drugs, 21 (10.2%) to X-rays, and 19 (9.3%) to infectious organisms or vaccines.

3. Thirteen patients (1.5%) with maternal diabetes mellitus.

4. Forty-four patients (5.0%) with an elevation of serum or amniotic fluid AFP. Generally the AFP assay was done "incidentally" during genetic amniocenteses performed elsewhere for other indications. Ultrasound examination at these clinics was unable to identify the cause of the AFP elevation.

Table 8.4. High-risk group 1: Family history that prompted selection for evaluation

1. Neural tube defects		n
		127
Anencephaly	20	
Spina bifida	86	
Encephalocele	6	
Unspecified NTD	15	
Hydrocephalus		37
Hydranencephaly		2
Dandy-Walker syndrome		2
Microcephaly		11
Arnold-Chiari complex		1
Congenital AV aneurysm		2
Total:		**182**

2. Gastrointestinal tract and anterior abdominal wall		n
Omphalocele		15
Gastroschisis		5
Diaphragmatic atresia with enterothorax		7
Esophageal atresia		3
Small bowel atresia		2
Duodenal stenosis		1
Malrotation I		1
Total:		**34**

3. Urogenital tract		n
Potter's syndrome		35
Cystic kidneys (Potter Type I)		15
Cystic kidneys (Potter type II)		7
"Bilateral cystic kidneys"		1
Prune-belly syndrome		7
Bilateral hydroureters and hydronephrosis		1
Urethral atresia		2
Wilms' tumor		2
Bladder ectopia		1
Total:		**71**

4. Heart defects		n
a) Left-sided obstruction		39
Aortic stenosis	3	
Supravalvular aortic stenosis	1	
Aortic arch atresia	2	
Coarctation of aorta	7	
Williams-Beuren syndrome	1	
Mitral stenosis	1	
Shone's complex	1	
Hypoplastic left heart	23	
b) Right-sided obstruction		18
Tetralogy of Fallot	13	
Tricuspid atresia	3	
Pulmonary atresia	1	
Hypoplastic right heart	1	
c) Shunt defects		31
Atrial septal defect	1	
Single atrium	1	
Truncus arteriosus	5	
Ventricular septal defect	17	
Single ventricle	7	

		n
d) Anomalous insertion of great arteries	21	22
Transposition of great arteries (double-outlet right ventricle)	1	
e) Miscellaneous		16
Complex defect	2	
Endocardial fibroelastosis	3	
Premature closure of foramen ovale	2	
Unspecified "serious defects"	9	
Total:		**126**

5. Skeletal system		n
Limb malformations		35
Facial clefts		27
Osteogenesis imperfecta congenitalis		11
Arthrogryposis multiplex congenitalis		2
Achondroplasia		5
Achondrogenesis type II		2
Chondrodysplasia (recessive type)		1
Diastrophic dysplasia		1
Camptomelic dysplasia		2
Ellis-van Creveld syndrome		1
Leri-Weill syndrome		1
Ribbing's disease		2
Thanatophoric dwarfism		9
Pseudoachondroplasia		1
Hypophosphatasia		3
Craniostenosis		1
Total:		**104**

6. Syndromes	n
Jeune	6
Meckel-Gruber	5
C. de Lange	3
P. Robin	4
Wiedemann-Beckwith	1
Smith-Lemli-Opitz	1
Laurence-Moon-Biedl-Bardet	1
Nail-patella	1
Nager	1
TAR	3
Klippel-Feil	3
EEC	1
Anophthalmia	1
Joubert	2
Lenz	1
Mohr (OFD II)	1
Fanconi	1
Arhinencephaly	1
Holoprosencephaly	3
Unidentified syndrome with facial cleft	1
Basal cell nevus syndrome	1
Ivemark	2
Goldenhar	1
Roberts	1
COFS	1
Acrocephalosyndactyly type III	1
Recklinghausen's disease	1
VACTERL	4
Total:	**53**

Table 8.5. Twenty-five fetuses (of 616 examined) with malformations

No.	History	Defect at birth	Ultrasound diagnosis True positive	False negative	Termination (× yes, − no)
1	Anencephalus	Anencephaly	16 w		×
2	Spina bifida aperta	Anencephaly	14 w		×
3	Spina bifida aperta	Anencephaly	14 w		×
4	Spina bifida aperta	Spina bifida aperta	20 w		−
5	Cystic kidneys (Potter type I)	Spina bifida aperta		1	−
6	Cystic kidneys (Potter type I)	Cystic kidneys (Potter type I)	after 23 w		−
7	Cystic kidneys (Potter type I)	Cystic kidneys (Potter type I)	after 23 w		−
8	Cystic kidneys (Potter type I)	Valvular pulmonary stenosis		1[a]	−
9	Ventricular septal defect	Valvular pulmonary stenosis		1[a]	−
10	Transposition of the great arteries	Small ventricular septal defect		1[a]	−
11	Hypoplastic left heart	Total anomalous pulmonary venous drainage		1[b]	−
12	Transposition of the great arteries	Endocardial fibroelastosis	22 w		×
13	Complex heart defect	Complex heart defect	22 w		×
14	Hypoplastic left heart	Complete AV canal		1	−
15	Multiple limb malformations	Biliary atresia		1[b]	−
16	Cleft hands	Cleft hands		1	−
17	Multiple limb malformations	Achondrogenesis type I	19 w		×
18	Pseudoachondroplasia	Pseudoachondroplasia	18 w		−
19	Chondrodysplasia punctata	Chondrodysplasia punctata	18 w		×
20	Ellis-van-Creveld syndrome	Ellis-van Creveld s.	19 w		×
21	Jeune's syndrome	Jeune's syndrome		1	−
22	Meckel-Gruber syndrome	Meckel-Gruber syndrome	18 w		×
23	COFS syndrome	COFS syndrome		1	−
24	Arhinencephaly syndrome	Arhinencephaly syndrome	23 w		×
25	Unidentified syndrome with facial cleft	Unidentified syndrome with facial cleft	22 w		×
	Total		15	5+3[a] +2[b]	11

[a] No severe, disabling malformations are present in these cases
[b] Prenatal ultrasound diagnosis is not possible in these cases

8.9.1 High-Risk Group 1: Family History of Malformations

Of the 616 fetuses in this group, malformations were present in 25 (4.1%) (Table 8.5). A correct prenatal sonographic diagnosis was made in 15 of these fetuses, with 13 diagnosed before 24 weeks. In 11 of these 13 cases, the pregnancy was terminated. In the remaining two (one fetus with spina bifida aperta and one with pseudo-achondroplasia), the parents accepted the anomaly and chose to continue with the pregnancy. In 10 cases no malformations were detected. At least three of these anomalies were classified as "inconsequential," and two others were judged not to be detectable prenatally with ultrasound. Malformations were "correctly" excluded in 591 fetuses (96%).

We shall now examine the capabilities and limitations of diagnostic ultrasound in these patients for the confirmation or exclusion of anomalies of specific fetal organ systems on the basis of our own clinical experience.

Malformations of the Central Nervous System. *Neural Tube Defects.* 127 of the 182 patients who were referred to us for exclusion of malformations of the fetal CNS had a family history of neural tube defect, including anencephaly, spina bifida, and encephalocele (Table 8.4). The recurrence risk following the previous birth of an affected child is reported to be approximately 5% in Great Britain (Brock 1979). The risk is considerably lower in the Federal Republic of Germany owing to the generally lower prevalence of neural tube defects [1:1,000 according to Warkany (1971) and only 0.4:1,000 according to Weitzel (1983) vs. 4.5:1,000 in Great Britain according to the Report of the U.K. Collaborative Study (1977)]. In our series the recurrence of a neural tube defect (three cases of anencephaly, one case of spina bifida aperta) was diagnosed sonographically before 24 weeks in all four patients with previously affected offspring (3.1%). It appears that spina bifida, which has the same incidence as anencephaly (Report of the U.K. Collaborative Study 1977), is almost never diagnosed during routine ultrasound examination.

In our series one case of lumbosacral spina bifida aperta was correctly diagnosed, and spina bifida was correctly excluded in the remaining 181 patients. The false-negative diagnoses of lumbosacral spina bifida in a patient who had been referred for exclusion of Potter type I cystic kidneys, and of sacral spina bifida aperta in a second patient who had been referred with suspected rubella in early pregnancy (see Sect. 8.9.2), illustrate the diagnostic difficulties involved.

For this reason, all patients with a family history of neural tube defect should undergo a serum AFP assay. Amniocentesis for amniotic fluid analysis may be dispensed with if the serum AFP is normal *and* a detailed ultrasound examination is performed by an experienced examiner under good conditions (adequate amniotic fluid volume, no obesity) shows no evidence of such defects (Gembruch et al. 1984).

Hydrocephalus. The prevalence of congenital hydrocephalus in the absence of spina bifida or other anomalies is 0.22–1.8:1,000, and the recurrence risk is 0.5–1.0% (Shannon and Nadler 1968). Exceptions are the extremely rare autosomal recessive form of hydrocephalus and X-linked aqueductal stenosis. Dandy-Walker syndrome has a somewhat higher risk of recurrence (Lehman 1981; Taybi 1983). It should be noted that the birth of a child with hydrocephalus signifies a 2 to 5 times higher risk of a neural tube defect in a subsequent child (Cohen et al. 1979). Conversely, a family history of neural tube defect is associated with an increased risk of hydrocephalus (Robertson et al. 1981). So far no recurrences have been observed in our patients at risk ($n = 37$).

Malformations of the Anterior Abdominal Wall and Gastrointestinal Tract. *Anterior Wall Defects.* The incidence of omphalocele is between 1 in 2,280 and 1 in 10,000 live births; gastroschisis is rarer still (Kirk and Wah 1983). The

recurrence risk for these defects is small, and a familial occurrence is observed only sporadically, unless the defect is part of a syndrome and follows its mode of inheritance (e.g., Wiedemann-Beckwith syndrome). To date we have diagnosed 20 of 22 omphaloceles in our study population. Thirteen were diagnosed before 24 weeks gestation, the earliest at 12 weeks (Hansmann 1984).

Bowel Obstruction. Esophageal atresia is detectable only indirectly with ultrasound through the presence of polyhydramnios and the inability to visualize the stomach and bowel loops. On the other hand, duodenal obstruction as seen with duodenal atresia, annular pancreas, or peritoneal cords is easily recognized by the "double-bubble sign," which is almost pathognomonic for that disorder (Hansmann 1981a). Atresias of other bowel segments and the anus can also be diagnosed using ultrasound (Bean et al. 1978; Hobbins et al. 1979). With duodenal atresia a chromosome analysis should be performed, since this condition is associated with trisomy 21 in 30% of cases (Jassani et al. 1982). None of the 34 newborns from the high-risk group had bowel malformations, and a correct negative prenatal diagnosis was made in all cases.

Malformations of the Urogenital Tract. Typical indications for the evaluation of the fetal urinary tract are: previous delivery of a child with Potter's syndrome or prune-belly syndrome; family history of cystic kidneys.

Potter's syndrome has an incidence of 1:3,000 to 1:4,000 (Hansmann et al. 1979) with a low recurrence risk (Carter et al. 1979). It tends to occur sporadically, although familial occurrences with Mendelian modes of inheritance have been described (Knöpfle et al. 1982). The cause is an absence of functioning kidneys, due to bilateral renal agenesis, cystic renal dysplasia, or complex urogenital malformations (Knöpfle et al. 1982).

Based on experience with two positive cases in our high-risk patients, it appears that autosomal recessive bilateral cystic kidneys (type 1) cannot be confidently excluded before 24 weeks. The resolution of ultrasound equipment is inadequate to demonstrate the small (1–2 mm) tubular cysts during the second trimester. The amniotic fluid volume in such cases may be completely normal initially (Weiss et al. 1981). So far, prenatal diagnosis in the third trimester has been based on markedly enlarged kidneys displaying patchy hyperechoic areas. This diagnosis was made in the 28th week in one of our at-risk patients, and shortly before delivery in another patient whose physician had considered earlier referral "unnecessary." The ratio of renal circumference to abdominal circumference is considered a particularly sensitive index of abnormal renal size and thus of type I cystic disease (Grannum et al. 1980).

On the other hand, type II cystic kidneys, which are not inherited, occur bilaterally in about 50% of cases, have associated anomalies in a similar percentage, and can be diagnosed in the second trimester owing to the larger size of the cysts. The kidneys themselves may be hypoplastic or enlarged. Type II cystic kidneys also occur in association with syndromes such as Meckel-Gruber, Dandy-Walker, prune-belly, and Ivemark's, and are thus subject to their modes of inheritance (Zerres and Födisch 1982).

The cysts in Potter type III polycystic kidneys, which have an autosomal dominant inheritance, are rarely recognizable prenatally and thus are not considered an indication for early detailed ultrasound evaluation (Weiss et al. 1981).

Prune-belly syndrome (the triad of abdominal muscle deficiency, urinary tract dysplasia, and cryptorchidism), has a generally low recurrence risk (Rehder 1982) and only rarely shows a familial incidence. Although a primary aplasia of the abdominal muscles (as described for Eagle-Barrett syndrome) cannot always be excluded, this appears to be a secondary condition in the great majority of cases. Thus, a variety of intraabdominal space-occupying processes can lead to prune-belly syndrome, including all forms of obstructive uropathy, polycystic kidneys, congenital cystic adenomatoid malformation of the lungs, and Hirschsprung's disease. The most common mechanism underlying prune-belly syndrome is the urethral obstruction malformation complex, caused by urethral obstruction in the form of valves, atresia, and, less frequently, anterior strictures and diverticula. Bladder distention and hypertrophy, dilated ureters, hydronephrosis, and even dysplastic kidneys may characterize the sonographic picture. In addition, intestinal and skeletal anomalies are present in up to 50% of fetuses with this complex (Pagon et al. 1979). Based on our experience ($n = 15$), prune-belly syndrome encompasses a range of obstructive uropathies in which the degree of obstruction and quality of renal function determine the severity of the syndrome (Hansmann 1984). For example, we have observed the complete picture of prune-belly syndrome as early as 15 weeks in a patient referred with suspicious sonographic findings. In another case we aspirated 1.5 liters of urine from a fetus at 21 weeks to reduce abdominal circumference prior to a pharmacologically induced abortion. In yet another case the fetal bladder was reported to be "abnormal" at 12 weeks (diameter 1.5 cm), and by 17 weeks the syndrome was fully developed. These and other observations (Pagon et al. 1979) point to an insidious pathogenesis that depends both on the degree and location of the obstruction and on the rate of fetal urine production. This raises the possibility of intrauterine therapy (repeated aspirations, placement of a shunt catheter, surgical procedures on the fetus), which should only be performed if postpartum correction is possible. Such procedures must be preceeded by detailed sonographic examination and serial observations which should identify the causative lesion, its extent, and the function of both kidneys and also exclude associated anomalies (e.g., chromosome aberrations). Cases involving unilateral involution of a kidney or ureter and a normal amniotic fluid volume have a good prognosis and prenatal therapy is not generally necessary.

Cardiac Malformations. Congenital cardiac malformations have an incidence of 0.7%–0.8%, with a recurrence risk between 1% and 4.4% depending on the type and frequency of the lesion in the general population (Keith et al. 1978). Genetic causes are predominant in 8% of cases, environmental factors in 2%, and 90% have a multifactorial etiology involving an interaction of genetic and exogenous factors (Nora and Nora 1978). In this group it is necessary to distinguish between low-risk and high-risk families and patients. The latter are predisposed to the development of cardiac defects on exposure to certain environmental influences, and it may in the future be possible to identify these patients on the basis of biochemical or immunologic parameters. When associated with a syndrome (Holt-Oram, Treacher-Collins, Goldenhar, Ellis-van Creveld, Smith-Lemli-Opitz, chondrodysplasia punctata, etc.), cardiac anomalies follow the mode of inheritance of that syndrome, though with varying penetrance. The likelihood of recurrence of cardiac defects is particularly high in families with autosomal recessive or autosomal dominant inheritance due to a single gene. This especially applies to cases of supravalvular aortic stenosis, atrial septal defect, familial cardiomyopathy, dextrocardia, situs inversus, endocardial fibroelastosis, and hypoplastic left heart (Keith et al. 1978)

The complex embryonic development of the heart and multifactorial pathogenesis of many cardiac defects explain why groups of defects have a familial incidence, and also why different defects can be observed in the same family. For example, closure of the ventricular septum relies on the precise fusion of the endocardial cushion, proximal bulbar septum, and interventricular septum at a given point in time. Accordingly, 30%–60% of affected first-degree relatives have a ventricular septal defect, while 40%–70% have other, often embryologically related cardiac anomalies (Nora and Nora 1978). In our patients with a family history of cardiac defects, two severe fetal heart anomalies were diagnosed with ultrasound at 22 weeks gestation (*Case 1:* Family history of atrial septal defect and partial anomalous pulmonary venous drainage in the first child, a lethal complex defect in the second child. Present diagnosis: complete AV canal with common atrium, common AV valve, and a large ventricular septal defect with a rudimentary interventricular septum. *Case 2:* Family history of transposition of the great arteries in the first child. Present diagnosis: marked left ventricular endocardial fibroelastosis and hypoplasia of the mitral valve and ascending aorta.) Both pregnancies were terminated at the request of the parents following consultation with a cardiac surgeon and a pediatric pathologist, and the prenatal diagnoses were confirmed at autopsy. Anomalous pulmonary venous drainage was overlooked in one patient whose first child had died of hypoplastic left heart syndrome. This anomaly, which is hemodynamically significant postnatally, is extremely difficult to detect sonographically even after birth. Prenatally, this malformation appears to be inaccessible to echocar-

diography, because due to shunting the blood bypasses the pulmonary circuit, and only 5%–10% of the cardiac output flows through the pulmonary veins. Also, the signs of right heart overload that are present postnatally are not observed in utero. Neither is prenatal Doppler flow analysis a very useful technique for evaluating the pulmonary veins. Accordingly, we have not yet been able to diagnose a case of anomalous pulmonary venous drainage antenatally. A small, hemodynamically insignificant ventricular septal defect was also missed in a patient who had previously delivered an infant with pulmonary stenosis. While easy to recognize in neonates, such lesions are extremely difficult to verify prenatally, even by Doppler flow analysis, due to shunting of blood by the ventricles and the resultant pressure equilibrium. The prenatal diagnosis of pulmonary stenosis is also difficult, especially if the condition is mild. This was the case in two fetuses, one of which was not specifically examined for cardiac anomalies because the purpose of the evaluation was to confirm or exclude type I cystic kidneys. Finally, a complete AV canal lesion could not be confidently diagnosed prenatally, although suggestive signs were present (suspicion of a common AV valve and septum primum defect on first examination; evidence of insertion of both AV valves at the same level of the septum with a suspected defect of the anterior mitral valve leaflet and septum primum defect on second examination).

In general, it is likely that many severe, incorrectable fetal cardiac defects are diagnosable prenatally, although the associated hemodynamic changes, consisting of excessive pressure or volume load and resulting hypertrophy or dilatation, rarely develop before birth due to the shunting of blood by the fetal ventricles. On the other hand, minor cardiac defects that involve minimal anatomic changes are not yet accessible to prenatal diagnosis. These include pulmonary and aortic stenosis and small atrial and ventricular septal defects.

Skeletal Malformations. With modern real-time scanners it is possible to measure the diaphyses of the long bones of the extremities from 11 weeks on (Schlensker 1981). The many types of dysmelia (amelia, phocomelia, micromelia, isolated radial and tibial aplasia, cleft hand and foot, oligo- and polydactyly) can be diagnosed using ultrasound (Hansmann 1981a, 1984). But bone length measurements require considerable experience, due in part to the physiologic curvature of the fetal limb bones. In addition, substantial differences may be noted between external measurements performed on aborted fetuses, sonographic measurements in vitro (water bath), and intrauterine sonographic measurements. These factors may well account for the discrepancies in the nomograms published by different authors (Schlensker 1981; Queenan et al. 1980; Filly et al. 1981; Hobbins et al. 1982a). For this reason it is best for each center to establish its own normal values. This is particularly important for early evaluation of high-risk pregnancies, which requires extremely accurate measurements. The difficulties involved are illustrated by the following observations: Hobbins et al. (1982a) found that femur lengths in chondroectogermal dysplasia (Ellis-van Creveld syndrome) and an autosomal dominant form of osteogenesis imperfecta were "small" at 17 and 18 weeks respectively, but not outside 95% confidence limits. Filly et al. (1981) even described one case of fetal achondroplasia in which femur lengths in the third trimester were only slightly shorter than the mean for gestation. By contrast, camptomelic and diastrophic dysplasia – two autosomal recessive forms of dwarfism – caused significant shortening of the long bones before 24 weeks gestation, at least in the cases diagnosed by Hobbins et al. (1982a). The same applies to Saldino-Noonan syndrome (Johnson et al. 1982). In our own patients at risk, recurrence of the following autosomal recessive disorders could be established: (1) chondrodysplasia punctata of the rhizomelic type at 18 weeks; (2) pseudo-achondroplasia at 18 weeks in a couple who already had two affected children and in this case elected not to continue the pregnancy; (3) achondrogenesis type I at 19 weeks; and (4) chondroectodermal dysplasia (Ellis-van Creveld syndrome) at 19 weeks in a patient who had previously delivered two affected children who did not survive. In all four cases the prenatal diagnosis was based on the demonstration of "short" diaphyses – not only in relation to gestational age, but also in terms of the relation of bone lengths to head and trunk diameters. This discrepancy was greatest in the fetus with achondrogenesis type I (19 weeks: humerus 12 mm, femur 14 mm, radius 17 mm, tibia

17 mm, BPD 47 mm, TTD 41 mm). The discrepancy was smallest in the fetus with Ellis-van Creveld syndrome (19 weeks: humerus 20 mm, femur 23 mm, ulna 19 mm, tibia 20 mm, BPD 44 mm, TTD 40 mm). In this case the long bone lengths at 16 weeks were still at the lower limit of the normal range. In 100 other patients at risk for fetal skeletal anomalies, one recurrence of a cleft hand was missed prenatally. In all others, recurrent anomalies were excluded by ultrasound. Remarkably, none of the 11 patients who had previously delivered children with type II osteogenesis imperfecta congenita (Sillence et al. 1979) had a second affected fetus, despite the autosomal recessive inheritance of the disorder. Similarly, Hobbins et al. (1982a) made only one positive diagnosis of fetal osteogenesis imperfecta in 13 patients at risk. It may be that some fetuses from earlier pregnancies were incorrectly diagnosed as malformed. Also, the lethal type of osteogenesis imperfecta is known to have several subtypes that may not be autosomal recessive.

Another large group was examined to exclude a facial cleft malformation (approximately 5% recurrence risk in first-degree relatives). The anomaly was correctly excluded in all 27 cases (Claussen and Hansmann 1984).

8.9.2 High-Risk Group 2: Exposure to Exogenous, Potentially Teratogenic Agents in Early Pregnancy

A total of 205 pregnant women exposed in early pregnancy to exogenous, potentially teratogenic agents were examined sonographically for fetal malformations. Anomalies were correctly excluded in 204 fetuses. Only one neonate from this group (0.5%) exhibited a malformation – a small spina bifida lesion in the lumbosacral region that was missed on scans performed for a suspected rubella infection. This very low incidence, which is even below the 2% overall risk for congenital malformations, is presumably a result of the small study population.

Drugs. The absence of fetal malformations in this group is due partly to the fact that the majority of our patients took only laxatives, antiemetics, flu remedies, antitussives, psychotropic drugs, hypnotics, and antibiotics during early pregnancy. Moreover, they often used them only once or for a short period, and some drugs were taken outside the sensitive phase of embryonic development from 3 to 7 weeks after conception. According to genetic opinion, the drug classes listed above are associated with only a minimal increase in teratogenic risk (further references in Kleinebrecht 1982). The difficulties in defining the risk of a fetal malformation are based on the combined effects of several factors (agent, dose, timing of exposure, duration of exposure, interaction with other agents, genotype) on the etiology of developmental anomalies. This also applies to female sex steroids, which some patients took for abortion prophylaxis and others used for contraception before knowing they were already pregnant. Although some studies claim to have demonstrated a statistical correlation between these drugs and various congenital anomalies (cardiovascular defects, neural tube defects, limb malformations, VACTERL syndrome), critical analysis refutes this, especially since the total incidence of malformations is not measurably increased (Nocke 1978). Only a small group of patients ($n = 29$) consumed known or probable teratogenic substances (Ramzin 1982) during early pregnancy in the form of alcohol, cytostatics, immunosuppressives, antiepileptics, and coumarin derivatives.

X-Rays. Radiologic diagnostic procedures must be used with caution in pregnant women, because there is no "threshold" dose below which an X-ray examination may be considered safe for the conceptus. However, due to repair mechanisms at the molecular level, teratogenicity may not be seen below an embryonic dose of 0.1 Gy, and doses of 0.2 Gy or higher are needed to produce a marked increase in the malformation rate. For radiologic examinations in pregnancy, the embryo or fetus usually receives a dose of less than 0.01 Gy. Generally the same applies to the use of radioisotopes in pregnancy, although ^{131}I should not be used due to its tendency to accumulate in the fetal thyroid (further references in Knorr 1983). A level of 0.01 Gy was not exceeded in any of our 21 patients exposed to ionizing radiation. In all cases fetal malformations were correctly excluded sonographically before 24 weeks.

Infectious Diseases. A viral infection or high fever in early pregnancy increases the risk of fetal abnormalities. The most notorious disease in this regard is rubella (Gregg's syndrome). The missed case of lumbosacral spina bifida in our series was referred to us with a suspicion of maternal rubella. In all other cases – two were vaccinated against poliomyelitis and yellow fever in early pregnancy – fetal anomalies were correctly excluded.

To critically review the results in the group of patients exposed to exogenous, potentially teratogenic agents in early pregnancy:

1. It is apparent that the selection of patients was too broad.

2. Accurate risk appraisal requires collaboration with experts, although given the multifactorial etiology of anomalies, it is often impossible to adequately quantify the risk in an individual patient (in doubtful cases, pragmatism is better).

3. On a more subtle level, the sonographic exclusion of fetal malformations unquestionably serves an important psychological purpose within the context of prenatal care. It was evident that the degree of anxiety in some of our patients had clinical significance. This anxiety could be partially or completely resolved by the patient's encounter with her child on the monitor screen.

8.9.3 High-Risk Group 3: Maternal Diabetes Mellitus

The risk of congenital anomalies in offspring of women with diabetes mellitus ranges from 4.5% to 9% (Kucera 1981; Malins 1978; Pedersen and Molsted-Pedersen 1981). As with spontaneous abortion, the incidence of fetal malformations increases with the duration and severity of the diabetes. This is especially true for pregnant women with class D and F diabetes (according to White's classification) who have longstanding insulin dependence and/or vascular complications (Artner et al. 1982).

While improvements in perinatal care have led to a marked decline of perinatal mortality and morbidity from respiratory distress syndrome, neonatal hypoglycemia, macrosomia, and cardiomegaly, they have only lessened the incidence of congenital malformations when effective prepregnancy management could be instituted (Artner et al. 1981; Pedersen and Molsted-Pedersen 1981).

The teratogenic agent of diabetes mellitus remains unknown. Vascular lesions, hypoglycemia, and other metabolic disturbances have been postulated. Whatever its nature, the agent must act between 3 and 6 weeks after conception, during the critical phase of teratogenesis (Mills et al. 1979). Although insulin is capable of producing congenital anomalies in laboratory animals, all studies indicate that therapeutic insulin doses are unlikely to be teratogenic in human fetuses (Malins 1978; Mills et al. 1979; Kleinebrecht 1982).

The fetal growth retardation recorded by Pedersen and Molsted-Pedersen (1981) on sonographic measurements of CRL between 7 and 14 weeks in diabetics, the association of this retardation with severe class D and F maternal diabetes, and the increased risk of malformations in these fetuses point to a common etiologic mechanism for early intrauterine growth retardation, abnormal embryogenesis, and perhaps also spontaneous abortion.

The majority of malformations in infants of diabetic mothers affect the heart, varying widely in severity. Since an increased incidence of neural tube defects is also observed serum AFP determination is imperative in all pregnant women with diabetes. Renal anomalies, caudal regression syndrome (agenesis or hypoplasia of the femora and agenesis of the caudal vertebral bodies), and situs inversus are readily accessible to early ultrasound diagnosis. In the 13 pregnant women with diabetes mellitus examined by us (two class A, five class B, six class C), fetal malformations were correctly excluded.

Thus, besides the determination of serum AFP, detailed ultrasound examination is recommended for all pregnant women with diabetes to rule out fetal malformations (Hansmann 1981 a, b). This examination should be an integral part of the management of these high-risk pregnancies. This is particularly important when one considers that good diabetic management can reduce all other aspects of perinatal mortality and morbidity, and presumably congenital malformations as well (Plotz et al. 1978).

8.9.4 High-Risk Group 4: Elevation of Serum or Amniotic Fluid AFP

An elevated level of AFP in the maternal serum and amniotic fluid is suggestive of the presence of neural tube defects, although the elevation may also be associated with other abnormalities (Brock 1979; Weitzel 1983). Because over 90% of neonates with neural tube defects have no apparent genetic risk, a program of mass prenatal screening of maternal serum AFP has been instituted in Great Britain, where the incidence of neural tube defects is high. In the Federal Republic of Germany only regional studies have so far been conducted (Fuhrmann 1983; Weitzel 1983). The use of serum AFP screening in pregnant women who have a family history of neural tube defects is an accepted practice, as the risk of such defects in these patients is markedly increased (Brock 1979).

The British AFP screening protocol (Leonard 1981; Second Report of U.K. Collaborative Study 1979) calls for an ultrasound examination to be performed after elevated serum AFP levels are measured on two occasions. The purpose of this examination is to exclude an error in dates, twins, intrauterine growth retardation and fetal death, as well as gross fetal malformations such as anencephaly and large abdominal wall defects. If no cause for the AFP elevation is found, an amniocentesis and amniotic fluid analysis is performed which should include determination of the neural-tube-specific isoenzyme acetylcholinesterase (Report of the Collaborative Acetylcholinesterase Study 1981).

Ultrasound in patients with elevated serum and amniotic fluid AFP levels is capable of identifying or excluding a causative defect (Gembruch et al. 1984; Hobbins et al. 1982b). Forty-four patients examined before 24 weeks were referred for evaluation of elevated serum or amniotic fluid AFP levels (Fuhrmann, Giessen; Weitzel, Hannover). A common feature of all these cases was that ultrasound examination performed elsewhere failed to disclose the cause of the AFP elevation. In 15 patients, serum AFP was determined for the purpose of screening. In 29 patients, amniotic fluid AFP was determined incidentally to amniocentesis for chromosome analysis. In 11 patients with an elevation of only the serum AFP, sonographic evaluation was normal. Of 33 patients with abnormal amniotic fluid AFP levels, 12 had fetal anomalies. All were correctly diagnosed by ultrasound – spina bifida aperta in eight fetuses, omphalocele in three fetuses, and gastroschisis in one fetus. The repeat amniocenteses performed in some patients and supplementary

Table 8.6. Ultrasound diagnosis of fetal malformations: summary of results, Bonn (up to October 1983). Excluded are fetuses with cardiac defects ($n > 30$), chromosome anomalies ($n > 45$) and nonimmunologic hydrops fetalis ($n > 70$)

Diagnosis	Total	Correct	Before 23 weeks	False +	False −
An-, ex-, iniencephalus	48	48	30	0	0
Spina bifida	30	23	12	0	7
Meningomyelo-encephalocele	14	11	3	0	(3)
Hydrocephalus (without spina bifida)	27	27	8	0	0
Microcephalus	11	11	2	0	0
Omphalocele	22	20	13	0	(2)
Eventration	7	7	3	0	0
Gastroschisis	4	4	2	0	0
Stenosis of GI tract	7	5	0	0	2
Bowel perforation	2	1	0	0	(1)
Biliary atresia	1	0	0	0	1
Potter syndrome	30	24	12	(1)	6
Prune-belly syndrome	15	14	12	0	(1)
Cystic kidneys (types 1–4)	15	12	2	1	(2)
Hydronephrosis	15	15	1	(1)	(2)
Other uropathies	12	10	0	0	1
Solid tumors: astrocytoma, rhabdomyoma, hamartoma, etc.	5	(5)	3	0	0
Sacral teratoma	5	5	1	0	0
Cystic tumors (e.g., ovarian)	6	(6)	3	0	0
Dysmelia/amelia	2	2	1	0	0
Achondrogenesis	3	2	1	0	1
Pseudoachondroplasia	1	1	1	0	0
Thanatophoric dwarfism	5	4	0	0	(1)
Thoracophagus	2	2	1	0	0
Arhinencephalus	1	1	1	0	0
Wiedemann-Beckwith syndrome	2	1	0	0	(1)
Chondrodysplasia punctata	1	1	1	0	0
COFS syndrome	1	0	0	0	1
Dandy-Walker syndrome	1	1	1	0	0
Ellis v. Crefeld syndrome	1	1	1	0	0
Jeune syndrome	1	0	0	0	1
Meckel-Gruber syndrome	3	2	2	0	1
Osteogenesis imperfecta	1	1	0	0	0
Cleft hand	1	0	0	0	1
VACTERL	2	1	0	0	1
Total:	304	268	117	(3)	23 + (13)

amniotic fluid acetylcholinesterase determinations also yielded some false-positive results (Gembruch et al. 1984). All 21 fetuses of the elevated AFP group that were classified as normal sonographically were found to have no malformations at birth.

These results show that biochemical studies of the serum and amniotic fluid, though widely used to screen for fetal malformations, do not enable a decision to be made regarding the continuation or termination of a pregnancy. Before elective termination can be considered on the basis of elevated amniotic fluid AFP levels, the patient should undergo detailed ultrasound evaluation at a specialized facility (Hansmann 1981a, b).

The prompt referral of patients to such a center obviates the need for a repeat amniocentesis in most cases. Besides spina bifida aperta and anencephaly, a large number of other fetal malformations associated with an elevation of AFP can be diagnosed sonographically, including omphalocele, gastroschisis, Meckel-Gruber syndrome, polycystic kidneys, and Potter's syndrome, and certain atresias of the gastrointestinal tract. The extemely rare autosomal recessive

Finnish type of congenital nephrosis cannot be excluded with ultrasound (Aula et al. 1978).

In 1980 the Federal Republic of Germany became the first country in the world to institute ultrasound screening of all pregnancies. Since that time, remarkable progress has been made in the diagnosis of fetal malformations, due largely to the fact that increasing numbers of patients are actually being referred to specialized (Stage II and III) centers because of suspicious findings on initial examination (Stage I). It is noteworthy that among our patients, more than 90% of all fetal malformations diagnosed prenatally are detected at the initial screening stage. This raises the question of whether specialized detailed evaluation is in fact necessary. We believe unequivocally that it is, because it serves different goals than screening, and because each patient must be viewed individually.

References

Artner J, Irsigler K, Ogris E, Rosenkranz A et al. (1981) Diabetes und Schwangerschaft. Z Geburtshilfe Perinatol 185:125

Aula P, Rapola J, Karjalainen O, Lindgren J, Hartikainen A, Seppälä M (1978) Prenatal diagnosis of congenital nephrosis in 23 high-risk families. Am J Dis Child 132:984

Bean WJ, Calonje MA, Aprill CN, Geshner J (1978) Anal atresia: A prenatal ultrasound diagnosis. J Clin Ultrasound 6:111

Brock DJH (1979) Prenatal diagnosis of neural tube defects. In: Weitzel HK, Schneider J (eds) Alpha-fetoprotein in clinical medicine. Thieme, Stuttgart New York, pp 1–7

Carter CO, Evans K, Pescia G (1979) A family study of renal agenesis. J Med Genet 16:176

Claussen U, Hansmann M (1984) Die „Pipettenmethode" zur schnellen Karyotypisierung bei sonographischen Verdachtskriterien für eine Chromosomenanomalie. Gynäkologe 17

Cohen T, Stern E, Rosenmann A (1979) Sib risk of neural tube defect: Is prenatal diagnosis indicated in pregnancies following the birth of a hydrocephalic child? J Med Genet 16:14

Filly RA, Golbus MS, Carey JC, Hall JG (1981) Short-limbed dwarfism: Ultrasonographic diagnosis by mensuration of fetal femoral length. Radiology 138:653

Födisch HJ (1982) Pathologisch-anatomische Mißbildungsdiagnostik – Heute. Verh Dtsch Ges Pathol 66:37

Födisch HJ, Knöpfle G (1984) Patho-anatomische Teratologie – eine aktuelle Herausforderung. Gynäkologe 17:2–12

Fuhrmann W (1983) Die Alpha-Fetoproteinbestimmung in der pränatalen Diagnostik und Vorsorge. Diagn Intensivther 6:1

Gembruch U, Venn HJ, Gembruch G, Hansmann M (1983) Ergebnisse der gezielten „frühen" pränatalen Ausschlußdiagnostik von Mißbildungen mittels Ultraschall. In: Otto RC, Jann FX (eds) Ultraschalldiagnostik 82, Interventionelle Sonographie. Thieme, Stuttgart New York, S 159–161

Gembruch U, Bellmann O, Hansmann M (1984) Die gezielte sonographische Mißbildungsdiagnostik bei Feten mit erhöhten Alpha-Fetoprotein-Konzentrationen. In: Lutz Reichel L (ed) Ultraschalldiagnostik 83, Drei-Länder-Treffen Erlangen 1983. Thieme, Stuttgart New York (in press)

Golbus MS, Holzgreve W, Harrison NR (1984) Intrauterine Direktbehandlung des Feten. Gynäkologe 17:62

Grannum P, Bracken M, Silverman R, Hobbins JC (1980) Assessment of fetal kidney size in normal gestation by comparison of ratio of kidney circumference to abdominal circumference. Am J Obstet Gynecol 136:249

Hansmann M (1981a) Nachweis und Ausschluß fetaler Entwicklungsstörungen mittels Ultraschallscreening und gezielter Untersuchung – ein Mehrstufenkonzept. Ultraschall 2:206

Hansmann M (1981b) Ultraschallscreening in der Schwangerschaft – Vorsicht vor übertriebenen Forderungen. Geburtshilfe Frauenheilkd 41:725

Hansmann M (1984) Möglichkeiten und Grenzen sonographischer Diagnostik bei fetalen Erkrankungen und Mißbildungen. In: INA 47: Kowalewski S (ed) 6. Symp. Pädiatr. Intensivmedizin. Thieme, Stuttgart New York

Hansmann M, Gembruch U (1984) Gezielte sonographische Ausschlußdiagnostik fetaler Fehlbildungen in Risikogruppen. Gynäkologe 17:19

Hansmann M, Niesen M, Födisch HJ (1979) Pränatale Ultraschalldiagnose des Potter-Syndroms. Gynäkologe 12:69

Hobbins JC, Grannum PAT, Berkowitz RL, Silverman R, Mahoney MI (1979) Ultrasound in the diagnosis of congenital anomalies. Am J Obstet Gynecol 134:331

Hobbins JC, Bracken MB, Mahoney MJ (1982a) Diagnosis of fetal skeletal dysplasias with ultrasound. Am J Obstet Gynecol 142:306

Hobbins JC, Venus I, Tortora M, Mayden K, Mahoney ML (1982b) Stage II ultrasound examination for the diagnosis of fetal abnormalities with an elevated amniotic fluid alpha-fetoprotein concentration. Am J Obstet Gynecol 142:1026

Jassani MN, Gauderer MWL, Fanaroff AA, Fletcher B, Merkatz IR (1982) A perinatal approach to the diagnosis and management of gastrointestinal malformations. Obstet Gynecol 59:33

Johnson VP, Petersen LP, Hozwarth DR, Messner FD (1982) Midtrimester prenatal diagnosis of short-limb dwarfism (Saldino-Noonan-syndrome). Birth Defects 18:133

Keith JD, Rowe RD, Vlad P (1978) Heart disease in infancy and childhood. Macmillan, New York

Kirk EP, Wah RM (1983) Obstetric management of the fetus with omphalocele or gastroschisis: A review and report of one hundred twelve cases. Am J Obstet Gynecol 146:512

Kleinebrecht J (1982) Arzneimittel in der Schwangerschaft. Deutscher Apotheker Verlag, Stuttgart

Knöpfle G, Födisch HJ, Hansmann M (1982) Das Potter-Syndrom. Prä- und postnatale Diagnostik. Verh Dtsch Ges Pathol 66:278

Knörr K (1983) Schwangerenvorsorge: Prävention für Mutter und Kind. Urban & Schwarzenberg, München Wien Baltimore

Kowalewski S (1984) Pränatale Diagnostik und symptomatische Therapie aus neonatologischer Sicht. Gynäkologe 17:56–61

Kucera J (1971) Rate and type of congenital anomalies among offspring of diabetic women. J Reprod Med 7:61

Lehman RM (1981) Dandy-Walker syndrome in consecutive siblings: Familial hindbrain malformation. Neurosurgery 8:717

Leonard CO (1981) Serum AFP screening for neural tube defects. Clin Obstet Gynecol 24:1121

Malins JM (1979) Congenital malformations and fetal mortality in diabetic pregnancy. J R Soc Med 71:205

Mills JL, Baker L, Goldman AS (1979) Malformations in infants of diabetic mothers occur before the seventh gestational week. Implications for treatment. Diabetes 28:292

Nocke W (1978) Sind weibliche Sexualsteroide teratogen? Rückblick – Zwischenbilanz – Konsequenzen. Gynäkologe 11:119

Nora JJ, Nora AH (1978) The evolution of specific genetic and environmental counseling in congenital heart diseases. Circulation 57:205

Pagon RA, Smith DW, Shepard TH (1979) Urethral obstruction malformation complex: A cause of abdominal muscle deficiency and the "prune belly". J Pediatr 94:900

Pedersen JF, Molsted-Pedersen L (1981) Early fetal growth delay detected by ultrasound marks increased risk of congenital malformation in diabetic pregnancy. Br Med J 283:269

Plotz EJ, Lang N, Hansmann M, Hinkers HJ, Garstka G, Niesen M, Bellmann O (1978) Diabetes mellitus und Schwangerschaft. Gynäkologe 11:67

Queenan JT, O'Brien GD, Campbell S (1980) Ultrasound measurement of fetal limb bones. Am J Obstet Gynecol 138:297

Ramzin MS (1982) Teratogene Wirkung von Medikamenten. Gynäkologe 15:136

Rehder H (1982) Fetalpathologie im Rahmen pränataler Diagnostik. Verh Dtsch Ges Pathol 66:58

Report of U.K. Collaborative Study (1977) on alphafetoprotein in relation to neural-tube defects. Maternal serum alpha fetoprotein measurement in antenatal screening for anencephaly and spina bifida in early pregnancy. Lancet I:1323

Report of the Collaborative Acetylcholinesterase Study (1981) Amniotic fluid acetylcholinesterase electrophoresis as a secondary test in the diagnosis of anencephaly and open spina bifida in early pregnancy. Lancet II:321

Robertson RD, Sarti DA, Brown WJ, Crandall BF (1981) Congenital hydrocephalus in two pregnancies following the birth of a child with neural tube defect: aetiology and management. J Med Genet 18:105

Schlensker KH (1981) Die sonographische Darstellung der fetalen Extremitäten im mittleren Trimenon. Geburtshilfe Frauenheilkd 41:366

Second report of the U.K. Collaborative Study (1979) on alpha-fetoprotein in relation to neural-tube defects. Amniotic fluid alpha-fetoprotein measurement in antenatal diagnosis of anencephaly and open spina bifida in early pregnancy. Lancet II:651

Shannon MW, Nadler HL (1968) X-linked hydrocephalus. J Med Genet 5:526

Sillence DO, Senn A, Danks DM (1979) Genetic heterogenity in osteogenesis imperfecta. J Med Genet 16:101

Taybi H (1983) Radiology of syndromes and metabolic disorders. Year Book Medical Publishers, Chicago London

Warkany J (1971) Congenital malformations. Year Book Medical Publishers, Chicago London

Weiß H, Zerres K, Hansmann M (1981) Pränatale Diagnose zystischer Nierenveränderungen mit Hilfe der Ultraschalltechnik. Ultraschall 2:205

Weitzel H (1983) Alpha-Fetoprotein in der Geburtshilfe. Gynäkologe 16:148

Zerres K, Födisch HJ (1982) Kongenitale Zystennieren. Probleme der Klassifikation aus morphologischer und humangenetischer Sicht. Verh Dtsch Ges Pathol 66:285

9 Rhesus Incompatibility and Nonimmunologic Hydrops Fetalis

9.1 Rh Incompatibility

Rh incompatibility provides a good example of how a disease process can be elucidated and to some extent controlled through interdisciplinary cooperation – in this case between obstetricians, pediatricians, and serologists. Within a period of 30 years it has been possible to explain the pathogenesis of this disorder, develop reliable diagnostic methods, and find effective therapeutic measures.

9.1.1 Definition and Pathogenetic Principle

Rh incompatibility, erythroblastosis fetalis, and Rh hemolytic disease are all terms applied to a disease of the fetus (and newborn) caused by the action of maternal immune antibodies on fetal red cells. The basis of the disease is maternal Rh sensitization and antibody production, usually as a result of the transplacental passage of Rh-positive fetal red cells into the mother during a previous pregnancy. The Rh isoantigen is genetically transmitted to the fetus by the father. The maternally formed IgG antibodies cross the placenta and produce in the fetus a variety of symptoms mainly related to the destruction of fetal red cells. It is believed that the antibody-coated red cells are destroyed by phagocytosis in the reticuloendothelial system.

The cardinal symptoms are anemia, icterus gravis, and hydrops fetalis. The development of hydrops fetalis is probably based on intrauterine cardiac failure secondary to severe chronic anemia. Hypoproteinemia (possible causes: reduced albumin production associated with massive hepatic erythropoesis, protein loss from the vascular system due to capillary hypoxia, or transsudation into tissue and body cavities with congestive failure) appears to be another important factor in the occurrence of hydrops. Without treatment, death will occur in about 20% of cases, or permanent brain damage will result. This pathogenesis was postulated in 1939 by Levine and Stetson and proved a short time later by Landsteiner and Wiener (1940) and Levine et al. (1941) following discovery of the Rh factor.

9.1.2 Diagnosis and Management

Available options for the prevention and treatment of Rh hemolytic disease can be ranked as follows in terms of their efficacy in reducing infant morbidity and mortality:

1. Prevention of Rh sensitization (by administration of Rh antibodies)
2. Exchange transfusion of the newborn
3. Elective preterm delivery, if fetal lung maturity permits
4. Intrauterine treatment in the form of fetal intraperitoneal or (with early, severe disease) intravascular transfusion

Other treatment options during pregnancy are intensive plasmapheresis to decrease the antibody content of the maternal blood (Hauth et al. 1981; Bowman and Manning 1983), the maternal administration of immunosuppressive drugs (Charles and Blumenthal 1982), or the administration of red cell extracts with Rh antigens (Bierme et al. 1979). When intrauterine treatment is necessary, these options are far less successful than intrauterine transfusion (IUT), although they can be useful as supportive measures (Bowman and Manning 1983).

The strategy for the prevention of Rh incompatibility is based on the pioneering research of Finn and Clarke in England (1961–1963), Freda, Gorman, and Pollack in the United States (1964), and Schneider and Preisler (1962–1969) in Germany. These authors succeeded in preventing the antigenic effect of Rh-positive red cells in Rh-negative persons by the injection of sera containing Rh antibodies (Schneider and Maas 1978).

According to Bowman 1984), the rate of Rh sensitization can be reduced to about $^1/_{10}$ by the rigorous use of this anti-Rh gamma globulin prophylaxis. However, up to 10% of Rh-negative women form Rh antibodies in their first pregnancy. Given this fact and the level at which Rh prophylaxis is currently being practiced, the sensitization rate of Rh-negative women is still approximately 20% of previous levels. It can only be reduced further if prophylactic anti-Rh gamma globulin is used at the end of the second trimester to prevent sensitization in the first pregnancy.

With 600,000 births annually in the Federal Republic of Germany, we may assume (based on gene frequencies) that the combination of an Rh-negative mother and Rh-positive fetus will exist in approximately 60,000 pregnancies, and that about 5% of these fetuses (3,000) may be affected by Rh disease – one-fifth (600) so severely that prenatal treatment will be required to prevent a lethal outcome. In practice, the number of deaths has been reduced by 80% through prophylaxis. At present about 100 cases of severe Rh disease are seen annually in the Federal Republic of Germany.

The basis for the successful treatment of Rh incompatibility is an accurate early diagnosis that will enable the severity of fetal disease to be assessed. The main criteria available for this purpose are:

History and physical examination
Serial testing for maternal antibodies
Monitoring of amniotic fluid bilirubin
Ultrasound
Cardiotocography (CTG)

The most important element of the patient's history is the presence of previous Rh-linked stillbirths or serious fetal disease. As a rule, the Rh-positive fetus in a subsequent pregnancy has no chance of surviving beyond the point at which the previous fetus died.

While the determination of Rh antibody titers in the maternal blood is the basic method of diagnosing sensitization, it is of little value in assessing the severity of fetal disease. An increase in antibody titers may be seen in an Rh-negative fetus, and low titers may be recorded in the presence of severe disease.

If significant levels of Rh antibodies are detected during pregnancy, the risk to the fetus should be determined by analyzing the amniotic fluid for bilirubin. Today the collection of amniotic fluid by transabdominal amniocentesis is a relatively safe procedure as long as the location of the placenta and fetus are known. Ultrasound is an indispensable adjunct to this procedure, since it can clearly demonstrate the fetus and the placenta. This is an important advantage when one considers that in about 50% of patients at least part of the placenta is implanted on the anterior uterine wall. Moreover, when the amniocentesis is performed during the second trimester (14–28 weeks), access is limited by the relatively large size of the placenta in relation to the uterus (Holzgreve and Hansmann 1984). Every transplacental amniocentesis carries the risk of fetomaternal transfusion, which is usually followed by a marked rise in maternal antibody titer. When amniocentesis is attempted without localization of the placenta, there is a 10% risk that the needle will traverse the placenta (Bowman 1984). The booster effect of a fetomaternal transfusion with the consequent rise in antibody titer, can increase the severity of fetal hemolytic disease.

The amniotic fluid sample is analyzed to determine the concentration of bilirubin, which provides an indirect measure of the degree of fetal red cell destruction. Because the bilirubin concentration in the amniotic fluid is extremely low, the earlier results of biochemical analysis were disappointing. The decisive breakthrough came when Liley introduced the spectrophotometric method in 1961. This method measures the rise in optical density at a wavelength of 450 nm, which corresponds to the concentration of bilirubin in the sample. Liley (1961) constructed a chart on which the rise in optical density is plotted against gestation in weeks (Fig. 9.11 a–c). The chart is divided empirically into three zones, with the low zone C indicating a mildly affected fetus, zone B a moderately affected fetus, and the high zone A a severely affected fetus. The downward slope of the zone boundaries reflects the normal decline of amniotic fluid bilirubin levels as gestation progresses. This method of predicting severity of hemolytic disease is reported to have an accuracy of between 64% (Liley) and 91% (Mast 1969). On the whole, however, the prediction is most accurate in cases of severe disease (Kopecky 1971). Kopecky found the highest percentage of inaccurate predictions in mildly affected and Rh-negative fetuses (22 incorrect interpretations in 55 analyses), which is consistent with our own experience. For the clinical management it is extremely important to consider the potential errors than can arise in spectrophotometric amniotic fluid analyses, because the therapeutic implications (early delivery or IUT) carry risks for the fetus. Thus, the examiner must be careful about "correcting" the ΔOD 450 value in amniotic fluid that is contaminated by meconium, which produces a secondary peak at 403 nm, or by blood, which produces peaks at 580 and 415 nm (Bowman 1984). When assessing the severity of disease, it is better to take the less favorable value.

Choosing the timing for a preterm delivery is difficult, because while the risk of intrauterine fetal death decreases the earlier the fetus is delivered, the risks of mortality and morbidity due to prematurity increase. This decision is further complicated by the fact that, according to Dewhurst et al. (1972), the gestational age in 20%–25% of cases cannot be accurately determined from the history and clinical findings. In these cases the earliest acceptable delivery date can be determined from sonographic measurements, which enable gestational age to be estimated with reasonable accuracy. Today, routine gestational age assessment during screening (see Chap. 14) has solved this problem for the majority of cases. If these data help in determining the earliest date at which the baby can be delivered with an acceptable chance of survival, then CTG and amniotic fluid analysis will decide how much longer the fetus can safely remain in utero.

The role of ultrasound in the prenatal monitoring of Rh incompatibility goes far beyond locating the placenta, determining its thickness (Fig. 9.5a, b), and recording fetal biometric parameters. It provides direct information on the severity of the disease, which bears critically on further therapeutic measures. The presence of hepato- and splenomegaly (Fig. 9.4), dilatation of the precardial veins (Fig. 9.3), ascites (Fig. 9.1), pericardial and pleural effusions (pleural effusion is seen only in the terminal stage of Rh hemolytic disease), and skin edema, which is responsible for the well-known "halo sign" in fully developed hydrops fetalis (Figs. 9.2, 9.5c), is indicative of cardiac decom-

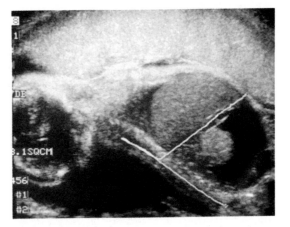

Fig. 9.1. Hydrops fetalis in Rh incompatibility. Longitudinal scan at 29 weeks: highly echogenic, hydropic anterior placenta, hepatomegaly, ascites

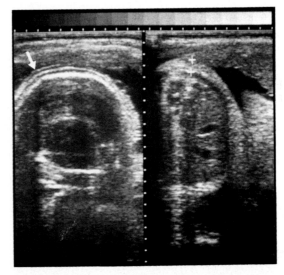

Fig. 9.2. Early hydrops fetalis in Rh incompatibility. *Arrow* points to edema of scalp. Edematous skin (*right*) is 10 mm thick (*crosses*). A conspicuous, crescent-shaped ascitic zone is visible between liver and abdominal wall

pensation in the presence of severe anemia. As in nonimmunologic hydrops fetalis, ascites and especially pericardial effusion are the earliest evidence of fetal fluid retention. Even a small fluid accumulation leads to distension of the pericardial cavity and can be demonstrated with fetal M-mode echocardiography before it becomes visible in B-scans (DeVore et al. 1982). Even before congestive phenomena appear, B-mode echocardiography can demonstrate the presence of cardiomegaly, diminished wall con-

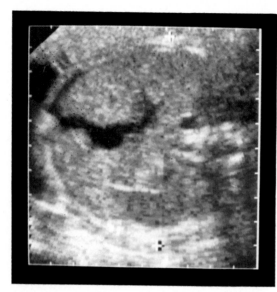

Fig. 9.3. Distended umbilical vein as a symptom of right-sided heart failure in Rh incompatibility at 27 weeks

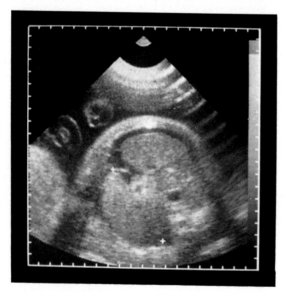

Fig. 9.4. Splenomegaly in Rh incompatibility at 31 weeks: transverse scan of trunk. Spleen lies between *markers*, spine is at 5 o'clock

tractility, and in increased end-systolic residual volume. M-mode echocardiography can then be used to quantitate the diameter of the heart and its chambers, wall thickness, and wall mobility (see Sects. 8.8 and 9.2 for details). Polyhydramnios may also present as an early sign of decompensation.

Diagnostic ultrasound yields crucial information on the severity of Rh hemolytic disease

and the risk of intrauterine fetal death, going well beyond the capabilities of amniotic fluid spectrophotometry, and provides an important basis for the management of these cases. This is particularly true if the ΔOD 450 reading is high in zone B (moderately severe fetal disease) or in zone A (severe fetal disease) on the Liley chart, as the amniotic fluid bilirubin concentration is only an indirect indicator of the severity of fetal hemolytic anemia. With polyhydramnios, for example, there is a diluting effect that renders the ΔOD 450 value less reliable than the Liley chart would indicate. Moreover, the degree of fetal anemia does not always correlate with the severity of the disease or the degree of fetal hydrops (Frigoletto et al. 1981), because other pathophysiologic mechanisms, such as secondary heart failure and hypoproteinemia, become operative in Rh incompatibility and profoundly affect the course of the disease. Once an IUT has been carried out, the ΔOD 450 value no longer reflects the severity of the disease or anemia, since this treatment suppresses the formation of Rh-positive blood by the fetus and thus reduces immediate hemolysis and bilirubin production. Even with severe fetal anemia and hydrops, the ΔOD 450 readings may fall below the "action line" in the Liley chart (Frigoletto et al. 1981). In cases such as this, ultrasound and CTG are the only diagnostic tools available for the monitoring of the fetus.

Approximately 20%–25% of affected fetuses become hydropic and are at high risk of intrauterine death (Bowman 1984). About half of these infants can be salvaged by early delivery. Recent advances in the intensive care of premature infants have greatly reduced their morbidity and mortality. We perform elective deliveries as early as 30 weeks, depending on the severity of disease, 48–72 h after administering corticosteroids to stimulate fetal lung maturation. Close cooperation between the neonatal and obstetric departments is essential in choosing the proper time for delivery and providing optimum perinatal care.

More than half of severely affected fetuses are threatened by intrauterine death prior to 30 weeks. Today, the majority of these infants can be saved by IUT, which may be performed by the intraperitoneal (IPT) or intravascular (IVT) route (Table 9.1). This procedure was first performed successfully in 1963 by the New

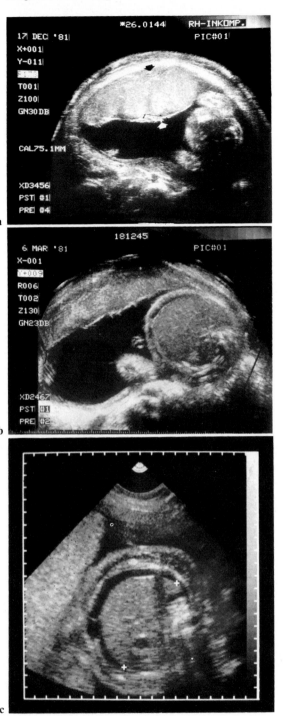

Fig. 9.5. a Transverse section: highly echogenic, hydropic anterior placenta in Rh incompatibility (thickness 7.5 cm). **b** Normal-appearing anterior placenta in Rh incompatibility with early decompensation. Increased intraamniotic pressure from polyhydramnios may prevent increase in placental thickness. Ascites and skin edema are obvious. **c** Complete picture of hydrops fetalis in Rh incompatibility at 26 weeks: hepatic diameter 8 cm (hepatomegaly), overall trunk diameter over 12 cm, trunk wall thickness 2 cm. Only a direct transfusion (intravascular or possibly intracardiac) can salvage a fetus in this condition

toneal cavity of the rabbit. Zimmermann repeated this experiment in 1921 and found that when nucleated avian red cells were used, only 15 min elapsed between injection and the appearance of the red cells in the peripheral circulation. In 1944 Hahn showed in human subjects that red cells with radiolabeled hemoglobin are preferentially absorbed in the region of the diaphragm through the peritoneal surface. Later a number of investigators were able to show that red cells are carried by lymphatics to the thoracic duct, from which they enter the circulation intact. The earliest report of an intraabdominal transfusion in man comes from Golgi and Raggi in 1888, who demonstrated a rise in hemoglobin following IPT of red cells. According to Liley's original technique (1963), a water-soluble contrast material (e.g., 10–20 ml Urovison) is first injected into the amniotic cavity. This material is swallowed by the fetus along with amniotic fluid (approx. 50 ml/24 h) and accumulates in the fetal bowel. Within 24–48 h the fetal peritoneal cavity can be visualized radiographically, and a needle is inserted into the fetal abdomen under radiographic control. Placement is checked by injecting a few milliliters of contrast material through the needle or a catheter threaded through the needle. Once correct placement is confirmed, between 10 and 100 ml (depending on fetal age) of group 0, Rh-negative packed red cells are instilled into the peritoneal cavity at an average rate of 2 ml/min.

Since 1963 numerous modifications of the IPT technique have been described, including transfusion via catheter (Queenan and Wyatt 1965), the two-needle technique (Queenan et al. 1966), and the use of image intensification fluoroscopy (Kwi and High 1974). The disadvantage of all these techniques is the necessity of fetal radiation exposure (genetic mutations, in-

Zealand obstetrician Liley, who transfused red blood cells into the fetal peritoneal cavity (IPT). The theoretical groundwork for the procedure dates back many years:

In 1863 von Recklinghausen reported on the absorption of defibrinated blood from the peri-

Table 9.1. IPT results from major centers (published since 1980)

Authors, period	n (total)	IPT n	Survivals n (%)	Without hydrops		With hydrops	
				Before 1st IPT n	Survivals n (%)	Before 1st IPT n	Survivals n (%)
Frigoletto et al. (1981)							
May 64–Dec 79 of which:	330	—[b]	142 (43)	258	137 (53)	72	5 (7)
Jan 78–Dec 79	35	87	17 (49)	21	13 (62)	14	4 (29)
Berkowitz and Hobbins (1981)							
Jun 76–Mar 80	17	37	12 (71)	10	8 (80)	7	4 (57)
Larkin et al. (1982)	16	36	12 (75)	11	9 (82)	5	3 (60)
Bowman and Manning (1983)							
Feb 78–Jun 80	21	53	11 (52)	14	8 (57)	7	3 (43)
Jul 80–Jun 82	24	64	22 (92)	16	16 (100)	8	6 (75)
UFK Bonn							
Jan 78–Apr 83	40	141	26 (65)	30	24 (80)	10	2 (20)

[a] After introduction of routine ultrasound guidance for intrauterine transfusions

[b] Not specified

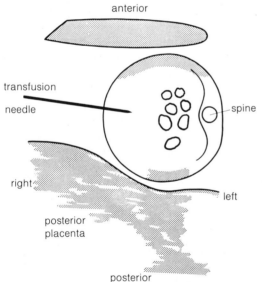
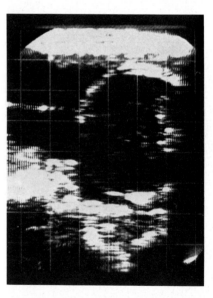

Fig. 9.6. Transverse section of fetal trunk showing placement of transfusion needle. Sectioned loops of bowel are visible posteriorly, needle anteriorly. Needle projects about 2 cm into peritoneal cavity and lies in an echo-poor ascitic zone. (From Hansmann and Lang 1972)

duction of malignant disease), amounting to 0.44–6.6 rad or 0.0044–0.066 Gy (Peddle and Campbell 1968; Hamilton 1977) per transfusion.

Hansmann and Lang (1972) first described the ultrasound guidance of IUTs (Fig. 9.6) as a means of eliminating fetal radiation hazard. Nearly 5 years passed before Hobbins et al. (1976) and Cooperberg and Carpenter (1977) published further reports on ultrasound-guided IUT. Today the majority of centers routinely perform IPTs under sonographic control. Some

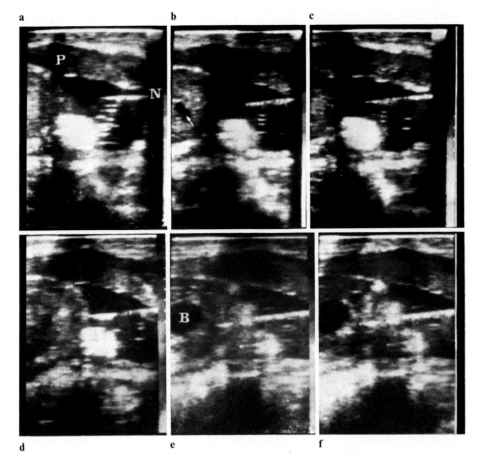

Fig. 9.7a–f. Frames from a videotape of an IPT performed under ultrasound guidance. **a, c** Needle inserted laterally from left (*right* in image), passing below anterior placenta. **b** *Arrow:* gallbladder. **d** Fetal abdominal wall reached. **e** Needle advanced in direction of bladder (*B*). **f** Instillation phase. (From Hansmann et al. 1980)

examiners obtain a single radiographic contrast film to confirm intraperitoneal placement of the transfusion needle (approx. 0.002 Gy; Berkowitz and Hobbins 1981; Clewell et al. 1981; Frigoletto et al. 1981; Harmann et al. 1983), while others (Bonn University Gynecologic Clinic; Grace Hospital, Vancouver; Larkin et al. 1982) avoid radiation altogether and rely for confirmation on lack of resistance to plunger motion, the presence of "microbubbles" during the injection of sterile saline and/or carbon dioxide (Fig. 9.7), and visualization of the catheter itself within the fetal peritoneal cavity.

The fetus is transfused with packed red blood cells [hematocrit (Hct) 80%–90%] that have been "washed" to remove leukocytes. This allows administration of large numbers of red cells in a small volume and reduction of absorption time (Harmann et al. 1983). A slow transfusion (1.5–2.5 ml/min) enables better adapta-

tion of the fetal intraabdominal pressure, core temperature, and umbilical venous blood flow, and is preferred to a bolus injection lasting 5–10 min. The following formula is generally used to calculate the necessary transfusion volume (after Bowman 1975): (gestation in weeks minus 20) × 10 ml. For example, in the 28th week the transfusion volume would be 8 × 10 ml = 80 ml. With severe fetal hydrops, the value should be increased by up to 25%. Fetal heart rate is monitored throughout the transfusion. The appearance of fetal bradycardia toward the end of the transfusion indicates immediate termination of the procedure (Bowman 1978). "Overtransfusion," which may cause interruption of blood flow in the umbilical vein, can be avoided by continuous fetal heart rate monitoring combined with a slow transfusion rate and, if necessary, a decreased transfusion volume. Since the introduction of

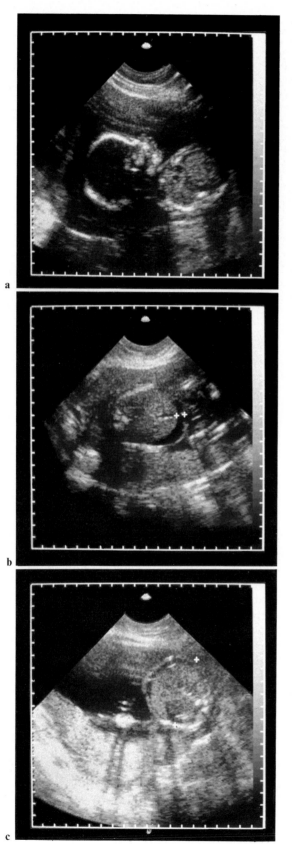

ultrasound for the monitoring of the transfusion procedure, the incidence of fetal trauma has been markedly reduced (Bowman and Manning 1983).

Maternal morbidity with IPT is very low, the principal risk being infection. When aseptic precautions are observed, the incidence of infection is less than 1%; there is generally no need for prophylactic antibiotics. Other risks associated with IPT are premature labor, premature rupture of membranes, abruptio placentae, maternal hepatitis, hematomas, and faulty insertion of the transfusion needle.

Fetal mortality within 48 h of the transfusion is usually a direct result of the procedure and is related to fetal or placental trauma. The risk of fetal mortality, according to recent studies, is between 3.6% and 9.3% (Berkowitz and Hobbins 1981; Clewell et al. 1981).

Increased incidence of malignancies in childhood as a consequence of X-ray exposure need no longer be feared since the introduction of sonographic guidance. Fetal graft-versus-host disease (Parkman et al. 1974) is extremely rare (use of washed or irradiated packed red cells) (Frigoletto et al. 1981; Larkin et al. 1982).

The postnatal development of infants treated by IPT has been investigated by several authors (White et al. 1978; Knobbe et al. 1979; Hardyment et al. 1979; Kowalewski et al. 1981). All conclude that there is no significant difference, in mental or motor development, from untreated children of equal birth weight, gestational age, and mode of delivery, except for a higher incidence of umbilical and inguinal hernias in children treated by IPT (White et al. 1978). It is very difficult to compare the success rates of IPTs performed at different centers, either because of low numbers of cases or because data from several decades generally cannot be adjusted for changes in neonatal care techniques or for the varying experience of the examiners. Some authors list cases of hydrops fetalis separately in their statistics, while others consider the presence of hydrops to be a contraindication to IPT. As some centers (Bonn University, London King's College), fetuses in very poor condition are transfused even prior

Fig. 9.8a–c. Status following IPT of 15 ml packed red cells at 20 weeks. **a** Longitudinal scan: fetal head. **b** Transverse trunk scan immediately after transfusion. **c** Transverse trunk scan 48 h after transfusion

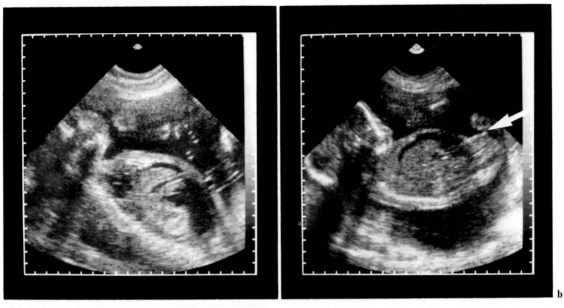

Fig. 9.9. a Frank hydrops in severe Rh incompatibility at 23 weeks: longitudinal scan. **b** Status following 2nd IPT (40 ml) at 24 weeks: longitudinal scan. Note marked reduction of skin edema following transfusion

to 20 weeks, while other centers reject this practice.

Besides the introduction of ultrasound monitoring, the use of improved needle and catheter designs (Bowman and Manning 1983) and of high-Hct red cell concentrates that are more rapidly absorbed (Bowman and Manning 1983), the experience of recent years has taught that the survival rate of fetuses with Rh disease can be increased only through careful planning and aggressive management. We recommend the following protocol:

The best results are achieved when monitoring is initiated early, i.e., when the first amniotic fluid bilirubin measurement is obtained before 20 weeks gestation. If a rising trend is noted on repeat amniocentesis 1–2 weeks later (Fig. 9.11 a–c), and extrauterine viability cannot be assumed, any ΔOD 450 reading above 0.2 is an indication for immediate IUT, regardless of gestational age. In our experience it is possible for the full picture of hydrops fetalis to develop within a period of 24–48 h, even if no congestive phenomena have been previously noted. The "action lines" in the Liley chart, which have been used, sometimes in a modified form, by other authors (Bowman and Manning 1983; Larkin et al. 1982; Berkowitz and Hobbins 1981), differ very little from our own approach. However, it should be noted that Rh-

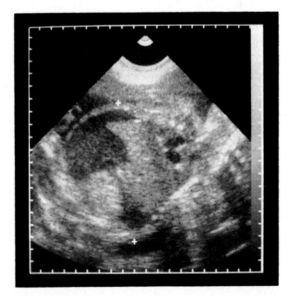

Fig. 9.10. Status 48 h after IPT in a hydropic fetus at 29 weeks. The mixture of packed red cells and ascitic fluid is markedly echogenic. Absorption of the red cells at this point is extremely unlikely

negative unaffected fetuses will occasionally have ΔOD 450 values of 0.20–0.25 early in the 21st–23rd week. In these cases a repeat amniocentesis within 7–10 days should differentiate between the Rh-positive affected fetus and the Rh-negative unaffected fetus (Bowman 1984).

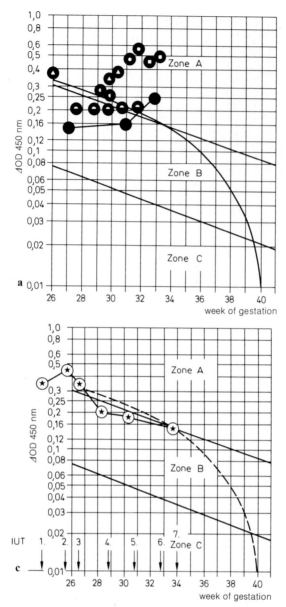

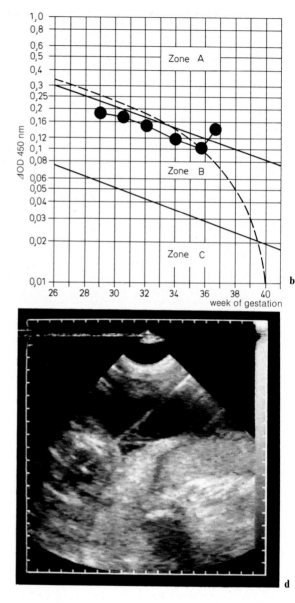

Fig. 9.11. a Liley chart with ΔOD 450 readings of six fetuses requiring intrauterine transfusion. **b** Liley chart with serial readings for one fetus. The fifth reading at 35 weeks is on the "action line" of Whitfield et al. (1972). Thereafter the ΔOD 450 shows a surprisingly sharp rise. The antibody titer during this period rose from 1:128 to 1:4096. The newborn had an anemia of 8.4%. **c** Liley chart for seven IUTs: Note the steady decline of ΔOD 450 readings over the observation period. At delivery the amniotic fluid was "clear," and the newborn had a hemoglobin of 16.4 g% with 99.8% Hb-A. **d** ICT with the needle in place (tip within right ventricle)

Also, if sonograms show evidence of early congestive phenomena in confirmed Rh incompatibility, IUT is indicated regardless of the result of the bilirubin assay, which, as stated earlier, may not always correlate with the severity of fetal disease (Frigoletto et al. 1981; Harman et al. 1983). Our approach is consistent with

the conclusion of recent studies recommending that IUT be started at 20 weeks (Fig. 9.8), especially if the fetus is hydropic (Frigoletto et al. 1981; Berkowitz and Hobbins 1981; Larkin et al. 1982; Harmann et al. 1983).

Serial ultrasound examinations will determine the management following IPT and

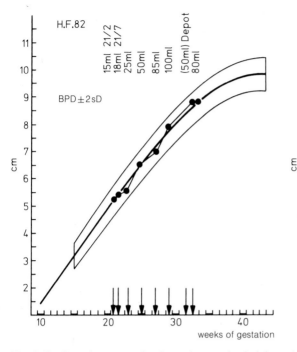

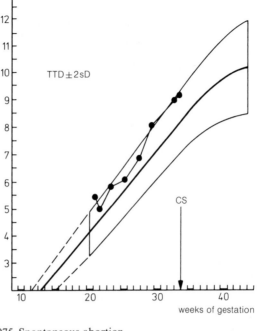

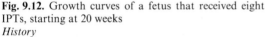

weeks of gestation

Fig. 9.12. Growth curves of a fetus that received eight
IPTs, starting at 20 weeks
History
Mother: Age 45 years, A Rh − ccdee
Father: B Rh +
1961 Stillbirth of hydropic fetus
1966 Cesarean birth at 35 weeks, infant survived 30 min

1975 Spontaneous abortion
1979 Elective abortion on advice of gynecologist
1982 Delivery at 34 weeks of baby treated in utero
(2,300 g/44 cm)
Apgar: 1 min = 4, 10 min = 10
Hemoglobin: 16.5 g%
Further development "excellent"

should be performed every 2–3 days for nonhydropic fetuses and daily for hydropic fetuses.
While the transfusion intervals for nonhydropic
fetuses are fairly standardized with only minor
variations (10–14 days until the second IPT,
26–30 days until the third IPT), the intervals
for hydropic fetuses are determined entirely by
the results of the sonographic examination
(Fig. 9.12). A progression of skin edema and
ascites (or increase of abdominal circumference), a decrease in fetal movements, and polyhydramnios are considered signs of impending
fetal death. If they are observed, a second IPT
is performed within 3–5 days, preceded if necessary by the aspiration of ascitic fluid. Even with
severe hydrops, a dramatic improvement of fetal condition may be noted in just 2–5 days,
as evidenced by a partial or complete clearing
of fluid collections and an increase of fetal
movements (Fig. 9.9a, b) as the transfused
blood is absorbed.

In contrast to Bowman and Manning (1983)
and Harmann et al. (1983), who reject other
treatment methods because of their positive ex-

perience with IPT, we believe that IPT is often
inadequate when dealing with severe hydrops
fetalis. The delay and occasional absence of red
cell absorption by the hydropic fetus (Fig. 9.10)
and the high risk of trauma from IPT prior
to 22 weeks are serious disadvantages of this
method.

Intrauterine exchange transfusion following
hysterotomy via the femoral vein (Freda and
Adamson 1964), saphenous vein and jugular
veins (Asensio et al. 1966), and a venous chorionic vessel (Seelen et al. 1962) had to be abandoned due to the almost inevitable precipitation
of labor and the very poor survival rates (only
5 of 30 fetuses so treated).

On the other hand, very good results have
been obtained with direct IVT by fetoscopy,
introduced by Rodeck et al. (1981). With this
method a needle is first inserted into the umbilical artery at the placental or fetal insertion of
the umbilical cord, and blood is drawn for biochemical analysis (blood grouping, Hct, reticu-
locyte count, antibody level, and bilirubin).
Based on the measured Hct a sufficient volume

of group 0, Rh-negative blood (Hct 60%–80%) is transfused to produce an Hct of 35%–40%. The most recent results of the London group (Rodeck and Nicolaides 1984) are encouraging. The IVT may be performed from 18 weeks onward if necessary. Of 24 fetuses that received IVTs before 25 weeks (15 with hydrops), 21 survived (88%), with 7 hydropic fetuses recovering in utero.

Recently we successfully treated a fetus at 25 weeks by intracardiac transfusion (ICT). The fetus was motionless, and its prone position in the uterus precluded puncture of the umbilical vein or vena cava. Because fetal death was imminent, we decided to attempt ICT as a last resort. The needle was introduced over the cardiac apex and into the right ventricle under sonographic vision. The initial hemoglobin of 4.4 g% rose to 14.5 g% following the infusion of 60 ml packed red cells (HCT 80%). Although the needle was in the heart for 30 min, no alteration of heart rhythm was observed. The clinical condition of the fetus improved immediately. The newborn survived and showed no evidence of injury.

In summary, our experience and that of other authors has led to the following basic changes in the management of Rh incompatibility:

1. An aggressive and successful treatment regimen must be based on early amniocentesis to determine the ΔOD 450 value. This should be done no later than at 20 weeks gestation.

2. Early IUTs are indicated even in boderline cases due to the often poor correlation between the ΔOD 450 value and the severity of Rh disease.

3. A gestational age below 25 weeks and/or the presence of hydrops fetalis do not contraindicate IUT.

4. With severe hydrops, or before 22 weeks, IVT offers significant advantages over IPT. Further research is required before final decisions on this technique and on ICT can be made.

5. The sonographic guidance of IPT can eliminate radiation hazard to the fetus and reduce the incidence of fetal trauma. Needle placement under radiographic guidance is considered obsolete.

References

Asensio SH, Figueroa-Longo JG, Pelegrina IA (1966) Intrauterine exchange transfusion. Am J Obstet Gynecol 95:1128

Berkowitz RL, Hobbins JC (1981) Intrauterine transfusion utilizing ultrasound. Obstet Gynecol 57:33

Bierme SJ, Blanc M, Abbal M, Fournie A (1979) Oral Rh-treatment for severely immunised mothers. Lancet I:604

Bowman JM (1975) Rh erythroblastosis 1975. Semin Hematol 12:189

Bowman JM (1978) The management of Rh-isoimmunization. Obstet Gynecol 52:1

Bowman JM (1984) Rhesus haemolytic disease. In: Wald N (ed) Antenatal and neonatal screening. Oxford University Press, Oxford New York Tokyo, p 314

Bowman JM, Manning FA (1983) Intrauterine fetal transfusions: Winnipeg 1982. Obstet Gynecol 61:203

Charles AG, Blumenthal LS (1982) Promethazine hydrochloride therapy in severely Rh-sensitized pregnancies. Obstet Gynecol 60:627

Clewell WH, Dunne MG, Johnson ML, Bowes WA (1981) Fetal transfusion with real time ultrasound guidance. Obstet Gynecol 57:516

Cooperberg PL, Carpenter CW (1977) Ultrasound as an aid in intrauterine transfusion. Am J Obstet Gynecol 128:239

De Vore GR, Donnerstein RL, Kleinman CS, Platt LD, Hobbins JC (1982) Fetal echocardiography. II. The diagnosis and significance of a pericardial effusion in the fetus using real-time-directed M-mode ultrasound. Am J Obstet Gynecol 144:693

Dewhurst CJ, Beazly JM, Campbell S (1972) Assessment of fetal maturity and dysmaturity. Am J Obstet Gynecol 113:141

Finn R, Clarke CA, Donohoe WTA, Connel RB, Sheppard PM, Lehane D, Kulke W (1961) Experimental studies on the prevention of Rh hemolytic disease. Br Med J I:1486

Freda VJ, Adamsons K (1964) Exchange transfusion in utero. Am J Obstet Gynecol 89:817

Freda VJ, Gorman JG, Pollack W (1964) Successful prevention of experimental Rh sensitization in man with an anti-Rh gamma 2 – globulin antibody preparation: A preliminary report. Transfusion 4:26

Frigoletto FD, Umansky I, Birnholz J, Acker D, Easterday CL, Harris GBC, Griscom NT (1981) Intrauterine fetal transfusion in 365 fetuses during fifteen years. Am J Obstet Gynecol 139:781

Hamilton EG (1977) Intrauterine transfusion. Safeguard or peril? Obstet Gynecol 50:255

Hansmann M, Lang N (1972) Intrauterine Transfusion unter Ultraschallkontrolle. Klin Wochenschr 50:930

Hansmann M, Paulussen F, Weiß H, Niesen M, Lang N, Plotz E-J (1980) Intrauterine Transfusion unter Real-Time-Ultraschall-Kontrolle. In: Hinselmann M, Anliker M, Meudt R (eds) Ultraschalldiagnostik in der Medizin. Thieme, Stuttgart New York, S 159

Hardyment AF, Salvador HS, Towell ME, Carpenter CW, Jan FE, Tingle AJ (1979) Follow-up of intrauterine transfused surviving children. Am J Obstet Gynecol 133:235

Harman CR, Manning FA, Bowman JM, Lange IR (1983) Severe Rh disease – Poor outcome is not inevitable. Am J Obstet Gynecol 145:823

Hauth JC, Brekken AL, Pollack W (1981) Plasmapheresis as am adjunct to management of Rh isoimmunization. Obstet Gynecol 57:132

Hobbins JC, Davis ED, Webster J (1976) A new technique utilizing ultrasound to aid in intrauterine transfusion. J Clin Ultrasound 4:135

Holzgreve W, Hansmann M (1984) Erfahrungen mit der „Free hand needle" – Technik bei 3,215 Amniozentesen im II. Trimenon zur pränatalen Diagnostik. Gynäkologe 17:77

Knobbe T, Meier P, Wenar C, Cordero L (1979) Psychological development of children who received intrauterine transfusion. Am J Obstet Gynecol 133:877

Kopecky P (1971) Zur Diagnostik und Therapie der Rhesus-Inkompatibilität und Untersuchungen zum fetalen Bilirubin-Metabolismus. Habilitationsschrift, RWTH Aachen

Kowalewski S, Kochs G, Kartheiser C, Hansmann M (1981) Untersuchungen zur Spätprognose von Kindern mit M. haemolyticus neonatorum (Rh) nach intrauterinen Transfusionen. 77. Tagung der Dtsch Ges Kinderheilk, Düsseldorf, 20.–23.09.1981

Kwi NK, High NK (1974) A simple technique of intrauterine transfusion of fetus in University Hospital. Kuala Lumpur. Med J Malaysia 28:287

Landsteiner K, Wiener AS (1940) An agglutinable factor in human blood recognized by immune sera for rhesus blood. Proc Soc Exp Biol Med 43:223

Larkin RM, Knochel JQ, Lee TG (1982) Intrauterine transfusions: New techniques and results. Clin Obstet Gynecol 25:303

Levine P, Stetson R (1939) An unusual case of intragroup agglutination. JAMA 113:126

Levine P, Katzin EM, Burnham L (1941) Isoimmunization in pregnancy: its possible bearing on the etiology of erythroblastosis fetalis. JAMA 116:825

Liley AW (1961) Liquor amnii analysis in the management of pregnancy complicated by rhesus sensitization. Am J Obstet Gynecol 82:1359

Mast H (1969) Morbus haemolyticus neonatorum. Z Geburtshilfe 170 (Beilageheft)

Parkman R, Mosier D, Umansky I, Cochran W, Carpenter CB, Rosen FS (1974) Graft-versus-host disease after intrauterine and exchange transfusions for hemolytic disease of the newborn. N Engl J Med 290:359

Peddle LJ, Campbell EM (1968) Radiation of the fetus in intrauterine transfusion. Am J Obstet Gynecol 100:366

Preisler O, Schneider J (1964) Versuche der Sensibilisierung Rh-negativen Frauen durch antikörperhaltige Seren zu verhindern. Geburtshilfe Frauenheilkd 24:124

Queenan JT, Wyatt RH (1965) Intrauterine transfusion of fetus for severe erythroblastosis fetalis. Am J Obstet Gynecol 92:375

Queenan JT, Anderson GG, Mead PB (1966) Intrauterine transfusion by the multiple needle technique. JAMA 196:664

Rodeck CH, Nicolaides KH (1984) Anwendung der Fetoskopie bei fetaler Therapie. Gynäkologe 17:52

Rodeck CH, Holman CA, Karnicki J, Kemp JR, Whitmore DN, Austin MA (1981) Direct intravascular fetal blood transfusion by fetoscopy in severe rhesus isoimmunisation. Lancet I:625

Schneider J, Maas DHA (1978) Rhesuserythroblastose. Klin Frauenheilkd III:164/1 (Ergänzung 1978)

Seelen J, Kessel, Hiam V, Eskes T, Leusden H v, Been K, Evers J, Genet D v, Peeters L, Velden W, Zonderland F vd (1966) A new method of exchange transfusion in utero. Am J Obstet Gynecol 95:872

White CA, Goplerud CP, Kisker CT, Stehbens JA, Kitchell M, Taylor JC (1978) Intrauterine fetal transfusion, 1965–1976, with an assessment of the surviving children. Am J Obstet Gynecol 130:933

Whitfield CR, Thompson W, Armstrong M, Reid McC (1972) Intrauterine fetal transfusion for severe rhesus haemolytic disease. Br J Obstet Gynaecol 79:931

9.2 Nonimmunologic Hydrops Fetalis

Hydrops fetalis is the term applied to excessive fluid accumulation in body cavities and soft tissue edema. If the cause of the hydrops does not relate to fetomaternal blood group incompatibility (isoimmunization), then the term nonimmunologic hydrops fetalis (NIHF) is used.

With the development of anti-D Rh prophylaxis programs in the major industrialized nations, the incidence of Rh isoimmunization has been substantially reduced, and NIHF has become the predominant form of fetal hydrops (Senft et al. 1982; Andersen et al. 1983). The reported incidence of NIHF is between 1 in 2,566 (Maidman et al. 1980) and 1 in 3,538 births (Macafee et al. 1970), and perinatal mortality from NIHF is between 50% (Etches and Lemons 1979) and 98% (Hutchison et al. 1982). Early prenatal diagnosis and specific treatment of fetuses and newborns have improved the chance of survival in NIHF for at least some of its etiologic subgroups. New approaches in diagnosis and therapy will result in further improvement in perinatal NIHF mortality.

9.2.1 Etiology and Pathogenesis
Etiology

Since Potter (1943) first described a case of fetal hydrops unrelated to isoimmunization, a large number of fetal, placental, and maternal disorders have been identified that may be associated with varying degrees of pericardial and pleural effusion, ascites, and soft tissue edema (e.g., Macafee et al. 1970; Etches and Lemons 1979; Maidman et al. 1980; Schwartz et al. 1981; Perlin et al. 1981; Davis 1982; Hutchison et al. 1982; Hansmann and Redel 1982).

Diseases associated with NIHF (Modified from Hutchison et al. 1982; Davis 1982; Hansmann and Redel 1982; Hansmann and Gembruch 1982)

A. *Fetal*

1. *Hematologic (anemia)*
   - Chronic transfusion
       fetomaternal
       fetofetal
   - Homozygous α-thalassemia
   - Glucose-6-phosphate dehydrogenase (G-6-PD)
     deficiency

2. *Cardiovascular*
   - Dysrhythmias
       tachyarrhythmias (SVT, atrial fibrillation and
       flutter)
       bradyarrhythmias (3rd-degree AV block)
       complex dysrhythmias
   - Premature closure of fetal blood passages
       foramen ovale
       ductus arteriosus
   - Myocardial disease
       endocardial fibroelastosis
       cardiomyopathies (e.g., diabetic cardiomyo-
       pathy)
       myocardial infarction from coronary artery
       thrombosis
       intrauterine myocarditis (e.g., cytomegalovirus)
   - Cardiac malformations (e.g., AV canal with mitral
     regurgitation, insufficiency or absence of pulmo-
     nary valve, tricuspid insufficiency, Ebstein's anom-
     aly, complex cardiac malformations)
   - Intracavitary space-occupying lesions (e.g., neo-
     plasm, thrombus)
   - Generalized arterial calcification
   - Any defect occurring in association with the fore-
     going causes, especially with dysrhythmias (e.g.,
     AV canal, tetralogy of Fallot, single ventricle, Eb-
     stein's anomaly)

3. *Pulmonary*
   - Cystic adenomatoid malformation of the lung
   - Pulmonary lymphangiectasis
   - Hemangioma of the lung
   - Pulmonary hypoplasia (diaphragmatic hernia)

4. *Gastrointestinal*
   - Bowel perforation (e.g., meconium peritonitis)
   - Cirrhosis and portal hypertension
   - Hepatic cirrhosis

5. *Urogenital*
   - Congenital nephrosis
   - Renal dysplasia
   - Prune-belly syndrome
   - Renal venous thrombosis
   - Ovarian cyst

6. *Intrauterine infection*
   - TORCH (**t**oxoplasmosis, **r**ubella, **c**ytomegalovir-
     us, **h**erpes simplex)
   - Leptospirosis
   - Congenital hepatitis
   - Chagas' disease
   - Syphilis

7. *Neurologic*
   - Tuberous sclerosis
   - Storage diseases (e.g., Gaucher's disease)
   - Neuroblastoma

8. *Multiple pregnancy*
   - Parasitic fetus
   - Fetofetal transfusion

9. *Chromosome abnormalities*
   - Turner's syndrome
   - Trisomy 18, 21
   - XX/XY mosaic
   - Triploidy (69XXX)

10. *Miscellaneous*
   - Sacrococcygeal teratoma
   - AV shunt
   - Disseminated intravascular coagulation (DIC)
   - Saldino-Noonan syndrome
   - Francois' syndrome type III
   - Osteogenesis imperfecta
   - Asphyxiating thoracic dysplasia

B. *Maternal*
   - Diabetes mellitus
   - Hypertension in pregnancy

C. *Placental*
   - Renal venous thrombosis
   - Chorionic venous thrombosis
   - Chorioangioma
   - Umbilical occlusion or stenosis
   - AV shunt

D. *Idiopathic*

Some of these diseases are incompatible with extrauterine life, some are amenable to medical or surgical treatment before or after birth, and others are of significance only in utero (e.g., placental and umbilical lesions, premature closure of fetal blood passages). Most nonimmunologic cases of fetal hydrops have cardiovascular disease as their underlying cause. Thus, Kleinman et al. (1982) were able to demonstrate cardiovascular anomalies in 10 of 13 fetuses with NIHF. Among the cases seen at our center from January 1979 to April 1982, cardiovascular disease was present in 20 of 40 fetuses (Hansmann and Redel 1982). In the 115 cases of NIHF examined through May of 1984, cardiovascular anomalies were the cause in 25% ($n = 29$) and chromosome abnormalities in 16% ($n = 18$).

Pathogenesis. Fetal fluid accumulation cannot always be explained in terms of "underlying disease" (malformation syndromes, renal venous thrombosis, etc.), because the presumed mechanisms of edema formation rarely occur in isolation and do not lead uniformly to hydrops fetalis. Edema may be the result of a low oncotic pressure, chronic anemia, obstructed venous return, intrauterine infection, a malformation of the lymphatic system, or cardiac failure. A reduced plasma colloid osmotic pressure occurs in hypoproteinemic states, such as congenital nephrosis with nephrotic syndrome (Senft et al. 1980), or in the presence of hepatocellular protein synthesis defects (Turski et al. 1975). Anemia and infections can cause increased capillary permeability through chronic tissue hypoxia, resulting in the extravasation of fluid. Obstructions of the umbilical vein, ductus, venosus, or vena cava can result from space-accupying lesions (e.g., neuroblastoma, cystic adenomatoid malformation of the lung) or from the thrombosis of these vessels. Besides chronic tissue hypoxia, intrauterine infections can also cause congestion as a result of myocarditis, hepatitis, or nephrotic syndrome. Fetal cystic hygromas, which usually affect the neck region, are believed to result from a lymphatic malformation. Some cases may be based on a absence of communication between the lymphatic and venous systems in the cervical region. The resulting fluid accumulation may remain localized or may progress to hydrops fetalis. If the jugular lymphatics of the fetus subsequently gain attachment to the jugular veins in utero, then, following this hypothesis, the cystic hygroma and edema could conceivably undergo a complete or partial (pterygium colli, edema of the dorsa of hand and foot in neonates with Turner's syndrome) regression (Chervenak et al. 1983). We have not yet observed this in any of our patients, although regression has frequently been observed with all degrees of cavitary effusion and with generalized skin edema. In most cases fetal heart failure is the underlying pathophysiologic mechanism of edema, although hypoproteinemia and anemia may have secondary significance. Fetal heart failure, whether of cardiac or extracardiac origin (chronic anemia, transfusion syndrome, arteriovenous fistula, sacrococcygeal teratoma), generally manifests itself as a right-sided failure owing to the peculiarities of the fetal circulation. With a high pulmonary vascular resistance, low pulmonary blood flow (only 5%–10% of the ejection fraction of both ventricles), and the shunting of blood by the ventricles (Rudolph 1974), pulmonary edema is unlikely to develop in the fetus, even with disease of the left heart. The common mechanism of all diseases that produce fetal cardiac failure is an excessive volume and pressure load on the right atrium (Kleinman et al. 1982). Besides the true fetal heart diseases (occlusion of fetal blood passages, dysrhythmias, myocardial disease), other cardiac malformations (see list on p. 294) can lead to hydrops fetalis, as can an AV canal in the presence of a left ventricular to right atrial shunt through an incompetent mitral valve. On the other hand, other cardiac malformations are compatible with the fetal circulation and do not cause problems prior to delivery (tetralogy of Fallot, truncus arteriosus, transposition of the great arteries, hypoplastic left heart, etc.) (Hansmann and Gembruch 1984). The compensatory mechanism of the fetal heart seems less competent to deal with pressure and volume loads than that of the adult heart (Rudolph 1974; Kleinman et al. 1982), with the result that even minor disturbances of the fetal circulation (e.g., SVT) can lead to cardiac failure and even intrauterine death. The rapidity with which right heart failure can progress to hydrops fetalis – in just 1–3 days – is another peculiarity of this condition. Conversely, the rapidity with which hydropic symptoms can regress following removal of the cause (e.g., cardioversion of fetal tachyarrhythmias) was initially surprising but is consistent with experience in neonates. In some cases edema will clear completely within in a matter of days, although it may require weeks or months if hydrops is advanced.

9.2.2 Diagnosis and Treatment

Diagnosis

Clinical signs suggestive of NIHF are polyhydramnios, decreased fetal movement (Hansmann and Redel 1982; Hutchinson et al. 1982; Kleinman et al. 1982), fetal dysrhythmias (Hansmann and Redel 1982), and, less frequently, maternal anemia and preeclampsia (Macafee et al. 1970; Hutchison et al. 1982). Today the prenatal diagnosis of hydrops fetalis relies entirely on sonography (Fleischer et al. 1981; Hutchison et al. 1982; Davis 1982; Hansmann and Redel 1982), with fetal skin edema, effusions in body cavities, and particularly ascites being the main criteria for this condition (Figs. 9.13 and 9.14). Hydramnios and placental edema are common associated findings.

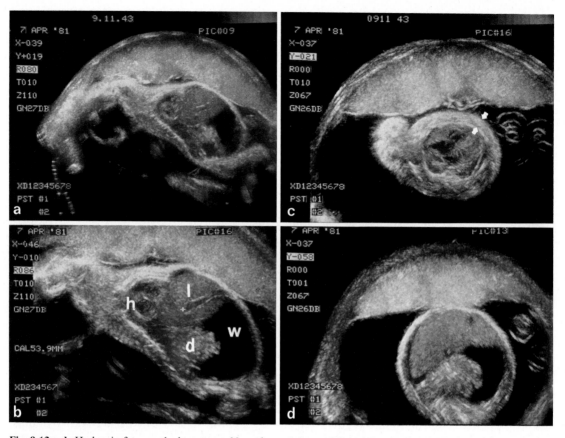

Fig. 9.13a–d. Hydropic fetus and placenta at 33 weeks secondary to anemia of unknown etiology (Hb 5.1 g%). **a** Longitudinal scan: fetus in breech presentation with large, hyperechoic placenta. **b** Detailed view (*h*, heart; *l*, liver; *d*, bowel; *w*, ascites). **c** Transverse scan: marked thoracic skin edema (*arrow*). **d** Transverse scan: hepatomegaly and ascites (spine at 6 o'clock)

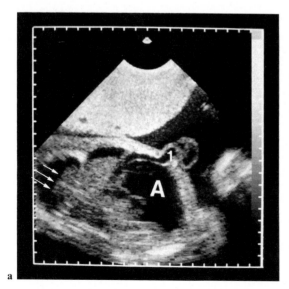

Fig. 9.14a, b. Hydrops fetalis with diaphragmatic defect at 29 weeks. **a** Longitudinal scan, (*A*, ascites; *arrows*, liver partially in hydrothorax; *1*, umbilical vein). **b** Same scan after ultrasound-guided aspiration of ascitic fluid (220 ml)

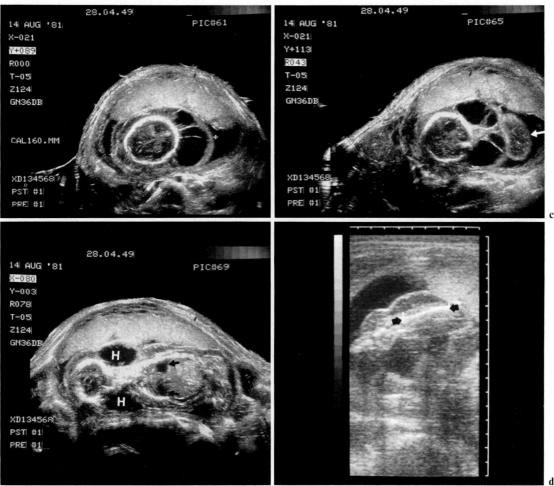

Fig. 9.15a–d. Hydropic fetus and placenta in Noonan's syndrome at 25 weeks: chromosomes 46 XY. **a** Cranial transverse scan: head surrounded by edematous skin and cystic hygroma. **b** Longitudinal scan: generalized skin edema, cystic hygroma (*H*), bilateral pleural effusions (*arrow*). **c** Transverse scan of head and neck region: typical septation of hygroma, extreme nuchal skin edema (*arrow*). **d** Same fetus: skin edema of forearm and hand (ulna 35 mm)

Since hydrops fetalis may be the result of a primary or secondary cardiac failure, we find that various sonographic parameters (B-mode and M-mode measurements) are useful in providing quantitative as well as qualitative information on cardiac decompensation and congestive phenomena (see table below). Increasingly, the quantification of fetal cardiac failure is becoming an essential prerequisite for assessing prognosis and determining the most suitable mode and timing of therapy. Quantitative data are also useful in evaluating treatment response.

Sonographic parameters for the qualitative and quantitative evaluation of fetal cardiac failure

A. *Examination of the heart*
1. Standard four-chamber view with evaluation of cardiac position, shape, and size
2. Measurement of transverse cardiac diameter on the short-axis plane at the level of the AV valves
3. Diameter of both ventricles in systole and diastole
   Diameter of right atrium
   Diameter of great vessels
   Thickness of septum and ventricle walls
   If indicated: quantitative assessment of the function of both ventricles, measurement of systolic interval

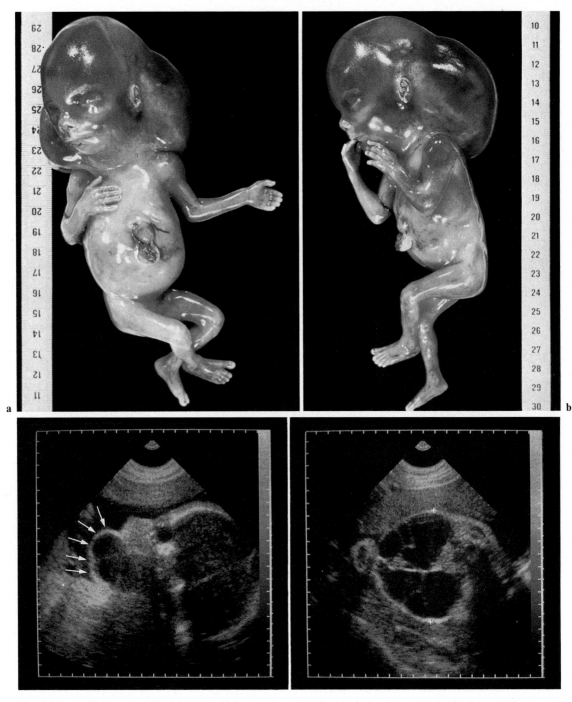

Fig. 9.16a–c. Phenotype of fetus with cystic hygroma, and partial ectopia cordis (23 weeks): Normal karyotype, 46 XX. **a** Frontal view. **b** Lateral view. **c** Isolated anterior cystic hygroma, longitudinal scan. **d** Same case, transverse scan: spine at 2 o'clock. (No other pathologic findings at birth, child doing fine after surgery)

of both ventricles (in conjunction with fetal ECG), etc.

B. Examination of other organs
1. Diameter of intra- and subhepatic veins
2. Diameter of umbilical vein

3. Qualitative and quantitative evaluation of:
   Pericardial effusion
   Ascites
   Pleural effusion
   Hepatomegaly
   Splenomegaly

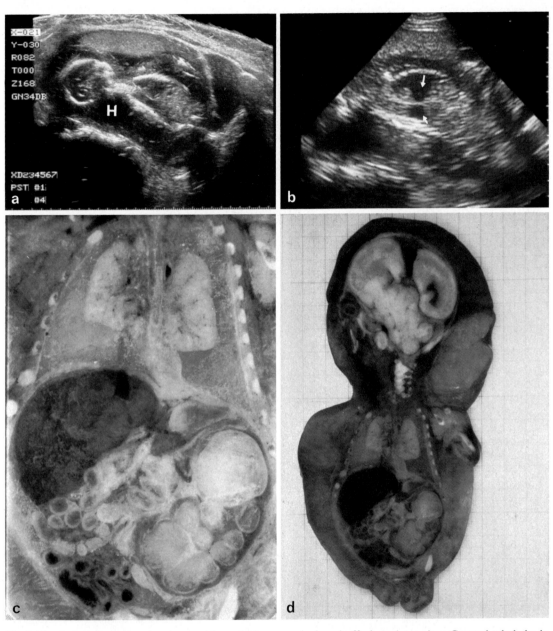

Fig. 9.17a–d. Lymphangiectatic edema with cystic hygroma and anhydramnios at 20 weeks in Turner's syndrome (45 XO). **a** Longitudinal scan: generalized edema and cystic hygroma (*H*). **b** Detail of thoracic scan: bilateral pleural effusions (*arrows*). **c** Coronal whole-body section: excessive skin edema. **d** Frozen section demonstrating pleural effusions

Skin edema
Hydramnios
Placental thickness and edema

Once the hydrops has been evaluated qualitatively and quantitatively, its etiology is sought. The steps in this process should be followed in strict sequence:

Examination protocol for the differential diagnosis of hydrops fetalis

1. Maternal blood studies
   a) Blood group and antibody screening test
   b) Serology
   c) TORCH infections
   d) AFP
   e) HbF cells (Kleinhauer technique)

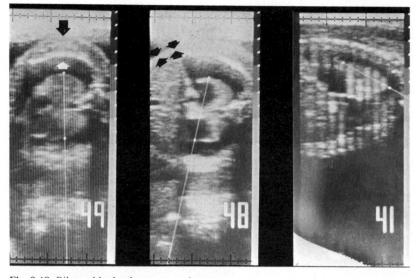

Fig. 9.18. Bilateral hydrothorax secondary to premature closure of foramen ovale, 31 weeks (case 1). *Left:* Transverse thoracic scan showing the heart, lungs, and skin edema (*arrows*). *Center:* Transverse scan on a more cau-dal plane showing basal pulmonary lobe and part of liver. Note absence of ascites and skin edema (*arrows*). Umbilical vein is at 9 o'clock. *Right:* Longitudinal scan with pulmonary lobe (41 mm)

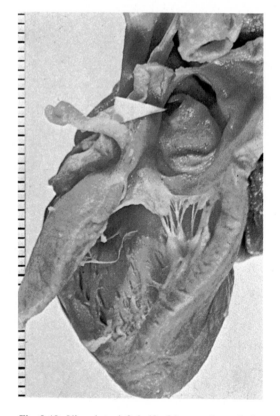

Fig. 9.19. View into left half of heart. *Arrow* indicates foramen ovale, which is narrowed to 2 mm. (From Hansmann et al. 1982)

    f) Oral glucose tolerance test (100 g)
    g) Hb electrophoresis (heterozygous α-thalassemia)
    h) Erythrocyte enzymes (heterozygous G-6-PD deficiency)

2. Ultrasound examination
    a) Evaluation for fetal malformations (detailed examination)
    b) Fetal echocardiography (two-dimensional pulsed Doppler echocardiography with integrated M-mode)

3. Amniocentesis for chromosome analysis, karyotyping, and biochemical amniotic fluid analysis

4. If indicated: fetal blood sampling [hemoglobin, protein, hemoglobin structure, specific IgM, erythrocyte enzyme determination (G-6-PD etc.), blood group (Rh)]

5. If indicated: fetoscopy (detection of malformations, aspiration of fetal blood)

The purpose of maternal blood grouping and antibody screening is to exclude Rh isoimmunization and confirm the diagnosis of NIHF. This is followed by tests for the exclusion of infectious diseases (TORCH = toxoplasmosis, rubella, cytomegalovirus, herpes simplex), AFP assay (e.g., chorioangioma), maternal HbF cell count (fetomaternal transfusion), Hb electrophoresis (heterozygous α-thalassemia), erythro-

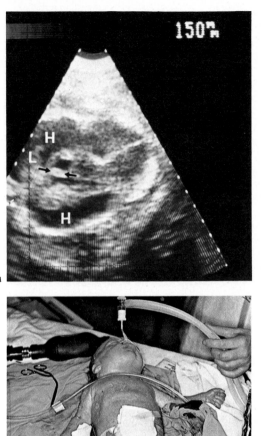

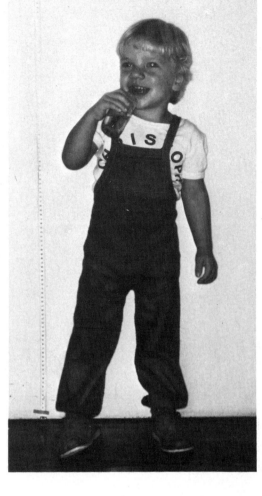

Fig. 9.20. a Hydrothorax secondary to premature closure of foramen ovale, 33 weeks (case 2). Note abnormally thick and rigid septum between atria (*arrows*) *L*, lung; *H*, hydrothorax. **b** Newborn following intrauterine pleural aspiration (120 ml) at 33 weeks (3,450 g, 43 cm; after clearing of edema, 2,350 g!). **c** Child at 2 years of age

cyte enzymes (heterozygous G-6-PD deficiency), etc.

The ultrasound examination is the most important step in the evaluation process. A detailed, specific examination for fetal malformations that includes fetal echocardiography can identify a great number of underlying fetal and placental disorders. In approximately two-thirds of cases, the cause of NIHF can be found in this way (Hansmann and Redel 1982; Kleinman et al. 1982).

The quantification of the degree of hydrops and cardiac function (see above) and the time of onset of intrauterine decompensation and its progression in stages are important prognostic criteria: An early onset of hydrops fetalis (before 24 weeks) is most commonly associated with chromosome abnormalities such as Turner's syndrome and trisomies (18, 21), and less frequently with triploidy. Hydrops secondary to fetal dysrhythmias tends to occur later (after 24 weeks), although we have seen and

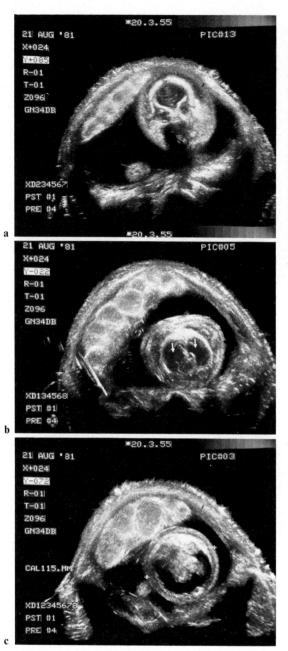

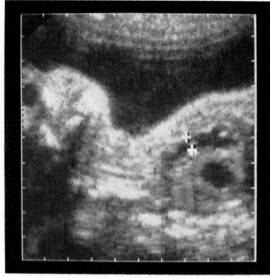

Fig. 9.22. Pericardial effusion as a symptom of cardiac decompensation (fluid layer 5 mm thick)

Fig. 9.21 a–c. Hydrops secondary to premature closure of foramen ovale, 33 weeks (case 3). **a** Head in frontal view with severe skin edema. **b** Thorax with excessive skin edema and bilateral pleural effusions (*arrows*). **c** Abdomen with mild skin edema and ascites. Secondary finding: mature placental appearance

successfully treated one patient referred to our center who presented with hydrops fetalis at 21 weeks and a tachyarrhythmia of 280–300 beats/min (see Sect. 8.8). The further differentiation of fetal brady- and tachyarrhythmias (paroxysmal SVT, atrial fibrillation and flutter) is aided by the use of M-mode ultrasound (DeVore et al. 1983). Whenever a fetal dysrhythmia is noted, even if hemodynamically insignificant, a careful search should be made for associated cardiac anomalies, particularly an AV canal, univentricular heart, tetralogy of Fallot, and Ebstein's anomaly (Redel and Hansmann 1984).

The discovery of a cystic hygroma of the neck (hygroma colli) is suggestive of a chromosome abnormality, especially Turner's syndrome (45X or 45X/46XX), although this condition may occur in isolation or in association with other anomalies, all trisomies, and even with a normal karyotype (Figs. 9.15–9.17).

Differential diagnosis is further aided by noting the distribution of fetal fluid accumulation. For example, when accumulation is confined to the upper half of the body (hydrothorax, skin edema), premature closure of the foramen ovale is the likely cause (Hansmann et al. 1982; Redel and Hansmann 1981) (Figs. 9.18–9.21). Isolated ascites and pericardial effusion are considered early symptoms of cardiac decompensation (DeVore et al. 1982; Fig. 9.22). Dilatation of the vena cava and intrahepatic veins is indicative of right-sided cardiac failure (Fig. 9.23). Isolated ascites is a feature of many other diseases, including infections, gastrointestinal perforation associated with mucoviscido-

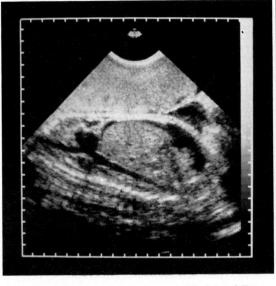

Fig. 9.23a, b. Sonographic features of right heart failure. **a** Longitudinal scan: dilatation of inferior vena cava as it enters right atrium. **b** Dilatation of hepatic veins before their entry into inferior vena cava

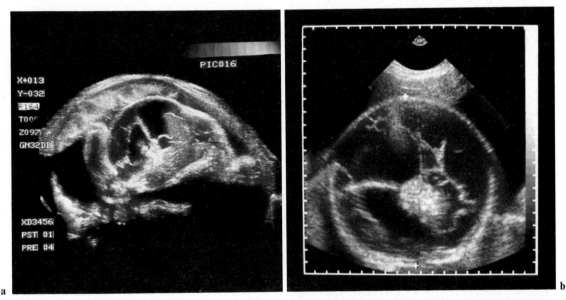

Fig. 9.24a, b. Fetal ascites secondary to bowel perforation in mucoviscidosis (case 1). Note septation caused by formation of adhesions in meconium peritonitis. Abdominal circumference (54 cm) was reduced prenatally by aspirating 1,100 ml fluid. Infant was treated surgically on 1st day of life

sis (Staab et al. 1984; Figs. 9.24, 9.25), diseases of the urogenital tract, and neoplasms. Although this form of isolated ascites does not constitute hydrops fetalis in the strict sense, the similarities are such that we recommend following the same diagnostic steps as for true NIHF.

In twin gestations, fetofetal transfusion through anastomosing placental vessels is almost always the cause of an observed NIHF. Both twins may develop cardiac failure as a result of volume overload in the recipient and chronic anemia in the donor. In the rare case of a parasitic fetus (e.g., acardius acephalus), both fetuses may become hydropic through mechanisms similar to those in fetofetal transfusion.

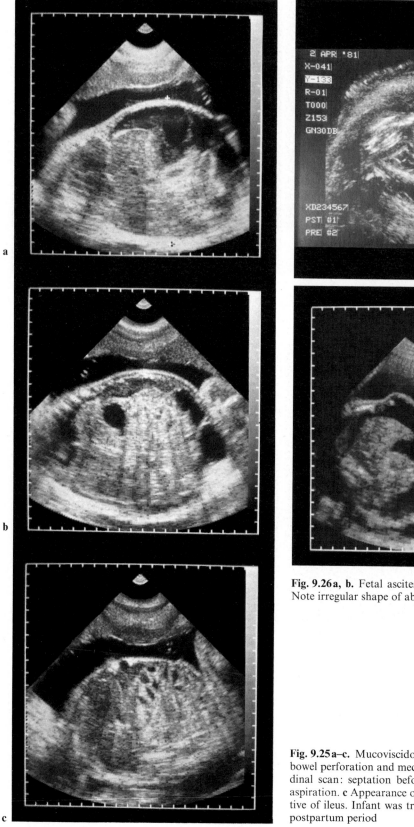

Fig. 9.26a, b. Fetal ascites in stage of recompensation. Note irregular shape of abdomen

Fig. 9.25a–c. Mucoviscidosis (case 2) with intrauterine bowel perforation and meconium peritonitis. **a** Longitudinal scan: septation before aspiration. **b** Status after aspiration. **c** Appearance of small bowel loops is suggestive of ileus. Infant was treated surgically in immediate postpartum period

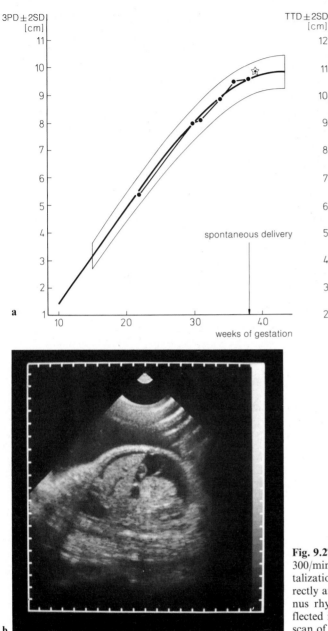

Fig. 9.27. **a** Growth curves: fetal tachycardia (*FFS;* 300/min) at 29 weeks. Ascites at this stage is severe. Digitalization and administration of propafenone, first directly and later transplacentally, effect conversion to sinus rhythm (*S*). Complete regression of ascites is reflected in fall of TTD to normal range. **b** Longitudinal scan of fetus at start of therapy

Another important diagnostic step is amniocentesis for the purpose of chromosome and biochemical analysis. The pipette method (Claussen and Hansmann 1984) offers the advantage of rapid karyotyping (5–6 days) and provides a practical basis for clinical decision-making even in the third trimester. If the pipette method is not available, or the etiology of the NIHF remains unclear, fetal blood sampling from the umbilical vein may be carried out under ultrasound or fetoscopic control (Daffos et al. 1983; Rodeck and Nicolaides 1984; Golbus 1984). This will enable a definitive diagnosis of α-thalassemia, G-6-PD deficiency, chronic anemia, and hypoproteinemia. Infection can also be diagnosed by the demonstration of specific IgM in the fetal blood. The determination of the karyotype from fetal lymphocytes is possible within 3 days after collection of the blood (Rodeck and Nicolaides 1984).

The use of all diagnostic steps in this protocol will help to establish the etiology of NIHF in

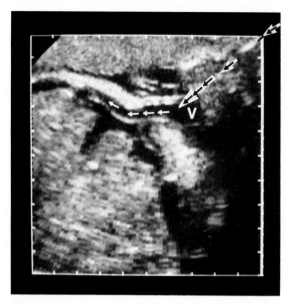

Fig. 9.28. Demonstration of umbilical vein at insertion of umbilical cord. Fixation of vein at site of entry enables direct i.v. injection of medication under ultrasound vision (*arrows*)

all but a few cases, which constitute the category of idiopathic hydrops fetalis.

Treatment. Only an accurate diagnosis of the underlying disease and knowledge of the prognosis will provide the information needed to develop an individual approach to the prenatal care in general and to intrauterine therapy in particular.

The efficacy of intrauterine treatment measures can be assessed sonographically using the parameters listed in p. 297. Quantitative changes in ascites, skin edema, and pleural and pericardial effusions are particularly useful indicators and are easy to measure (Fig. 9.26). An important prognostic sign is the irregular outline of the abdomen (Fig. 9.26) resulting from the decrease in intraabdominal pressure with improvement of ascites. It is indicative of compensation.

The principles of the intrauterine treatment of NIHF may be summarized as follows:

1. Only in cases where there appears to be an immediate threat to fetal life (possibly in connection with other measures such as cell sampling for chromosome analysis, exclusion of anemia or hypoproteinemia, or therapeutic aspiration) is it reasonable to administer drugs directly to the fetus (intravenous, intramuscu-

lar, intracavitary, or intracardiac) under ultrasound guidance. In most cases it is sufficient to treat the fetus transplacentally through the administration of drugs to the mother, e.g., for the conversion of fetal dysrhythmias with digoxin and various antiarrhythmic agents or to treat a heart failure of cardiac or extracardiac origin (complete AV block, fetal anemia, sacrococcygeal teratoma, fetofetal transfusion syndrome) with digoxin (Kleinman et al. 1983; Redel and Hansmann 1984; further details in Sect. 8.8).

2. Aspiration to remove fluid from the abdominal, pleural, and pericardial spaces and to relieve hydramnios is of only temporary benefit and is indicated only as a supportive measure if there is response to pharmacologic decompression, or immediately before delivery to facilitate postnatal resuscitation (pulmonary expansion; Hansmann and Redel 1982). Otherwise aspiration may seriously exacerbate an existing hypoproteinemia.

3. The intrauterine transfusion of red cells into the fetal peritoneal cavity or directly into a fetal vessel is the causal treatment for chronic anemia secondary to fetomaternal transfusion or other causes.

4. Intravascular infusion of albumin under fetoscopic control has been successfully used to treat hydrops in fetuses with confirmed hypoalbuminemia (Rodeck and Nicolaides 1984).

5. Elective preterm delivery should be considered if there is suspicion of impending fetal demise, i.e., if there is rapid worsening of the hydrops.

If the fetus is judged to have an acceptable potential for survival, an elective cesarean birth is generally preferred to vaginal delivery, because the sometimes extreme placental edema in these cases may lead to fetal asphyxia in labor.

6. Elective abortion should be considered only if severe fetal malformations are detected. This group includes chromosome abnormalities, which are commonly associated with the early appearance of hydrops.

Besides the cause of the NIHF, the distribution and volume of the hydropic fluid and gestational age are factors that affect the prognosis. Whereas NIHF secondary to fetal dysrhythmias can and should be treated in utero even with a massive fluid volume, other causes are amenable to intrauterine treatment only in exceptional cases. In the often difficult differential diagnosis and management of NIHF, the best results are achieved through consultation and cooperation with a range of specialties (neonatologist, pediatric cardiologist, radiologist, pediatric surgeon, pediatric pathologist, etc.).

For the future, it is hoped that progress in research related to the etiology, pathogenesis, diagnosis, and management of NIHF will further reduce the high perinatal mortality associated with this condition (Figs. 9.27 and 9.28).

References

Andersen HM, Drew JH, Beischer NA, Hutchison AA, Fortune DW (1983) Non-immune hydrops fetalis: Changing contribution to perinatal mortality. Br J Obstet Gynaecol 90:636

Chervenak FA, Isaacson G, Blakemore KJ, Breg WR, Hobbins JC, Berkowitz RL, Tortora M, Mayden K, Mahoney MJ (1983) Fetal cystic hygroma. Cause and natural history. N Engl J Med 309:822

Clausen U, Hansmann M (1984) Die „Pipettenmethode" zur schnellen Karyotypisierung bei sonographischen Verdachtskriterien für eine Chromosomenanomalie. Gynäkologe 17:33

Daffos F, Capella-Pavlovsky M, Forestier F (1983) Fetal blood sampling via the umbilical cord using a needle guided by ultrasound: Report of 66 cases. Prenat Diagn 3:271

Davis CL (1982) Diagnosis and management of nonimmune hydrops fetalis. J Reprod Med 27:594

DeVore GR, Donnerstein RL, Kleinmann CS, Platt LD, Hobbins JC (1982) Fetal echocardiography. II. The diagnosis and significance of a pericardial effusion in the fetus using real-time-directed M-mode ultrasound. Am J Obstet Gynecol 144:693

DeVore GR, Siassi B, Platt LD (1983) Fetal echocardiography. III. The diagnosis of cardiac arrhythmias using real-time-directed M-mode ultrasound. Am J Obstet Gynecol 146:792

Etches PC, Lemons JA (1979) Nonimmune hydrops fetalis: Report of 22 cases including three siblings. Pediatrics 64:326

Fleischer AC, Killam AP, Boehm FH, Hutchison AA, Jones TB, Shaff MI, Barrett JM, Lindsey AM, James AE (1981) Hydrops fetalis: Sonographic evaluation and clinical implications. Radiology 141:163

Golbus MS (1984) The status of fetoscopy and fetal tissue sampling. Prenat Diagn 4:79

Hansmann M (1981) Nachweis und Ausschluß fetaler Entwicklungsstörungen mittels Ultraschallscreening und gezielter Untersuchung – ein Mehrstufenkonzept. Ultraschall 2:206

Hansmann M, Redel DA (1982) Prenatal symptoms and clinical management of heart disease. In: 1er symposium international d'echocardiologie foetale. Strasbourg 1982, p 137

Hansmann M, Gembruch U (1984) Symptome und Behandlung möglicher fetaler Herzkrankheiten. 93. Tagung der Nordwestdeutschen Gesellschaft für Gynäkologie und Geburtshilfe. Alete Wissenschaftlicher Dienst, München, S. 56

Hansmann M, Redel DA, Födisch HJ (1982) Premature obstruction of the foramen ovale detected, treated and reconfirmed by help of ultrasound. In: Burruto F, Hansmann M, Wladimiroff JW (eds) Fetal ultrasonography: The secret prenatal life. Wiley, Chichester New York, p 151

Hutchison AA, Drew JH, Yu VYH, Williams ML, Fortune DW, Beischer NA (1982) Nonimmunologic hydrops fetalis: a review of 61 cases. Obstet Gynecol 59:347

Kleinman CS, Donnerstein RL, DeVore GR, Jaffe CC, Lynch DC, Berkowitz RL, Talner NS, Hobbins JC (1982) Fetal echocardiography for evaluation of in utero congestive heart failure. N Engl J Med 306:568

Kleinman CS, Donnerstein RL, Jaffe CC, DeVore GR, Weinstein EM, Lynch DC, Talner NS, Berkowitz RL, Hobbins JC (1983) Fetal echocardiography. A tool for evaluation of in utero cardiac arrhythmias and monitoring of in utero therapy: Analysis of 71 patients. Am J Cardiol 51:237

Macafee CAJ, Fortune DW, Beischer NA (1970) Nonimmunological hydrops fetalis. Br J Obstet Gynaecol 77:226

Machin GA (1981) Differential diagnosis of hydrops fetalis. Am J Med Genet 9:341

Maidman JE, Yeager C, Anderson V, Makabali G, O'Grady P, Arce J, Tishler DM (1980) Prenatal diagnosis and management of nonimmunologic hydrops fetalis. Obstet Gynecol 56:571

Perlin BM, Pomerance JJ, Schifrin BS (1981) Nonimmunologic hydrops fetalis. Obstet Gynecol 57:584

Potter EL (1983) Universal edema of the fetus unassociated with erythroblastosis. Am J Obstet Gynecol 46:130

Redel DA, Hansmann M (1981) Fetal obstruction of the foramen ovale detected by two-dimensional doppler echocardiography. In: Rijsterborgh H (ed) Echocardiology. Nijhoff, The Hague Boston London, p 425

Redel DA, Hansmann M (1982) Prenatal diagnosis and treatment of heart disease. In: 1er symposium international d'echocardiologie foetale. Strasbourg 1982, p 137

Redel DA, Hansmann M (1984) Fetale Echokardiographie – ihre Anwendung in Diagnostik und Therapie. Gynäkologe 17:41

Rodeck CH, Nicolaides KH (1984) Die Anwendung der Fetoskopie bei fetaler Therapie. Gynäkologe 17:52

Rudolph A (1974) Congenital diseases of the heart. Year Book Medical Publishers, Chicago

Schwartz SM, Viseskul C, Laxova R, McPherson EW, Gilbert EF (1981) Idiopathic hydrops fetalis. Report of 4 patients including 2 affected sibs. Am J Med Genet 8:59

Senft HH, Födisch HJ, Hansmann M (1982) Hydrops fetalis. Fragen der prä- und postnatalen Diagnostik sowie der Pathogenese. Verh Dtsch Ges Pathol 66:164

Staab D, Schlemminger R, Emons D, Hansmann M, Kowalewski S (1984) Darmperforation als Ursache des fetalen Aszites. INA Bd 47. Kowalewski S (ed) Pädiatrische Intensivmedizin VI. Thieme, Stuttgart New York, S. 86

Turski DM, Shahadi N, Viseskul C, Gilbert E (1978) Non-immunologic hydrops fetalis. Am J Obstet Gynecol 131:586

10 Phenotype and Rare Syndromes

With the development of high-resolution equipment, there have been dramatic improvements in many areas of ultrasound diagnosis, including the diagnosis of congenital anomalies. Today a specific search for fetal anomalies can be made in patients who are at high risk on grounds of family or obstetric history. In addition, studies of fetal behavior, patterns of fetal movement, and particularly of fetal physiognomy can be useful diagnostically. This requires an examiner who has enough experience to be able to delineate and evaluate a normal facial profile (Fig. 10.1a, b).

At this point one has to consider whether it would be possible antenatally to detect changes of phenotype or behavior that are characteristic of specific abnormalities.

It should be noted that the primary function of diagnostic ultrasound in this context is not to replace karyotyping in high-risk patients, but rather to seek grounds for suspicion of an anomaly in patients not assigned to a high-risk group.

Whenever a fetal abnormality is detected by ultrasound, the fetal karyotype should be determined as rapidly as possible. These cases do not primarily involve women who from the outset are candidates for a prenatal cytogenetic evaluation, but women in whom ultrasound scans have demonstrated abnormalities. Many of these pregnancies are past 20 weeks, and a chromosome analysis of cultured amniotic cells is usually not available. But even beyond 20 weeks, a knowledge of fetal karyotype can have an important bearing on the management of the pregnancy. Thus, for example, a patient who goes into preterm labor can be spared the ordeal of cerclage or tocolysis if it is known that her fetus has an abnormal karyotype. To shorten the interval between amniocentesis and the result of the chromosome analysis, Claussen developed the pipette method (Claussen 1980).

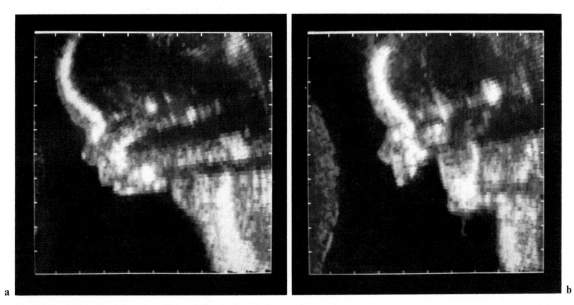

a   b

Fig. 10.1a, b. Normal face (profile). **a** Mouth closed; **b** mouth open

Table 10.1. Results of chromosomal analyses in fetuses with sonographic evidence of a chromosome abnormality

Case no., initials and age of patient, referred for … (week/day of pregnancy)	Findings of ultrasound examination at UFK Bonn	Time of amniocentesis (week/day)	Interval from sampling to reporting of result (days)	Result of chromosome analysis	Remarks and management
1. (K.R.) 40 Prior amniocentesis at 20 weeks; hydrops; ascites (22/3)	1. Ascites (massive) 2. Skin edema 3. Heart defect (AV canal) 4. Shortened diaphyses, prox. more than distal 5. Round skull 6. Abnormal facial profile *Consistent with diagnosis of:* trisomy 21	(22/3)	5	47XX, +21	Termination of pregnancy; the result of the chromosome analysis by conventional technique was not available
2. (U.B.) 36 Abnormal placenta (21/6)	1. Placenta large, multiple cysts 2. Oligohydramnios 3. Disproportionate IUGR 4. Spina bifida with small sac in lumbosacral region *Consistent with diagnosis of:* chromosome abnormality	(21/6)	4	69XXX	Termination of pregnancy
3. (C.F.) 20 Hydramnios (34/6)	1. Polyhydramnios 2. Extreme IUGR 3. Stomach not demonstrable 4. Heart defect (VSD) 5. Suspected esophageal atresia 6. Small interocular distance 7. Radial aplasia *Consistent with diagnosis of:* chromosome abnormality	(35/4)	5	47XY, +18	Premature rupture of membranes; no cesarean birth; spontaneous breech stillbirth
4. (J.P.) 27 Oligohydramnios; suspected Potter's syndrome (19/2)	1. Extreme IUGR 2. Large placenta 3. Anhydramnios 4. Spina bifida in lumbosacral region *Consistent with diagnosis of:* chromosome abnormality	(19/2)	7	69XXX	Termination of pregnancy

Patient	Ultrasound findings / diagnosis			Karyotype	Outcome
5. (U.D.) 23 Bradycardia (25/5)	1. Sinus bradycardia 80/min 2. Suspected hypoplastic left heart with mitral atresia 3. Situs inversus ambiguus *Conclusion:* exclusion of chromosome abnormality	(26/4)	6	46XY	Elective cesarean birth at 37 weeks; infant died at 8 weeks from cardiac defect
6. (H.H.) 36 Polyhydramnios; IUGR (32/3)	1. Polyhydramnios 2. Moderate IUGR 3. Stomach not demonstrable 4. Suspected esophageal atresia *Consistent with diagnosis of:* trisomy 18	(32/— amniography)	6	47XX, +18	Premature rupture of membranes; spontaneous delivery at 33 weeks
7. (A.O.) 34 Gestational age? Double bubble in pelvis (16/7)	1. Severe disproportionate IUGR 2. Microcephaly 3. Microphthalmia 4. Facial dysmorphia 5. Bilateral hydronephrosis with ureteropelvic stenosis 6. Excessive uncoordinated movements *Consistent with diagnosis of:* complex malformation syndrome, possibly a chromosome abnormality	(26/7)	8	46XX, inv.	Delivery following rupture of membranes at 27 weeks; complex malformation syndrome of undetermined etiology
8. (G.K.) 26 IUGR (23/2)	1. Disproportionate IUGR with greater shortening of proximal than distal diaphyses 2. Heart defect (AV canal) 3. Facial cleft *Consistent with diagnosis of:* trisomy 13	(23/5)	8	47XX, +13	Termination of pregnancy
9. (M.K.) 38 Advanced age (16/1)	1. IUGR 2. Cystic hygroma 3. Heart defect (AV canal) *Consistent with diagnosis of:* trisomy 21	(16/4)	6	47XY, +21	Termination of pregnancy
10. (G.V.) 32 Suspected encephalocele (20/1)	1. Moderate IUGR 2. Hydrops fetalis 3. Pleural effusion 4. Excessive skin edema 5. Suspected cardiac defect *Consistent with diagnosis of:* chromosome abnormality	(20/4)	6	47XY, +2	Intrauterine fetal death at 20 weeks

Table 10.1 (continued)

Case no., initials and age of patient, referred for … (week/day of pregnancy)	Findings of ultrasound examination at UFK Bonn	Time of amniocentesis (week/day)	Interval from sampling to reporting of result (days)	Result of chromosome analysis	Remarks and management
11. (S.B.) 36 Hydrops fetalis (22/1)	1. Hydrops fetalis 2. Shortened diaphyses 3. Right lung enlarged and hyperechoic 4. Suspected cardiac defect *Consistent with diagnosis of:* chromosome abnormality	(22/1)	6	47XY, +21	Termination of pregnancy
12. (I.L.) 24 Twin gestation, one fetus with IUGR (26/1)	Fetus I: normal Fetus II: 1. IUGR 2. Cardiac defect 3. Hydrocephalus *Conclusion:* exclusion of chromosome abnormality	(26/1) (26/1)	5 5	46XX 46XX	Abnormal twin: ultrasound findings confirmed. Neonatal death
13. (G.H.) 28 Polyhydramnios, hydrothorax (31/1)	1. Polyhydramnios 2. Cardiac defect 3. Ectocardia 4. Pleural effusion 5. Suspected esophageal atresia *Consistent with diagnosis of:* trisomy 21	(31/1)	4	47XX, +21	Intrauterine fetal death at 31 weeks

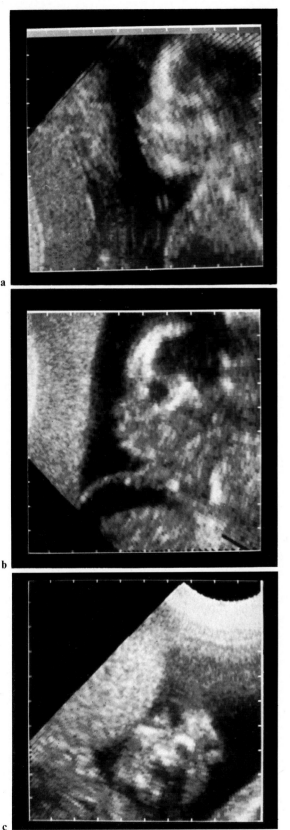

Today this method is fairly well standardized and can be used both routinely and individually. In a pilot study, the pipette method of rapid chromosome analysis was used in 13 patients who had sonographic evidence of a fetal chromosome abnormality (Claussen and Hansmann 1984). The sonographic signs, the gestational age at amniocentesis, the interval between fluid sampling and reporting of the result, the findings, and the outcomes in this series are summarized in Table 10.1.

The average interval between sampling and reporting in this series was only 5.8 days. This means that the pipette method enables routine genetic testing at any time beyond 20 weeks. It is recommended that blood from both parents be drawn for chromosome analysis, in addition to the amniocentesis, as this will enable certain features of the fetal karyotype to be evaluated without loss of time. The relatively short period between amniocentesis and chromosome analysis opens up many areas of application for the pipette method. In high-risk cases where medical attention is sought late in pregnancy, and in cases where ultrasound scans suggest a fetal chromosome abnormality, the conventional strategy has been either to dispense with chromosome analysis altogether or to attempt chromosome analysis from fetal blood. The pipette method offers a new alternative. While it is true that a fetal blood chromosome analysis will yield a result 2–3 days after sampling, this procedure is far less attractive than amniocentesis because it carries a greater than 2% risk of precipitating labor. Moreover, fetal blood sampling can presently be done at only a few specialized centers, and the delay involved in scheduling and travel negates the theoretical time advantage over the pipette method.

At our center, ultrasound examinations have invariably enabled a refined differentiation of findings compared with the diagnosis at referral (see Table 10.1). In cases 1, 6, 8, 9, and 13, a presumptive diagnosis of a specific chromo-

Fig. 10.2. a Profile of normal fetus: straight, high forehead, well-modeled nose, and prominent chin (21 weeks). **b** Profile of fetus with trisomy 21: moderately high forehead, round, flat nose, and receding chin; pleural effusion is also evident (21 weeks; case 1 from Table 10.1). **c** Trisomy 21: frontal view of face, which appears coarse and has sloping lid axes

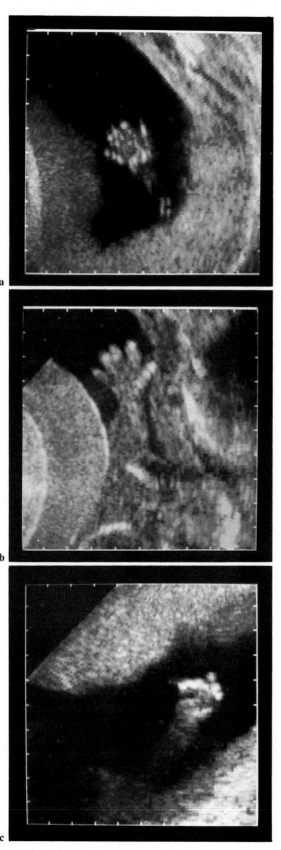

some abnormality could be expressed on the basis of ultrasound findings. In each case the presumptive diagnosis was confirmed by karyotyping. It should again be emphasized that we do not propose replacing the chromosome analysis with a detailed sonographic evaluation. In all cases a definitive diagnosis must await karyotypic analysis. Our intent, rather, is to show that the capabilities of diagnostic ultrasound go beyond the recognition of gross malformations to the discernment of relatively subtle deviations of phenotype and behavior that may be useful diagnostically.

This is particularly true in the case of *trisomy 21* (Down's syndrome), which manifests a number of subtle changes such as a characteristic profile (Fig. 10.2b, c), a round skull, and plump hands with short or even crossed fingers (Fig. 10.3b, c), possibly associated with a congenital heart defect (ventricular septal defect, AV canal; Fig. 10.4). Of course, it must be understood that a variety of sonographic findings can characterize trisomy 21. Intrauterine growth retardation is not often seen. Of the five cases presented here (see Table 10.1), growth retardation was present in only two (cases 9 and 10). At the same time, all five fetuses with trisomy 21 had demonstrable cardiac defects. In affected newborns, there is about a 40% likelihood that a cardiac defect will be present; this percentage may be higher earlier in gestation. Fetuses with trisomy 21 are subject to a selection process in utero that may culminate in fetal death, depending on malformations. This means that fetuses with cardiac defects are at greatest risk for intrauterine death. Thus, defects are probably much more common in a second-trimester fetus with trisomy 21 than in a newborn with the same syndrome. It is anticipated that fetal and pediatric pathologists will soon be able to provide more detailed data on the prevalence of malformations at different stages of gestation in infants with chromosome abnormalities. The series of fetuses with trisomy 21 presented here is too small to be representative. Also, it is possible that affected fetuses having no recognizable symptoms were excluded from our series.

Fig. 10.3. **a** Normal slender hand. **b** Trisomy 21: hand wide and pawlike with relatively short digits (19 weeks; case 10 from Table 10.1). **c** Trisomy 21: clinodactyly

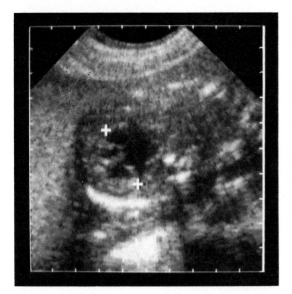

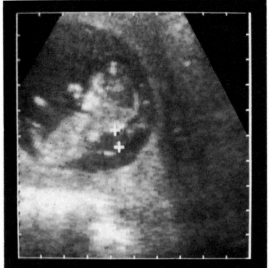

Fig. 10.4. Trisomy 21: four-chamber view demonstrating a common AV canal, a typical defect in this anomaly

Fig. 10.5. Trisomy 18 (14 weeks), hygroma colli. Fetus is growth-retarded. Paucity of body movements was another anomalous sign

With trisomy 18 or 13, a presumptive ultrasound diagnosis is somewhat less difficult to make than with trisomy 21. This is because the suggestive signs of these syndromes are more numerous and conspicuous.

In *trisomy 18* (Figs. 10.5–10.9), however, specific diagnosis is made difficult by the variability of fetal malformations. The two trisomies may show similarities in the symptoms that are accessible to ultrasound detection, and are also similar in their poor prognoses and in their outcomes. The prenatal sonographic diagnosis of trisomy 18, based on a combination of hydramnios, micrognathia, low-set ears, hand deformities, flexion deformities of the fingers, absent umbilical artery and moderate growth retardation, was also described by Staudach et al. (1984) (Figs. 10.9, 10.10). A presumptive ultrasound diagnosis of chromosome abnormality is always an indication for karyotypic analysis.

In *trisomy 13*, 60%–80% of affected newborns have a cleft lip and palate (Fig. 10.11 a, b) (Smith 1982). These clefts are easily visualized by ultrasound (Fig. 10.12 a–e) (Hansmann 1984). The choice of scanning plane is critical. If a facial cleft is noted incidentally on ultrasound scans, further evaluation at a specialized center is indicated. The presence of associated anomalies should be excluded. If it can be established through ultrasound and karyotypic

analysis that the facial cleft is an isolated anomaly, the outlook becomes more favorable, and an effort should generally be made to preserve or engender a positive motivation toward accepting the pregnancy. It should be noted in this regard that cleft lip and palate can be reliably excluded or established with ultrasound, provided the examination is properly timed (second trimester). Invasive fetoscopy can no longer be justified for this purpose.

The presumptive ultrasound diagnosis of triploidy is based largely on two sets of findings: (1) early intrauterine growth retardation with malproportions, and (2) a large, vacuolated placenta in the presence of oligohydramnios (see Table 10.1, Figs. 10.13, 10.14). As the table indicates, the presumptive sonographic diagnosis of a fetal chromosome abnormality was always based on the presence of multiple symptoms.

The criteria arousing suspicion of a fetal chromosome abnormality may be summarized as follows:

1. Early growth retardation
2. Malproportions (e.g., shape of skull, microcephaly, shortened diaphyses; Figs. 10.6 a, b, 10.7 a–c)
3. Facial dysmorphisms (profile, retrognathia, microphthalmia, cleft; Fig. 10.18 a, b)

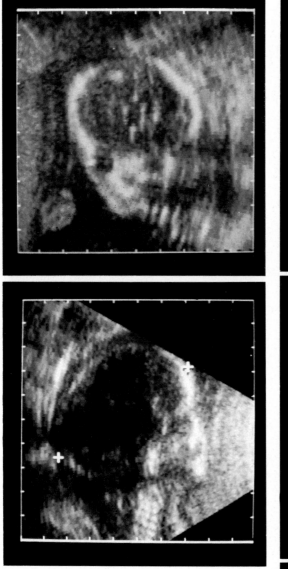

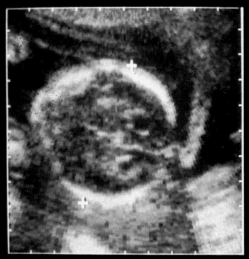

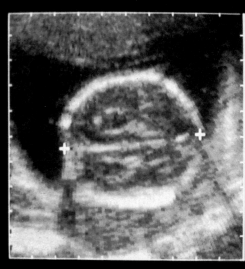

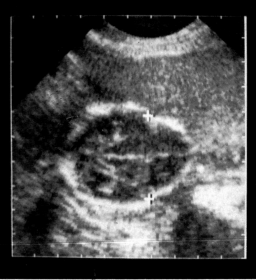

Fig. 10.6a, b. Trisomy 18: **a** Frontal view of typically small face. **b** Profile: face is flat and retrognathia is present

Fig. 10.7a–c. Trisomy 18. **a** Brachycephaly: BPD 5.7 cm (25 weeks). **b** Same head, same plane of section: OFD only 5.7 cm. **c** Scaphocephaly is typical

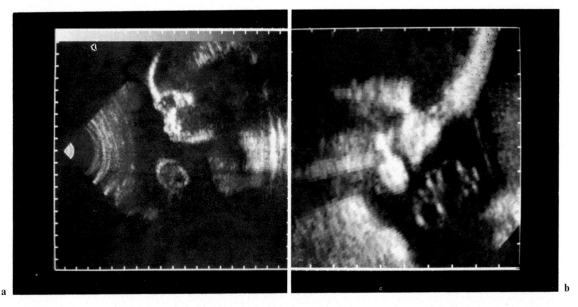

Fig. 10.8. a Trisomy 18 (case 6 from Table 10.1): nasal bridge depressed, chin poorly developed. **b** Trisomy 13 at 35 weeks: nose almost completely absent, chin poorly developed; profile has abnormal appearance

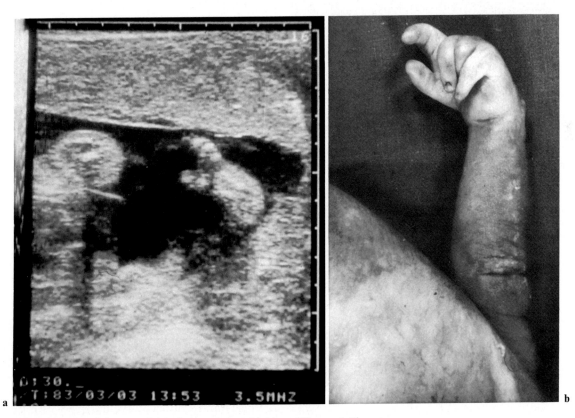

Fig. 10.9 a, b. Trisomy 18. **a** Typical abnormal positioning of fingers. **b** Phenotype

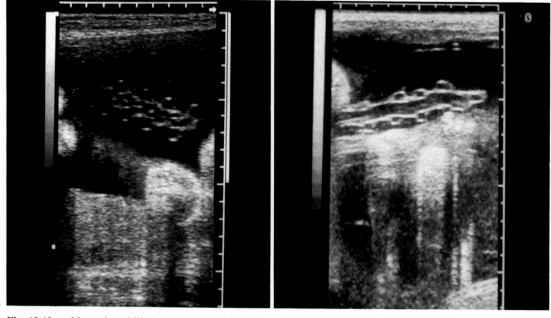

Fig. 10.10. a Normal umbilical cord: one vein and two arteries. **b** Trisomy 18: only one artery winds around umbilical vein

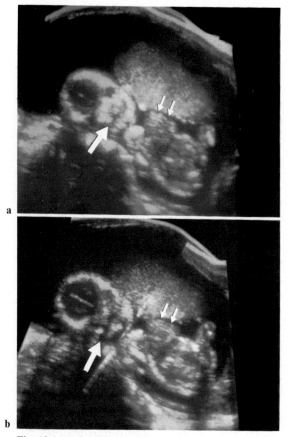

Fig. 10.11a, b. Trisomy 13 at 25 weeks: longitudinal scans. Growth retardation, cleft lip and palate (*single arrow*) omphalocele (*arrows*)

4. Hydrops fetalis (skin edema, hygroma colli, ascites; Fig. 10.5)
5. Cardiovascular abnormalities (e.g., single umbilical artery, VSD, truncus arteriosus, AV canal, single ventricle, ectopia)
6. Limb malformations (e.g., polydactyly; Fig. 10.19) and malformations of internal organs and systems (Figs. 10.11a, b, 10.20)
7. Large placenta with inhomogeneous or "honeycomb" structure (Fig. 10.13a–c)
8. Anomalous amniotic fluid volume (oligohydramnios or polyhydramnios)
9. Anomalous fetal behavior (alternating episodes of hyperactivity and immobility)

The peculiar clinical circumstances of these cases, and particularly the late recognition of symptoms, have frequently led clinicians to dispense with chromosome analysis. The reason for this lay in the long waiting period associated with conventional laboratory analysis, which often was incompatible with, and irrelevant to, the needs of clinical decision making. However, it has been our experience that rapid chromosome analysis, which generally allows a definitive prognosis, is indeed a great asset to clinical decision making. For example, many patients have been spared the necessity of late cervical cerclage and tocolysis by the discovery of a lethal fetal karyotype. In the future we intend

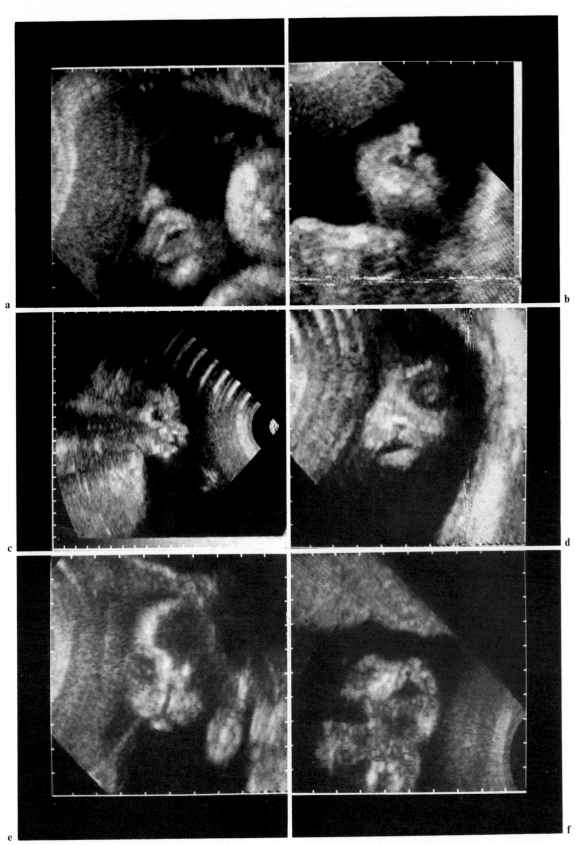

Fig. 10.12. a Tangential scan through normal face: both nostrils seen, complete contour of upper lip visible. **b** Typical appearance of cleft lip and palate (zoom magnification): harelip defect well depicted. **c–f** Trisomy 18: cleft lip and palate. **c, d** Profile and frontal view; **e, f** different planes of section

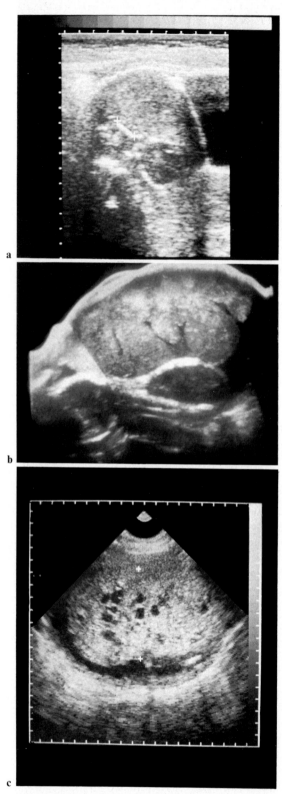

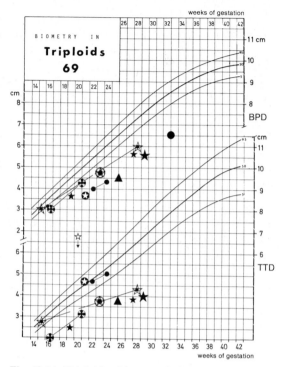

Fig. 10.14. Triploidy: biometry indicates early, severe growth retardation

to work closely with geneticists to develop a more differentiated approach to the clinical management of the high-risk pregnancy.

The special problems and limitations of the sonographic diagnosis of fetal malformations were illustrated in one patient whose fetus was examined for exclusion of autosomal COFS (cerebro-oculo-facio-skeletal) syndrome. Three separate examinations between 17 and 23 weeks gestation failed to disclose any anomalies other than the presence of "small but not very small" orbits (Jeanty et al. 1982). On pediatric evaluation on the first day of life, the male infant was declared to be normal. It was only during a later ophthalmologic examination that micro-ophthalmia and mature cataracts were detected, signifying a recurrence of COFS syndrome, although the child had no other commonly associated anomalies such as growth retardation (birth weight 3,850 g, length 51 cm, HC 36 cm). Cases of this type underscore the need to apprise parents not only of the capabilities of ultrasound for the exclusion or confirmation of a syndrome or individual symptoms, but also of its limitations.

A major limitation of ultrasound stems from variations in the genetic penetrance and expres-

Fig. 10.13a–c. Triploidy. **a** 69XXX at 19 weeks: anhydramnios, early growth retardation. **b** Abnormal placental structure: 12 cm thick (!) and hyperechoic. **c** Placenta: large, hyperechoic, multiple cystic areas

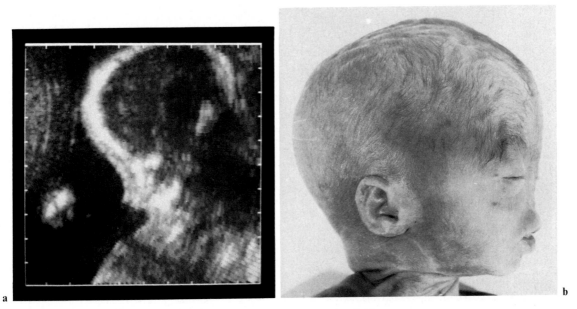

Fig. 10.15a, b. Arhinencephaly. **a** Median profile view: absence of nose. **b** Phenotype

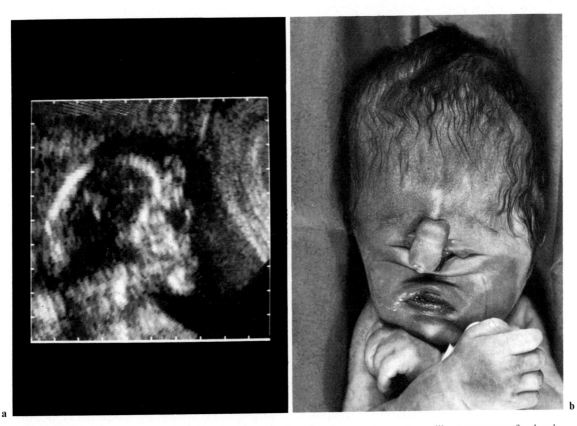

Fig. 10.16a, b. Cyclops. **a** Median profile view: abnormal orbits, absence of nose, tumorlike structure on forehead. **b** Phenotype

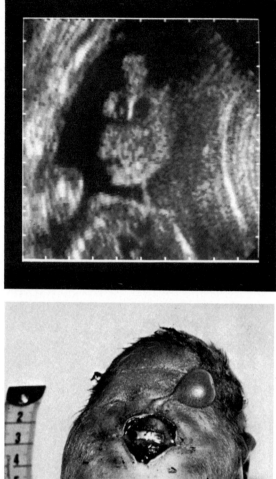

Fig. 10.17a, b. Cyclops. **a** Frontal scan through face: medial displacement of orbits. **b** Phenotype of cyclops in trisomy 18 (different case)

sivity of individual symptoms. An understanding of this fact should make the physician wary about definitively excluding the recurrence of a syndrome based on the apparent absence of symptoms in sonograms.

Some years ago we failed to recognize a recurrence of the autosomal recessive Jeune's syndrome (asphyxiating thoracic dysplasia). It re-

mains unclear whether the long, narrow thorax and/or short limbs are so pronounced before 24 weeks as to provide sonographic criteria for confirmation or exclusion. Another complicating factor is the variation in the expressivity of individual symptoms. Diagnosis in high-risk cases may be aided by the demonstration of facultative anomalies, such as renal cysts or a

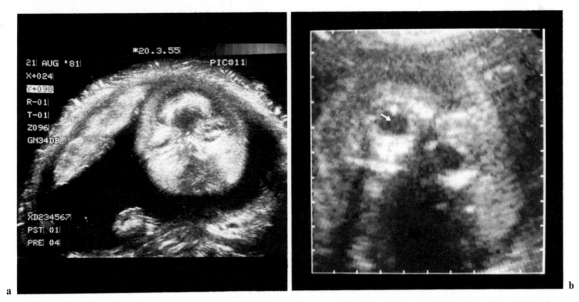

Fig. 10.18a, b. Hydrops. **a** Frontal scan through face: note "moon facies" and marked skin edema in region of forehead. **b** Frontal scan through upper portion of face: eye visible within right orbit (*arrow*)

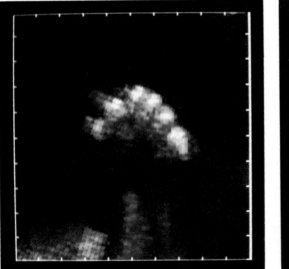

Fig. 10.19. Hexadactyly in hydramnios

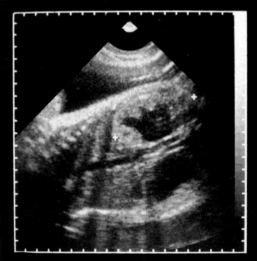

Fig. 10.20. Hydronephrosis in trisomy 21

situs inversus in Jeune's syndrome (Taybi 1983). In many other syndromes where we feel that the sonographic demonstration of one or more facultative or obligatory symptoms will allow a prenatal diagnosis in selected patients, we have correctly excluded a recurrence by early ultrasound evaluation. In patients who do not have a high-risk history, syndromes and rare malformations can be detected only by thorough careful anatomic screening of the fetus. The importance of evaluating the facial soft tissues is again emphasized. Arhinencephaly (Fig. 10.15a, b) and cyclopia (Figs. 10.16, 10.17) are "easy" to recognize in theory because of their distinctive pathomorphologies, but in practice this is true only if the evaluation of facial morphology is included in the screening process. As we saw in Sect. 8.5 (Table 8.5), chromosome defects are frequently associated with genitourinary anomalies. In the case shown in Fig. 10.20, the typical picture of hydronephrosis was the primary finding. Because no sonomorphologic substrate for the hydronephrosis could be found, karyotyping was done, leading to a diagnosis of trisomy 21.

A discussion of the complete range of diagnosable symptoms would exceed the scope of this book. Major syndromes are illustrated and described in Sect. 8.9.

References

Claussen U (1980) The pipette method: a new rapid technique for chromosome analysis in prenatal diagnosis. Hum Genet 54:277

Claussen U, Hansmann M (1984) Die „Pipettenmethode" zur schnellen Karyotypisierung bei sonographischen Verdachtskriterien für eine Chromosomenanomalie. Gynäkologe 17

Hansmann M (1984) Möglichkeiten und Grenzen sonographischer Diagnostik fetaler Erkrankungen und Mißbildungen. In: Kowalewski S (ed) Pädiatrische Intensivmedizin VI. Thieme, Stuttgart New York

Jeanty P, Dramaix-Wilmet M, Gansbecke D van, Regemorter N van, Rodesch F (1982) Fetal ocular biometry by ultrasound. Radiology 143:513

Smith DW (1982) Recognizable patterns of human malformations. Sounders, London Toronto Mexico City Rio de Janeiro Sydney Tokio

Staudach A, Laßmann R, Rosenkranz W, Engels M, Joos H, Rücker J (1984) Pränatale Diagnose fetaler Entwicklungsstörungen – das Modell eines interdisziplinären Teams. In: Kowalewski S (ed) Pädiatrische Intensivmedizin VI. Thieme, Stuttgart New York

Taybi H (1983) Radiology of syndromes and metabolic disorders. Year Book Medical Publishers, Chicago London

11 The Placenta

In Cooperation with R. Terinde

Visualization of the placenta with B-mode ultrasound is superior to all other imaging techniques (Doppler method, radiographic placentography or arteriography, thermography, scintigraphy). It is the simplest means of establishing the topographic relation of the placenta to the uterine wall and cervix. This makes sonography the method of choice for localizing the placenta (excluding placenta previa) and for evaluating the separation of a normally positioned placenta. Localization of the placenta is an essential part of routine obstetric examinations. With the development of high-resolution gray-scale equipment, tissue differentiation of the placenta has become possible, although the correlation between ultrasound appearance and pathologic anatomy is not entirely clear. Ultrasound may be of value in the assessment of placental maturity and the recognition of a growth-retarded (SGA) fetus. It appears that the combination of clinical and sonographic data (hypertension, gestational age, growth retardation) can also provide a basis for predicting placental function in cases of accelerated placental maturation. Research into these areas is made all the more urgent by the disappointing results of hormonal methods for the diagnosis of placental insufficiency.

11.1 Sonographic Placental Development

Initially, the entire surface of the implanted chorion is covered with villi. As the conceptus grows and expands, a nutritional disparity arises which favors development of the basal portion of the trophoblast adjacent to the endometrium over development of the capsular portion. The polar discrepancy in the growth of the gestational sac leads to the development of the villous placenta (chorion frondosum) and to a loss of villi in the remainder of the chorion (chorion laeve). With high-resolution B-mode ultrasound this process can be clearly followed from 7 to 11 weeks gestation (Fig. 11.1, 11.2). After 12 weeks the chorion frondosum is well defined on ultrasound and can be separated into three main areas: the basal plate, the placental substance, and the chorionic plate (Fig. 11.3). The barely perceptible line of the basal plate, the finely homogeneous placental substance, and the thin, smooth line of the chorionic plate characterize the immature placenta (grade 0 of Grannum et al. 1979 or score 3 of Koslowski et al. 1980). A change in the echo pattern of these structures may or may not be observed as pregnancy progresses. With modern instrumentation the placenta can generally be differentiated from the uterine musculature without difficulty from 12 weeks on, making it possible to distinguish the placenta from a local uterine contraction (Fig. 11.4). The danger of mistaking a contraction of the lower uterine segment for a placenta previa or a submucous or intramural myoma can be avoided by prolonged observation with real-time ultrasound. Disorders of placentation that are associated with vaginal bleeding may produce areas of hemorrhage between the chorion laeve and

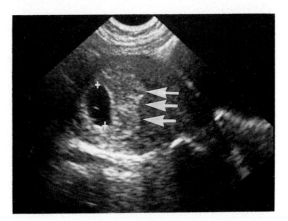

Fig. 11.1. Chorion frondosum (*arrows*) at 7 weeks

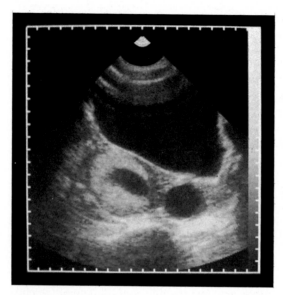

Fig. 11.2. Placenta at 11 weeks: placenta distinguished from myometrium by its greater echogenicity. Left adnexal cyst

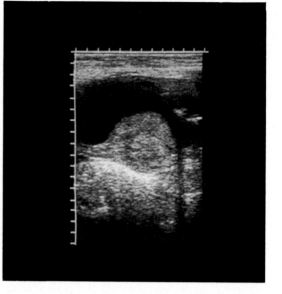

Fig. 11.4. Contraction of posterior uterine wall mimicking increase in placental thickness

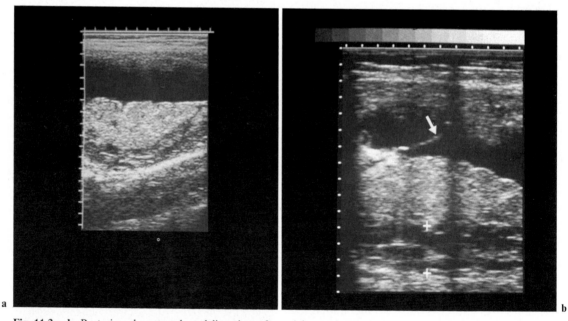

a   b

Fig. 11.3a, b. Posterior placenta: clear delineation of retroplacental vascular bed. a 21 weeks; b 29 weeks. Note retroplacental vascular space (diameter 29 mm) and intraamniotic band (*arrow*)

uterine wall. These areas should not be mistaken for a second gestational sac (see also Figs. 4.29, 4.30, and Chap. 5). With a viable embryo and a hematoma in the region of the chorion laeve, there is a favorable prognosis for continuation of the pregnancy.

11.2 Localization of the Placenta

Demonstration and delineation of the placenta as an organ has become an integral part of routine obstetric sonography. As a rule, the placenta can be cleary seen with respect to sur-

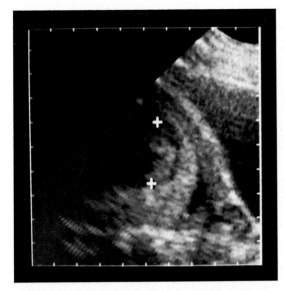

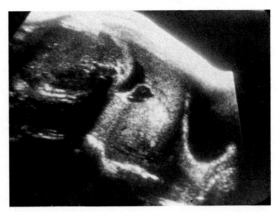

Fig. 11.7. Complete placenta previa at term with transverse fetal lie. Hypoechoic area in region of chorionic plate corresponds to umbilical cord insertion

Fig. 11.5. Placenta overlying internal cervical as at 9 weeks. Note echo-free zone in region of internal os in this patient, who had symptoms of threatened abortion

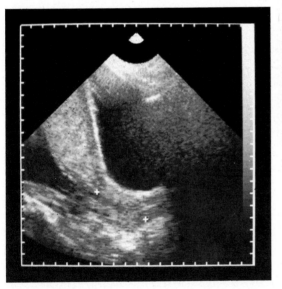

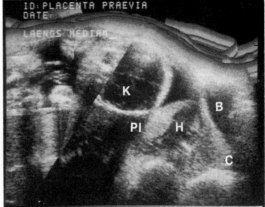

Fig. 11.8. Longitudinal scan through lower uterine segment (B, bladder) in a patient with posterior placenta previa. Placenta (Pl) and a retroplacental hematoma (H) separate fetal head (K) from cervix (C). Note acoustic shadowing behind head

Fig. 11.6. Low-lying anterior placenta with visualization of cervix (length 4.5 cm)

rounding portions of the chorion by 12 weeks menstrual age owing to disparities of echo density. Fine delineation of the placenta with respect to the uterine wall is made difficult by the relatively poor demonstrability of the basal plate, which presents as a thin, broken line. On the other hand, the chorionic plate, which interfaces with the amnion, is easily distinguished owing to the different acoustic impedances of the placental tissue and amniotic fluid. In some cases the impedance differences between the placenta and the chorion laeve or decidua may be so slight that accurate delineation of the placenta is impossible even after 12 weeks. But on the whole, sonographic localization of the placenta is satisfactory for clinical demands. Special indications for placental localization are:

1. Bleeding in the second and third trimesters
2. Transabdominal amniocentesis and other intrauterine procedures at any time during pregnancy
3. Evaluation of placental margins and area of placental attachment to exclude abruption

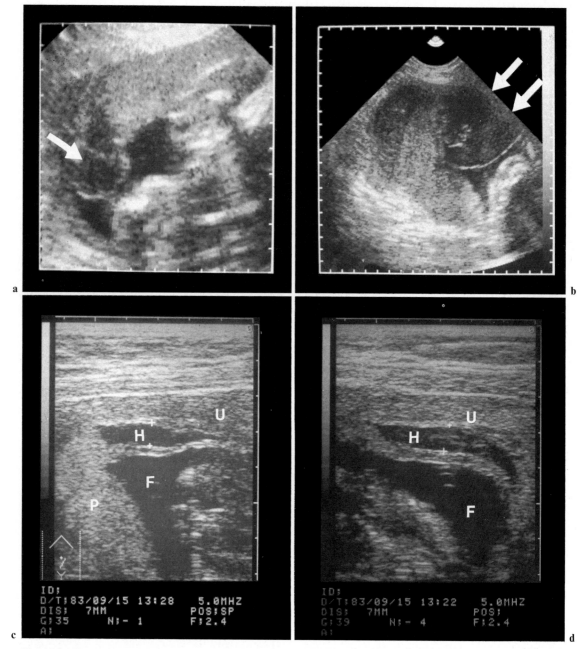

Fig. 11.9 a–d

A placenta implanted on the posterior wall of the uterus can be difficult to image due to shadowing from the fetal skeleton. Thus, as gestation progresses, increasingly greater portions of the posterior uterine wall become inaccessible to ultrasound.

It can also be difficult to demonstrate a placenta which is low-lying or which covers all or part of the internal cervical os. These placentas can be imaged only if the maternal bladder is well filled, so that an acoustic window is created anterior to the lower uterine segment (Figs. 11.5–11.8). While a low-lying placenta can be readily diagnosed following suitable preparation of the patient, it may be difficult to distinguish the various degrees of placenta previa by sonographic examination alone, and management should be guided by clinical findings.

The ability to demonstrate the premature

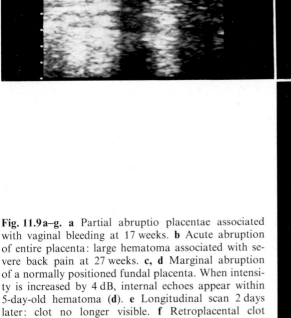

e

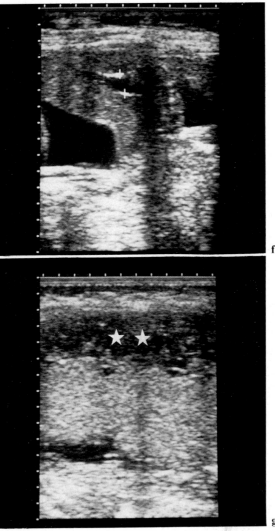

f

g

Fig. 11.9a–g. a Partial abruptio placentae associated with vaginal bleeding at 17 weeks. b Acute abruption of entire placenta: large hematoma associated with severe back pain at 27 weeks. c, d Marginal abruption of a normally positioned fundal placenta. When intensity is increased by 4 dB, internal echoes appear within 5-day-old hematoma (d). e Longitudinal scan 2 days later: clot no longer visible. f Retroplacental clot (12 mm) of small abruptio placentae: uterine bleeding, abdominal pain. *P*, placenta; *F*, amniotic fluid; *U*, myometrium; *H*, hematoma

separation of a normally positioned placenta (abruptio placentae) depends on the stage of the process. Fresh, unclotted blood appears in sonograms as a largely echo-free zone (Figs. 11.9a–e, 11.10), whereas older, more organized clots are more echogenic and can be extremely difficult to distinguish from placental tissue (Fig. 11.9f). Thus, the only direct sonographic evidence of a retroplacental hemorrhage is the presence of an echo-free zone between the placenta and uterine wall. A fresh bleed from the placental margins presents as a largely or completely echo-free, crescent-shaped area between the placenta, fetal membrane, and uterine wall. Clinically, tenderness to pressure may be noted over the area of sonographic change. The suspicion of a placental

hematoma should not prompt intervention unless clinical symptoms are present; sometimes the condition is found to be resolved when the examination is repeated. Abruption of the placenta should be differentiated from large sinusoids at the uteroplacental junction (Fig. 11.3, 11.9g).

When bleeding occurs during the second half of pregnancy, the placenta should be localized sonographically with the bladder filled before a vaginal examination is performed. Under these conditions total placenta previa can be diagnosed with a reported accuracy of 95% (Schlensker 1976). Cesarean birth is the only acceptable mode of delivery in such cases. Obstetric textbooks recommend that the cervix first be examined with a speculum after the pa-

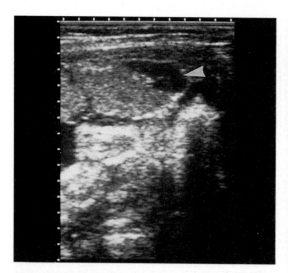

Fig. 11.10. Echo-free, blood-filled space (*S*) in marginal region of placenta (*Pl*)

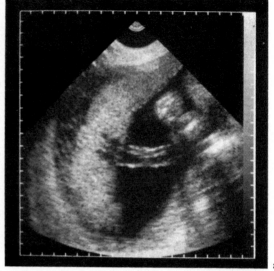

tient is prepared for surgery, on the chance that favorable findings might warrant a postponement of the operation. The sonographic differentiation between a marginal and partial placenta previa is not meaningful from a clinical standpoint. The severity of hemorrhage, progress of the delivery, and condition of the infant will determine the course of the parturition.

If a placenta previa is diagnosed in the absence of overt bleeding, a passive (though watchful) approach may be taken, with the consent of the patient and her physician, until the third trimester. After that time the patient may be hospitalized for further supervision.

If scans reveal a placenta previa prior to 20 weeks [incidence of 20% according to Lee et al. (1981)], it is common for this condition to resolve spontaneously by the start of the third trimester. The incidence at term is only 0.5%! This apparent change, sometimes referred to as "placental migration," is the result of growth of the lower uterine segment combined with lateral expansion and slight rotation.

While the uterine circumference continues to increase even after 32 weeks, the area of placental attachment ceases to grow after that time. An abnormal implantation of the placenta is

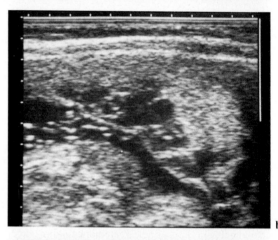

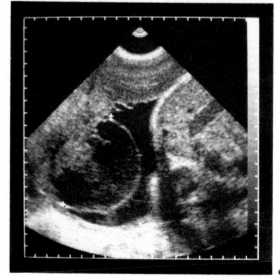

Fig. 11.11. a Central insertion of umbilical cord in a fundal placenta at 28 weeks. **b** Needle within follicle. **c** Cystic placental tumor at 34 weeks: no signs of placental dysfunction, healthy child delivered spontaneously at term

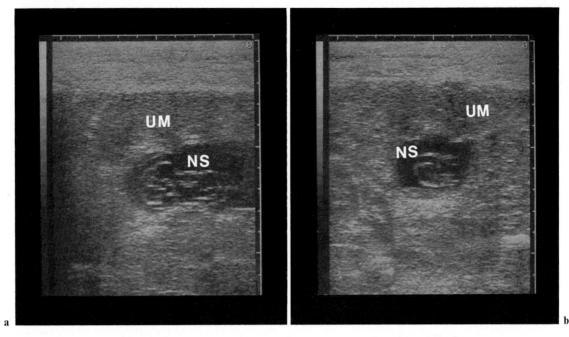

Fig. 11.12. Loop of umbilical cord in lower segment of a fibroid uterus: cord prolapse following premature rupture of membranes. **a** Longitudinal scan through cervical region; **b** tranverse scan. *UM*, uterine muscle with fibroids; *NS*, umbilical cord

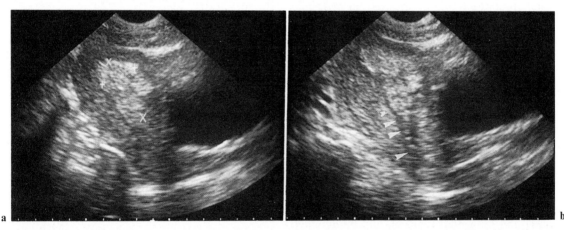

Fig. 11.13. a Longitudinal scan 2 weeks post partum: retained placental products (22 × 37 mm) within uterus. **b** Fluid (blood) track within uterus

commonly associated with malpresentation of the fetus (25% of transverse lies).

In the past, little clinical importance was attached to ultrasound imaging of the umbilical cord. This may have been due largely to the poor resolution of older real-time scanners, since visualization of the cord with a compound scanner is possible but very time-consuming. Today, technical improvement in instrumentation permits visualization of the cord insertion,

the umbilical vein, the umbilical arteries, and the Wharton's jelly (Fig. 11.11). The insertion of the cord into the placenta, like its insertion into the fetal abdomen, is an appropriate site for puncture of the umbilical vein – a procedure of growing importance in prenatal diagnosis and therapy. The potential importance of the cord insertion site is illustrated by the case in Fig. 11.12. The umbilical cord presented in the lower uterine segment, which was narrowed by fibroids. The patient was hospitalized immediately after the ultrasound scan at 33 weeks. Premature rupture of the membranes and cord prolapse occurred on the day of admission. The patient was delivered by cesarean birth of a healthy infant. The fibroid uterus had to be extirpated.

The search for retained products of conception following delivery can have clinical significance. With the maternal bladder filled, the uterine cavity can be visualized, and blood clots can be distinguished from placental tissue (Figs. 13.2, 13.3). The longer the retained tissue remains in utero, the more organized and echogenic it becomes. The heavily vascularized uterine musculature in the presence of a hydatidiform mole can mimic the tissue structure of a homogeneous placenta (Fig. 11.13 b).

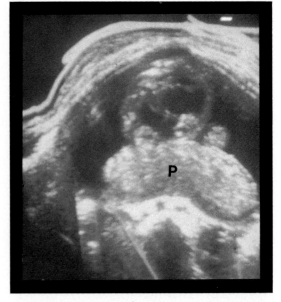

Fig. 11.14. Thick placenta (*P*) associated with nonimmunologic hydrops fetalis and hydramnios at 27 weeks

11.3 Evaluation of Placental Growth

11.3.1 Placental Thickness

The observation of an increase in placental thickness was attributed greater clinical significance in the early days of obstetric ultrasound than it is today. Holländer and Mast (1968) reported an upper normal limit of 4.5–4.7 cm after 34 weeks gestation. According to Schlensker (1976), placental thickness increases continuously, to an average maximum value of 3.6 ± 0.5 cm, until 36 weeks. Difficulties arise when one considers that the gray-scale equipment available at that time was generally incapable of resolving the exact boundary between the placenta and the uterine wall. The location of the placenta and the plane of the scan (oblique and tangential scans should be avoided) also contribute to errors of placental measurement. We share the opinion of Grannum and Hobbins (1983) that a placental thickness greater than 5 cm is not necessarily pathologic. The calculation of mean placental thickness from multiple cross-sectional images confirms the claim of Holländer and Schlensker that placental thickness increases up to 36 weeks. Clinical observation that placental thickness greater than 5 cm before 27 weeks in patients with Rh incompatibility indicates a poor prognosis still has validity today, although placental findings should always be evaluated in relation to find-

ings in the liver (hepatomegaly), skin (edema) and abdomen (ascites). The appearance of the placenta in nonimmunologic hydrops (Fig. 11.14) differs from the normal placenta in its greater echogenicity (see also Fig. 9.13). A thick placenta that shows accelerated maturation (see below) may be indicative of gestational diabetes, in which case a glucose tolerance test is advised (Grannum and Hobbins 1983). Thin, expanded placentas are most commonly seen in connection with polyhydramnios.

11.3.2 Placental Attachment Area, Surface Area, and Volume

In 1970 Hellmann et al. described a simple geometric model for the estimation of placental volume. On the basis of that model, it was concluded that placental volume continued to increase beyond term. However, longitudinal studies by Bleker et al. (1977) showed that placental volume frequently attains a maximum well before the end of pregnancy. In an attempt to clarify these contradictory reports, we investigated the following questions (Koslowski et al. 1980):

1. How does placental growth correlate with gestational age in the third trimester?

2. What is the relationship between placental growth and fetal size as determined by ultrasound?
3. What is the relationship between placental surface parameters (surface area, area of attachment) and placental volume?
4. Do these parameters correlate with placental function?
5. Do intrauterine measurements of placental size differ between normal and abnormal pregnancies?

The placenta was scanned and graphically recorded in a total of 285 examinations conducted in 171 pregnant women with anterior placentas. To avoid the errors of a geometric model, each placenta was examined with a series of longitudinal and transverse scans. The scanning planes were spaced 2 cm apart to ensure the imaging of peripheral areas. Knowing the spacing of the planes, it was possible to calculate the volume of the placenta from the areas of the individual sectional images. The examinations were performed with a Diasonograph NE 4102 compound scanner (Nuclear Enterprises, Edinburgh), which was calibrated in B-mode to a sound velocity of 1546 m/s corresponding to human soft tissue.

Volumetric analysis was done according to a fixed scheme. The individual sectional images were recorded on punched tape, and a computer program used to calculate values for the area of placental attachment, total placental surface area, and placental volume. Another programm was used to display the longitudinal and transverse images graphically in a three-dimensional coordinate system so that the images could be studied in their topographic context. The heavy lines in Fig. 11.15 represent the lines of uteroplacental attachment. Each display was accompanied by the fetal ultrasound parameters obtained during this examination.

The intraexaminer error was less than 5% for volume and area of placental attachment; the interexaminer error was 8.6% for volume and 4.4% for area of attachment.

In Fig. 11.16 the growth of placental volume is plotted against gestational age, with fitted curves representing the mean values and simple standard deviation. The normal population was comprised of pregnancies with known dates in which nondiabetic mothers were delivered of mature infants with a birth weight greater than

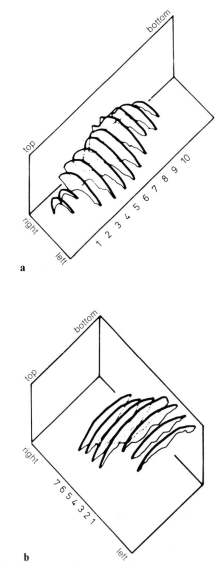

Fig. 11.15a, b. Biometry of placenta from a series of cross-sectional images, shown here in a three-dimensional coordinate system. **a** Transverse sections 1–10; **b** longitudinal sections 1–7. *Heavy line,* line of uteroplacental attachment

2,700 g. None of the three parameters exhibited further growth after 34 weeks gestation.

The individual values of two abnormal groups were plotted on a similar graph. Twenty-three volume measurements were performed in a group of ten pregnancies with maternal diabetes mellitus (B, C, or D White class). A second group comprised nine pregnancies in which fetal growth retardation was diagnosed prenatally and confirmed postpartum; 15 measurements were recorded for this group.

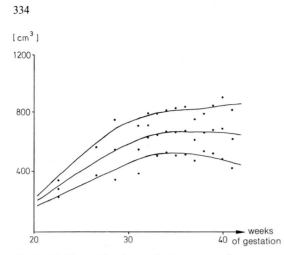

Fig. 11.16. Placental volumes during course of pregnancy: computer-fitted curve of mean values $+/-$ one standard deviation

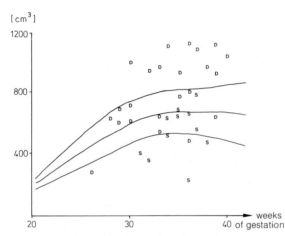

Fig. 11.17. Individual values of abnormal groups shown in relation to mean and SD placental volume curve. *D*, diabetes type B, C, or D; *S* growth-retarded fetuses (term newborn weighing less than 2,700 g)

Figure 11.17 shows the normal growth curve and individual measured values, with D indicating the diabetic group and S the group with an SGA fetus. The volumetric values for the diabetic group tend to lie above the mean for the normal population, while the values for the SGA group are below the mean in all cases but one. To obtain further information, we examined the ratio of placental volume to area of placental attachment. This ratio provides indirect information on the increase in placental thickness; its change during the course of pregnancy was determined in all three patient groups. The ratio is 1.9 between 20 and

24 weeks gestation and increases to 2.3 at 32nd weeks, with no further increase afterwards.

Analogous to the ratio of placental weight to birth weight obtained post partum, we calculated the ratio of the sonographically determined placental volume to the estimated weight of the fetus. Fetal weight was estimated from the biparietal diameter (BPD) and transverse trunk diameter (TTD), using the nomogram of Hansmann and Voigt (1973). The ratio decreases to 0.54 by 30 weeks, and after 40 weeks is only 0.21. Thus, placental growth in the third trimester decreases almost linearly in relation to fetal growth, with no growth after 34 weeks. There is little point in comparing intrauterine and postpartum measurements because the blood-filled intrauterine placenta is in no way comparable to the delivered placenta. The questions posed above can now be answered as follows:

1. The growth curves for placental volume, area of attachment, and surface area are similar. None of these parameters exhibits an increase beyond 34 weeks (Bleker et al. 1977). The results of Hellmann et al. (1970) were obtained in a cross-sectional study, which may account for the observation of continuous growth up to 40 weeks. Of course, the placental growth curves obtained post partum are also cross-sectional and therefore not applicable to the conditions in utero.

2. Individual measurements of placental volume show a greater variation than the area of placental attachment, indicating that the variations of placental volume for the same gestational age are based less on differences in area of attachment than on differences in placental thickness. The ratio of volume to area of attachment may be taken as an approximate measure of mean placental thickness, and it may well provide a means of diagnosing a placenta which is abnormally thick. Compared with the thickness curves of Holländer and Mast (1968) and Schlensker (1976), the ratio of volume to area of attachment usually became maximal 32 weeks rather than at 36 weeks.

3. The placentas of growth-retarded fetuses show smaller volumes and areas of attachment than the normal population. Most are below the mean and thus are generally smaller, although the difference was not statistically significant. The ratio of volume to area of attachment in these fetuses does not differ from controls.

4. On comparing the individual placental volumes and areas of attachment of diabetic mothers with the mean values of normal controls, the tendency toward greater volume in the diabetic pregnancies with virtually no increase in the area of attachment is apparent, indicating that the volume increase is mainly mediated by an increase of placental thickness. However, the size of individual placentas cannot be correlated with the function of the organ.

11.4 Ultrasound Structure of the Placenta

Kratochwil in 1975 and Schlensker in 1976 reviewed the relationship between placenta and uterine muscle, and identified the sonographically visible line of placental attachment as Nitabuch's layer.

The characteristic age-dependent changes in the placenta were first described by Winsberg (1973) in serial studies. The echo-free areas "lakes" that appear in the placenta after 28 weeks gestation can be identified in the freshly delivered placenta as blood-filled cavities devoid of villi. The higher-level echoes that appear in the placental substance during the final weeks of pregnancy are identified by X-rays and pathological investigation as calcium and fibrin deposits infiltrating the connective tissue septa of the lobules. Echo-free areas located immediately below the chorion are described as chorionic cysts.

On several occasions we have observed protrusions in the region of the chorionic plate (Figs. 11.18–11.20). We were able to demonstrate conspicuous flow phenomena within these echo-poor and sometimes loculated areas. Serial studies showed a subsequent collapse of the protrusions with a marked reduction in their size. These phenomena might represent hematomas, since in some cases they were associated with vaginal bleeding or elevated levels of amniotic fluid AFP. They should be differentiated from intraamniotic bands (Fig. 11.21).

Koslowski et al. (1980), in a prospective study, evaluated placental tissue by ultrasound. They sought to relate the nature and extent of tissue changes during pregnancy to the condition of the newborn infant. Five tissue features were each evaluated according to a 4-point scale:

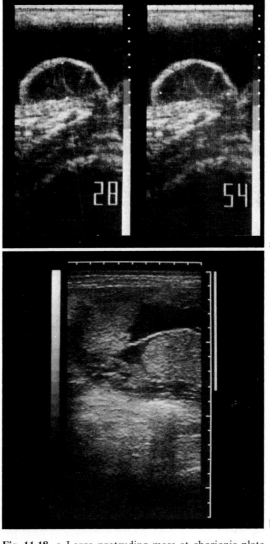

Fig. 11.18. a Large protruding mass at chorionic plate with sonographic evidence of flow phenomena, 27 weeks. **b** Same case 11 weeks later: mass has collapsed, a small, echo-free area is still visible at placental margin. No clinical symptoms occurred

Basal plate (uteroplacental attachment):
1. Visible but interrupted
2. Solid and thin
3. Solid and thick for up to 50% of its length
4. Solid and thick for 50%–100% of its length, with formation of arcade-like structures toward the fetal side

Peripheral zones:
1. Poorly defined
2. Thin and solid

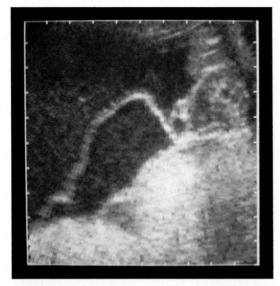

Fig. 11.19. Separation of amnion from chorionic plate with hematoma formation

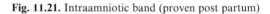

Fig. 11.21. Intraamniotic band (proven post partum)

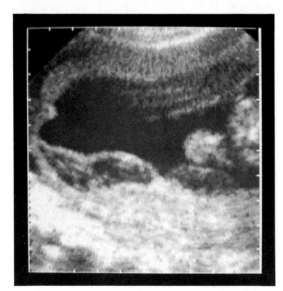

Fig. 11.20. Residual form of a hematoma originally similar to that shown in Fig. 11.19

3. Thickened on one side, echogenic
4. Thick and solid on both sides

Placental substance:
1. Finely homogeneous
2. Scattered streak-like echogenic areas up to 5 mm in length
3. Inhomogeneous with echogenic areas up to 1 cm in length

4. Scattered plate-like echogenic densities over 1 cm in diameter

Avillous spaces:
1. None
2. Limited
3. Extensive
4. Demarcated, echo-free, intraplacental areas surrounded by echogenic borders

Sinusoids (echofree areas just below the chorion):
1. None
2. Small
3. Extensive
4. Large and confluent

For clinical evaluation of these features, two groups of pregnancies were compared: (a) patients with a normal history and physical examination, a normal course of labor and delivery, and normal outcome, and (b) patients with complications in pregnancy, labor, or delivery involving fetal distress, operative delivery (for fetal indication), fetal growth retardation, and/or intrauterine fetal death. Of the five features that were scored, three – thickening of the peripheral zones, avillous spaces, and large sinusoids – showed no relevance to fetal outcome. A different picture emerged when placental substance and basal plate were analyzed. In cases

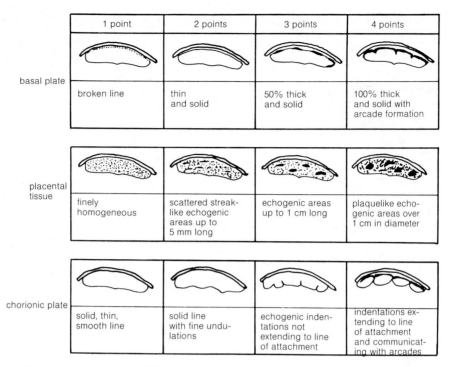

Fig. 11.22. Placental score. (After Koslowski et al. 1980)

Table 11.1. The Grannum scheme of placental grading. (After Grannum et al. 1979)

Region	Grade 0	Grade I	Grade II	Grade III
Basal layer	No densities	No densities	Linear arrangement of small echogenic areas (basal stippling)	Larger and partially confluent echogenic areas
Placental substance	Finely homogeneous	Few scattered echogenic areas	Linear echogenic densities (commalike densities)	Circular densities with central echopoor areas
Chorionic plate	Straight and well-defined	Subtle undulations	Early demarcation of cotyledons in the direction of the basal layer	Septation of cotyledons extending to the basal layer

where 75% or more of the scans of the placental tissue were judged to be grossly inhomogeneous and permeated by echogenic densities 1 cm or more in diameter, a statistically significant difference was apparent between the fetal outcomes of the two groups. The appearance of the basal plate showed a similar correlation with pregnancy outcome.

From these results we developed our own system for the evaluation of placental tissue (Fig. 11.22) in which a third feature, the chorionic plate, is added to the basal plate and placental substance.

Placental grading (0-III) by the method of Grannum et al. (1979) corresponds to our 4-point scoring system and is based on comparable sonographic features. Grannum (Table 11.1 and Figs. 11.23–11.26) suggested that the pulmonic maturity of the fetus as measured by the lecithin/sphingomyelin (L/S) ratio increases with placental grade. In the 86 cases he observed, he found that a grade I placenta was associated with an L/S ratio of 2.0 in 68%, grade II in 88%, and grade III in 100%. This finding was contradicted by Harman et al. (1982) in an extensive series. These authors

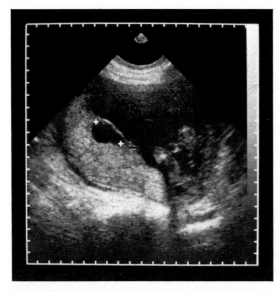

Fig. 11.23. Posterior placenta, Grannum grade 0, with echo-free cyst in region of basal plate. Associated finding: elevated amniotic fluid AFP with no apparent abnormality

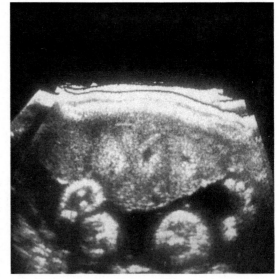

Fig. 11.25. Anterior placenta, Grannum grade II

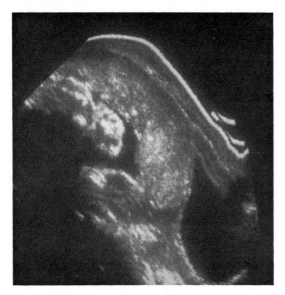

Fig. 11.24. Anterior placenta, Grannum grade I: placenta previa

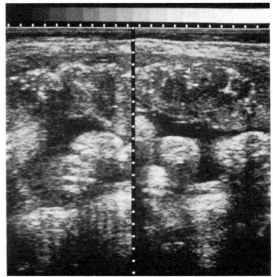

Fig. 11.26. Anterior placenta, Grannum grade III

found that a grade III placenta was associated with an immature L/S ratio in 7% of cases, and concluded from this that placental grading cannot replace amniocentesis as a standard technique for assessing pulmonic maturity. Without citing statistical data, Quinlan and Cruz (1982) confirm this observation. On the other hand, Petrucha et al. (1982) support the findings of Grannum. Clair et al. (1983) confirmed the Grannum scheme in high-risk pregnancies (e.g., diabetes) and found that a grade III placenta was indeed associated with fetal lung maturity, even if the L/S ratio indicated otherwise. In our opinion, it is not the purpose of placental grading to ascertain fetal age and maturity. Placental grading assumes clinical im-

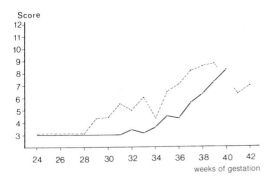

Fig. 11.27. Mean placental score during course of pregnancy in women smoking ten or more cigarettes per day (-----) and in nonsmokers (——)

portance only when interpreted on the basis of a known or established gestational age (initial examination). For example, we have found that the observation of a grade III placenta at 30 weeks gestation may be associated with subsequent fetal growth retardation, even though fetal biometry at this stage may indicate normal growth.

A major difficulty of previous studies on placental grading and fetal pulmonary maturity is based on a common error – the attempt to compare two different methods of assessing fetal pulmonic maturity. It should be pointed out that no method is 100% accurate in the prediction of lung maturity, and that it is entirely possible for respiratory distress syndrome to develop in a neonate with a grade III placenta.

Kazzi et al. (1983) used placental grading as a means of detecting intrauterine growth retardation. They report that the sensitivity of this screening method is 66%. Their results show that the sonographic demonstration of accelerated placental maturation in these fetuses correlates with the known anatomic phenomenon of premature ageing of the placenta. Thus, in cases where a small fetus is identified, placental grading may be helpful as an additional factor in the diagnosis of intrauterine growth retardation.

We conducted a prospective study in which placental scores were evaluated in relation to the risk factor of cigarette smoking during pregnancy. The group of smokers comprised 40 pregnant women who smoked 10 or more cigarettes per day and underwent a total of 85 ultrasound examinations. The control group

consisted of 44 pregnant nonsmokers who had 95 examinations. In Fig. 11.27 the mean values of the placental scores of both groups are plotted as a function of gestational age.

In the nonsmoking women, all placental features are very weakly expressed up to 30 weeks gestation, after which the scores increase to 7.3 (38 weeks) and 8.3 (39 weeks), with a mean score of 4.3 (35 weeks). In the smoking group, we observed a similar rise of placental scores (3.0 up to the 27 weeks, 4.3 at 28 weeks, and 7.1 at 35 weeks), but it begins about 4 weeks earlier than in the nonsmokers. The groups showed no significant differences with regard to pregnancy outcome.

So far, little research has been done on the anatomic causes of the sonographic changes in the placenta. Winsberg (1973) interpreted the appearance of "ring-like features" as a normal accompaniment of placental ageing. Hackelöer and Nitschke (1975) investigated 150 cases in which placental changes "garland echoes" were seen by ultrasound, but they were unable to establish a clinical relation on the basis of their material. Stein et al. (1976) detected radiologic microcalcifications in placentas described as having a "honeycomb" ultrasound pattern. Good agreement with sonograms was found in comparable sections. Our own observations confirm these findings (Fig. 11.28). Hoogland (1982) states that small calcium deposits on the basal plate and within the placental substance produce an increase in echogenicity. On the other hand, fibrin deposition can cause both an increase and a decrease of echogenicity. Because virtually no comparative studies have been done on the relationship of sonography and morphology, we must continue to rely on speculation when considering the possible causes of sonographic changes. Regarding the changes in the chorionic plate and placental substance, it is known that a slowing of blood flow in the intervillous space creates areas of turbulence and stasis which facilitate the deposition of fibrin thrombi, especially in the peripheral areas and subchorial space. This in turn promotes the occurrence of small, or, if fibrin deposition is extensive, large infarctions. The slowing of blood flow is initially manifested in a loss of echogenicity (Fig. 11.29). Fibrin deposits of macroscopic dimensions present as hyperechoic streaks, spots, or plaques in the sonogram of the placenta. The echogenic junction

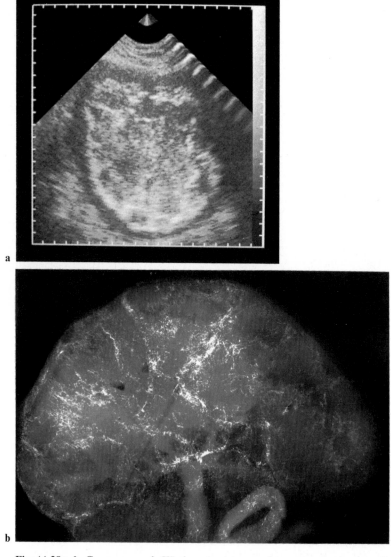

Fig. 11.28a, b. Grannum grade III placenta at term. **a** Sonogram; **b** corresponding radiograph showing microcalcifications

between uterus and placenta (basal plate) may well correspond to the trophoblastic shell, which normally becomes eroded toward the end of pregnancy and is replaced by a narrow fibrin layer.

Placental tumors such as chorioangiomas, hemangiomas, teratomas, and partial moles can usually be distinguished readily from normal placental tissue (Fig. 11.30). Depending on its homogeneity, the tumor may appear weakly echogenic and show encapsulation (chorioan-

gioma), or it may present as a mixed mass with multiple internal echoes caused by calcium deposition (teratoma). The typical "snowstorm" appearance of hydatidiform mole is easily differentiated from the tissue of the normal placenta.

The observation of sonographic placental changes provides a means of monitoring the intrauterine maturation of the placenta. An acceleration of placental maturation may be viewed as a pathologic sign if associated with

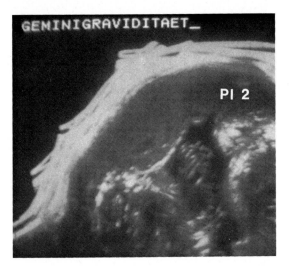

Fig. 11.29. Twin pregnancy with one dead fetus, whose unperfused placenta (*Pl 2*) is hypoechoic

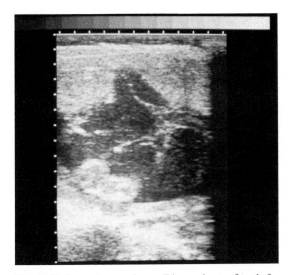

Fig. 11.30. Large hemangioma. Diagnosis at referral: fetal malformation, possibly omphalocele. Placental function was not impaired. Cesarean birth at 38 weeks

other pathologic findings and requires further studies.

References

Bleker OP, Kloosterman GJ, Breur W, Mieras DJ (1977) The volumetric growth of the human placenta: A longitudinal ultrasonic study. Am J Obstet Gynecol 127:657–661

Clair MR, Rosenberg E, Tempkin D, Andreotti RF, Bowie JD (1983) Placental grading in the complicated high-risk pregnancy. J Ultrasound Med 2:297

Fischer CC, Garrett W, Kossoff G (1976) Placental aging monitored by gray scale echography. Am J Obstet Gynecol 124:483–488

Gottesfeld KR, Thompson HE, Homes JH et al. (1966) Ultrasonic placentography – a new method for placental localization. Am J Obstet Gynecol 96:538

Grannum P, Hobbins JC (1983) The placenta. In: Callen PW (ed) Ultrasonography in obstetrics and gynecology. Saunders, Philadelphia, p 141–157

Grannum P, Berkowitz RI, Hobbins JC (1979) The ultrasonic changes in the maturing placenta and their relation to fetal pulmonic maturity. Am J Obstet Gynecol 133:915–922

Hackelöer BJ, Nitschke S (1975) Placental changes during pregnancy. V. European Congress on Ultrasound in Medicine, München

Hansmann M (1974) Kritische Bewertung der Leistungsfähigkeit der Ultraschalldiagnostik in der Geburtshilfe heute. Gynäkologe 7:26–39

Hansmann M, Voigt U (1973) Ultrasonic fetal thoracometry: an additional parameter for determing fetal growth. Excerpta Medica (Abstr), 2nd World Congress on Ultrasonics in Medicine, Rotterdam

Harman CR, Manning FA, Stearns E, Morrison I (1982) The correlation of ultrasonic placental grading and fetal pulmonary maturation in 563 pregnancies. Am J Obstet Gynecol 143:941–943

Hellmann LM, Koboyashi M, Tolles WE, Cromb E (1970) Ultrasonic studies on the volumetric growth of the human placenta. Am J Obstet Gynecol 108:740–745

Holländer HJ (1975) Ultraschalldiagnostik in der Schwangerschaft. Urban & Schwarzenberg, München Berlin Wien

Holländer HJ, Mast H (1968) Intrauterine Dickenmessungen der Plazenta mittels Ultraschall bei normalen Schwangerschaften und bei Rh-Inkompatibilität. Geburtshilfe Frauenheilkd 28:662–668

Hoogland HJ (1982) Ultrasonic placental morphology. Gynecol Obstet Invest 14:81–89

Kazzi GM, Gross TL, Sokol RJ, Kazzi NH (1983) Detection of intrauterine growth retardation: A new use for sonographic placental grading. Am J Obstet Gynecol 145:733–737

Koslowski P, Terinde R, Schmidt H (1980) Bestimmung des Plazentawachstums aus Ultraschallschnittbildern. Ultraschall 1:116–132

Kratochwil A (1975) The state of ultrasound diagnosis in perinatal medicine. J Perinat Med 3:75

Kurjak A, Barsic B (1977) Changes of placental site diagnosed by repeated ultrasonic examination. Acta Obstet Gynecol Scand 56:161–165

Petrucha RA, Golde SH, Platt LD (1982) Real-time ultrasound of the placenta in assessment of fetal pulmonic maturity. Am J Obstet Gynecol 142:463–467

Quinlan R, Cruz A (1982) Ultrasonic placental grading and fetal pulmonary maturity. Am J Obstet Gynecol 142:110

Schlensker KH (1976) Ultraschallplazentographie. Gynäkologe 9:156–165

Stein WW, Krämer A, Halberstadt E (1976) Mikrokalzifikation der Plazenta. In: Haller U (ed) Ultraschalldiagnostik. Thieme, Stuttgart, New York, S 51

Winsberg F (1973) Echographic changes with placental aging. J Clin Ultrasound 1:52

12 The Cervix

In contrast to the diagnosis of cervical carcinoma (Sect. 16.2), where ultrasound has not demonstrated significant value, sonography plays an important role in monitoring the progress of abortion or labor, evaluating cervical incompetence, selecting patients for surgical correction, and evaluating the correction (Ulbrich 1982; Zemlyn 1981; Bernstine et al. 1981; McGahan et al. 1981; Sarti et al. 1979).

Data on the prevalence of true cervical in-

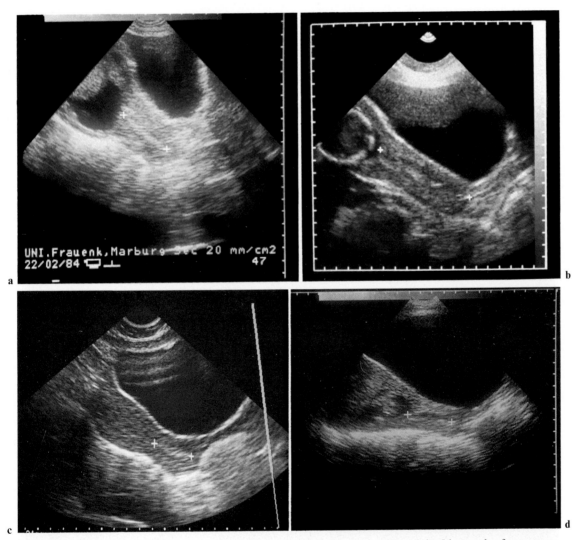

Fig. 12.1. a Normal cervix (47 mm) early in 3rd trimester. **b** Long cervix (84 mm) in 5th month of pregnancy. **c** Cervix (31 mm) of normal nonpregnant uterus: homogeneous echogenic structure. **d** Pregnant uterus: together with cervix, hyporeflective cervical canal is visible

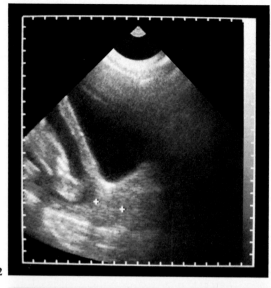

12.2

Fig. 12.2. Shortened cervix (22 mm) with formation of a funnel, 28 weeks

Fig. 12.3a, b. Vaginal examination was unremarkable: cervical incompetence was detected incidentally at 13 weeks. **a** Prolapsed membranes in cervical canal. **b** Protrusion of fetal head into funnel 30 min later. Fetus aborted 2 days later

Fig. 12.4. Longitudinal (*left*) and transverse (*right*) scans: early dilatation of cervical canal, with membranes at external cervical os (confirmed by speculum examination). U, uterus; E.C., cervical canal; C, cervix; V, vagina; B, bladder

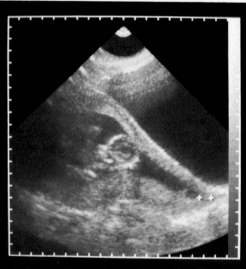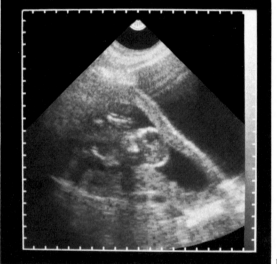

12.3 a   b

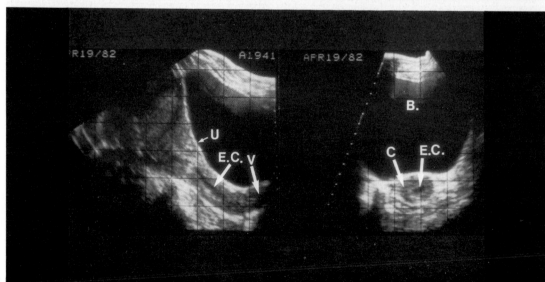

12.4

competence vary greatly. The most probable incidence is approximately 1 in 1,000 pregnancies. To diagnosis this condition, it is necessary to demonstrate the cervix (Fig. 12.1) and document cervical shortening (Fig. 12.2). In our experience the cervical length should be at least 3 cm. Serial measurements are more informative than a single examination. It should be recognized that the degree of bladder filling may influence this measurement. It is also important both diagnostically and therapeutically to assess the gestational sac. Ultrasound can provide evidence of cervical incompetence earlier than vaginal examination (Fig. 12.2), and may even help in predicting the future course of the pregnancy (Fig. 12.3a, b).

The advantage of this is that the indication for cerclage is then not based solely on history and the personal impression gained from vaginal examination, but on somewhat more objective and complex criteria.

With ultrasound, even subtle dilatation of the cervical canal can be demonstrated (Fig. 12.4), and the placement of the cerclage can be checked (Fig. 12.5). With an unsuccessful cerclage, the progress of the abortive process can be monitored (Fig. 12.6), and prompt clinical management initiated. This process may culminate in prolapse of the membranes (Fig. 12.6b), in which case ultrasound permits early observation of the protrusion into the cervical canal (Fig. 12.3a) and the vagina (Fig. 12.6b).

Patients who have had previous uterine surgery, such as cesarean birth, may manifest special problems. In the case shown in Fig. 12.7, the cervix of the patient having uterine contractions appears closed (a), but there is scar contracture of the uterine wall (b) secondary to a prior cesarean birth and ballooning of the lower uterine segment, a situation which cannot be appreciated by digital palpation.

Thus, sonographic evaluation of the cervix has become a valuable technique, especially in

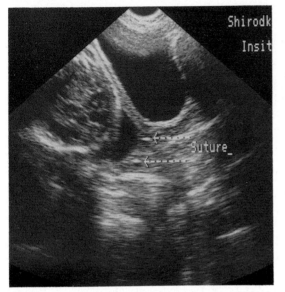

Fig. 12.5. Longitudinal scan of cervical cerclage (Shirodkar technique)

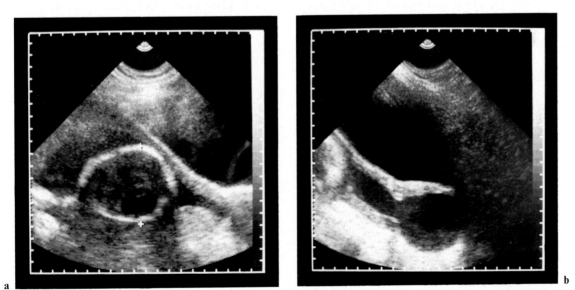

Fig. 12.6. a Dilated cervical canal with cerclage in place at 25 weeks. **b** Same case 30 min later: membranes prolapsing into vagina (hourglass herniation)

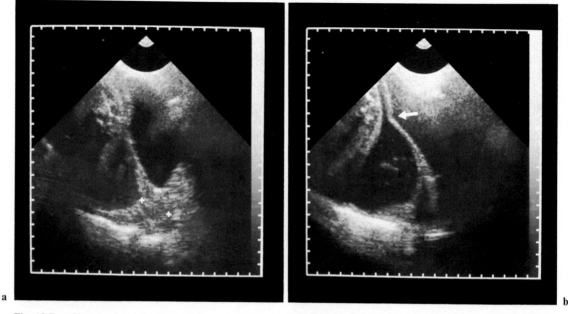

Fig. 12.7. a Shortened cervix (24 mm) in a patient with previous cesarean birth. **b** Marked retraction of uterine wall in region of scar

high-risk pregnancies. It enables more accurate selection of candidates for surgical correction and provides a means of distinguishing nonprogressive shortening of the cervix from true progressive cases through serial observations.

References

Bernstine RL, Lee Sh, Crawford WL et al. (1981) Sonographic evaluation of the incompetent cervix. J Clin Ultrasound 9:417–420

McGahan JP, Philips HE, Bowen MS (1981) Prolapse of the amniotic sac ("hourglass membranes"): Ultrasound appearance. Radiology 140:463–466

Sarti DA, Sample WF, Hobel CJ et al. (1979) Ultrasonic visualization of a dilated cervix during pregnancy. Radiology 130:417–420

Ulbrich R (1982) Ein neues Verfahren zur Beurteilung der Zervix bei Cerclageoperationen. In: Kratochwil A, Reinold E (eds) Ultraschalldiagnostik 81. Thieme, Stuttgart New York

Zemlyn S (1981) The length of the uterine cervix and its significance. J Clin Ultrasound 9:267

13 Postpartum Ultrasound

Increasingly, indications are arising for the use of diagnostic ultrasound in the puerperium, mainly in relation to the uterus, the upper abdomen (gallstones), and the kidneys (hydronephrosis). In the uterus, typical features of involution can be recognized (Fig. 13.1), and retained placental tissue or blood clots can be demonstrated (Figs. 13.2, 13.3). Because the uterus normally remains enlarged for 4–8 weeks post partum, a full bladder is not always necessary for the examination. The ultrasound examination is relatively simple and brief and, in our opinion, is used far too seldom.

The uterine muscle is markedly hypertrophic and thus easily visualized. The endometrium is usually visible as a central line (Fig. 13.1), but the presence of small blood clots may be normal during the first 1–3 days. Marked distension of the uterine cavity may indicate lochial retention (Fig. 13.2). This condition can usually be managed conservatively with oxytocic agents; curettage is usually not necessary.

The situation is different when scans reveal irregular, high-level echoes and no regular endometrial line or normal cavity echo is demonstrated (Fig. 13.3a, b). This signifies retained products of conception, and is an indication for evacuation of the uterus.

Frequently, scarring of the anterior uterine wall can be demonstrated following a cesarean birth (cf. Fig. 12.7), and retained placental tissue may be adherent on these sites.

It is clear that the demonstration of small placental polyps may not always be possible several weeks after delivery. However, retained products of conception are relatively easy to identify, even following an incomplete abortion, because their echo pattern differs so markedly from that of the myometrium (Fig. 13.4; see also Fig. 11.13).

Robinson (1972) and Malvern et al. (1973) had differing results when they compared abnormal ultrasound scans with histologic findings. Thus, we can say only that a sonographi-

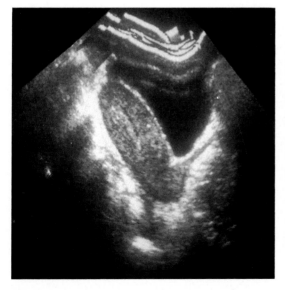

Fig. 13.1. Normal involution, 4th postpartum day

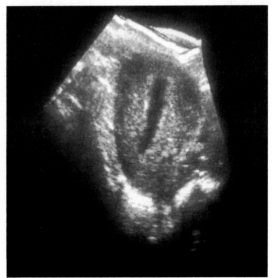

Fig. 13.2. Lochial retention: fluid in uterine cavity

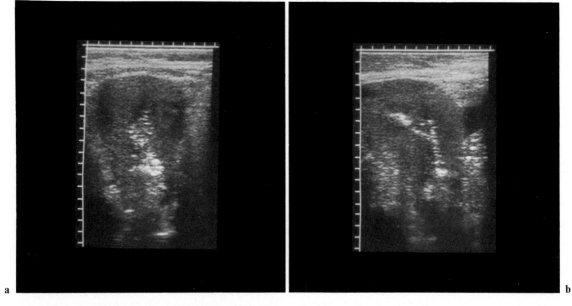

Fig. 13.3a, b. Residual placental tissue (hyperechoic) within uterus

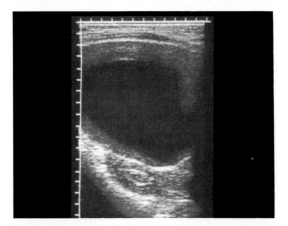

Fig. 13.4. Small postabortal uterus with retained products of conception (hyperechoic)

cally "empty" uterus indicates with *virtual* certainty that no retained products of conception are present.

References

Malvern J, Cambell S, May P (1973) Ultrasonic sanning of the puerperal uterus following secondary postpartum haemorrhage. Br J Obstet Gynecol 80:320

Robinson HP (1972a) Sonar in the management of abortion. J Obstet Gynecol Br Commonw 79:90

Robinson HP (1972b) Sonar in the puerperium. Scott Med J

Sanders RC (1980) Post-partum diagnostic ultrasound. In: Sanders RC, James E (eds) Ultrasonography in obstetrics and gynecology, 2nd edn. Appleton-Century-Crofts Medical, New York, p 311 ff

14 Ultrasound Screening

The revised Prenatal Care Guidelines of the Federal Republic of Germany, issued on 31 October, 1979, call for two ultrasound examinations for the screening of pregnant women on a nationwide basis. With this strategy, a significant step has been taken in the right direction. Some critics feel it might still have been too early to institute such a program. While there is no question that the necessary equipment is already on the market and available in quantities sufficient to screen 600,000 pregnancies per year in the FRG, there is less confidence concerning the competence of physicians in regard to diagnostic ultrasound. Even today, physicians often enter practice as "self-taught" individuals with no specialized training in ultrasound. On the one hand, the Polaroid pictures that are given to pregnant women by their doctors bear witness to the questionable quality of the sonograms being produced. On the other hand, the media present carefully selected images obtained by ultrasound professionals with highly sophisticated equipment at great cost in terms of both time and money. In the middle is the patient, wondering whether her doctor has really made sure that "everything is there," and if so, why his "best" picture shows so little evidence of it.

A dilemma exists in many respects. The guidelines describe the responsibilities of the physician only in general terms: "Two ultrasound examinations shall be performed to evaluate the pregnancy (development of the pregnancy, intrauterine location of the pregnancy, blighted ovum, fetal head, presentation, number of fetuses, placental localization, etc.). If possible, these examinations shall be done between 16 and 20 weeks and between 32 and 36 weeks gestation. Indications for further ultrasound examinations are accepted only as specified in Section B4a."

Section B4a contains the currently approved list of such indications (Appendix to 1979 Prenatal Care Guidelines):

A. *First trimester*
1. Suspicion of abnormal intrauterine pregnancy (e.g., presence of IUCD, uterine fibroids, adnexal mass, bleeding)
2. Strong suspicion of ectopic pregnancy
3. Discrepancy between uterine size and gestational age
4. Accidents, injuries, and poisoning that may jeopardize the pregnancy

---

B. *Second trimester*
5. As a necessary adjunct to other diagnostic procedures (e.g., amniocentesis)
6. Suspicion of intrauterine fetal death

C. *Third trimester*
7. Rh incompatibility (evaluation of placenta)
8. Suspicion of intrauterine growth retardation (e.g., hypertension)
9. Suspicion of hydramnios
10. Diabetes mellitus
11. Premature labor, cervical incompetence
12. Abnormal fetal presentation (only after completion of second routine examination)

D. *Any stage of pregnancy*
13. Antepartum hemorrhage

The exact manner in which the examinations are to be conducted has never been described in detail. In our view, the formidable problem of effective antenatal screening can be solved only within the framework of a multistage concept.

14.1 The Multistage Concept

The multistage concept recognizes the different levels of skill and training and provides for a division of responsibility in three stages, from the physician in the office to the highly trained specialist in the hospital (Hansmann 1981a), as described below.

Stage I. Stage I encompasses the screening of all pregnancies. The screening examination should be kept simple and brief, due in part to limitations of equipment and personnel. The basic instrument for Stage I examinations is the real-time scanner with a frequency range of 3–5 MHz, an acceptable gray-scale range (16), and an adequate image width (at least 10 cm at a depth of 6 cm). The examiner at Stage I is expected to know the ultrasound anatomy of the normal pregnancy and the basics of fetal biometry.

The minimum requirements for a Stage I examination are:

1. Detection of fetal life, with evaluation of fetal cardiac activity (rhythm and rate)
2. Confirmation or exclusion of multiple gestation
3. Complete evaluation of the fetus in longitudinal scans (only in first screening),
4. Measurement of biparietal diameter
5. Measurement of a cross-section of the trunk in a defined plane (e.g., transverse or anteroposterior at the level of the ductus venosus)
6. Placental localization (tentative on first screening, definitive on second screening)
7. Classification of amniotic fluid volume in three categories:
   a) present in "average volume"
   b) present in "decreased volume" or is "almost completely absent"
   c) present in "increased volume" [a second fetus would fit within the uterus = Holländer's definition of polyhydramnios (1972)]
8. Recognition of other obvious signs suggestive of a fetal malformation or disease (see list below).

Signs Suggestive of the Presence of a Fetal Malformation

- An- or oligohydramnios on 1st screening
- An-, oligo- or polyhydramnios at any time during pregnancy
- "Early" growth retardation with confirmed gestational age (e.g., BBT, pregnancy test, ultrasound)
- Anomalies of body contour (e.g., head cannot be delineated as an oval)
- Structural anomalies in the fetus or its organs (e.g., cysts, effusions)
- Abnormal relationship between individual parts or dimensions of the body
- Abnormal pattern of fetal activity (e.g., immobile, excessive)

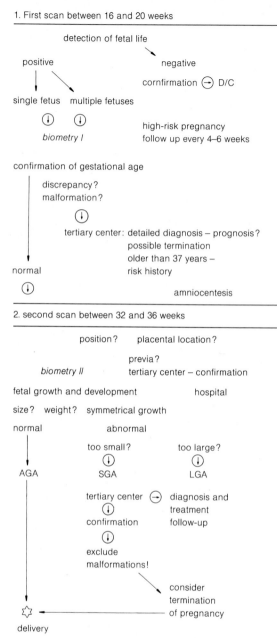

Fig. 14.1. Flowcharts for ultrasound screening

If abnormalities are noted or if the information anticipated from the examination cannot satisfactorily be obtained, a follow-up examination should be scheduled at once (not 4 weeks later) and should follow the Stage II protocol (Fig. 14.1).

Stage II. The Stage II ultrasound examination imposes greater demands on examiner and apparatus. Generally it should be conducted in a hospital setting. The examiner should have several years' experience in this area of diagnostic ultrasound, and at least two types of imaging system (e.g., a linear and a sector scanner) should be available, in addition to equipment for video documentation. The examiner must be familiar with the principal features of pathologic anatomy of the fetal organs (Hansmann 1981 a, b).

Biometric analyses at this stage may include measurements of circumference, area, and volume in addition to simple diameters.

The facilities for Stage II examinations can only be organized on a regional level. Physicians are usually well aware which site will offer the best facilities.

Stage III. Stage III usually deals with problems not resolved in Stages I and II and also performs certain specialized functions. These include the specific exclusion of rare disorders in high-risk pregnancies. It is important to recognize that experience with rare anomalies (incidence of 1 in 5,000 to 1 in 50,000) can only accumulate in these centers through the concentration of these abnormal cases by selective referral from the large pool of all pregnancies. Genetic institutes and counseling centers play a key role in this process. They know the individuals who are at risk for autosomal recessive disorders such as osteogenesis imperfecta, Potter type I cystic kidneys, and various forms of dwarfism, some of which have widely varying prognoses. In our experience the offer of a diagnostic service to these groups has an effect comparable to the offer of prenatal diagnosis in the area of cytogenetics: It fosters the motivation to accept a planned or existing pregnancy.

Other important tasks of Stage III centers include interdisciplinary collaboration in the conduct of rational intrauterine therapy and the assurance of adequate postnatal care for newborns with malformations or diseases. Finally, Stage III centers should be active in research for the advancement of knowledge in all related fields.

14.2 Ultrasound Anatomy

The clear depiction of anatomic details is the basis of all ultrasound diagnosis. Besides delineating the outline of the fetal body, modern ultrasound can provide detailed images of internal fetal organs. These images form the basis for plane selection in all areas of biometry and are the key to diagnosing fetal malformations. Basically, every ultrasound examination should begin with a careful inspection of the general fetal anatomy before specific measurements are sought. Even a general survey can yield important information regarding amniotic fluid volume and fetal position, number, appearance, and viability. If these findings are normal, the routine imaging of standard planes (BPD and transverse abdomen in Stage I) may commence. Stage II and III examinations include additional detailed anatomic and biometric evaluation. In the head area, for example, these examinations would focus on head shape, head size (with an estimation of head circumference), and the evaluation of intracranial structures including the cerebral ventricles. For the specialist, profile and frontal views of the face can provide important clues to underlying fetal pathology (see Chap. 10).

In the skeletal system, echogenicity and proportions can be used diagnostically. Special attention is given to the spine, as well as to the shape and length of the diaphyses of all the long bones. Even the number of fingers and toes, their position, and their mobility can be evaluated with ultrasound. However, these studies are justified only in the evaluation of pregnancies at risk (e.g., for Ellis-van Crefeld or Meckel-Gruber syndrome), or if there is the suggestion of anomalies.

In the region of the trunk, the diagnosis of effusions (peritoneal, pleural, or pericardial) is of clinical significance. The search for foreign contents in the thorax (e.g., stomach, bowel, or liver herniating through a diaphragmatic defect) is a service of the Stage III center.

A major organ of interest is the fetal heart. Its position, size, and shape can be accurately assessed by the 18th week of pregnancy. The basic plane for evaluating the fetal heart is the standard four-chamber view. If this cannot be obtained, a more detailed examination should be done at a Stage III center with appropriate subspecialization (i.e., one having the services of a pediatric cardiologist). This examination includes evaluation of the septa, the foramen ovale, the great vessels, and the valves. Doppler flow measurements supplement the examination.

Indications for a prenatal echocardiographic examination are risk factors in family history and evidence on screening of congenital heart disease such as hydrops (ascites, skin edema, thick placenta), cardiomegaly, or dysrhythmias.

14.3 Diagnosis of Fetal Malformations

The timing, specificity, and reliability of diagnosis are the essential criteria for the detection of fetal malformations, which has become an important secondary aspect of screening and a major focus of interest since screening was introduced. The most important sign suggestive of a malformation is an abnormal amniotic fluid volume. Thus, the inability to detect free amniotic fluid on initial screening at 19 weeks is highly indicative of pathology (Hansmann 1981a). The most common cause of anhydramnios is decreased fetal urine excretion secondary to a urogenital tract anomaly (e.g., Potter's syndrome, prune-belly syndrome), although a severe disturbance of placental maturation or chromosome abnormality (e.g., triploidy) may also be causative. Because the absence of amniotic fluid seriously hampers analysis of organ structures and functional dynamics, referral of the patient to a center is urgently indicated. The presence of polyhydramnios is equally relevant.

So far (1985) approximately 50% of cases referred to the authors with suspicion of a fetal malformation have proved to be negative. Of the remaining 50% with positive findings, half were found to have disorders that contradicted the diagnosis at referral. There is no question that this is a "dangerous" situation for the affected fetuses. There are many examples of misdiagnoses involving urogenital tract disease. In some cases, outflow obstructions with a relatively favorable prognosis (e.g., urethral valves with hydronephrosis and hydroureters) have been misinterpreted as cystic kidneys, while in other cases prognostically grave Potter type I cystic kidneys have gone undetected. Finally, we have seen several cases where a cystic, dysplastic kidney was correctly diagnosed, but the presence of a healthy contralateral kidney was overlooked. These examples underscore the importance of checking the relevance of a suspicious finding before expressing a presumptive diagnosis that may cause needless parental distress.

Increasingly, the diagnosis of a fetal malformation is raising therapeutic options that go well beyond elective abortion. The experience of recent years indicates that more fetuses can be salvaged than is generally supposed. Intrauterine therapy should be considered in all cases where it might be successful, such as fetal heart disease, urinary tract obstructions, and many other disorders.

When intrauterine therapy is not possible but a viable fetus is present, an accurate diagnosis will decide the course of further management. It improves the newborn's chances by enabling the selection of a suitable timing and mode of delivery and allowing preparations for appropriate postnatal care by specialists (neurosurgeon, pediatric surgeon, pediatric cardiologist). This should improve the infant's chances not only in terms of survival, but also in terms of sequelae and the quality of life in general.

14.4 Determination of Gestational Age, Growth Monitoring, and Weight Assessment

The previous discussion of ultrasound screening in pregnancy may have created the impression that screening primarily involves the exclusion of fetal malformations. This is by no means the case. The main intent of the first screening is to establish gestational age. This leads to significant corrections in 15%–20% of cases. The main aim of the second screening is the assessment of fetal growth, i.e., the detection of intrauterine growth retardation. The latter requires accurate knowledge of gestational age.

14.4.1 Gestational Age

If dates are unclear on the basis of history and clinical findings, gestational age should be established as early as possible by ultrasound. This need not be done within the period specified for the first screening; the German guidelines provide for earlier first-trimester examinations where special indications exist.

The period between 9 and 13 weeks of menstrual age is the most advantageous for estimating gestational age. The crown-rump length can generally be measured without difficulty at this time. Measurements of head and trunk diameters and femur length are possible alternatives in most cases. These parameters should provide an estimate of gestational age accurate enough to serve as a basis for the second screening between 31 and 35 weeks.

14.4.2 Growth Monitoring and Weight Assessment

In the second screening, fetal biometric evaluation is performed to assess the quality of somatic development. Data are compared with standard growth charts in which time (gestational age) is an independent variable on the x axis. The parameters most commonly measured are the biparietal diameter and the transverse trunk diameter at the level of the ductus venosus. The most important anatomic landmark is the umbilical vein. The circumference or area of this structure may also be measured as an alternative. The inclusion of trunk size has led to a marked improvement in the diagnosis of fetal growth disturbances (e.g., retardation from placental insufficiency or macrosomia in maternal diabetes). The accuracy rate in the detection of intrauterine growth retardation has increased from 60% to 90% through the use of fetal trunk measurements (Hansmann 1983).

References

Grennert L, Persson PH, Gennser G (1978) Benefits of ultrasonic screening of a pregnant population. Acta Obstet Gynecol Scand [Suppl] 78:5–14

Hackeloer B-J (1981) Die Rolle der Ultraschalldiagnostik bei der Erkennung fetaler Gefahrenzustände. Z Geburtshilfe Perinat 183:73–80

Hansmann M (1981a) Ultraschallscreening in der Schwangerschaft – Vorsicht vor übertriebenen Forderungen. Geburtshilfe Frauenheilkd 41:725–728

Hansmann M (1981b) Nachweis und Ausschluß fetaler Entwicklungsstörungen mittels Ultraschallscreening und gezielter Untersuchung – ein Mehrstufenkonzept. Ultraschall 2:206–220

Hansmann M (1982) Bestimmung des Gestationsalters und -gewichtes mittels Ultraschall unter Berücksichtigung seiner Bedeutung für das klinische Management. In: Huch A, Huch R, Doc G, Rooth G (eds) Klinisches Management des „kleinen" Frühgeborenen (1 500 g). Thieme, Stuttgart New York, S 31–54

Hansmann M (1983) Die Wertigkeit der Ultraschalldiagnose. Ultraschallscreening eine zuverlässige Methode? Arch Gynecol 235:522–534

14.5 Patterns of Fetal Activity and Their Relevance for the Assessment of Fetal Wellbeing

B.K. WITTMANN and A.G. ROSS

The introduction of real-time ultrasound (RTUS) into obstetrics has revolutionized our understanding of the fetus and its behavioral patterns. Based on the premise that a decrease or absence of fetal activity reflects fetal compromise, research in animals and humans was initiated in an attempt to unveil the secrets of fetal behavior. In the late 1960s Holländer (1979) and Reinold (1979) were the first to engage in dynamic evaluation of the fetus in the early second trimester (Vidoson, Siemens), and to show correlation between abnormal movement patterns and impending death. Since then rapid progress in electronics and computer technology has provided us with sophisticated ultrasound equipment of superior resolution. We can now observe generalized movements in the early embryo (7 weeks gestation), follow fetal developmental differentiation into detailed extremity movements (from 10 weeks on), breathing, yawning, sucking, swallowing, hiccoughs, and bladder emptying (de Vries et al. 1982). These various expressions of fetal activity appear to occur throughout the second trimester at random; however, toward the end of pregnancy they show coordination and organization into behavioral states. Some of these patterns of activity were suggested as tests for the recognition of the compromised fetus, and were enthusiastically introduced into obstetric practice without the benefit of basic research and controlled clinical evaluation. Critical review of the literature indicates that at present only fetal body and extremity movements, breathing, and possibly hiccoughs may be of any clinical importance. Understanding of the variability of these patterns throughout pregnancy in healthy subjects is required before they can be applied to the fetus at risk.

14.5.1 Patterns of Fetal Activity in Normal Pregnancy

Body and Extremity Movements. Fetal movements have been recorded as gross movements or movement episodes and as isolated movements. Observation of isolated movements over 1 h (20–42 weeks gestation) clearly shows that the normal fetus is very active, with 120 movements/h (mean) at 20 weeks. Over the next few weeks the number of movements per hour decreases to 80, and remains between 60 and 80 in the third trimester. With the beginning of labor, the number of movements decreases further to 40/h, and a strong association ($p < 0.001$) between movements, fetal heart rate accelerations, and contractions was noted (Wittmann et al. 1979).

Patrick et al. (1982) evaluated the physiological background of fetal activity in continuous 24-h studies by recording gross fetal movements. He noted the presence of movements for about 10% of the time, and a circadian rhythm with a significant increase between 22:00 and 02:00. The number of gross movements was not affected by meals, glucose, or alcohol.

Breathing Movements. Fetal breathing can be recognized without difficulty and with considerable accuracy with RTUS (Wittmann et al. 1981). In the second trimester it can be seen for 5 to 17% of the observation time (Wittmann and Brown 1982; Natale et al. 1983). After 28 weeks the incidence of breathing increases to approximately 30% of the time (Patrick 1980a, b), and it becomes episodic and more regular in amplitude and frequency. In labor, fetal breathing is rarely seen (Richardson et al. 1979; Wittmann et al. 1979). In the healthy fetus, episodes without any breathing of up to 2 h occur, and an increase in the incidence is seen with glucose and after meals. Nicotine and drugs have a variable effect on the incidence of breathing.

Hiccoughs. From 12 weeks on, abrupt thoracic and abdominal movements simulating hiccoughs can be observed in the human fetus. These movements, together with body and breathing movements occur in episodes lasting from 1 to 25 min and are repeated up to six times per 24 h (Patrick et al. 1980b; Wittmann et al. 1983a). Since enlargement of the fetal stomach has been observed in association with these movements, it is likely that they are related to swallowing.

Fetal Behavioral States. Research in human fetuses indicates that after 30 weeks gestation fetal movements and breathing become coordinated and occur in episodes lasting 20–60 min. These specific behavioral patterns are comparable to those seen in newborns (Campbell 1980). By synchronous observation of eye, body, and breathing movements and fetal heart rate with two RTUS units and a cardiotocograph, Awoust and Levi (1984) found specific patterns of behavior already at 30 weeks, while Nijhuis (1982) noticed no defined patterns before 36 weeks.

14.5.2 Patterns of Fetal Activity in Complicated Pregnancy

Maternal Observation of Fetal Activity. In spite of the availability of a variety of biochemical and biophysical tests for the recognition of fetal compromise, the time-honored evaluation of fetal movements by the mother continues to play a prominent role in prenatal care. Although it is not at all clear how much an individual fetus should move, there is general agreement that a decrease or absence of fetal movements may indicate compromise (Mathews 1973; Sadovsky and Yaffe 1973). In an attempt to quantify the maternal assessment of fetal activity, Sadovsky and Yaffe recommended the maternal recording of fetal movements for 30–60 min in the supine position, three times a day. Should the mother record less than three movements in 1 h, then continuous recording for 6–12 h should be performed. The number of recorded movements in different fetuses has a wide range; however, in individual fetuses it should remain constant. A definite decrease or cessation for 1 day is considered an "alarm signal," and delivery should be contemplated.

We tested the accuracy of maternal perception of *single* movements against RTUS observation, and found poor correlation. However, a significant correlation between maternal and RTUS recording was seen when *episodes* of movements were used instead of single movements (Wittmann et al. 1983b). It is our impression that the counting of episodes of fetal movements is easier for the mother and will improve compliance.

RTUS Observation of Fetal Activity. *Body Movements.* Observation of fetal body and extremity movements by RTUS in complicated pregnancy has shown that independant of maternal complications the number of movements remains in the normal range as long as the fetus itself is not compromised. Roberts et al. (1980) showed this in women with diabetes, and Wittmann and Brown (1982) in women with a multitude of other complications (hypertension, diabetes, growth retardation without asphyxia, hemorrhage, preterm labor, preterm rupture of membranes). If however, the fetus suffers severe asphyxia or acute infection, few if any movements are noted. Movement patterns in fetuses with severe abnormalities may be abnormal in number and character, and long periods without any movements have been noted. If we consider the episodic nature of fetal behavioral patterns and observe the fetus over sufficiently long periods of time, then RTUS counting of single movements or movement episodes should provide us with a test for fetal wellbeing. However, further research in patients with complicated pregnancies is required to confirm these findings.

Breathing Movements. Animal research has shown that in fetuses with severe asphyxia, apnea, abnormal breathing movements, and gasps occur, while the results of mild asphyxia are less obvious (Towell and Salvador 1974). Extrapolation to the human fetus was attempted by Boddy (1975), who was the first to use ultrasound (A-mode) for the evaluation of fetal breathing, and to correlate the findings with the fetal state. Unfortunately, the artifacts inherent in this technique prevented collection of reliable data. With the advent of RTUS an accurate tool for the evaluation of fetal breathing became available and was widely used for clinical research in complicated pregnancies. Initial enthusiasm has been replaced by a more critical assessment of the value of breathing as a test for fetal wellbeing. Although the presence of breathing probably indicates a healthy fetus, its absence has little clinical significance in view of the low incidence of breathing in the second trimester and the long episodes of apnea (up to 120 min) at any time in pregnancy (Patrick 1982).

Combinations of Patterns of Fetal Activity
When it was recognized that it is extremely difficult to evaluate fetal wellbeing from fetal breathing or fetal movements alone, more emphasis was placed on research directed toward the overall evaluation of fetal activity patterns.

Manning et al. (1980) developed a biophysical profile where five different tests are performed and evaluated on a scale from 0 (abnormal) to 2 (normal). The maximum score of 10 can be achieved when the following criteria are fulfilled:

Fetal breathing movements:	An episode of 30 s uninterrupted breathing in a 30-min observation period
Fetal movements:	Minimum of three movement episodes in 30 min
Tone:	A minimum of one rapid flexion/extension movement of one extremity
Cardiotocography:	At least two fetal heart rate accelerations in 40 min
Qualitative evaluation of amniotic fluid:	An amniotic fluid pocket with diameter at least 2 cm

If the score is between 8 and 10, then the test is considered normal and repeated in 3–6 days. A score of 7 or less is considered abnormal, and either the study is repeated within 24 h or delivery is considered.

In a large prospective study involving patients with complicated pregnancies, a significant decrease in perinatal mortality was achieved. In addition, in some of these patients previously unrecognized fetal abnormalities were diagnosed.

Our own research also shows that no single type of fetal activity can be used in isolation as a reliable test for the evaluation of fetal wellbeing. For this reaseon, we evaluated not only the overall fetal activity patterns, but also the duration of episodes without any movements at all. We found in fetuses with severe abnormalities that frequently no breathing was noted, the number of movements was decreased, and episodes without any movements often extended beyond 10 min.

From these data we felt that optimal surveillance of the fetus should include, in addition to the well-established cardiotocography, maternal and ultrasound observation of fetal activity, with emphasis on total activity patterns and length of episodes without any activity. Future research is necessary to further define fetal activity patterns and the changes related to fetal compromise. Van Vliet et al. (1984) used eye movements, body movements, and cardiotocography to observe states of fetal behavior in patients with intrauterine growth retardation. In comparison with normal fetuses, they found that although the patterns of behavior were disturbed, acceleration in the maturation of these behavioral processes was not observed.

14.5.3 Summary

With ongoing pregnancy the maturation of the central nervous system is reflected by the increased coordination of patterns of fetal movement and behavior. These states of behavior become more apparent in the last weeks of pregnancy, can be recognized in labor (Griffin et al. 1984), and are comparable to the behavioral states of the newborn. With increased recognition of the fetus as an individual and a person, it should be possible to relate subtle changes of these behavioral states to the fetal state of health.

References

Awoust I, Levi S (1984) New aspects of fetal dynamics with a special emphasis one eye movements. Ultrasound in Med Biol 10:107

Boddy K, Dawes GS (1975) Fetal breathing. Br Med Bull 31:3

Campbell K (1980) Ultradian rhythms in the human fetus during the last ten weeks of gestation: a review. Sem in Perinatol 4:301

deVries JIP, Visser GHA, Prechtl HFR (1982) The emergence of fetal behaviour. I. Qualitative aspects. Early Hum Dev 7:301

Griffin RL, Caron FIM, Geijn HP van (1984) Behavioural states in the human fetus during labour. Proceedings, 1st conference, The Society for the Study of Fetal Physiology, Oxford

Holländer H-J (1979) Historical review and clinical relevance of real-time observations of fetal movements. Contr Gynec Obstet 6:26

Manning FA, Platt LD, Sipos L (1980) Antepartum fetal evaluation: development of a fetal biophysical profile. Am J Obstet Gynecol 136:787

Mathews DD (1973) Fetal movements and fetal wellbeing. Lancet 1:1315

Natale R, Nasello C, Turliuk R (1983) Patterns of gross fetal body movements and fetal breathing activity in human fetuses at 24–31 completed weeks gestation. Proceedings, 10th conference on fetal breathing movements and other fetal measurements, Malmö

Nijhuis JG, Prechtl HFR, Martin CB, Bots RSGM (1982) Are there behavioural states in the human fetus? Early Hum Dev 6:177

Patrick J (1982) Fetal breathing movements. Clin Obstet Gynecol 25:787

Patrick J, Campbell K, Carmichael L et al. (1980a) A definition of human fetal apnea and the distribution of fetal apneic intervals during the last ten weeks of pregnancy. Am J Obstet Gynecol 136:471

Patrick J, Campbell K, Carmichael L et al. (1980b) Patterns of human fetal breathing during the last 10 weeks of pregnancy. Obstet Gynecol 56:24

Patrick J, Campbell K, Carmichael L et al. (1982) Patterns of gross fetal body movements over 24-hour observation intervals during the last 10 weeks of pregnancy. Am J Obstet Gynecol 142:363

Reinold E (1979) New trends in real-time ultrasound in early pregnancy. Contr Gynec Obstet 6:123

Richardson B, Natale R, Patrick J (1979) Human fetal breathing activity during electively induced labor at term. Am J Obstet Gynecol 133:247

Roberts AB, Stubbs SM, Mooney R et al. (1980) Fetal activity in pregnancies complicated by maternal diabetes mellitus. Br J Obstet Gynecol 87:485

Sadovsky E, Yaffe H (1973) Daily fetal movement recording and fetal prognosis. Obstet Gynecol 41:845

Towell ME, Salvador HS (1974) Intrauterine asphyxia and respiratory movements in the fetal goat. Am J Obstet Gynecol 118:1124

van Vliet MAT, Martin CB, Nijhuis JG, Prechtl HFR (1984) Behavioural state in growth-retarded human fetuses. Proceedings, 1st conference, The Society for the Study of Fetal Physiology, Oxford

Wittmann BK, Brown S (1982) Real-time ultrasound observation of fetal activity between 20 and 30 weeks gestation. 9th conference on fetal breathing and other fetal movements, London, Ontario

Wittmann BK, Davison BM, Lyons E et al. (1979) Real-time ultrasound observation of fetal activity in labour. Br J Obstet Gynecol 86:278

Wittmann BK, Rurak DW, Gruber N, Brown S (1981) Real-time ultrasound observation of breathing and movements in the fetal lamb. Am J Obstet Gynecol 141:807

Wittmann BK, Brown S, Davison B, Marguilies N (1983a) Observation of fetal hiccoughs in normal and abnormal pregnancy. Proceedings, 10th conference on fetal breathing movements and other fetal measurements, Malmö

Wittmann BK, Brown S, Davison BM (1983b) Maternal and ultrasound observation of fetal movements. Proceedings, Symposium on perinatal physiology and behaviour, Melbourne

14.6 The Psychological Impact of Ultrasound Scanning in Pregnancy

D.N. Cox and B.K. Wittmann

Although the diagnostic benefits of ultrasound scanning (USS) in obstetrics are well established, little attention has been given to its psychological impact, other than anecdotal observations (Treichel 1982; Fletcher and Evans 1983) and concern expressed over the increasing use of technology in prenatal care and obstetric services generally (MacIntyre 1977). Real-time USS allows for observation of fetal activity and behavior before fetal movement is experienced, or in those instances in which there is an insensitivity to such movement (Hertogs et al. 1979). Fetal movement perception is important in preparing women for birth and the subsequent separation from the neonate (Cohen 1979), as through it one becomes aware of the increasingly autonomous status of the fetus (Klaus and Kennel 1976). Feedback on the fetus via USS early in the pregnancy may have analogous effects to fetal movement perception while anticipating and augmenting the awareness resulting from this experience. This feedback of internal physiological activity, otherwise outside of conscious awareness, may be associated with behavioral and psychological changes of clinical significance through enhancing the perceived salience and relevance of the event.

In order to ensure the optimum intrauterine environment, women are required to observe a wide range of health care behaviors relating to concerns such as smoking, alcohol, nutrition, drugs, and clinic attendance. However, maternal adherence to prenatal health care recommendations is frequently less than ideal. Many women will continue to smoke during their pregnancy despite advice and evidence to the contrary (Butler et al. 1972; Wainright 1983; Sexton and Hebel 1984). Alcohol abuse is increasing amongst pregnant women and is expected to continue to do so, again despite overwhelming data concerning its impact (Abel 1980, 1982; Lamanna 1982; Kuzma and Sokol 1982; Rosett et al. 1983). A substantial proportion of women fail to attend for prenatal care until late in their pregnancy (McKinlay 1970). Also, there is a compelling literature associating maternal anxiety and stress during pregnancy with complications of pregnancy and delivery. Elevations in self-reported anxiety consistently emerges as a factor distinguishing obstetrically normal and abnormal groups (McDonald 1968; Crandon 1979; Reading 1983). A reason for increased anxiety early in the pregnancy is frequently concern over the viability and health of the fetus (Kumar and Robson 1982). The implications are that the more prenatal care a woman is involved in, the fewer will be her problems during the pregnancy and delivery and the more likely it will be that her baby will be born healthy. In this context, the possibility that USS in pregnancy may increase adherence to health care recommendations and decrease maternal anxiety takes on a greater meaning, particularly in view of indications that there is a high probability of compliance in those situations in which the cues to comply are highly specific and visible, whereas if they are invisible or ambiguous the probability is low (Zifferblatt 1975). While the implications of noncompliance or elevated anxiety are physiological, the origins of the problem may be psychological.

It was against this background that systematic evaluation of the psychological impact of USS in pregnancy was initiated (Reading and Cox 1982). This research was carried out in the Department of Obstetrics and Gynaecology at King's College Hospital in London, England, with the support of Prof. S. Campbell. Reports on subjective reactions to USS have indicated positive attitudes toward the experience (Kohn et al. 1980; Milne and Rich 1980). However, this was the first attempt to objectively investigate attitudinal and behavioral responses as a consequence of USS during pregnancy.

In the project we made use of the routine USS program available to women attending prenatal clinics in King's College Hospital. It provided for USS at three stages of pregnancy, approximately 10 weeks, 17 weeks, and 32 weeks. The study consisted of a prospective evaluation of 133 Caucasian primiparae aged between 18 and 22 years in stable relationships. High-risk pregnancies were excluded. At their first clinic visit women were randomly assigned to two conditions of real-time USS: (a) high feedback ($n = 67$), in which women were shown the monitor screen and provided with standardized visual and verbal feedback as to fetal size, shape, and movement; (b) low feedback ($n = 62$), in which women received a similar examination except that they were unable to see the monitor screen and received only verbal feedback linked to the visual image. At subsequent clinic visits USS examinations were performed using compound scanning. Prior to and following the scan, women rated their feelings toward being pregnant and toward the fetus. On completion of the USS they rated their attitudes toward the procedure itself, their emotional state at the time of the USS, and their anxiety levels, both currently and in anticipation of future events in the pregnancy.

With regard to the short-term effects of USS, there was no evidence that the procedure gave rise to maternal distress, although the emotional impact was influenced by the level of feedback provided. Women in the high feedback condition displayed uniformly more positive attitudes towards USS and the fetus. For example, when asked to select the single descriptor which best reflected their emotional state during the USS, the high feedback group showed considerable consensus, as 74% nominated "wonderful", as compared to 11% in the low feedback group. The results suggest USS is informative as well as emotionally rewarding when specific and detailed feedback is made available. In this initial phase of our evaluation (Campbell et al. 1982), we demonstrated the potential short-term impact of USS, with the implication being that feedback should become an integral part of the procedure in order to maximize its impact.

In the next phase of the project the effect of these initial results on longer term concerns such as adherence to prenatal health care recommendations was evaluated (Reading et al. 1982). In this regard, women were assessed prior to their second USS. In considering the results it is important to be aware that the women did not know that they had been assigned to conditions of high and low USS, and also that no attempt was made to relate the real-time USS experience to behavior change. In spite of this, exposure to high feedback USS was consistently related to more appropriate behavior change. Most importantly, women in this group were more likely to have shown decreases in smoking and alcohol consumption since their initial visit. Other behavioral changes were also noted as a function of the level of feedback provided. For example, women in the high feedback group were more likely to have visited the dentist and altered their style of dress.

With regard to the assessment of maternal anxiety, women in the high feedback group had a lower level of state anxiety after real-time USS, although this difference was not significant (Reading and Cox 1982). Both groups displayed a low level of state anxiety following

the USS which was similar to that of a no-USS control group ($n = 55$) included at this point to provide a comparison. The absence of elevated post-USS anxiety levels in both feedback groups further confirms the acceptability of USS in this context. There were minimal differences in reported anxiety in anticipation of future events such as fetal movement, contractions, and delivery, although events later in the pregnancy, potentially associated with greater concern, attracted higher scores, lending support to the validity of this measure of anticipatory anxiety. The control subjects did indicate higher ratings on anticipation of fetal movement, raising the possibility that USS may desensitize women to anxiety surrounding this experience.

Patient acceptability of the procedure was also assessed beyond the attitude change previously described. Fifty percent of the women nominated the first real-time USS as the most important of the three they received, with women in the high feedback condition being significantly more likely to choose the first USS. In further explaining their reaction to USS, the majority of the women referred either to the reassurance it provided or to the realization that they were definitely pregnant. In those instances in which the spouse attended the USS this was almost uniformly perceived as positive by the women due to the "involvement" and "sharing" of the experience it engendered. Regret was frequently expressed among those women whose spouse did not attend. When asked to indicate their intention to accept USS in subsequent pregnancies none of the women responding reported in the negative.

In summary, it was our intention in this project to study an integral part of prenatal care, USS, in order to objectively evaluate the optimal psychological contribution such a procedure can have. Although many involved with USS would insist we have only demonstrated the obvious, it is important to document its impact empirically. The results indicate an enhancement of effect contingent upon receiving extensive feedback, which may not currently be provided in many instances. Our evaluation of the psychological impact of USS in an obstetrically normal population provided normative data and some validation for our questionnaire procedures.

Recently, this research was extended by examining the impact of USS in high-risk pregnancies. This study was carried out in the high-risk clinic of the Grace Hospital in Vancouver, Canada. The sample ($n = 50$) was drawn from women attending for dating scans prior to amniocentesis. A low risk group ($n = 50$) was included to serve as a control group within this study and as a comparison for the first project. As in the previous research, the level of feedback provided was manipulated consecutively across the two groups. In the high feedback group the women and their partners, if they attended, again received extensive verbal and visual feedback through viewing the monitor screen, whereas in the low feedback condition visual access to the screen was denied and subjects received limited verbal evaluation. In those instances in which the partner attended he was included in the assessment and filled out questionnaires evaluating his response to USS. The dependent variables included measures of maternal anxiety, maternal and paternal attitudes towards the pregnancy, the fetus, and the procedure itself, and the emotional experience during the scan.

Preliminary results indicate a significant decrease in state anxiety and confirm the acceptability of USS in this context. The level of state anxiety experienced by high-risk women was not significantly different from that of low-risk subjects prior to the scan. This may be unique to the population we studied. For example, women having amniocentesis may not be as anxious at this point in their pregenancy as they will be following the amniocentesis itself. The greatest decreases in maternal anxiety, regardless of risk condition, were associated with the high feedback condition, again confirming the importance of providing feedback to enhance the psychological impact of USS. Attitude change in the two conditions, in both the women and their partners, has yet to be examined. However, it is interesting to note that significantly fewer men attended in the high-risk group. At a speculative level, this might reflect some apprehension on the part of the partner to become involved in the pregnancy until its viability is further confirmed.

This latter study is serving to document the psychological impact of USS on high-risk populations where greater concern over the pregnancy and the health of the fetus may be evidenced. Collectively, the two studies have extended our understanding of the positive psychological impact USS can have and moved our knowledge from the realm of anecdote to that of empirical data.

References

Abel EL (1980) Fetal alcohol syndrome: behavioral teratology. Psychol Bull 87 (1):29–50

Abel EL (1982) In utero alcohol exposure and developmental delay of response inhibition, Alcoholism Clin Exp Res 6 (3):369–376

Butler NR, Goldstein H, Ross EM (1972) Cigarette smoking in pregnancy: its influence on birthweight and perinatal mortality. Br Med J 2:127–130

Campbell S, Reading AE, Cox DN, Slemere CM, Mooney R, Chudleigh P, Beedle J, Ruddick H (1982) Ultrasound scanning in pregnancy: the short-term psychological effects of early real-time scans. J Psychosom Obstetr Gynecol 1:57–61

Cohen RL (1979) Maladaption to pregnancy. Semin Perinatol 3:15–24

Crandon AJ Maternal anxiety and obstetric complications. J Psychosom Res 23:190–111

Fletcher JC, Evans MI (1983) Maternal bonding in early fetal ultrasound examinations. N Engl J Med 308 (7):392–393

Hertogs K, Roberts AB, Cooper D, Griffen DR, Campbell S (1979) Maternal perception of fetal motor activity. Br Med J 2:1183–1186

Klaus M, Kennel J (1976) Maternal infant bonding. Mosby, St. Louis

Kohn CL, Nelson A, Weiner S (1980) Gravidas responses to real-time ultrasound fetal image. J Obstetr Gynecol Nurs March/April:77–80

Kumar R, Robson KM (1982) Previous induced abortion and anti-depression in primipare. Psychol Med 8:711–715

Kuzma JW, Sokol RJ (1982) Maternal drinking behavior and decreased intrauterine growth. Alcoholism Clin Exp Res 6 (3):396–402

Lamanna M (1982) Alcohol related birth defects: implications for education. J Drug Educ 12:113–123

Milne LS, Rich OJ (1980) Cognitive and affective aspects of the responses of pregnant women to sonography. Matern Child Nurs J March:15–39

McDonald RL (1968) The role of emotional factors in obstetric complications: a review. Psychosom Med 30:222–234

MacIntyre S (1977) The management of childbirth: a review of sociological research issues. Soc Sci Med 11:477

McKinlay J (1970) The new late-comers for antenatal care. Br J Soc Prevent Med 24:502–510

Reading AE (1983) The influence of maternal anxiety on the course and outcome of pregnancy: a review. Health Psychol 2 (2):187–202

Reading AE, Cox DN (1982) The effects of ultrasound examination on maternal anxiety levels. J Behav Med 5 (2):237–247

Reading AE, Campbell S, Cox DN, Shedmere CM (1982) Health beliefs and health care behaviors in pregnancy. Psychol Med 12:379–383

Rosett HL, Weiner L, Lee A, Zuckerman B, Dooking E, Oppenheimer E (1983) Patterns of alcohol consumption and fetal development. Obstetr Gynecol 61 (5):539–546

Sexton M, Hebel JR (1984) A clinical trial of change in maternal smoking and its effect on birth weight. JAMA 251 (7):911–935

Treichel JA (1982) More uses of ultrasound safety. Science News 121:398

Wainright RL (1983) Change in observed birth weight associated with change in maternal cigarette smoking. Am J Epidemiol 117 (6):668–674

Zifferblatt SM (1975) Increasing patient compliance through applied analysis of behavior. Prevent Med 4:173–182

14.7 Conclusions

It is still too early to assess the efficacy of ultrasound screening definitively. Already, however, some effects are being felt, as our own record in the diagnosis of anencephaly shows. Before ultrasound screening was introduced in 1980, only 4 of 13 cases were diagnosed before 24 weeks gestation. In 1980 the proportion increased to three of six, and in 1981, to six of nine. Since January 1982, 15 of 17 anencephalic fetuses were referred prior to 24 weeks with a suspicion of that anomaly.

In summary, we believe that the introduction of routine ultrasound screening is a welcome development, and that we will be increasingly successful in the early detection and prevention of dangers to mother and fetus. The scope and degree of this success will depend largely on the average quality of the examinations. To effect improvement in this regard, it is necessary to provide definition, direction, monitoring, and an appropriate fee base. Because the last-named must be acceptable, some limitations have to be imposed. It is our opinion that the multistage concept presented here has the potential of providing appropriate access to diagnostic ultrasound for all patients without producing exorbitant training and operating costs. The basis of the concept is a productive division of work and responsibility between the physician in his office and the hospital-based expert, with the former noting and referring cases with suspicious findings with a relatively limited investment of time and capital, and the latter sorting, differentiating, and *taking responsibility for further evaluation and its consequences*. If this concept is adhered to, there should be no problems concerning capacity or in striking a favorable balance between cost and benefit. In this way the patient is offered a maximum of diagnostic service on which management decisions can be based.

15 Sonographic Aspects of the Menstrual Cycle

Based on its ability to demonstrate the pelvic organs (Kratochwil et al. 1972; see Chap. 3), sonography can be utilized to monitor the changes that occur in the uterus, ovaries, and blood vessels (but not the fallopian tubes) during the normal menstrual cycle. Our earlier experience in patients undergoing hormonal therapy (Hackelöer and Hansmann 1976; Hackelöer et al. 1977) indicated that it was possible to demonstrate ovarian follicles, measure their size, and monitor their growth by ultrasound. These results were later confirmed (Hackelöer and Robinson 1978; Hackelöer et al. 1979; Hackelöer and Nitschke-Dabelstein 1980) in women with normal menstrual cycles.

Initially, ultrasound visualization of the uterus served only as an aid to orientation, and imaging of the endometrium was not possible due to the limited resolution of the instruments. Today this situation has changed, and we begin this chapter with a discussion of the sonographic features of the endometrium. The endometrium should always be evaluated *before* the ovary is scrutinized; otherwise, the observation of a large follicle, for example, might bias evaluation of the endometrial phase.

15.1 Endometrium, Follicles, Blood Vessels

15.1.1 Endometrial Changes

The examination begins with a longitudinal scan between the umbilicus and symphysis. This will demonstrate the uterus in virtually all cases.

After uterine size and shape have been evaluated, a scan is performed over the longitudinal axis of the uterus to document the central uterine echo.

In the early proliferative phase of the cycle, the endometrium appears as a thin, continuous line (Fig. 15.1).

Our investigations and those of other authors indicate that the endometrium has as many as six different sonographic patterns during the menstrual cycle (Bald 1983; Bald and Hackelöer 1983; Fleischer et al. 1983; Fig. 15.8b).

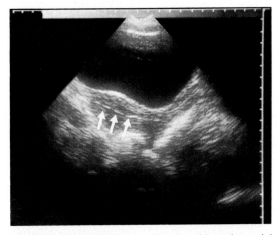

Fig. 15.1. Longitudinal scan of uterus: thin endometrial line (*arrows*) is characteristic of early proliferative phase (type 1/2)

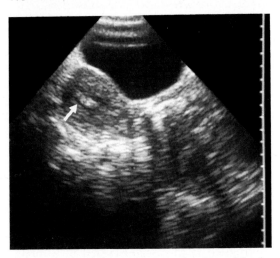

Fig. 15.2. Longitudinal scan: loss of endometrial echo in lower uterine segment. "Plump" endometrial echo with hypoechoic border (*arrow;* edema of superficial cells, late proliferative phase, type 3/4)

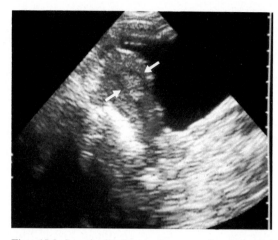

Fig. 15.3. Longitudinal scan: increase of endometrial thickness to 14 mm (*arrows*) 1–2 days before ovulation (type 4/5)

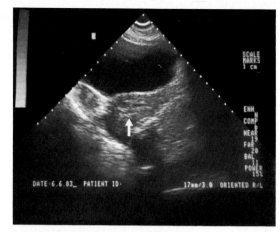

Fig. 15.5. Further dilatation of the uterine cavity, immediately before ovulation (type 5/6)

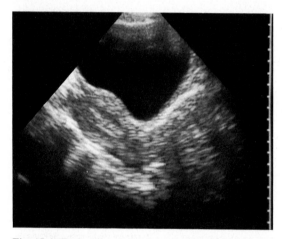

Fig. 15.4. Early dilatation of uterine lumen, preovulatory (type 5)

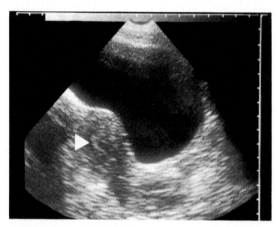

Fig. 15.6. Earliest appearance of ring sign (type 6). This is a periovulatory feature

These changes in the endometrium correlate well with maternal plasma estradiol and progesterone levels.

The late proliferative phase is characterized by an increase in endometrial thickness but a loss of the continuous endometrial line. Edema of the superficial cells is accompanied by the appearance of a fluid collection, which is visible as a hypoechoic area (Fig. 15.2). As the cycle progresses, a strong and easily measured proliferation occurs (Fig. 15.3). The preovulatory period (about 18 h) is characterized by a dilatation of the uterine cavity (Fig. 15.4) which progresses (Fig. 15.5) to a ring-like structure. This occurs concurrently with the rise in progester-

one and may represent the earliest sign of ovulation (Figs. 15.6, 15.7).

We do not yet know the precise mechanism by which this ring is produced. We believe that the pre- and postovulatory rise in progesterone may be associated with an abrupt increase in fluid secretion by the endometrium. This creates relatively large "impedance jumps" and results in a distinct ultrasound pattern. This hypothesis is supported by water-bath experiments on extirpated uteri, in which all patterns observed preoperatively could be reproduced except for the ring (Type 4). It would appear that this phenomenon is highly unstable. The ring also occurs in association with ectopic

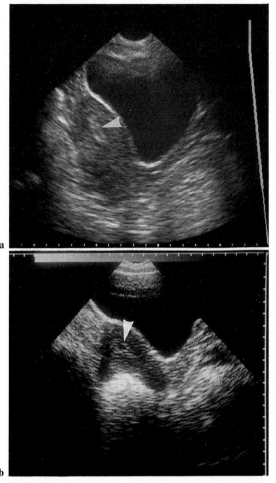

a

b

Fig. 15.7a, b. Periovulatory ring sign (*arrow*). **a** Shortly before ovulation. **b** Possibly shortly after ovulation (high progesterone)

pregnancies, where it again correlates closely with progesterone levels (Figs. 4.40, 4.41).

Care must be taken not to confuse the ring sign of the endometrial cycle with an early intrauterine pregnancy. Since as a rule the ring does not form in the absence of ovulation [early luteinization, luteinized unruptured follicle (LUF) syndrome], the presence of a ring may be taken as a sign that ovulation has occurred.

During normal menstruation the endometrium has an irregular appearance and contains numerous hypoechoic areas (Fig. 15.8a).

15.1.2 Follicular Growth

Ovarian follicles can be visualized with ultrasound after they have reached a diameter of 3–5 mm (see Sect. 3.1). They appear as echo-

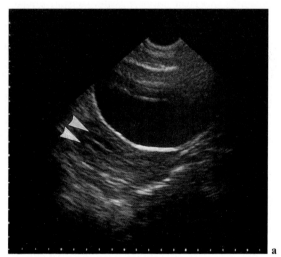

a

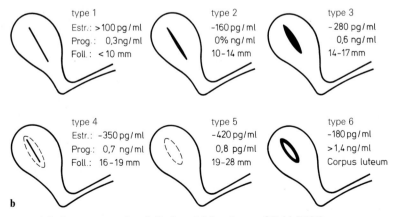

b

Fig. 15.8. a Fluid (*arrows*) in cavum uteri during menstruation. **b** Endometrial patterns of Bald (1983)

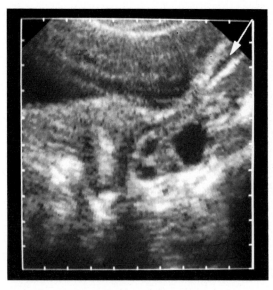

Fig. 15.9. Transverse scan showing three ovarian follicles: one dominant follicle 18 mm in diameter and two smaller than 10 mm. *Arrow* indicates an ovarian blood vessel in infundibulopelvic ligament

free structures within the more echogenic ovarian tissue.

Follicles are usually circular in shape, but they may appear elongated or distorted due to variations of internal pressure and bladder filling (Fig. 15.9). The technique for measuring the follicle is not standardized, but most workers measure the internal follicular diameter in three planes (longitudinal, transverse, sagittal) and calculate the average. The greatest apparent diameter should be taken on each plane, and only the purely cystic part of the follicle (i.e., inside to inside) should be measured.

Usually several follicles less than 10 mm in diameter can be demonstrated in each ovary on day – 10 (i.e., 10 days *before* ultrasound evidence of ovulation); later (day – 5) one follicle usually becomes dominant (Figs. 15.9 and 15.10). Hackelöer and Robinson (1978) found that the rate of growth was linear from day – 5 to ovulation and that the mean preovulatory follicular diameter was 20.2 mm (range from 18 to 24 mm; Fig. 15.29) Terinde et al. (1979), Queenan et al. (1980), Fleischer et al. (1981), and Bryce et al. (1982) report similar values (see Table 15.1). Follicular growth in stimulated cycles is discussed in Sect. 15.2.

The ovaries are not always easy to visualize. Our experience indicates that in 2%–5% of cases, one ovary – usually the left – cannot be

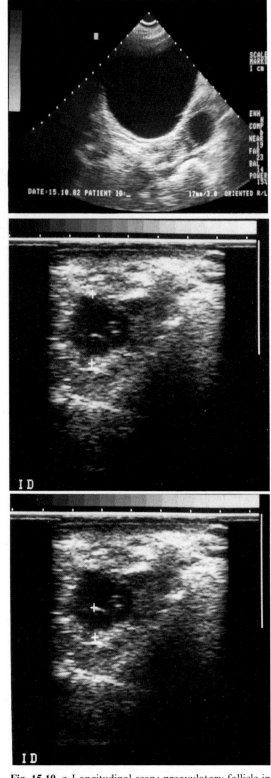

Fig. 15.10. a Longitudinal scan: preovulatory follicle in right ovary; below it, internal iliac artery. **b** Vaginal scan: preovulatory follicle (22 mm). **c** Same follicle: cumulus oophorus

Table 15.1. Size of preovulatory (Graafian) follicle in normal menstrual cycle. (Modified from Nitschke-Dabelstein 1981)

Authors	Size [mm]	Cycles (n)	Pa-tients (n)	Measuring technique	Ultrasound equipment
Bryce et al. (1982)	24.6 ± 2.3 (SD)[b]	24	14	mD	Compoundscanner
Fleischer et al. (1981)	20.0	15	15	$\bar{m}$D	Compound and sector scanner
Hackelöer et al. (1979)	20.0 ± 0.9 (SEM)[c]	14	25	mD (l, t, s)	Compoundscanner
Kerin et al. (1981)	23.2 ± 0.3 (SEM)	6	56	mD	Compoundscanner
Nilsson et al. (1982)	21.4 ± 0.8 (SD)	16	?	k.A.	Compoundscanner (2.5 MHz)
	19.3 ± 1.1 (SD)	10	?	k.A.	
Nitschke-Dabelstein et al. (1981)	20.9 ± 0.9 (SEM)	8	6	mD (l, t, s)	Compoundscanner (2.5 + 3.5 MHz)
O'Herlihy et al. (1980)	20.1 ± 1.6 (SD) 0.22 (SEM)	53	33	mD (l, t, s)	Real-time scanner (corresponds to nine cycles studied with compound instrument)
Queenan et al. (1980)	21.1 ± 3.5 (SD)	18	?	mD (l, t, s)	Sector scanner
Renaud et al. (1980)	27 ± 0.3 (SEM)	10	10	mD (l, t, s)	Compoundscanner (2 MHz)
Robertson et al. (1979)	25.0	12	11	mD	Compoundscanner
Smith et al. (1980)	25.5 ± 0.1 (SEM)	19	?	k.A.	Compoundscanner

[5] mD maximum diameter ($\bar{m}$D mean value); mD (l, t, s) mean value of maximum longitudinal, transverse and sagittal diameter; k.A. not specified

demonstrated, as it is covered by a loop of sigmoid colon.

In such cases real-time equipment should be used to differentiate fluid- or gas-filled loops of bowel from an ovarian follicle by searching for peristaltic motion.

15.1.3 Intrafollicular Structures

At one time we dismissed intrafollicular structures as artifacts. However, we now know that the cumulus oophorus can be visualized (Fig. 15.11a, b), as it only appears at a certain point in the menstrual cycle, and its size and appearance are always the same.

Bomsel-Helmreich et al. (1981) noted good correlation between the sonographic and histologic appearance of the cumulus oophorus in 12 sheep follicles and 3 human follicles. They concluded that sonographic visualization is made possible or at least facilitated by the dissociation of the cumulus mass just prior to ovulation. This result has particular relevance to the recovery of oocytes for in vitro fertilization.

In the postovulatory period, one or more of the following observations may be made:

1. The sudden "disappearance" of the follicle
2. The appearance of internal echoes caused by blood clotting and/or the invasion of the follicle by capillary endothelium and fibroblasts (Figs. 15.15–15.17)
3. Collapse of the follicle, creating the impression that the follicle is septated or that two follicles are present (Fig. 15.12)
4. The appearance of a "fluid track" leading from the ovary to the cul-de-sac, and the presence of free fluid in the culd-de-sac (Figs. 15.12, 15.13, 15.14)

Not all follicles mature to the point of ovulation, and some regress. Among the findings indicative of ovarian disorder are the appearance of internal echoes before the follicle is ruptured (LUF) or continuous growth of the follicle to 30 or 40 mm in diameter with the formation of a cyst.

During the midluteal phase the mature corpus luteum can be demonstrated as an elliptical structure 30–35 mm long and 20–25 mm wide (Figs. 15.16, 15.17). It consists of three concentric areas with different acoustic properties: a central echo-free area (possibly blood), an intermediate hypoechoic area (possibly luteal tissue), and a peripheral echogenic area composed of stromal tissue (Figs. 15.12–15.17) or solid material (Fig. 15.18).

The corpus luteum is more easily demonstrated in hormone-induced cycles. It usually

Fig. 15.11a, b. Longitudinal scans. **a** Preovulatory follicle in left ovary with early dissociation of cumulus mass (*arrow*). **b** Mature follicle with cumulus oophorus

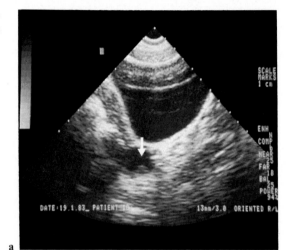

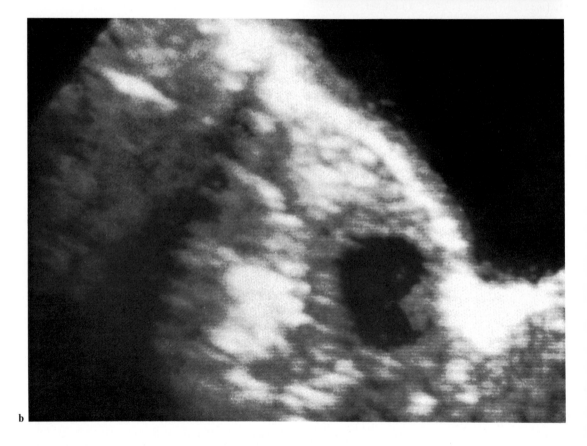

disappears before the onset of menstruation, but its persistence on day +12 or beyond may be the first sign of a successful implantation, which can be confirmed by the β-HCG test. Corpus luteum cysts are also more common in stimulated cycles (Fig. 15.19). Marked enlargement of the ovaries independent of the menstrual cycle is typical for Stein-Leventhal syndrome (Fig. 15.20).

15.1.4 Blood Vessels

The ovarian blood vessels were discussed in Chap. 3 (Figs. 3.11, 3.12). Traditionally they have served as landmarks for localization of the ovaries (Figs. 15.8, 15.9), but they also may be used for blood flow measurements with a combination of real-time and Doppler techniques (see also Figs. 15.32–15.34).

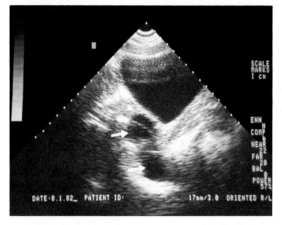

Fig. 15.12. Longitudinal scan immediately after ovulation: follicle (*arrow*) is collapsed; there is fluid in cul-de-sac

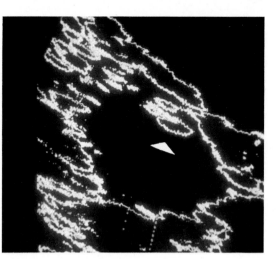

Fig. 15.15. Preovulatory follicle with cumulus mass (*arrow*): postprocessed image

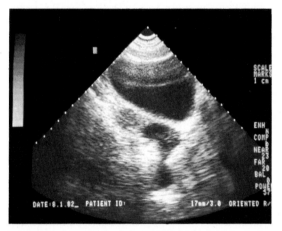

Fig. 15.13. Longitudinal scan: follicle is almost empty. Note fluid track

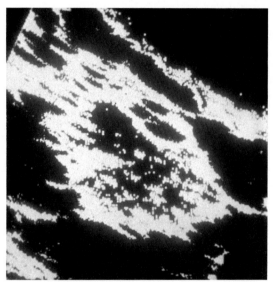

Fig. 15.16. Same follicle as in Fig. 15.15, 12 h later: echoes in follicle represent early corpus luteum

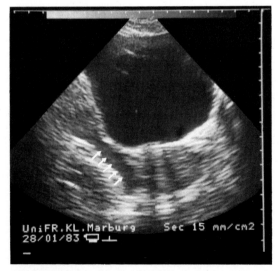

Fig. 15.14. Ovary largely echogenic, "fluid track" still visible: ovulation has occurred within past 12 h

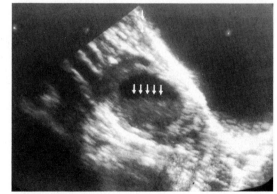

Fig. 15.17. Follicle with echogenic structure representing corpus luteum. Note blood vessels (*arrows:* ovarian artery and vein)

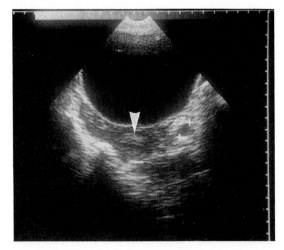

Fig. 15.18. Transverse scan: corpus luteum within left ovary. Note large secretory endometrium (*arrow*)

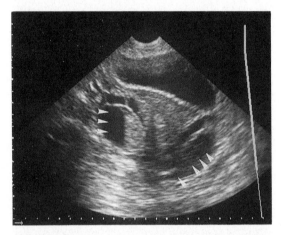

Fig. 15.19. Transverse scan in a patient stimulated with HMG and HCG: bilateral cystic corpora lutea (*arrows*)

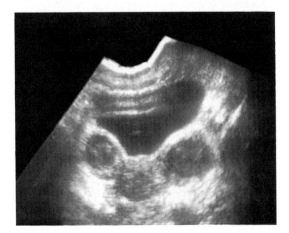

Fig. 15.20. Transverse scan: enlarged ovaries in Stein-Leventhal syndrome

References

Baird DT, Fraser IS (1974) Blood production and ovarian secretion rates of estradiol and estrone in women throughout the menstrual cycle. J Clin Endocrinol Metab 38:1009

Bald R (1983) Studien über die sonographische Endometriumdarstellung. Med Diss, Marburg

Bald R, Hackelöer BJ (1983) Ultraschalldarstellung verschiedener Endometriumformen. In: Otto R, Jan FX (eds) Ultraschalldiagnostik 82. Thieme, Stuttgart New York

Bomsel-Helmreich O, Bessis R, Lan Vu Huyen (1982) Cumulus oophorus of the preovulatory follicle assessed by ultrasound and histology. In: Christie AD (ed) Ultrasound and infertility. Chartwell-Bratt, Bromley, pp 105–119

Bryce RL, Shuter B, Sinosich MJ et al. (1982) The value of ultrasound gonadotrophin and oestradiol measurements for precise ovulation prediction. Fertil Steril 37:42–45

Fleischer A, Daniel J, Rodier J et al. (1981) Sonographic monitoring of ovarian follicular development. J Clin Ultrasound 9:275–280

Fleischer AC, Pittaway DE, Beard L (1983) Sonographic depiction of endometrial changes in spontaneous and stimulated cycles. 28. Jahrestagung der Amerikanischen Gesellschaft für Ultraschall (AIUM) New York

Heckelöer BJ (1984) The role of ultrasound in female infertility management. Ultrasound in Med & Biol 10:35–50

Hackelöer BJ, Hansmann M (1976) Ultraschalldiagnostik in der Frühschwangerschaft. Gynäkologe 9:108

Hackelöer BJ, Robinson HP (1978) Ultraschalldarstellung des wachsenden Follikels und Corpus luteum in normalen physiologischen Zyklus. Geburtshilfe Frauenheilkd 38:163–168

Hackelöer BJ, Fleming R, Robinson HP et al. (1979) Correlation of ultrasonic and endocrinologic assessment of human follicular development. Am J Obstet Gynecol 135:122–128

Hackelöer BJ, Nitschke-Dabelstein S (1980) Ovarian imaging by ultrasound: an attempt to define a reference plane. J Clin Ultrasound 9:275–280

Kerin JF, Edmonds DK, Warnes GM et al. (1981) Morphological and functional relations of Graafian follicle growth to ovulation in women using ultrasonic, laparoscopic and biochemical measurements. Br J Obstet Gynaecol 88:81–90

Kratochwil A, Urban G, Friedrich F (1972) Ultrasonic tomography of the ovaries. Ann Chir Gynecol 61:211–214

Leyendecker G, Wildt L, Hansmann M (1980) Pregnancies following chronic intermittent administration of Gn-Rh by means of a portable pump („Zyklomat"). J Clin Endocrinol Metab 51:1214–1216

McNatty KP, Baird DT, Bolton A, Chambers P, Corker CS, McLean H (1976) Concentration of östrogens and androgens in human ovarian venous plasma and follicular fluid throughout the menstrual cycle. J Endocrinol 71:77

Nilsson L, Wikland M, Hamberger L (1982) Recruitment of an ovulatory follicle in the human following follicle-ectomy and luteectomy. Fertil Steril 37:30–34

Nitschke-Dabelstein S (1983) Monitoring of follicular development using ultrasonography. In: Insler V,

Lunenfeld B (eds) Infertility – male and female. Churchill-Livingstone, Edinburgh

Nitschke-Dabelstein S, Hackelöer BJ, Sturm G (1981) Ovulation and corpus luteum formation observed by ultrasonography. Ultrasound in Med & Biol 7:33–39

O'Herlihy C, de Crespigny LHCh, Robinson HP (1980) Monitoring ovarian follicular development with real time ultrasound. Br J Obstet Gynaecol 87:613–618

Queenan JT, O'Brien GD, Bains LM et al. (1980) Ultrasound scanning of ovaries to detect ovulation in women. Fertil Steril 34:99–105

Renaud RL, Macklem J, DeVain et al. (1980) Echographic study of follicular maturation and ovulation during the normal menstrual cycle. Fertil Steril 33:272–276

Robertson RD, Picker R, Wilson PC, Saunders DM (1979) Assessment of ovulation by ultrasound and plasma estradiol determinations. Obstet Gynecol 54:686–691

Sanyal MK, Berger MJ, Thompson IF, Taymor MI, Horne HW (1974) Development of Graafian follicles in adult human ovary. I. Correlation of estrogen and progesterone concentration in antral fluid with growth of follicles. J Clin Endocrinol Metab 38:828

Strott CA, Yoshimi T, Ross GT, Lipsett MB (1969) Ovarian physiology: relationship between plasma LH and steroidogenesis by the follicle and corpus luteum; effect of HCG. J Clin Endocrinol Metab 19:1157

Terinde R, Distler W, Freundl G, Herberger J (1979) Hormonelle und ultrasonographische Kontrolle der spontanen Ovulation bei Patientinnen mit primärer und sekundärer Sterilität. Arch Gynäkologie 228:168–169

15.2 Applications of Ultrasound in Endocrinology

In Cooperation with W. FEICHTINGER

15.2.1 Monitoring of Gonadotropin Therapy

This clinical application of ultrasound formed the basis for ultrasound imaging of the follicles, which is essential in view of the multifollicular growth that is frequently produced by gonadotropin therapy. Sallam et al. (1983) reported that 37% of their patients treated with clomiphene and 63% treated with gonadotropin developed two or more follicles larger than 18 mm, with the dominant follicles exhibiting linear growth curves. Thus, a high percentage of these patients experienced multiple ovulations with a significant risk of hyperstimulation and multiple pregnancy. These cases were associated with a typical "cartwheel" appearance of the ovary (Figs. 15.21–15.23).

Fig. 15.21. Transverse scan: "cartwheel" phenomenon as an expression of multifollicular growth resulting from hormonal stimulation for ovulation induction (five follicles)

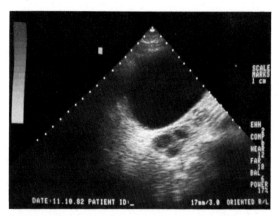

Fig. 15.22. Longitudinal scan: three follicles in a stimulated ovary

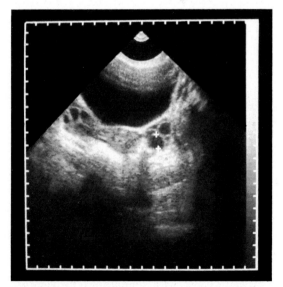

Fig. 15.23. Transverse scan of the uterus and ovaries: bilateral follicular growth. Follicle on right (crosses) measures 10 mm in diameter

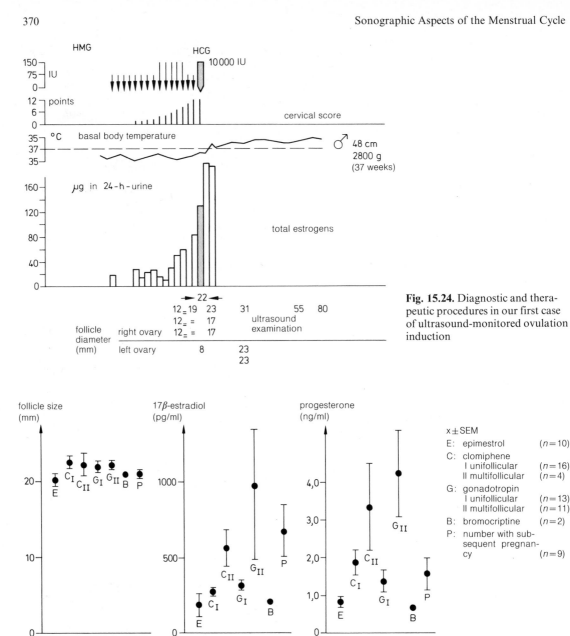

Fig. 15.24. Diagnostic and therapeutic procedures in our first case of ultrasound-monitored ovulation induction

Fig. 15.25. Comparison of follicular diameter, plasma estradiol, and plasma progesterone in stimulated cycles on day before ovulation

Figure 15.24 shows the first case in which we used ultrasound to monitor ovulation induction with gonadotropins. Today ultrasound is used mainly in two ways for the monitoring of fertility therapy:

1. In conjunction with hormonal monitoring, which is usually performed by means of daily plasma E_2 measurements or 24 h total urinary estrogen assays, with sonography providing a supplementary parameter (Fig. 15.25). With

this combination the response to pulsatile GnRH treatment can also be monitored (Fig. 15.26). This has resulted in a decline in the incidence and severity of hyperstimulation syndrome (Fig. 15.27) and multiple pregnancy rates (Hackelöer et al. 1977; Ylöstalo et al. 1981; Siebel et al. 1981; Fink et al. 1982).

2. As the sole monitoring technique, owing to the good correlation that exists between follicular diameter and plasma E_2 (Hackelöer

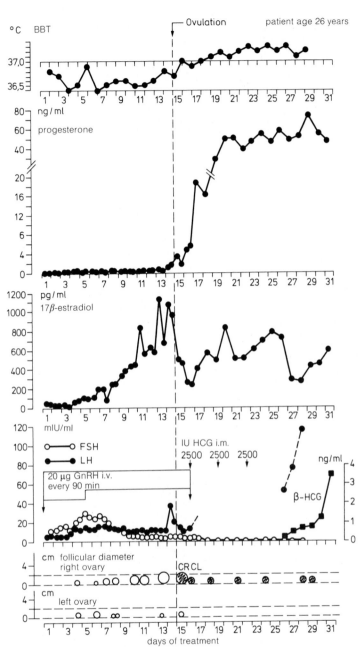

Fig. 15.26. Typical scheme of infertility therapy with pulsatile GnRH. Hormonal profiles and follicular measurements for comparison

1979; Vargyas et al. 1982; Figs. 15.28–15.30). HMG is administered for a specified period, and follicular growth is monitored with ultrasound. HCG is administered when one or two follicles reach the optimum diameter of 20–25 mm. If more than two follicles reach 20 mm, the cycle is abandoned and no HCG is given; in addition, contraceptive measures are recommended.

Although the combined monitoring method would obviously be ideal, our experience indicates that ultrasound monitoring alone is at least as successful as plasma estradiol assays in the prevention of multiple pregnancies and hyperstimulation syndrome (Fig. 15.25). Sallam et al. (1983) showed that the cumulative pregnancy rate after 9 months was higher in the ultrasound-monitored group than in the estradiol-monitored group.

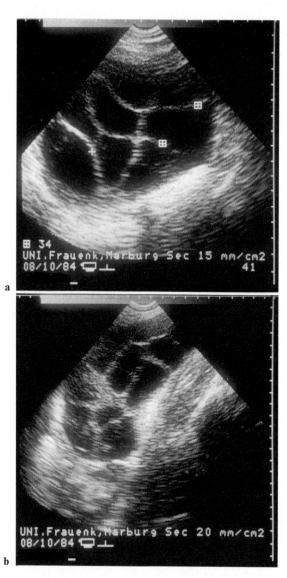

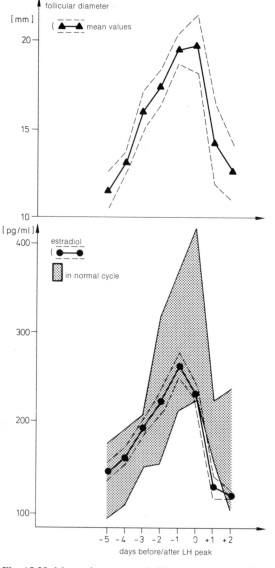

Fig. 15.27. a, b. Hyperstimulation, multifollicular development. **a** Transverse scan; **b** longitudinal scan

Fig. 15.28. Mean plasma estradiol levels and mean follicular diameter ($\pm$ SEM) in spontaneous cycles in relation to day of plasma LH peak

15.2.2 Monitoring of Clomiphene Citrate Therapy

Vargyas, in 1982, described the successful monitoring of patients treated with clomiphene and reported good correlation between follicular diameters and plasma estradiol. The same observations can be made as with the HMG/HCG therapy and in addition ultrasound can be used to time the administration of HCG to induce ovulation in patients who do not ovulate spontaneously (O'Herlihy et al. 1982).

The superiority of ultrasound to basal body temperature is well documented (Fig. 15.31).

15.2.3 Oocyte Collection for In Vitro Fertilization

Ultrasound can once again be used in two ways:

1. As the sole method of timing oocyte recovery. Usually the patient is stimulated with clomiphene citrate (100–150 mg/day), monitored

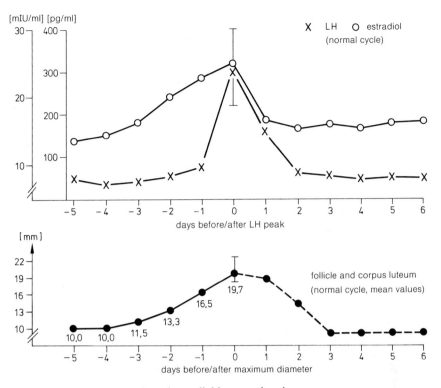

Fig. 15.29. Comparison of follicular diameter, LH peak, and estradiol in normal cycle

with ultrasound, and HCG is administered when one or more follicles reach a size of 20 mm or greater. Oocyte collection is attempted 32–36 h later (Wood et al. 1981; Hoult et al. 1981). The reported rate of oocyte recovery with this method is 80%–90%, although the rate of fertilization is low. This led Buttery et al. (1983) to conclude that sonography should not be used as the sole timing method. However, more recent results from Feichtinger (personal communication 1984) appear to refute this conclusion.

2. In combination with hormonal monitoring. This is now thought to be the method of choice for achieving a high rate of continuing pregnancies (Johnston et al. 1981; Trounson and Conti 1982). Ultrasound is used in conjunction with LH or estradiol to time the oocyte collection. If spontaneous cycles are used, ultrasound will assist in deciding when to initiate LH assays; in stimulated cycles it will aid in timing the administration of HCG. For example, Trounson and Conti report that HCG is administered as soon as the plasma estradiol reaches 1.8 nmol/l per *visible* follicle. In all cases ultrasound can assist in determining the loca-

tion, number, and size of the growing follicles and help to eliminate unnecessary laparoscopies.

According to recent studies on the measurement of blood flow through the ovarian vessels, the combined use of Doppler and real-time ultrasound may provide an even more accurate means of predicting time of ovulation and recognizing disorders of ovarian function (Figs. 15.32–15.34).

Lenz and Lauritsen (1982) and Wikland et al. (1983) reported on the collection of oocytes by the transvesical ultrasound-guided needle aspiration of follicles. No deleterious effects were reported, and at least one pregnancy was achieved. Feichtinger et al. (1981, 1982) have the greatest experience in the aspiration of follicles under sonographic guidance, and describe the following outpatient technique:

We perform the aspiration under local anesthesia, having sedated the patient with 10 mg diazepam and 30 mg pentazocine. A broad-spectrum penicillin is given for prophylaxis. The urinary bladder is filled spontaneously rather than by catheter. One ampule of atropine is administered i.v. as premedication for the sedation. Ultrasound scans are performed with a 2.5-MHz Kretz

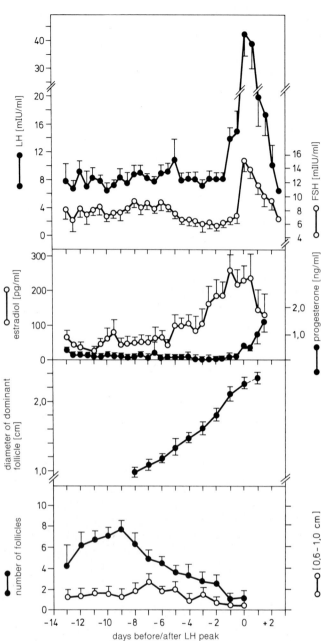

Fig. 15.30. Comparison as in Fig. 15.29 (Wildt et al., Bonn)

Combison 100 sector scanner. First the follicles are localized and measured on transverse and longitudinal scans. Our regimen of stimulation with clomiphene citrate and HMG followed by induction of ovulation with HCG yields an average of four preovulatory follicles per patient, with a range of one to ten.

Oocyte recovery is attempted 35 h after the injection of HCG. The scanner is covered with coupling agent while the puncture site on the lower abdomen is prepared with antiseptic solution. The area is draped with sterile towels, and the transducer is covered with a sterile plastic bag. A needle guide (supplied by the ultrasound manu-

facturer) is attached to the transducer to ensure that the needle will be inserted in the proper direction. The area of the plastic bag overlying the transducer is again covered with sterile coupling agent (a fixative-free gel or filtered sterile mineral oil). Then the follicle is visualized at an angle which is displayed on the monitor screen and corresponds to the puncture line. The puncture site on the abdomen is anesthetized with 1% lidocaine, taking care to infiltrate the entire abdominal wall up to and including the anterior bladder wall. Then an aspirating needle of 1.4 mm external diameter is introduced into the needle guide. The needle is connected to an oocyte collecting system of the type used for laparoscopy (see Feichtinger et al. 1981). With a rapid motion the needle is inserted through the abdominal wall and into the bladder. At this point the needle image is checked to confirm alignment with the puncture line on the screen; it is then advanced into the follicle with another

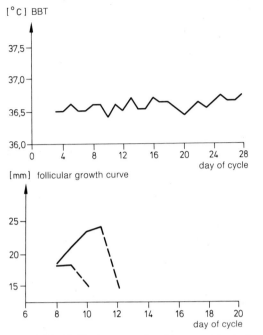

Fig. 15.31. Follicular growth with monophasic basal body temperature (*BBT*)

rapid motion. The aspiration of follicular fluid may commence at once using a pressure of about 100 mmHg (13.3 kPa), which is regulated by an electronic aspiration apparatus. With correct technique, clear follicular fluid should flow immediately into the collecting tube. The fluid is examined under a microscope for the presence of an oocyte. If an oocyte is not found in the first aspirate, the follicle is flushed through the tubing with heparinized irrigating solution, and the fluid is aspirated back into a test tube and examined for the presence of an oocyte. The aspiration or collapse of the follicle and its refilling with irrigating solution are readily observed on the monitor. The irrigation process is repeated several times if necessary. If multiple follicles are to be aspirated and are not in line, the needle should be completely withdrawn and realigned so that the puncture line is over the next follicle before reinserting the needle. When the procedure is completed, the bladder is emptied by catheter. Following 1–2 h observation postoperatively, the patient may be discharged home (Figs. 15.35a–i, 15.36a, b).

Feichtinger reports (personal communication 1984) that at present, the oocyte recovery rate (and thus the number of embryo transfers and the pregnancy rate) is still poorer than with laparoscopy, but he believes that this will improve as experience is gained.

In fact, the oocyte recovery rate with ultrasound-guided aspiration already began to approach that of laparoscopy toward the end of 1982, indicating that this technique is likely eventually to replace laparoscopy in many cases

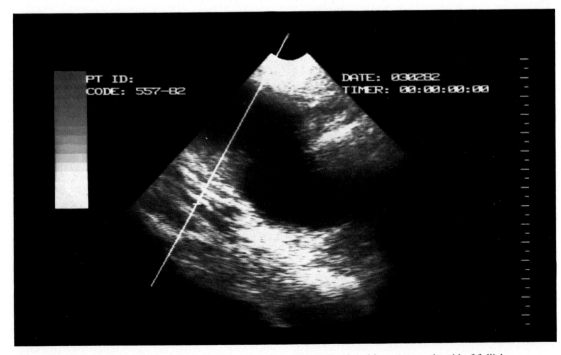

Fig. 15.32. Scan of ovarian blood vessels with superimposed Doppler signal in an ovary devoid of follicles

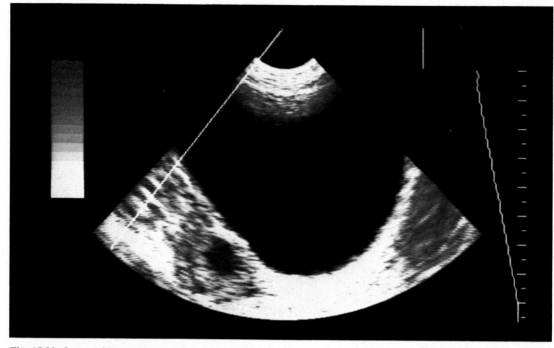

Fig. 15.33. Ovary with preovulatory follicle and Doppler signal

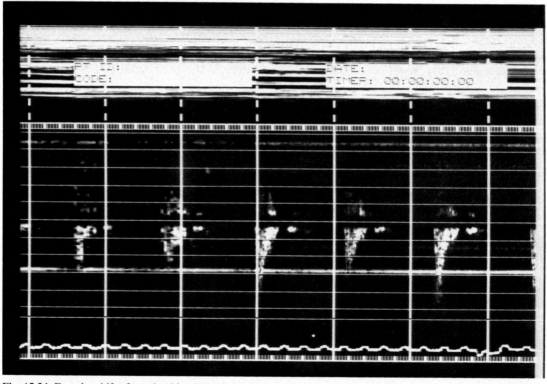

Fig. 15.34. Doppler shift of ovarian blood vessels

Fig. 15.35a, b. Follicular aspiration. **a** Right follicular aspiration: *1* Needle in urinary bladder; *2* needle aimed at follicle; *3* needle pierces follicle; *4, 5* needle in follicle, aspiration begins; *6* follicle collapses; *7* follicle is eva-cuated; *8* next follicle in line with first, can be pierced by simple advancement of needle; *9* needle pierces sec-ond follicle; *10* second follicle collapses and is evacuated. **b** see page 378

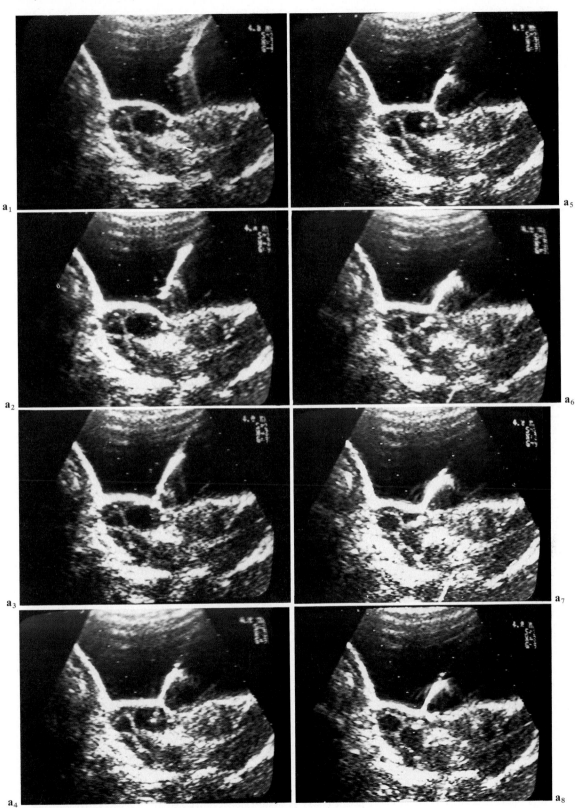

Fig. 15.35

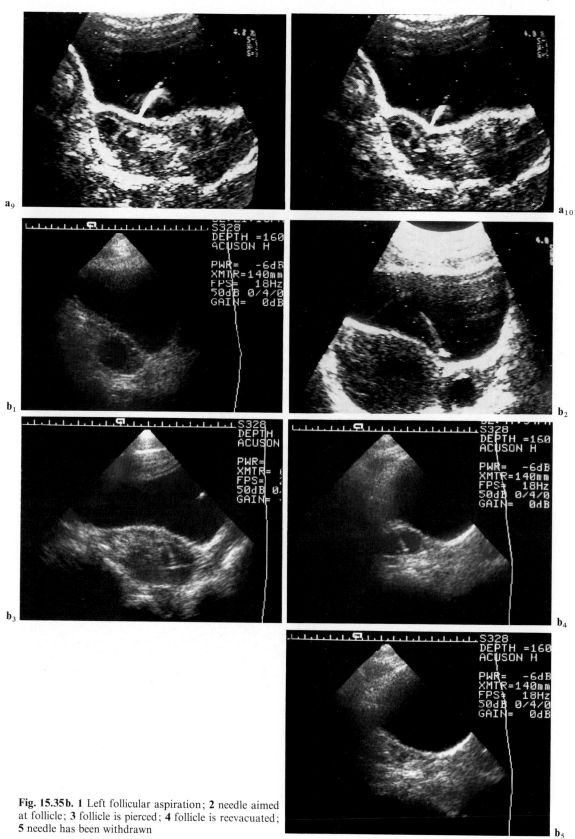

Fig. 15.35b. 1 Left follicular aspiration; **2** needle aimed at follicle; **3** follicle is pierced; **4** follicle is reevacuated; **5** needle has been withdrawn

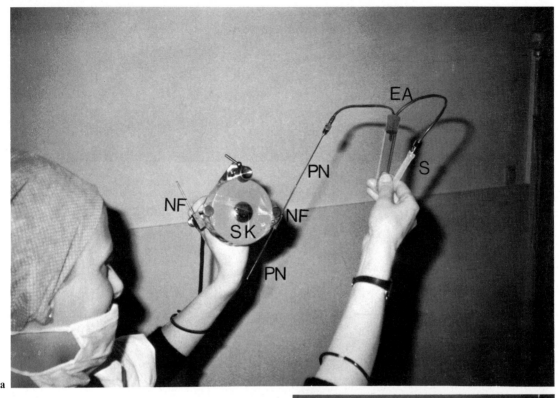

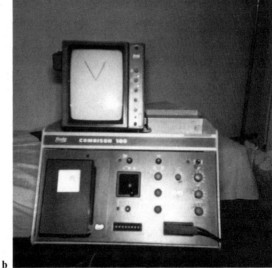

Fig. 15.36. a Apparatus for follicular aspiration (*SK* transducer, *NF* needle guide, *PN* aspirating needle, *EA* oocyte collecting vessel, *S* suction tubing). **b** The puncture line on the monitor screen aids in directing the aspirating needle to its target and corresponds precisely to the angle of the needle guide on the transducer

for the harvesting of oocytes. In special indications it may be of advantage to use a vaginal approach toward follicle aspiration under abdominal or vaginal ultrasound guidance.

A special indication for ultrasound-guided follicular aspiration already exists in patients who have had multiple prior intraabdominal operations that impede laparoscopic visualization of the ovaries, but in whom ultrasound-guided aspiration is still possible.

We feel that the laparoscopic aspiration of follicles will remain the procedure of choice in cases where diagnostic information from intraabdominal inspection is desired in addition to oocyte recovery.

Finally, reimplantation of the fertilized ovum

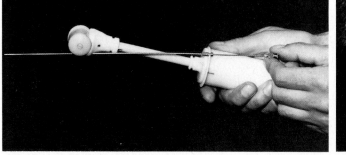

Patients	3
Follicles	12
Ova	11
Fertile	9
c Pregnancies	1

Fig. 15.37. a Vaginal scanner with needle. **b** Vaginal follicular puncture. **c** First results (Feichtinger and Kemeter 1984)

represents another possible application of ultrasound in in vitro fertilization and embryo transfer programs.

15.2.4 Timing the Postcoital Test

Only optimum timing of the postcoital test will ensure good results. Ultrasound can assist interpretation and help to differentiate between an abnormal test due to poor mucus production (e.g., in the presence of a mature follicle) or one due to faulty sperm transport. Studies of the cervical mucus and of sperm-mucus interaction may be performed concurrently.

15.2.5 Luteal Phase Defects

Ultrasound can have many uses in patients with luteal phase defects. It can determine the precise length of the luteal phase, thereby aiding the interpretation of hormonal or histologic findings. In addition, Coutts et al. (1981) found, instead of solid corpus luteum structures, increased incidence of cystic ovarian changes in cycles with a low luteal phase progesterone. Further research in this area is needed.

References

Buttery B, Trounson A, McMaster R, Wood C (1983) Evaluation of diagnostic ultrasound as a parameter of follicular development in an in-vitro fertilization program. Fertil Steril 39:458–463

Coutts JRT, Adam AH, Fleming R (1981) Ovarian ultrasound and endocrine profiles in women with unexplained infertility. In: Christie AD (ed) Ultrasound and Infertility. Chartwell-Bratt, Bromley (Kent), pp 89–99

Dornbluth NC, Potter JL, Shepard MK, Balmacedo JP, Siter-Khodr TM (1983) Assessment of follicular development by ultrasonography and total serum estrogen in HMG-stimulated cycles. U Ultrasound Med 2:407

Feichtinger W, Szalay S, Beck A, Kemeter P, Janisch H (1981) Results of laparoscopic recovery of preovulatory human oocytes from non-stimulated ovaries in an ongoing in vitro fertilization program. Fertil Steril 36:707

Feichtinger W, Szalay S, Kemeter P, Beck A, Bieglmayer C, Riss P, Kratochwil A, Janisch H (1982) The preovulatory follicle and oocyte. In: Edwards RG, Purdy GM (eds) Human conception in vitro. Academic Press, London, p 73

Fink RS, Bowes LP, Mackintosh CE et al. (1982) The value of ultrasound for monitoring ovarian responses to gonadotropin stimulated therapy. Br J Obstet Gynaecol 89:856–861

Fleisher AC, Daniell J, Rodier J, Lindsay A, James AE Jr (1981) Sonographic monitoring of ovarian follicular development. J Clin Ultrasound 9:275–280

Hackelöer BJ, Robinson HP (1978) Ultraschalldarstellung des wachsenden Follikels und corpus luteum in normalen physiologischen Zyklus. Geburtshilfe Frauenheilkd 38:163–168

Hackelöer BJ, Nitschke S, Daume E et al. (1977) Ultraschalldarstellung von Ovarveränderungen bei Gonadotropin-Stimulierung. Geburtshilfe Frauenheilkd 37:185–190

Hackelöer BJ, Fleming R, Robinson HP et al. (1979) Correlation of ultrasonic and endocrinologic assessment of human follicular development. Am J Obstet Gynecol 135:122–128

Hoult IJ, Crespigny LCh de, O'Herlihy C et al. (1981) Ultrasound control of clomiphene human chorionic gonadotropin stimulated cycles for oocyte recovery and in vitro fertilization. Fertil Steril 36:316–322

Johnston I, Lopata A, Speirs A et al. (1981) In-vitro fertilization: the challenge of the eighties. Fertil Steril 36:699–706

Lenz S, Lauritsen JG (1982) Ultrasonically guided percutaneous aspiration of human follicles under local anaesthesia: a new method of collecting oocytes for in-vitro fertilization. Fertil Steril 38:673–677

O'Herlihy C, Crespigny LJC de, Robinson HP (1980) Monitoring ovarian follicular development with real time ultrasound. Br J Obstet Gynaecol 87:613–618

O'Herlihy C, Pepperell RJ, Robinson HP (1982) Ultrasound timing of human chorionic gonadotropin administration in clomiphene stimulated cycles. Obstet Gynaecol 59:40–45

Sallam HN, Whithehead MI, Collins WP, Campbell S (1983) A retrospective analysis of two methods of monitoring gonadotropin therapy. Paper present at the IXth World Congress on Fertility and Sterility, Dublin

Siebel MM, McArdle CR, Thompson IE et al. (1981) The role of ultrasound in ovulation induction: a critical appraisal. Fertil Steril 36:573–577

Trounson A, Conti A (1982) Research in human in-vitro fertilisation and embryo transfer. Br Med J 285:244–248

Vargyas J, Marrs R, Kletzky O, Mishell DR Jr (1982) Correlation of ultrasonic measurement of ovarian follicle size and serum estradiol levels in ovulatory patients following clomiphene citrate for in-vitro fertilization. Am J Obstet Gynaecol 144:569–573

Wikland M, Nilsson L, Hansson R et al. (1983) Collection of human oocytes by the use of sonography. Fertil Steril 39:603–608

Wood C, Trounson A, Leeton J et al. (1981) A clinical assessment of nine pregnancies obtained by in-vitro fertilization and embryo transfer. Fertil Steril 35:502–508

Ylöstalo P, Lindgren PG, Nillius SJ (1981) Ultrasonic measurement of ovarian follicles, ovarian and uterine size during induction of ovulation with human gonadotrophins. Acta Endocrinol (Copenh) 98:592–598

16 Pathology of the Genital Tract

An understanding of the findings presented in Chap. 3 is fundamental to the diagnosis of female genital tract pathology. While 90% of publications on ultrasound prior to 1980 dealt with obstetrics, increasing attention is being focused on the importance and potential applications of ultrasound in gynecology, owing mainly to technical improvements in ultrasound instrumentation.

Holländer's recommendation that a vaginal examination be performed concurrently with real-time ultrasound as a means of resolving equivocal findings has particular relevance to gynecologic studies. Diagnostic ultrasound becomes a "seeing finger," and while every medical examination should be predicated on a proper indication, there is no reason why ultrasound should not be used even in cases without a specific indication.

16.1 Capabilities and Limitations of Sonographic Diagnosis

Uterine anomalies such as the double uterus (Fig. 16.1a, b) are manifested by the presence of two endometrial echoes. White and Lawson (1978) state that anomalies of this type are associated with other organ malformations. The bicornuate uterus (Fig. 16.1c) cannot always be reliably diagnosed with ultrasound, except with coexisting pregnancy (see Sect. 4.4), and other methods of diagnosis, such as hysteroscopy and hysterosalpingography, are superior in these cases.

Fibroids, on the other hand, are easily diagnosed with ultrasound. They occur in 20% of all women over the age of 35. Approximately 95% of fibroids are in intramural location in the uterine fundus. Although all fibroids originate intramurally, they are classified by their subsequent growth and extension as being subserous (Fig. 16.2), intramural (Fig. 16.3), or submucous (Sect. 4.4, Fig. 4.50). Often these tumors do not present as discrete foci, but instead produce a general enlargement of the uterus (Fig. 16.4). This presentation, together with palpatory findings, should be sufficient to establish a diagnosis of fibroid uterus. Although in general fibroids can be associated with the uterus (Fig. 16.5), occasionally doubts remain as to whether the uterus or the adnexa are involved. Often these doubts can be resolved by concurrent bimanual examination. In our experience, only 60%–70% of lower abdominal masses can be definitively assigned to a particular organ based on sonographic criteria alone.

Gross et al. (1983) report a sensitivity of 60% in prospective studies of 41 fibroids and 78% in retrospective evaluation, which is consistent with our experience. Kratochwil (1976) emphasized the problems involved in the evaluation of masses that have both cystic and solid components (Fig. 16.6). Palpation is even less accurate than ultrasound and will correctly assign the mass in only 40%–50% of cases. In ovarian masses tested by various investigators, we found size discrepancies of 20%–200% based on palpatory findings as compared to 80%–120% based on sonography. Similar accuracies were achieved in identifying the involved organs. However, the accuracy of sonography fell below 30% when examinations were performed by less experienced operators and when real-time linear scanners were used.

Surprisingly, nonneoplastic inflammatory lesions of the tubal region can be well visualized, even though the normal fallopian tubes are not demonstrable because of their shape and position. In cases of acute adnexitis we often find conspicuous fluid collections and distinct organ boundaries (Fig. 16.7). This is valuable, because suspicious palpatory findings are often associated with normal laboratory findings (white blood count, ESR, CRP), and symptoms regress relatively quickly after the start of thera-

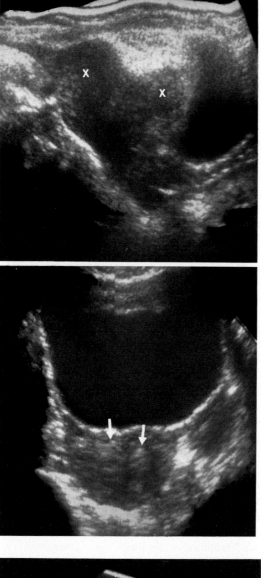

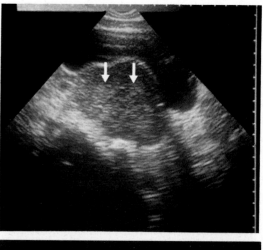

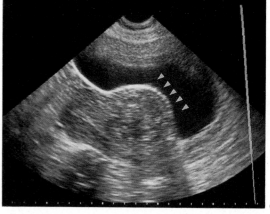

Fig. 16.1.a Longitudinal scan of a double uterus (*x-x*). **b** Transverse scan: *arrows* mark endometrial echoes. **c** Bicornuate uterus. **d** Hematoma following curettage mimicking a fibroid or a bicornuate uterus (*arrows*)

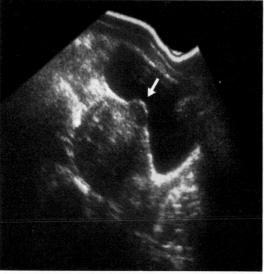

Fig. 16.2. Longitudinal scan: marked widening of uterine fundus with a small subserous fibroid on its anterior wall

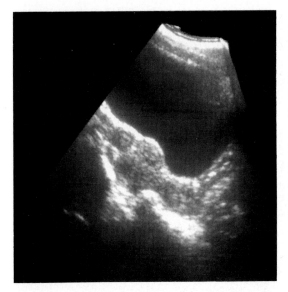

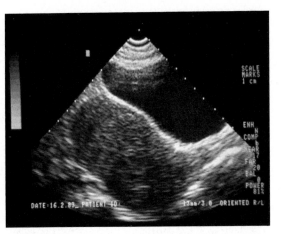

Fig. 16.4. A fibroid uterus showing marked general enlargement (width over 5 cm, length over 10 cm)

Fig. 16.3. Intramural fibroids causing minimal uterine enlargement

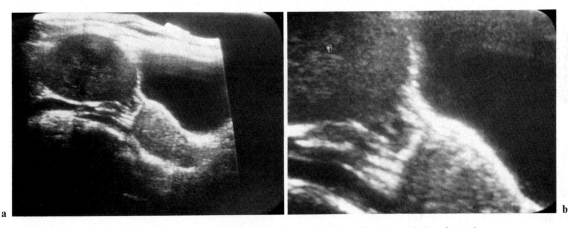

Fig. 16.5. a Longitudinal scan: large, subserous fibroid of uterus. **b** Magnified view of site of attachment

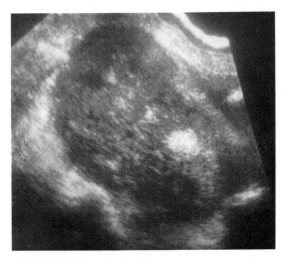

Fig. 16.6. Fibroid uterus filling lower abdomen, with hyperechoic and hypoechoic zones (calcification and degeneration)

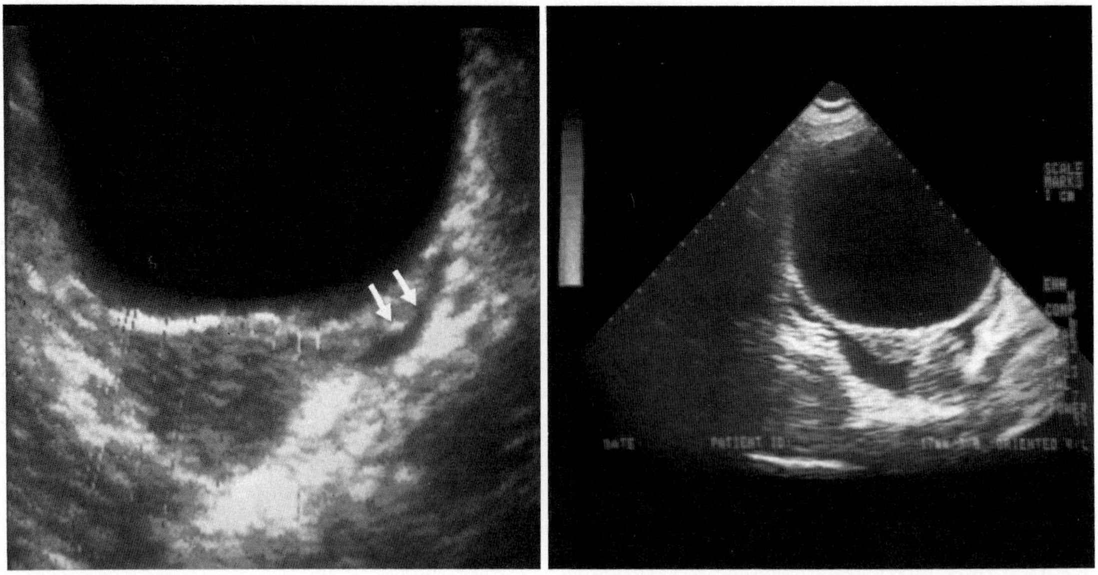

a b

Fig. 16.7a, b. Transverse scans. **a** Uterus and left fallopian tube with a fluid collection in acute left-sided adnexitis. **b** Fluid collections in both adnexal regions and cul-de-sac with bilateral adnexitis

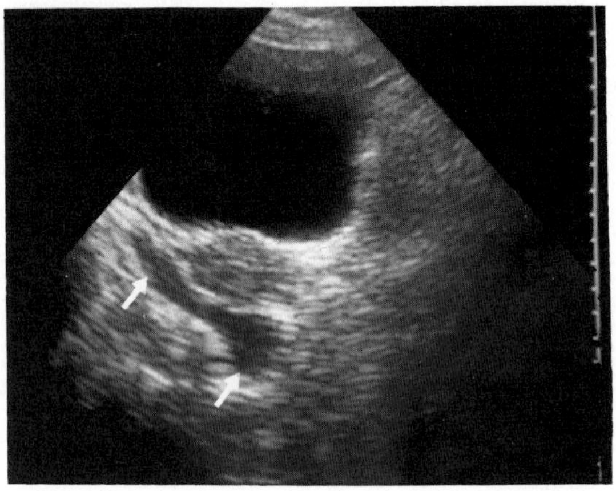

Fig. 16.8. Transverse scan: left fallopian tube is markedly thickened, fluid-filled and rigid; chronic adnexitis

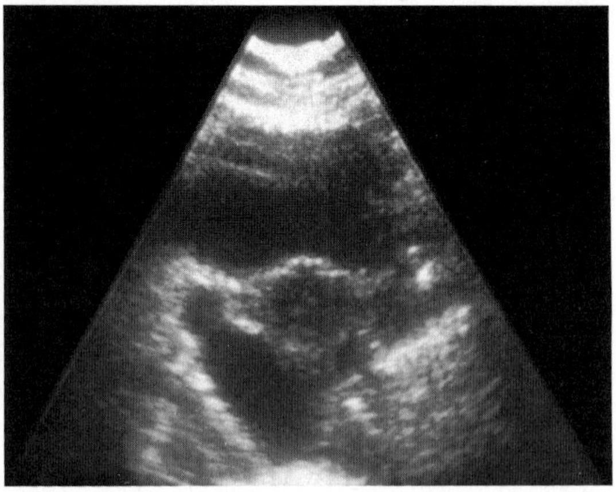

Fig. 16.9. Transverse scan: cystic dilatation of right fallopian tube in hydrosalpinx

py, raising questions of diagnosis that ultimately may have to be resolved by laparoscopy. Noninvasive, risk-free sonography can eliminate the need for more invasive procedures in many patients.

If the inflammation goes untreated for a prolonged period, the adnexal region becomes more difficult to evaluate with ultrasound, although individual portions of the fallopian tubes can be demonstrated (Fig. 16.8). Visualization of pyo- and hydrosalpinx (Fig. 16.9) is easier due to their favorable acoustic properties.

Tuboovarian abscesses are well visualized owing to their cystic components, with echoes in the mass showing the presence of purulent material (Fig. 16.10). In such cases it is important to perform serial examinations while anti-inflammatory therapy is being administered. Sometimes the presence of a capsule-like border can mimic an ovarian cyst or tumor, providing an incorrect indication for surgery. These cases show again that sonographic findings alone cannot always be considered specific.

Often situations arise that require differentia-

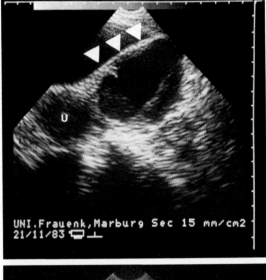

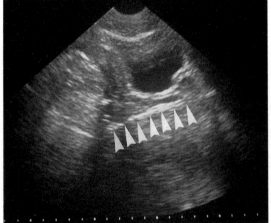

Fig. 16.10. a Transverse scan: fluid collection with internal echoes. Left tuboovarian abscess (*arrows*) *U*, uterus. **b** Following drainage of abscess of cul-de-sac: catheter still in place (*arrows*)

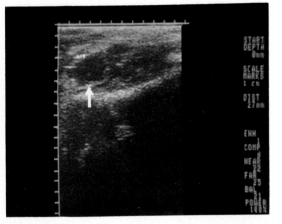

Fig. 16.11. Longitudinal scan. Patient had pain in the lower right quadrant. Adnexa appear normal. A cystic area (diameter (27 mm) is visible over psoas muscle. Periappendiceal abscess associated with appendicitis

tion between adnexitis and appendicitis. If adnexal findings are negative in these cases, the psoas region should be examined for a periappendiceal abscess (Fig. 16.11). Abscesses descending from a more cranial area into the pelvis can lead to false interpretations.

Although the diagnosis of large endometriomas (Fig. 16.12a) is usually straightforward, more subtle findings, especially in the region of the cul-de-sac, may be difficult to differentiate from other lesions, artifacts, and bowel loops (Fig. 16.12b). If the findings are confirmed, follow-up studies should be scheduled to monitor the efficacy of surgical or hormonal therapy. Ultrasound is not a satisfactory prima-

ry modality for confirming endometriosis, however (Walsh et al. 1979).

Next to inflammatory changes, ovarian cysts are the most common pathologic finding in the pelvis. They are relatively easy to diagnose with ultrasound owing to their well-defined borders and secondary acoustic phenomena (see Chaps. 3, 4, 15). There is no need to discuss the broad range of simple paraovarian and ovarian cysts, which cannot always be differentiated. It should be noted that functional follicular and corpus luteum cysts are indistinguishable sonographically from true neoplasms. Internal echoes may be a feature of corpus luteum cysts, endometriomas, and abscesses, as well as tumors. The indication for surgery should thus not rest on sonographic findings alone.

Ovarian cystadenomas (Fig. 16.13) are an absolute indication for surgery, not only because of their size, but also because of their partially solid contents. Dermoids or dermoid cysts can vary greatly in their composition, and in extreme cases are indistinguishable from simple cysts. They account for 20% of all ovarian cysts and 10% of ovarian tumors, and usually give the appearance of a very homogeneous, dense, solid, echogenic mass surrounded by a less echogenic capsule (Fig. 16.14). The back wall of the mass may not be demonstrated due to acoustic absorption, or it may cast a distinct acoustic shadow (Fig. 16.15). This feature is highly characteristic, because the masses associated with hemorrhagic cysts, endometriosis,

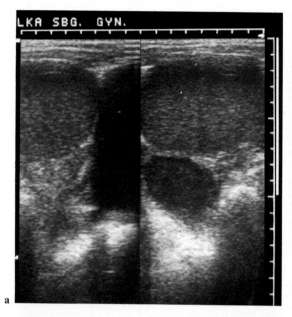

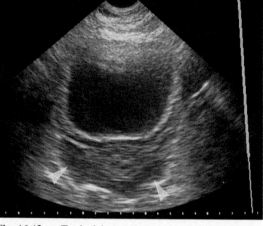

Fig. 16.12. a Typical internal structure of an endometrioma (chocolate cyst): second cyst of equal size located behind first appears "emptier" because of echo absorption by first cyst. **b** Longitudinal scan: poorly defined, irregular, hypoechoic areas behind uterus and in cul-desac (*arrows*) in endometriosis

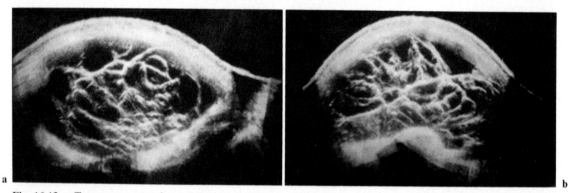

Fig. 16.13. a Transverse scan of a multilocular cystic mass filling abdomen: ovarian cystadenoma. **b** Longitudinal scan of same mass

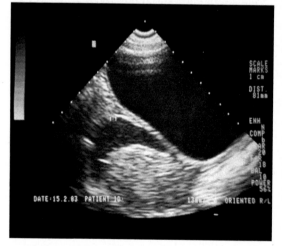

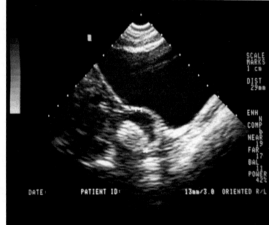

Fig. 16.14. Longitudinal scan showing a highly echogenic ovarian mass with less echogenic capsule: dermoid (diameter 81 mm)

Fig. 16.15. Longitudinal scan depicting a small mass (29 mm) with an echo pattern similar to that in Fig. 16.14: dermoid

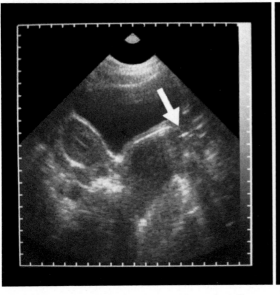

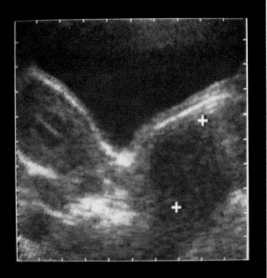

Fig. 16.16. a Longitudinal scan showing marked distension (*arrow*) of vagina (diameter 3.6 cm) in hematocolpos: neglected vaginal tampon. Uterine cavity is dilated. b Magnified view of affected area

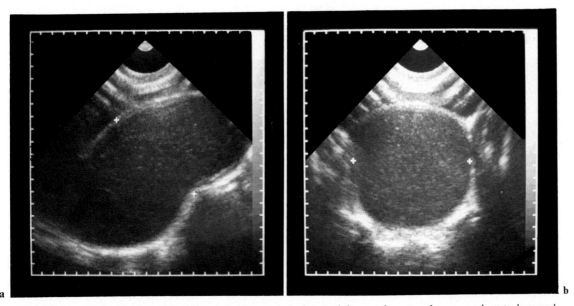

Fig. 16.17. a Longitudinal scan showing a complex mass in lower abdomen: hematocolpos secondary to hymenal atresia. b Same case: transverse scan (diameter 9.9 cm)

ectopic pregnancy, and tuboovarian abscess can be very similar in appearance to dermoid cysts, but none produces an acoustic shadow. Benign solid ovarian tumors are rare, and it is clear that ultrasound cannot distinguish benign from malignant lesions in the case of a dermoid cyst or any other mass.

Cystic masses, even if large, do not necessarily involve the uterus or adnexa. Hematocolpos can have varying causes and degrees. Figure 16.16 shows a case resulting from a neglected vaginal tampon. The uterine cavity is distended, and the fluid collection is almost 4 cm in diameter (Fig. 16.16b). The patient had

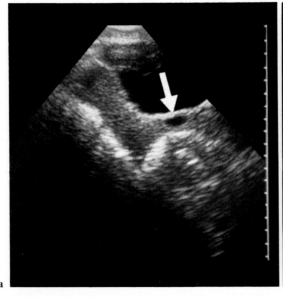

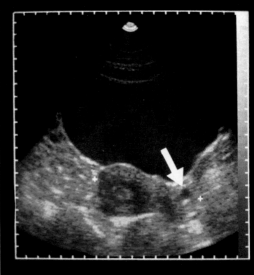

a   b

Fig. 16.18. a Longitudinal scan of uterus showing a small cystic mass (*arrow*) in vaginal wall: Gartner's duct cyst.

b Longitudinal scan showing similar cystic area (*arrow*) in cervix: Naboth's follicle

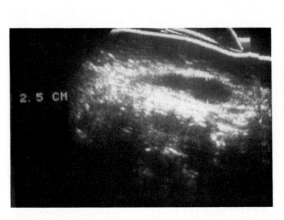

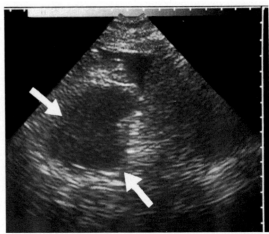

Fig. 16.19. Longitudinal scan of an abdominal wall hematoma (diameter 2.5 cm) following laparotomy

Fig. 16.20. Longitudinal scan of an intraabdominal hematoma (*arrows*) following laparotomy

severe complaints, as did the patient with hematocolpos secondary to hymenal atresia (Fig. 16.17). This problem is by no means rare, and sonography in such cases is an excellent adjunct to gynecologic examination (Seiler 1979).

The solitary use of ultrasound in such cases might prompt suspicion of a complex lower abdominal mass (in this case 10 cm) and result in an unnecessary laparoscopy.

The imaging of cysts in the vagina and cervical region (Fig. 16.18) serves less as an indication for surgery than as a means of demonstrating the capabilities of ultrasound. The sonographic appearance of the Gartner's duct cyst (Fig. 16.18a) supplements and confirms palpatory findings, while the cervical inclusion cyst (Fig. 16.18b) tends to be an incidental finding.

The postoperative use of ultrasound is of definite value when there is suspicion of an abdom-

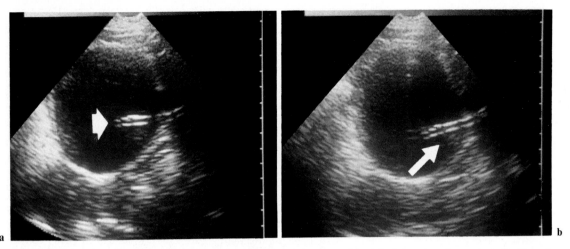

Fig. 16.21 a, b. Longitudinal scans. A bladder catheter indicates urethrovesical junction (*arrows*). **a** Resting; **b** straining. There is little descent of urethrovesical junction (normal case)

inal wall hematoma (Fig. 16.19) or an intraabdominal hematoma (Fig. 16.20). Serial observations in such cases is easily accomplished even in critically ill patients and can greatly assist surgical decision making. Possible coexisting conditions, such as hydronephrosis from ureteral obstruction, can also be evaluated.

White et al. (1980) and Bernaschek et al. (1981) report the use of ultrasound in patients with urinary stress incontinence. Scans of the urethrovesical junction may be particularly use-ful and demonstrate typical changes in the incontinent patient (Figs. 16.21 and 16.22); we have been able to confirm this in our own studies. Evidence indicates that sonography may be just as accurate as radiography in depicting the posterior urethrovesical junction, and offer the additional advantage of demonstrating coexisting lesions such as fibroids. Presumably, diagnostic ultrasound could also aid in the selection and monitoring of continence-restoring operations.

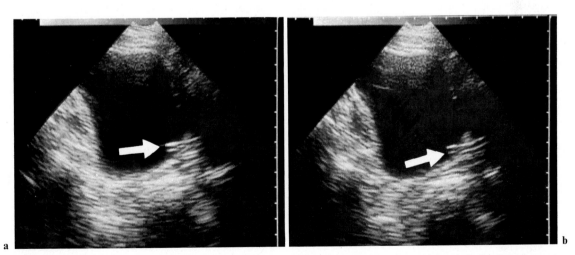

Fig. 16.22. a–e Longitudinal scans. **a** Urethrovesical junction is already low at rest (*arrow*). **b** Straining causes marked descent (*arrow*).

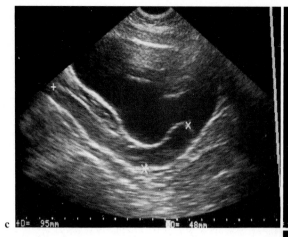
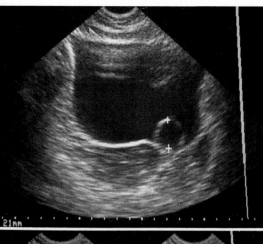
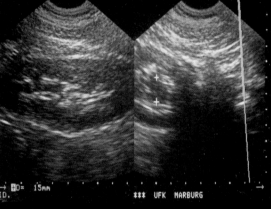

Fig. 16.22c–e. c Englarged ureterocele on right. **d** Transverse scan: ureterocele within urinary bladder (21 mm). **e** Longitudinal scan: normal left kidney, hydronephrosis of right kidney

References

Bernaschek KG, Spernol R, Wolf G, Kratochwil A (1981) Vergleichende Bestimmung des Urethra-Blasenwinkels bei Inkontinenzfällen mittels Ultraschall und lateralem Urethrozystogramm. Geburtshilfe Frauenheilkd 41:339

Fleischer AC, James AE, Krause DA, Millis JB (1978) Differential diagnosis of pelvic masses by grey scale ultrasound. Am J Radiol 131:469

Gross BH, Silver TM, Jaffe MH (1983) Sonographic features of uterine leiomyomas. U Ultrasound Med 2:401

Kratochwil A (1976) Ultraschalldiagnostik in der Gynäkologie. Gynäkologe 9:166

Micsky L von (1977) Sonographic study of uterine fibromyomata in the non-pregnant state and during gestation. In: Sanders RC, James AE (eds) Ultrasonography in obstetrics and gynecology. Appleton-Century-Croft, New York, pp 297

Morley P, Barnett E (1980) The ovarian mass. In: Sanders R, James E (eds) Ultrasonography in obstetrics and gynecology, 2nd edn. Appleton-Century-Crofts, New York

Seiler JF (1979) Hematometra and hematocolpos: ultrasound findings. Am J Radiol 132:1010

Ulrich PC, Sanders RC (1976) Ultrasonic characteristics of pelvic inflammatory masses. J Clin Ultrasound 4:199

Walsh JW, Taylor KJW, Wasson JFM, Schwartz PE, Rosenfield AT (1979) Gray-scale ultrasonography in the diagnosis of endometriosis and adenomyosis. Am J Radiol 132:87

White JL, Lawson TL (1978) Congenital uterine anomaly with renal agenesis. J Clin Ultrasound 6:117

White RD, McQuown D, McCarthy T, Ostergard DR (1980) Real-time ultrasonography in the evaluation of urinary stress incontinence. Am J Obstet Gynecol 138:235

16.2 Applications of Ultrasound in Oncology

The early detection of gynecologic tumors is not possible with ultrasound. While this statement is basically true, it requires qualification. Campbell et al. (1982) used compound and real-time scanners to measure ovarian volumes in the hope that comparison of both ovaries would permit the early detection of unilateral changes. Structural changes indeed occur very early in some cases (Fig. 16.23a), but primary attention should be given to marked ovarian enlargement in postmenopausal women (Fig. 16.23b). On the other hand, structural anomalies can be seen in association with certain chromosome disorders (Turner's syndrome; Fig. 16.23c).

With improved resolution, it has become possible to delineate even small cystic masses (Fig. 16.23b). This is important, because ca. 94% of all carcinomas contain cystic components, and the majority of epithelial tumors (about 85% of all malignant ovarian tumors) are cystic (McGrowan 1978; Fig. 16.24a). Whether early solid tumors that invade the ovarian capsule are detectable with ultrasound remains to be determined. It is known that asymmetry of the ovaries can be detected early by the measurement of ovarian volumes. In a prospective screening study of 1,084 postmenopausal women, Campbell et al. (1982) and Goswamy et al. (1983) obtained useful information from ovarian scans in 1,077 of them. Gross obesity, dense adhesions, tiny ovaries, and inability to fill the bladder adequately were reasons for failure to demonstrate the ovaries. 1,041 subjects were found to be normal, while 15 had "abnormal" ovarian findings which prompted surgical procedures to obtain a histologic diagnosis. Besides one true carcinoma (FIGO stage 1), there were at least nine lesions (serous cysts with adenofibromatous nodules, mucinous cystadenomas, dermoid cysts, papillary serous cystadenomas) that had to be classified as potentially malignant. Based on these results, Campbell performed a cost-benefit analysis and was able to confirm the efficacy of a screening program for Great Britain.

This approach is undoubtedly more promising than the postprocessing that is sometimes used as an adjunct to tumor imaging by ultrasound (Fig. 16.24b, c). A computer can only process the information that is supplied to it by the equipment, and an abundance of solid material in a cystic mass (Fig. 16.25) is highly suggestive of a malignancy with or without postprocessing.

We know of no case in which postprocessing disclosed information about a tumor that could not have been derived from the unprocessed image. Neither have transvaginal or transrectal

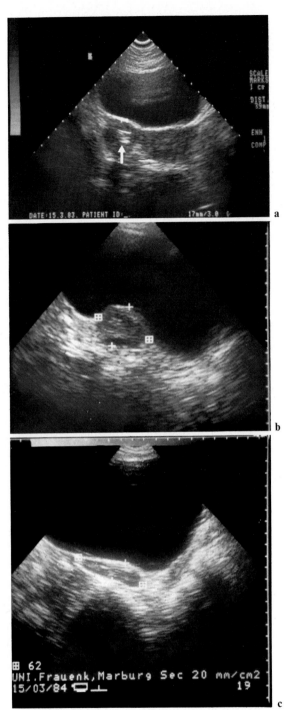

Fig. 16.23. a Transverse scan of a 55-year-old woman with marked enlargement of right ovary (3.9 cm), which shows solid components: right ovarian carcinoma, acoustic shadowing (*arrow*). **b** Longitudinal scan of an enlarged ovary (3.7 × 4.8 cm) in a 49-year-old menopausal woman: ovarian carcinoma. **c** Longitudinal scan of an ovary in Turner's syndrome (XO): both ovarian shape (6.2 × 1.9 cm) and hyperechoic capsule are abnormal

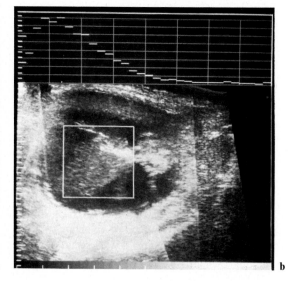

a

c

Fig. 16.24. a Longitudinal scan showing predominantly cystic mass over uterus: ovarian carcinoma. **b** Transverse scan: "area histogram" of an ovarian carcinoma (postprocessing). **c** Same case: "internal surface" (postprocessing)

probes been effective in improving ultrasound diagnosis. It is possible that intraoperative ultrasound in cases identified by Campbell's proposed screening procedure can provide a means for the early detection of ovarian carcinoma.

Some investigators have attempted a differentiation of benign and malignant tumors on the basis of ultrasound findings. So far these studies have not yielded useful results, because the appearance of carcinomas may range from predominantly cystic to completely solid.

In patients with ovarian carcinomas treated primarily with cytostatics or in cases of recurrence after surgery, ultrasound can be used to determine the extent of the tumor and the approximate relation of cystic to solid components. Progression or regression of the tumor can be verified by examinations at intervals of 1–3 months, depending on the extent of the tumor and the condition of the patient. With ap-

propriate documentation of findings, the progress of the disease can be closely monitored, and treatment can be modified. We have seen cases of apparent clinical regression in which sonograms demonstrated only a reduction of the cystic components of the tumor relative to its solid components (or vice versa), raising doubt as to whether a regression had really occurred.

The endometrial evaluation presented in Chap. 15 can also be useful in the detection of uterine cancer. Thus, the demonstration of menstrual-cycle-like endometrial changes in postmenopausal women would be highly suggestive of carcinoma and should be evaluated by D & C (Fig. 16.26a–c). Polyposis may be a precancerous stage and, in the present case, was found during the course of a tumor search. A corpus carcinoma was already present (Fig. 16.26d, e). Kratochwil, in 1976, pointed

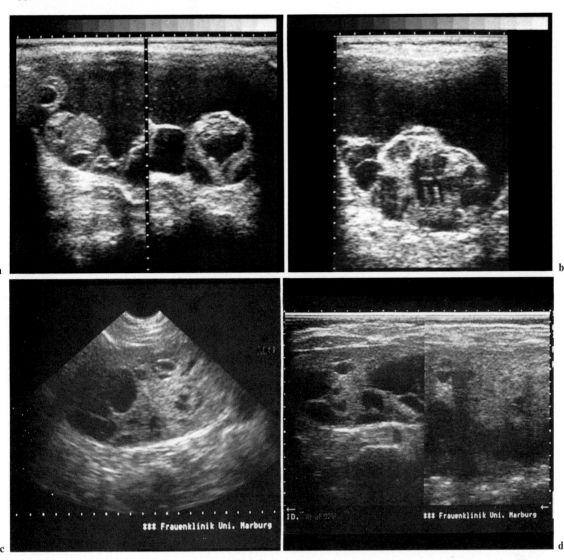

Fig. 16.25a, b. Typical ovarian carcinoma with cystic and solid components and internal echoes from viscous contents. **c, d** Adreoblastoma, partially malignant

out the value of ultrasound in planning the radiotherapy of cervical and other carcinomas.

Of course, sections through the whole body of patients with gynecologic tumors can be performed only with compound scanners. The sonograms obtained provide accurate information on the depth of the tumor, its extent, and its relationship to adjacent organs. Ultrasound can also aid in the planning of intracavitary radiotherapy. It can assist in choosing the most appropriate applicator for a given uterus and can determine the distance of the radiation sources from the bladder and rectal wall so that

the doses delivered to these organs can be accurately calculated (Brascho and Kim 1978).

In some cases endometrial changes have been observed with ultrasound following irradiation therapy of the uterus (Fig. 16.27).

When a palpable mass is noted on gynecologic examination, an ultrasound scan of the pelvis may yield surprising results in other organs (Fig. 16.28), which again underscores the value of the supplementary ultrasound examination.

The demonstration of cervical carcinoma is limited to advanced cases (Fig. 16.29) and so

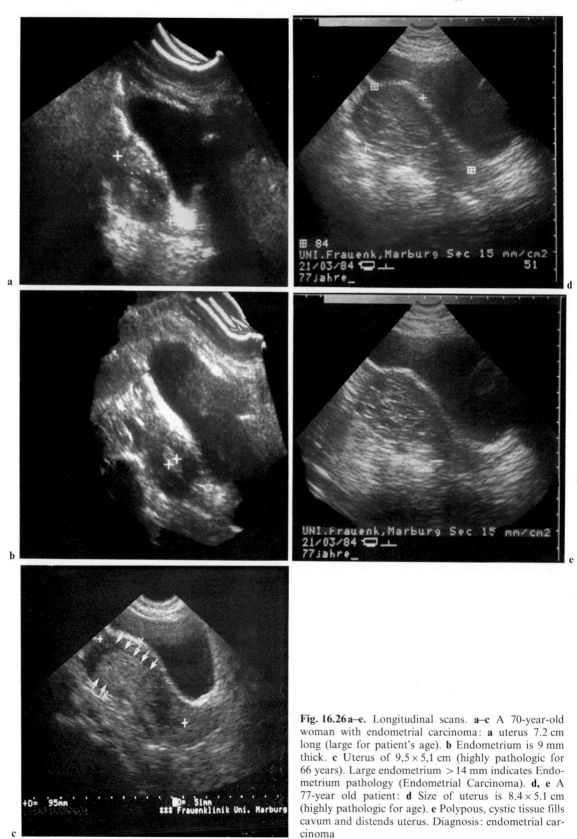

Fig. 16.26a–e. Longitudinal scans. **a–c** A 70-year-old woman with endometrial carcinoma: **a** uterus 7.2 cm long (large for patient's age). **b** Endometrium is 9 mm thick. **c** Uterus of 9,5 × 5,1 cm (highly pathologic for 66 years). Large endometrium > 14 mm indicates Endometrium pathology (Endometrial Carcinoma). **d, e** A 77-year old patient: **d** Size of uterus is 8.4 × 5.1 cm (highly pathologic for age). **e** Polypous, cystic tissue fills cavum and distends uterus. Diagnosis: endometrial carcinoma

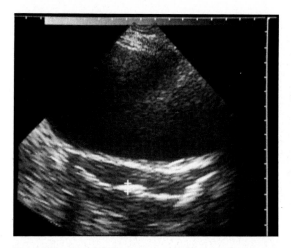

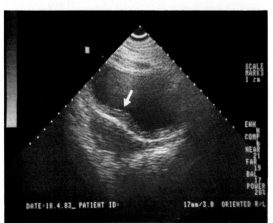

Fig. 16.27. Longitudinal scan: endometrial changes (5 mm thick, highly echogenic) following radium insertion and subsequent external megavoltage irradiation for endometrial carcinoma

Fig. 16.28. Longitudinal scan. Diagnosis at referral: adnexal mass. Findings: Uterus and adnexa unremarkable, abnormal echogenic structures in urinary bladder. Final diagnosis: bladder carcinoma

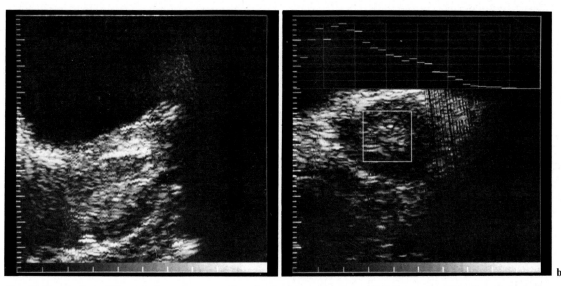

Fig. 16.29a, b. State III cervical carcinoma. **a** Longitudinal scan: tumor well delineated within distended cervix. **b** Transverse scan: area histogram (echo distribution in tumor)

far has not contributed to preoperative tumor staging. Infiltration of the parametria cannot be reliably diagnosed with ultrasound, whereas tumor recurrences or involved pelvic wall lymph nodes can be visualized before they are palpable clinically (Fig. 16.30). Coexisting venous or ureteral changes are also demonstrable (Fig. 16.31a, b). Besides visualization of the tumor, the observation of other related intraabdominal structures is important. The greater omentum is demonstrable in normal cases (Fig. 16.32) and is even more obvious when thickened as a result of infiltration or metastasis (Fig. 16.33).

Visualization is enhanced in the presence of ascites, which is easily seen between the abdominal wall and bowel loops and often cannot be demonstrated clinically, especially in obese patients. This problem frequently arises in oncologic aftercare. With benign ascites, change of the position of the patient will cause shifting of the ascites and movement of the bowel loops,

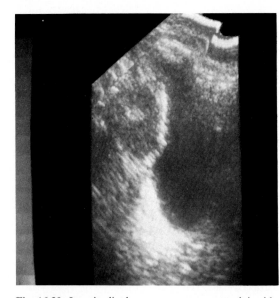

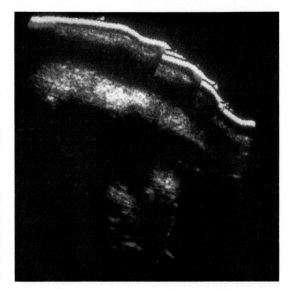

Fig. 16.30. Longitudinal scan: recurrence at pelvic side wall following radical hysterectomy for cervical carcinoma

Fig. 16.32. Longitudinal scan: greater omentum

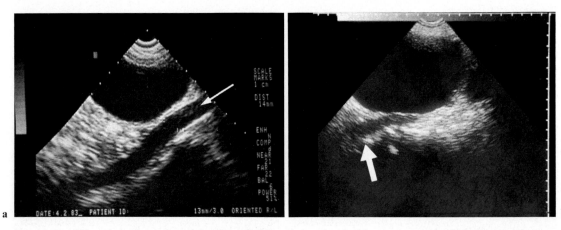

Fig. 16.31. a Distended vein at the pelvic side wall (14 mm) associated with tumor recurrence. **b** Obstructed ureter (*arrow*)

which float freely on the ascitic fluid. With carcinoma-associated ascites, on the other hand, there may be adhesions of the bowel loops, which in turn are fixed at the mesenteric root so that they no longer float freely on the fluid surface, but appear like a "mushroom cloud" (Kratochwil 1976) surrounded by fluid. If there is loculation of the ascites, ultrasound plays a role not only in the detection of the ascites, but also in its aspiration. Especially after multiple aspirations, there is likely to be adhesion of the bowel loops to the abdominal wall and

loculation of the ascites, in which case ultrasound can contribute to a successful aspiration (Figs. 16.34 and 16.35).

With a suspected tumor or unexplained ascites, it is always wise to examine the upper abdomen, specifically the liver, to ensure that metastases (Figs. 16.36–16.38) or pleural effusion (Fig. 16.39) are not overlooked.

Regular sonograms of the liver are an essential part of cytostatic therapy and follow-up after oncologic treatment. Liver scans also provide an indirect means of monitoring treatment

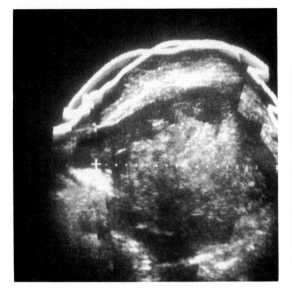

Fig. 16.33. Transverse scan: large, solid lower abdominal mass (ovarian carcinoma) of 18.5 cm diameter, over which omentum is visibly thickened

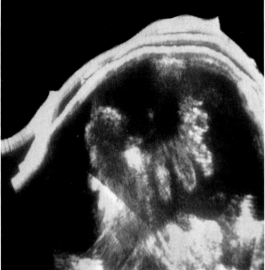

Fig. 16.35. Transverse scan through middle of abdomen in ovarian carcinoma. Note "fingerlike" loops of bowel within ascites

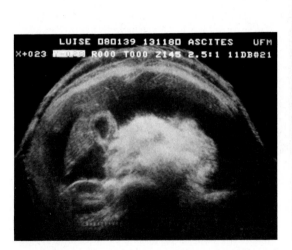

Fig. 16.34. Transverse scan at junction of middle and upper quadrants in ovarian carcinoma: ascites, fixed loops of small bowel, parts of liver and gallbladder, right kidney

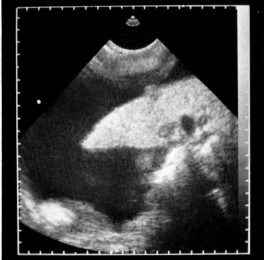

Fig. 16.36. Liver scan in ovarian carcinoma: multiple hypoechoic areas (metastases) and ascites

response, especially in patients with breast carcinoma (see also Chap. 18).

On the whole, we feel that the safety and capability of ultrasound give it an important role in oncologic diagnosis and treatment. Recurrences following primary surgical treatment can be detected earlier than with clinical methods. Infiltration of the bladder is readily identifiable even in a very early stage, whereas rectal involvement is demonstrable only occasionally. Serial sonographic monitoring is also appropriate for postsurgical or postirradiation pa-

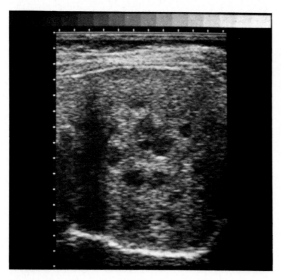

Fig. 16.37. Liver with multiple hypoechoic areas (metastases) in a patient with ovarian carcinoma

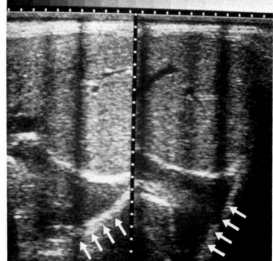

Fig. 16.39. Sagittal scan: liver unremarkable, but large pleural effusion visible (*arrows*)

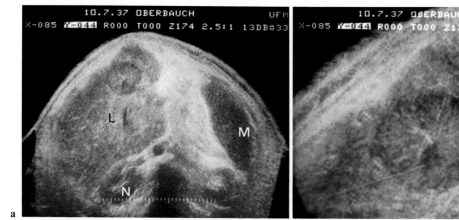

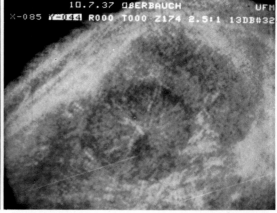

Fig. 16.38a, b. Transverse whole-body scan of a 21-year-old woman: spleen (*M*), liver (*L*), both kidneys (*N*). Echogenic area with hypoechoic border represents metastasis from breast carcinoma. Liver and spleen are enlarged

tients in whom extreme shortening of the vagina or scar formation prevent adequate gynecologic examination.

References

Blake D (1979) Transrectal ultrasonography in the evaluation of cervical carcinoma. Obstet Gynecol 53:105–108

Brascho D (1975) Radiation therapy planning with ultrasound. Radiol Clin North Am 13:505–521

Brascho D (1977) Tumor localization and treatment planning with ultrasound. Cancer 39:697–705

Brascho D, Kim R (1978) Use of ultrasonography in planning intracavitary radiotherapy of endometrial carcinoma. Radiology 129:163–167

Campbell S, Goessens L, Goswamy R, Whitehead MI (1982) Real-time ultrasonography for determination of ovarian morphology and volume. A possible early screening test for ovarian cancer. Lancet I:425–426

Doll R, Muir C, Waterhouse J (1970) Cancer incidence in five continents. International Union Against Cancer, vol II. Springer, Berlin Heidelberg New York

Donald I (1963) Use of ultrasonics in diagnosis of abdominal swellings. Br Med J II:1154–1155

Fleischer AC, Wentz ACC, Jones HW, Everette-James A Jr (1983) Ultrasound evaluation of the ovary. In: Hobbins JC, Winsberg F, Berkowitz RL (eds) Ultrasonography in obstetrics and gynecology, 2nd edn. Williams & Wilkins, London, pp 209–225

Goldberg B, Goodman C, Clearfield H (1970) Evaluation of ascites by ultrasound. Radiology 96:15–22

Goswamy RK, Campbell S, Whitehead MI (1983) Screening for Ovarian Cancer. In: Campbell S (ed) Clinics in obstetrics and gynaecology, vol 10 No 3. Saunders, London, p 621

Koyabashi M (1967) Use of diagnostic ultrasound in trophoblastic neoplasm and ovarian tumors. Cancer 38:441–452

Kratochwil A (1970) Ultrasonic diagnosis in pelvic malignancy. Clin Obstet Gynecol 13:898–909

Kratochwil A (1976) Ultraschalldiagnostik in der Gynäkologie. Gynäkologe 9:166–180

Lawson T, Albarelli J (1977) Diagnosis of gynecologic pelvic masses by gray scale ultrasonography: analysis of specificity and accuracy. Am J Roentgenol 128:1003–1006

Levi S, Delval R (1976) Value of ultrasonic diagnosis of gynecologic tumors in 370 surgical cases. Obstet Gynecol Scand 55:261–266

McGrowan L (1978) Ovarian Cancer. In: McGrowan (ed) Gynecologie oncology. Appleton-Century Crofts, New York, pp 283–299

Meire HB, Farrant P, Guha T (1978) Distinction of benign from malignant ovarian cysts by ultrasound. Br J Obstet Gynaecol 85:893–899

Morley P, Barnett E (1970) The use of ultrasound in the diagnosis of pelvic masses. Br J Radiol 43:602–616

Parker RT, Parker CH, Wilbanks GD (1970) Cancer of the ovary. Survival studies based upon operative therapy, chemotherapy and radiotherapy. Am J Obstet Gynecol 108:878–888

Paling MR, Shawker TH (1981) Abdominal ultrasound in advanced ovarian carcinoma. J Clin Ultrasound 9:435

17 Intrauterine Contraceptive Devices

The intrauterine contraceptive device (IUCD) is considered to be the second most effective method of preventing pregnancy after oral contraceptives. However, several studies (Schmidt et al. 1978; Meyenburg et al. 1981; Bernascheck 1981) indicate that this efficacy depends (1) on the type of IUCD, (2) on the uterine anatomy of the user, and (3) on the interaction between the IUCD and the user, and is therefore subject to variation. Displacement of the IUCD is responsible for approximately 30% of contraceptive failures in these patients. The position of the IUCD can be checked using ultrasound, with attention directed to several points.

First, the portion of the device visible within the uterus should be measured (Fig. 17.1). A useful parameter is the measurable distance between the fundal end of the IUCD and the surface of the uterine fundus (Fig. 17.2a). As a rule, this distance should not exceed 2 cm.

However, this measurement does not take into account the individual thickness of the uterine wall, and so it is not always clear how the IUCD is actually positioned within the uterus. This led Bernascheck (1981a) to propose a formula that corrects for the thickness of the uterine wall. According to this formula, the IUCD is correctly positioned only if the distance between the uterine fundus and the fundal end of the IUCD is less than

$$\frac{\text{anterior wall thickness} + \text{posterior wall thickness}}{2} \cdot \frac{4}{3}$$

This formula appears to be practical, especially for examiners who are experienced enough to obtain truly accurate measurements of the uterine walls (Fig. 17.2b).

With some IUCDs it is necessary to confirm intrauterine extension of the lateral arms, requiring that both longitudinal and transverse scans be obtained (Figs. 17.3, 17.4). As Kratochwil noted in 1976, a perforating IUCD can usually be demonstrated only if some portion of it remains in utero. An IUCD that has perforated into the peritoneal cavity cannot be visualized.

An IUCD that has been displaced into the lower uterine segment (Fig. 17.5) should definitely be removed. We have seen cases in which IUCD displacement was a recurring problem. In these patients the length of the endometrial cavity should be determined with ultrasound, and an IUCD of appropriate size and configuration selected.

We recommend checking the position of the IUCD during the first days after insertion and again after the first or second menstruation. We have found that these are the times when most displacements occur. Additional scans at 6-month intervals are recommended.

When intrauterine pregnancy occurs in a patient with an IUCD, the position of the IUCD should be checked in relation to the gestational

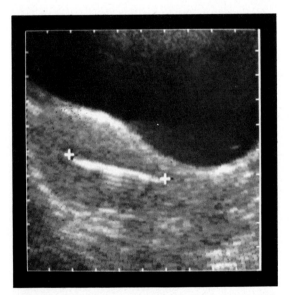

Fig. 17.1. Position check: longitudinal scan. IUCD, with a length of 41 mm, is correctly positioned within uterine cavity

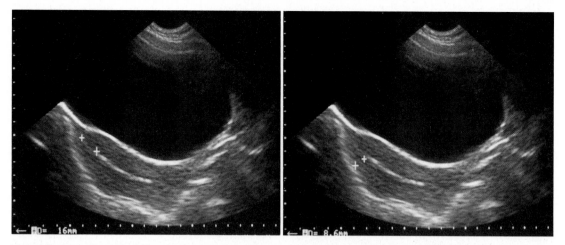

Fig. 17.2. a Position check: longitudinal scan. Measurement of fundus-IUCD distance (16 mm). **b** Measurement of myometrial thickness (8.6 mm)

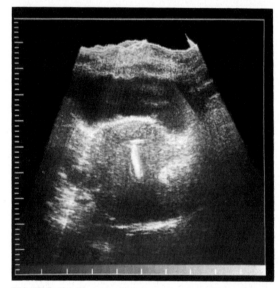

Fig. 17.3. Position check: transverse scan. Lateral arms of T-shaped IUCD are extended

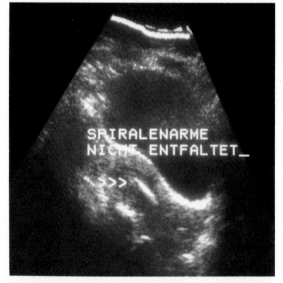

Fig. 17.4. Longitudinal scan: lateral arms of IUCD are not extended

sac (Figs. 17.6, 17.7). If the IUCD is immediately adjacent to the gestational sac (Fig. 17.8), removal may pose an increased risk to the pregnancy. However, if the IUCD is already in the cervix and the gestational sac is high in the fundus (Fig. 17.9), it should be possible to remove the device without disturbing the pregnancy.

As in ultrasound examinations in early pregnancy, retroflexion of the uterus can sometimes be a problem when attempting to demonstrate an IUCD. This is especially true when real-time linear scanners with high-resolution transducers are used, for the depth of penetration of these devices is often inadequate to delineate the re-

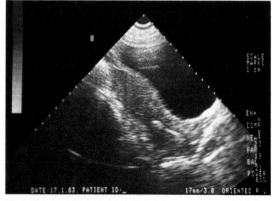

Fig. 17.5. IUCD has been displaced into lower uterine segment and is partly intracervical

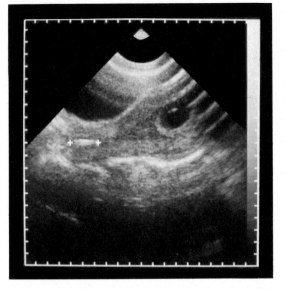

Fig. 17.6. Longitudinal scan: IUCD has been expelled almost into vagina, and there is an intrauterine gestational sac (7 weeks)

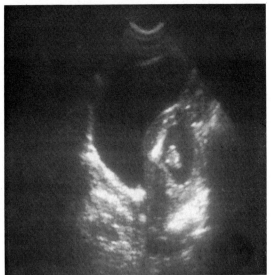

Fig. 17.8. Longitudinal scan: intact intrauterine pregnancy (8 weeks) with an IUCD directly adjacent to gestational sac

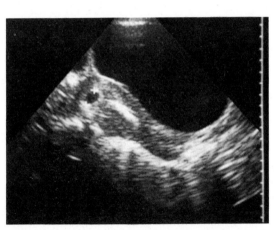

Fig. 17.7. Longitudinal scan: IUCD is seen immediately adjacent to an empty gestational sac (6 weeks; blighted ovum)

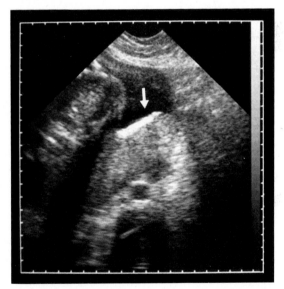

Fig. 17.9. Longitudinal scan of an intact pregnancy (24 weeks): IUCD (*arrow*) is adjacent to posterior placenta for its full length

troflexed uterus and the IUCD within it. In these cases, as in almost all gynecologic investigations, the sector scanner is preferred.

Given the relatively high incidence of ectopic gestation in patients with IUCDs [accounting for 50% of all pregnancies in IUCD users, (FDA 1978)], every ultrasound examination should include an evaluation of the adnexal region. In addition, consideration should be given to the possibility of partial or complete duplication of the uterus, where the IUCD can be located in one horn and the pregnancy in the other (see Fig. 4.54).

References

Bernascheck G, Endler M, Beck A (1981a) Zur Lagekontrolle von Intrauterinpessaren. Geburtshilfe Frauenheilkd 41:566

Bernaschek G, Spernol R, Beck A (1981b) IUD – Lage bei intrauterinen Schwangerschaften. Geburtshilfe Frauenheilkd 41:645

Cochrane WJ, Thomas MA (1972) The use of ultrasound B-mode scanning in the localization of intrauterine contraceptive devices. Radiology 104:623–627

Ianniruberto A, Mastroberadino A (1972) Ultrasound loclization of the Lippes Loop. Am J Obstet Gynecol 114:78–82

Kratochwil A (1976) Ultraschalldiagnostik in der Gynäkologie. Gynäkologe 9:166–180

McArdle CR (1978) Ultrasonic locallization of missing intrauterine contraceptive devices. Obstet Gynecol 51:330–333

The Medical Device and Drug Advisory Commitees of Obstetrics and Gynecology (1978) Second Report on Intrauterine Contrazeptive Devices. Department of Health. Education and Welfare – Food and Drug Administration, Washington, D.C.U.S.

Meyenburg M, Höbich D, Hein H-W (1981) Sonographische Darstellung von Cu-T-Intrauterinpessaren. Ultraschall 2:153

Nelson LH, Miller JB (1979) Real-time ultrasound in locating intrauterine contraceptive devices. Obstet Gynecol 54:711–714

Nemes G, Kerenyi TD (1971) Ultrasonic localization of the IUCD: A new technique. Am J Obstet Gynecol 109:1219–1220

Ory HW (1981) Ectopic pregnancy and intrauterine contraceptive devices: New perspectives. Obstet Gynecol 57:137–144

Schmidt EG, Wagner H, Quackernack K, Beller FK (1979) Ergebnisse der Lageüberwachung von Intrauterinpessaren durch Ultraschall. Geburtshilfe Frauenheilkd 39:138

Winters HS (1966) Ultrasound detection of intrauterine contraceptive devices. Am J Obstet Gynecol 95:880–882

Wittmann BK, Chow TS (1976) Diagnostic ultrasound in the management of patients using intrauterine contraceptive devices. Br J Obstet Gynaecol 83:802

18 Diagnosis of Breast Disease

Imaging of the female breast with ultrasound was first performed in the early 1950s by Wild and Neal (1951, 1952), but the method did not gain wide acceptance due to the need for specially designed machines that were not available commercially. Only after ultrasound diagnosis became firmly established in other areas were special breast scanners developed, most notably through the efforts of the Japanese groups of Kobayashi (1974) and Wagai et al. (1967) and the Australian groups of Kossoff and Jellins (from 1971 to 1975). The introduction of the gray-scale technique by the same groups, combined with the use of automated water-bath scanners, provided greatly enhanced images of the female breast. It must be emphasized, however, that while instruments have been specially developed for breast examination, their capabilities are not inherently superior to those of good real-time scanners, because they have the same limitations of resolution. Nevertheless, the over view provided by immersion-type scanners is a definite advantage. There is no *one* breast scanner that is ideal in all situations. Today ultrasound has two principal applications in the diagnosis of breast disease:

1. The separation of palpable masses into cystic and solid and the guidance of fine-needle aspiration. This can be done with almost any conventional compound and real-time scanner, with or without water coupling.

2. Structural examination of the breast in an attempt to characterize tissues. Only automated water-bath scanners are satisfactory for this purpose. Since so far no instrument can provide true early detection of breast carcinoma, this should be attempted only at specialized centers and on a research basis.

Our own experience is based on real-time examinations performed since 1975 and on systematically evaluated examinations with a modern water-bath scanner since 1979. We use the U.S. Octoson, which has the capability of performing compound scans with one to eight transducers and single scans with one transducer only. During this time we have examined more than 1,400 patients, in whom more than 300 carcinomas and several hundred benign lesions have been histologically confirmed.

18.1 Normal Structures

The immersion method is preferred for the depiction of breast anatomy, as it avoids deformation of the breast (Fig. 18.1). The following structures can be identified:

1. Nipple
2. Skin
3. Subcutaneous fat
4. Glandular tissue
5. Chest wall with pectoralis muscle

Additional breast structures may sometimes be visualized (Fig. 18.2):

1. Lactiferous duct
2. Lactiferous sinus
3. Montgomery's gland
4. Subcutaneous vein

Based on our experience (Duda and Hüneke 1982), four main types of glandular tissue can be demonstrated with ultrasound:

1. Tissue with strong central acoustic absorption (Fig. 18.3a; unfavorable for evaluation)
2. Homogeneously dense tissue (Fig. 18.3b; favorable)
3. Partially involuted tissue (Fig. 18.3c; relatively unfavorable due to fatty infiltration)
4. Involuted tissue (Fig. 18.3d; hypoechoic fat hampers detection of pathologic processes)

Our experience also indicates that the majority of women have breasts of the homogeneously dense or partially involuted type, and thus that the conditions for sonographic examination are favorable in most patients.

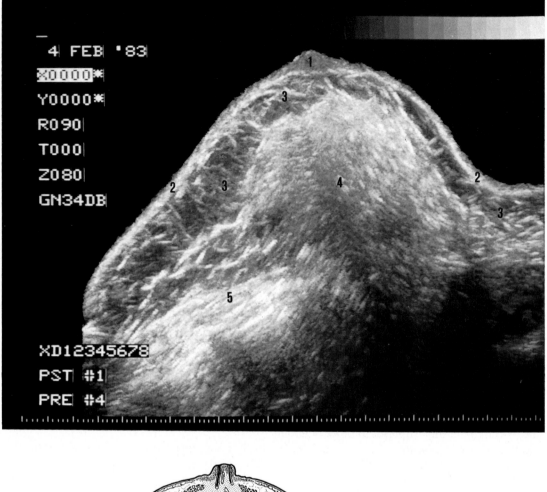

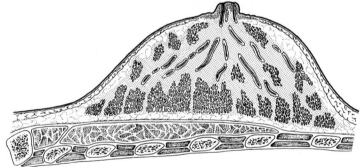

Fig. 18.1. a Ultrasound anatomy of normal female breast: *1* nipple, *2* skin, *3* subcutaneous fat, *4* glandular tissue, *5* chest wall. **b** Anatomic drawing

18.2 Pathologic Structures

18.2.1 Duct Ectasia

Normal lactiferous ducts are visible with ultrasound (Fig. 18.2a), and ectatic ducts are quite conspicuous. One might assume that carcinomas or other solid masses could be easily identified within the dilated ducts, but this is not the case, because the relatively thick cross-sectional image leads to superimpositions that mimic the appearance of solid structures projecting into the lumina (Fig. 18.4a–c).

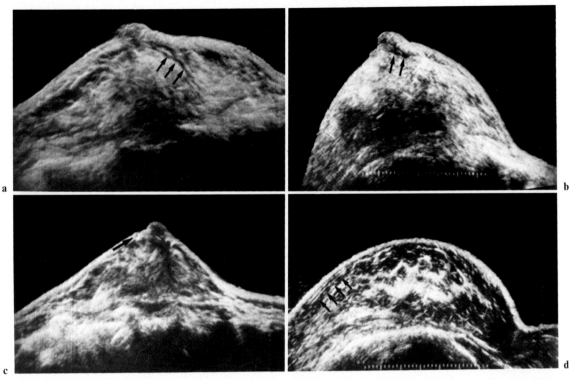

Fig. 18.2. a Lactiferous duct; **b** lactiferous sinus; **c** Montgomery's gland; **d** cutaneous vein

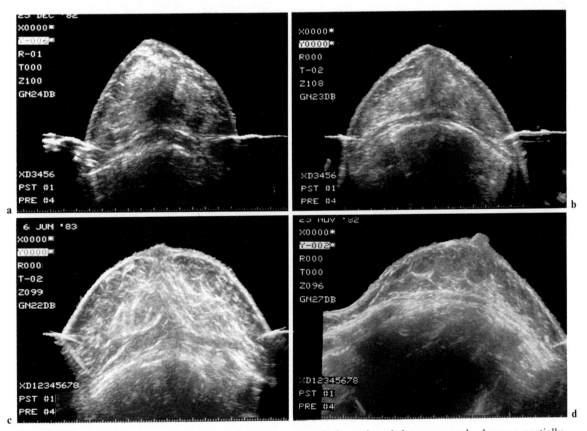

Fig. 18.3a–d. Sonographic types of glandular tissue: **a** central absorption; **b** homogeneously dense; **c** partially involuted; **d** involuted

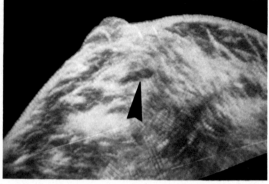

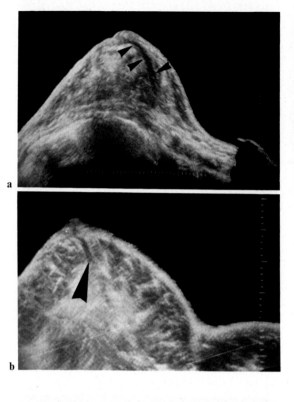

Fig. 18.4. a–c. Duct ectasia. **a** Markedly ectatic lactiferous duct. **b** Lactiferous duct with internal echoes in presence of histologically confirmed duct papilloma. **c** Lactiferous duct with internal echoes mimicking intraductal mass

18.2.2 Cysts

Evaluation of cystic masses has been the cardinal application of diagnostic ultrasound (Figs. 18.5–18.7), and many authors have noted its usefulness in this regard (e.g., Jellins et al. 1975). The typical ultrasound features of a cyst are:

1. A circular, echo-free area
2. Sharply defined front and back walls
3. Back-wall acoustic enhancement
4. Lateral shadowing

Cysts can have a variety of ultrasound patterns, however. Bleeding into a cyst or the presence of cellular debris can create the appearance of a solid mass (Fig. 18.7b). Loculated cysts and intracystic papillomas have a distinctive pattern (Fig. 18.7a). A distinctive crescent-shaped pattern is likewise produced by pneumocystography, which is usually done following the aspiration of a cyst (Fig. 18.5b). Occasionally the aspiration of a cyst leaves behind a residual mass that, although invisible on X-ray, is palpable clinically and can be demonstrated as a cystic mass by ultrasound (Fig. 18.6a, b).

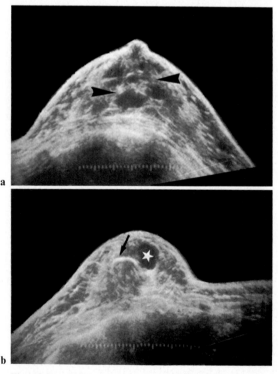

Fig. 18.5. a Polycystic changes of glandular tissue of breast. **b** Breast cyst (*star*) with hyperechoic crescent following aspiration of cyst and subsequent air insufflation (*arrow*)

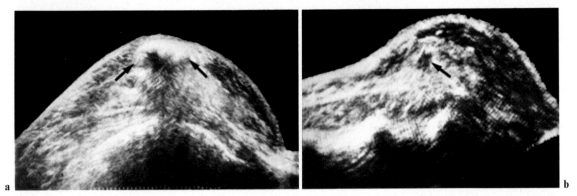

Fig. 18.6. a Cloudy, hyperechoic structure and an anechoic area in region of a partially aspirated cyst. **b** Residuum of an aspirated cyst

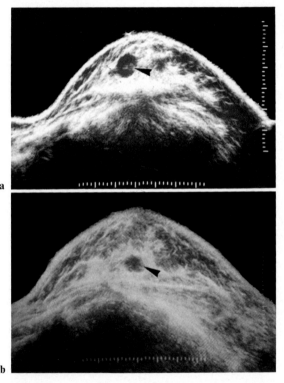

Fig. 18.7. a Intracystic papilloma (*arrow*): histologically confirmed. **b** Cyst with internal echoes (aspiration yielded a highly viscous material)

18.2.3 Acoustic Shadowing

In addition to back-wall acoustic enhancement, which is typical of cystic masses, acoustic shadowing plays an important role in the evaluation of the breast. Only in the diagnosis of calculi (gallbladder, kidney) does acoustic shadowing assume comparable significance.

Acoustic shadowing is caused by special reflective processes that occur when sound waves have a strictly parallel incidence, by strong reflection due to high acoustic impedance (e.g., calcium), and by strong acoustic absorption in a tissue. The explanation why this tissue factor occurs particularly in breast carcinomas may lie in the amount of connective tissue present. We distinguish between lateral shadowing and central shadowing.

Lateral shadowing occurs at the borders of cysts and fibroadenomas (Figs. 18.9, 18.27), while central shadowing is typical of scirrhous carcinomas (Fig. 18.8d). However, this does not mean that lateral shadowing is pathognomonic of benign lesions while central shadowing indicates malignancy, because both phenomena can have various causes. For example, the nipple normally casts a distinct central shadow (Fig. 18.8a). Acoustic enhancement has been associated with cysts as well as carcinomas (Fig. 18.17).

18.2.4 Fibroadenomas

Fibroadenomas are the most common benign tumors of the breast. We have observed them in women between 18 and 70 years of age, with a peak incidence between the ages of 20 and 50. The typical ultrasound features of fibroadenoma are:

1. Regular, homogeneous internal echoes (ca. 70%–80% of cases)
2. Smooth borders that compress adjacent tissues (ca. 60%–70%)
3. Lateral shadowing (ca. 30%–40%)

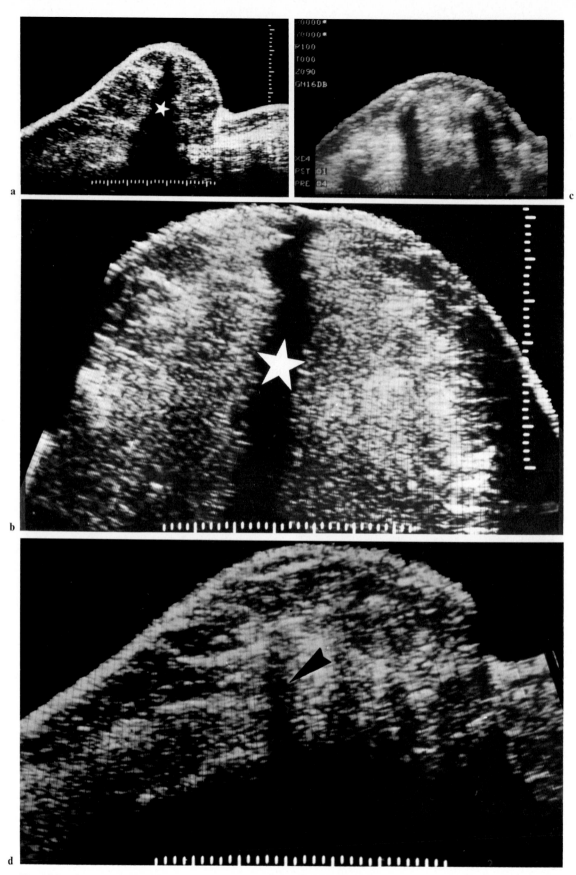

Fig. 18.8a–d. Acoustic shadowing due to various causes. **a** Normal nipple shadow; **b** mastitis; **c** calcified fibroadenoma; **d** scirrhous carcinoma

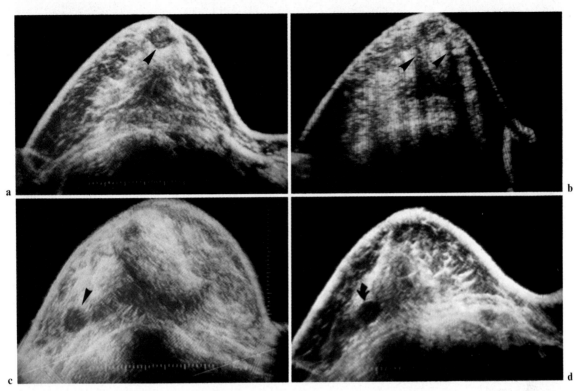

Fig. 18.9a–d. Typical sonographic presentation of fibroadenoma. **a** Compound scan: smooth borders, homogeneous internal echo structure. **b** Single scan: lateral shadowing (*arrows*). **c** Fibroadenoma that is difficult to visualize with mammography due to its eccentric location (confirmed by aspiration histology). **d** Fibroadenoma not demonstrable by mammography, located close to chest wall in dense glandular tissue (*arrow*)

Besides the typical cases described above (Figs. 18.9a–d, 18.10a–b), there are also fibroadenomas that show features characteristic of malignant tumors, such as ill-defined borders, irregular and inhomogeneous internal echoes, and central shadowing. We have never observed "broom-straw" or "fir-tree" patterns in fibroadenomas, however (see Sect. 18.2.5). The presence of a central shadow may be evidence of a carcinoma coexisting with the fibroadenoma (Fig. 18.11). Thus, even with a sharply outlined fibroadenoma, it is always recommended that a portion of the surrounding tissue be removed for pathologic study.

Cysts with internal echoes and masses associated with fat necrosis can mimic the sonographic appearance of fibroadenomas (Fig. 18.7b). Carcinomas, too, may develop forms that closely resemble fibroadenoma (Figs. 18.12, 18.13). A special transitional or borderline form between benign and malignant tumors is cystosarcoma phylloides (Fig. 18.14), which constitutes a polycystic, multilobulated mass that has well-defined borders and a fairly regular echo pattern (Fig. 18.14a). Lateral shadowing is visible in single-pass compound scans. In the case depicted, the knob of tissue growing into the superior part of the mass showed a degree of malignant change on histopathologic examination.

Various authors (Harper and Kelly-Frey 1980; Jellins et al. 1978) report that the diagnosis of benign lesions, particularly fibroadenoma, is possible in almost all cases by ultrasound. We have been able to confirm that sonography is superior to radiography in patients with fibroadenoma in its ability to demonstrate the tumor and identify it as benign (Hüneke 1982). Whenever fibroadenoma or cysts are suspected on clinical grounds, or whenever a dense breast is noted in a young woman, it is appropriate to precede radiography with ultrasound. This is not to say that we dispense with X-ray mammography or biopsy in doubtful cases, but only that sonography appears to be superior to radiography in many of these cases.

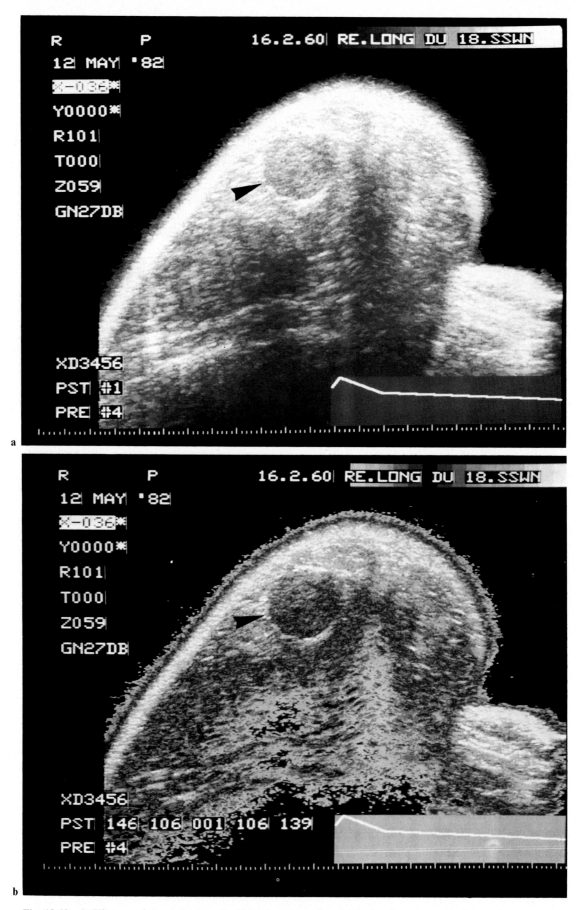

Fig. 18.10a, b. Ultrasound mammogram of a fibroadenoma. **a** Regular image; **b** postprocessed image

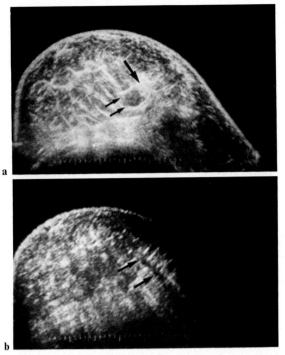

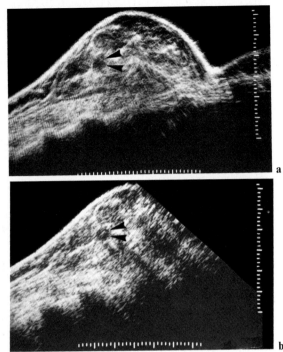

Fig. 18.11 a, b. Fibroadenoma in dense glandular tissue. **a** Compound scan. **b** Single scan (one transducer) demonstrates shadowing from an adjacent carcinoma

Fig. 18.13 a, b. Carcinoma with a circular contour. **a** Compound scan; **b** single scan

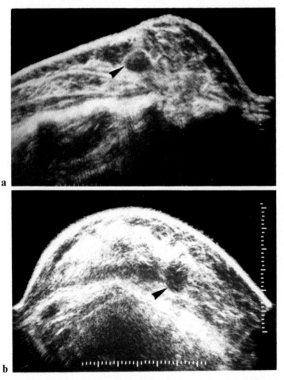

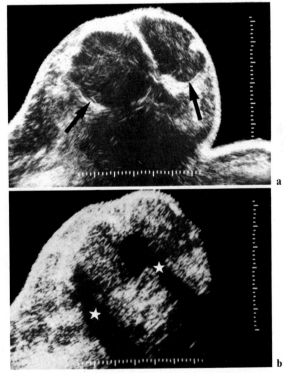

Fig. 18.12 a, b. Two carcinomas resembling fibroadenomas in their margination and internal echoes

Fig. 18.14 a, b. Cystosarcoma phylloides. **a** Compound scan showing lobulated surface of mass (*arrows*). **b** Single scan with lateral shadowing

Fibroadenomas that are confirmed by biopsy but not treated operatively can be monitored by ultrasound. In this regard we point to the great importance of mammary pathology as a reference point for physicians dealing with breast disease. Ultrasound, mammography, and the diagnosis of breast disease in general yield good results only when there is close cooperation with a specialized mammary pathologist.

18.2.5 Carcinomas

The major question in the diagnosis of carcinomas by ultrasound concerns their amenability to early detection, i.e., detection at a stage when the tumor is less than 10 mm or even less than 5 mm (microcarcinoma) in diameter.

It appears that sonography is not effective as an early screening test for breast carcinoma, and that X-ray mammography is the dominant modality in this regard [for example, sonograms do not demonstrate microcalcifications; although one author (Mulz 1981) makes a claim to the contrary, we have not been able to reproduce these findings, and more recent studies (Lambie et al. 1983) also refute them (see Fig. 18.29a,b)]. Nevertheless, we feel that it is worthwhile to examine the typical ultrasound features of carcinomas in general and their correlation with specific histologic findings. For the group of adenocarcinomas, we distinguish two basic ultrasound patterns.

The first is a focal mass with indistinct margins and inhomogeneously irregular or weak internal echoes. Often there are echogenic extensions from the mass, creating a broom-straw pattern (Fig. 18.15a, c). The skin overlying the tumor is flattened or retracted (Figs. 18.15a, 18.18a); this flattening of the skin can be an important early warning sign. The acoustic shadowing described by many authors as the most important feature of carcinoma is frequently present (Fig. 18.15b). The back-wall acoustic enhancement characteristic of cysts is never observed with these lesions. This pattern is seen in approximately one-third of cases (Fig. 18.16).

The second pattern, with an incidence of 10%–15%, is nonspecific, more difficult to appreciate in sonograms, and harder to differentiate from benign conditions. We often find a

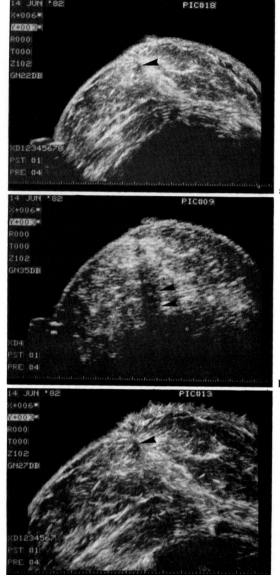

Fig. 18.15a–c. Carcinoma exhibiting "broom-straw" pattern. **a** Compound scan; **b** single scan (*arrows:* shadowing); **c** magnification

poorly outlined mass with weak internal echoes that shows no acoustic shadowing or enhancement (Figs. 18.12, 18.13).

Taking all carcinomas together, the structural features typical of malignancy are reported in the literature to occur with the following frequencies:

1. Indistinct outline: 84%
2. Broom-straw pattern (echogenic extensions): 60%–70%

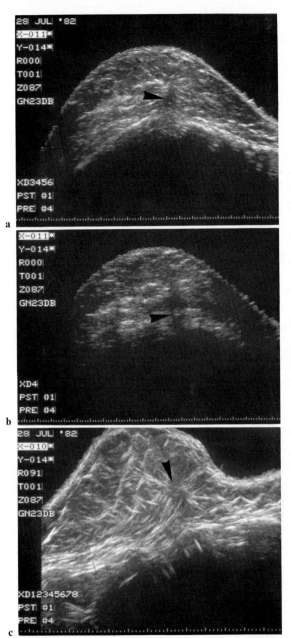

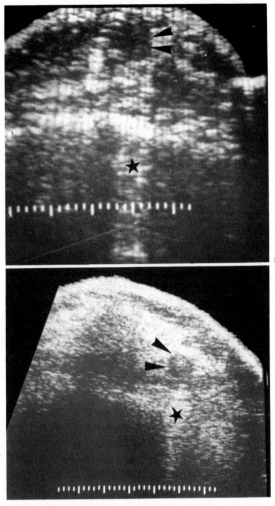

Fig. 18.17a, b. Two carcinomas with circular contours (*arrows*) and acoustic enhancement (*stars*)

Fig. 18.16a–c. Carcinoma exhibiting "broom-straw" pattern. **a** Compound scan; **b** single scan (*arrows*: shadowing); **c** magnification

3. Inhomogeneous, irregular internal echoes: 60%–70%
4. Acoustic shadowing (central shadowing): 70%–80%
5. Fir-tree pattern: ca. 25%

Many types of carcinoma show mixed features, ranging from partially smooth borders and somewhat regular internal echoes to markedly irregular internal echoes and a fir-tree pattern.

Acoustic enhancement and shadowing are observed. However, shadowing can be misleading since it may also result from calcified fibroadenomas and scar tissue (Fig. 18.8c). Almost 20% of carcinomas show acoustic enhancement at the posterior edge of the tumor. Every necrotic carcinoma may show acoustic enhancement, but it is often also found in medullary carcinomas and mucinous carcinomas (Fig. 18.17a, b).

Besides the primary tumor, ultrasound can record other changes that may accompany breast carcinoma (Fig. 18.18):

1. Flattening or retraction of the skin
2. Cutaneous lymphedema (orange-peel skin)
3. Cancer en cuirasse

The concomitant visualization of the axilla (Fig. 18.19a), which generally requires immer-

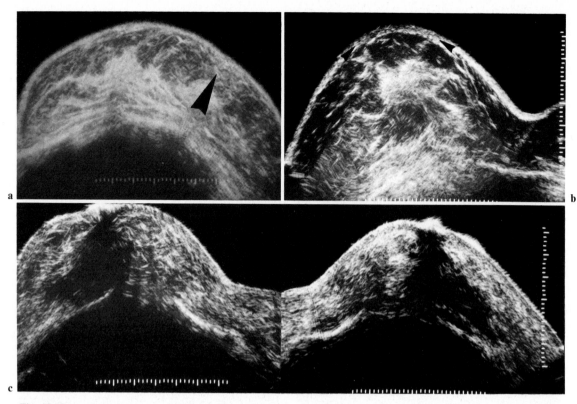

Fig. 18.18a–c. Cutaneous signs. **a** Flattening; **b** cutaneous lymphedema; **c** both breasts of a patient with cancer en cuirasse

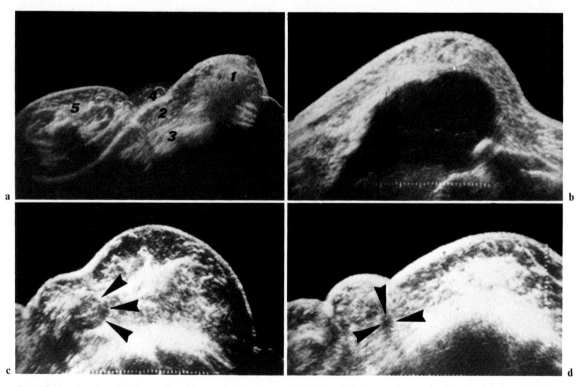

Fig. 18.19a–d. Visualization of axillary structures. **a** Overview: *1*, glandular tissue; *2*, axilla; *3*, chest wall; *4*, axillary hair; *5*, upper arm. **b** Neoplastic process that has invaded breast from thorax. **c** Calcified axillary lymph node (*arrows*) secondary to tuberculosis. **d** Axillary lymph node metastases (*arrows*) in breast carcinoma

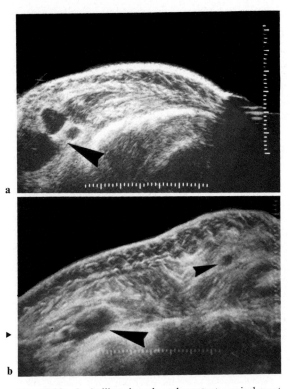

Fig. 18.20 a, b. Axillary lymph node metastases in breast carcinoma. **a** Mass of axillary nodes (*arrow*). **b** Large axillary node metastasis (*large arrow*) from a small primary focus (*small arrow*)

The presence of scar tissue is a serious obstacle to the clinical, radiographic and sonographic diagnosis of carcinoma. In some cases abnormal findings could be identified as scar tissue only by histopathologic examination and could not otherwise be differentiated from carcinoma by noninvasive means.

18.2.6 Mastopathies

In our experience with mastopathies (Prechtel grades I–III), we have found grades I and II to be associated with suspicious findings in approximately 60% of cases, and grade III in almost 90% of cases. Given the potential of grade III mastopathy for degenerative change (Bässler 1978), ultrasound assumes an important role in these cases. Unfortunately, the degree of histologic differentiation cannot be established from the sonographic appearance of mastopathic lesions. Both grade II and grade III disease can produce findings suspicious of malignancy (Fig. 18.21 a–f). In difficult cases it may remain unclear whether the original sonographic findings correspond to the intraductal carcinoma that is later diagnosed or to the surrounding grade III mastopathy. Nevertheless, we feel that ultrasound is an important guide to more detailed diagnostic evaluation of these cases. Beyond this, the mastopathies may present a range of patterns that are difficult to evaluate in patients with suspicious breast masses (Figs. 18.22, 18.23).

18.2.7 Mastitis

Distinctive ultrasound patterns are produced by inflammatory processes that have undergone liquiefaction or abscess formation (Fig. 18.24 a–d). Inflammation unassociated with liquefaction produces a nonspecific pattern. Of particular interest is the possibility of demonstrating abscess formation by ultrasound before clinical symptoms appear.

18.2.8 Implants

Large silicone implants produce a cyst-like pattern in sonograms (Fig. 18.25 a). The smooth outline of the implant is clearly demonstrated,

sion, offers advantages over both X-ray mammography and real-time ultrasound. Complications associated with neoplasms, e.g., abscesses and hematomas (Fig. 18.19 b), as well as lymph nodes, can be demonstrated with this method (Fig. 18.19 c, d). Nothing can be inferred about the origin of the primary tumor, but sometimes the axillary mass may be larger than the primary tumor (Fig. 18.20 a, b) or may have relevance to preoperative planning.

The smallest carcinoma that we have been able to detect as a discrete lesion had a histopathologic diameter of 6 mm. Comparable results were achieved by Harper and Kelly-Frey (7 mm; 1980) and Jellins et al. (5 mm, 1975). However, our experience indicates that the main radiographic sign for the early detection of carcinoma (microcalcifications with a particle diameter of 0.2–0.8 mm) is not accessible to ultrasound. As far as early detection is concerned, radiography is superior to sonography and will continue to be the mainstay in the diagnosis of breast disease.

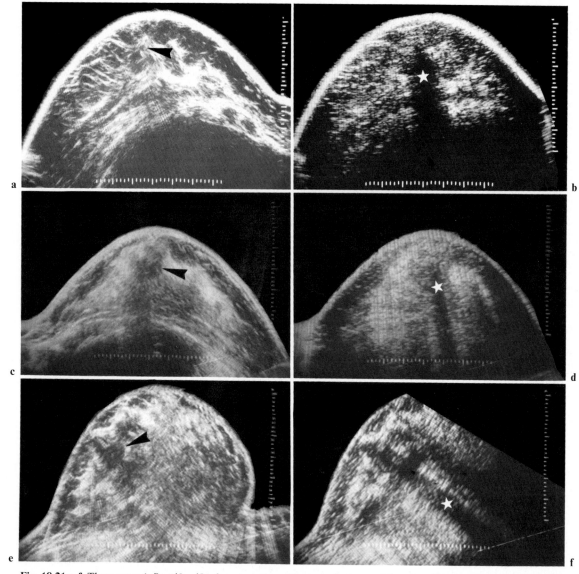

Fig. 18.21 a–f. Three cases (**a/b; c/d; e/f**) of mastopathy with increasingly suspicious focal findings (**e** fir-tree pattern) and acoustic shadowing (*stars* in **b, d, f**)

which is very difficult to do with X-ray mammography. However, proliferative tissue growth is sometimes indistinguishable from acoustic artifacts (reverberation). Retromammary implants (Fig. 18.25b) permit good visualization of breast tissue.

18.2.9 Gynecomastia

Our experience with ultrasound in gynecomastia confirms the observation of Jellins et al.

(1975) and Wigley et al. (1981) that a basic distinction can be made between a focal type of gynecomastia (Fig. 18.26c, d) and a more diffuse type (Fig. 18.26a, b).

18.3 Real-Time Scans

While it is true that high-resolution real-time scanners produce images similar to those obtained with special breast scanners (Fig. 18.27a–g), some differences are relevant

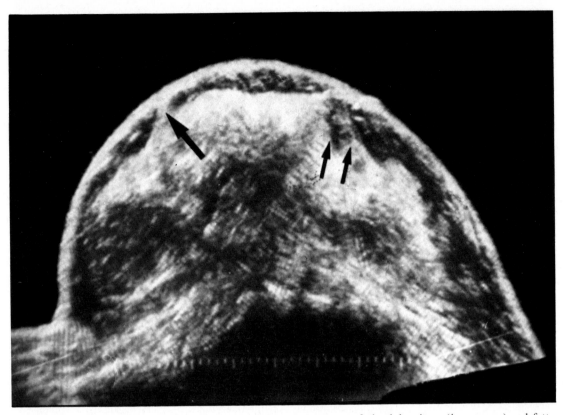

Fig. 18.22. Scan in patient with palpable breast masses: displacement of glandular tissue (*large arrow*) and fatty infiltration (*small arrows*)

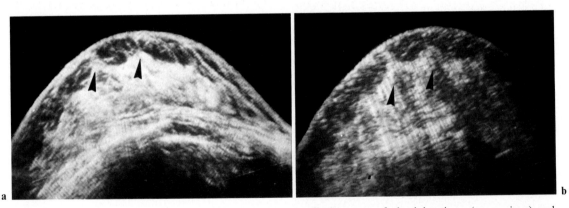

Fig. 18.23a, b. Scan in patient with palpable breast masses: displacement of glandular tissue (*arrows* in **a**) and acoustic shadowing (*arrows* in **b**)

to diagnosis. Above all, real-time scans portray only a limited region of the breast and so do not permit an overall assessment of breast architecture. However, this is important, especially in the detection of very small lesions, for observation of a discontinuity of breast architecture often prompts a selective search which then verifies a small mass that would easily have been overlooked in a more limited scan (Fig. 18.27f, g). Comparison of Octoson scans with real-time scans have shown differences in their diagnostic capabilities.

Particularly in a structure as inhomogeneous as the breast, it appears necessary to use every

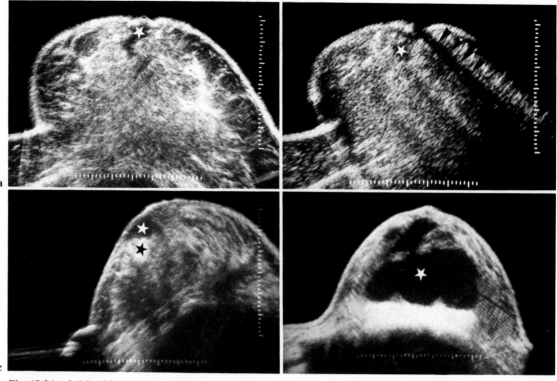

Fig. 18.24a–d. Mastitis with abscess formation. **a** Non-puerperal mastitis: compound scan (*star*, abscess cavity). **b** Nonpuerperal mastitis: single scan (*star*, abscess cavity; *arrows*, shadowing behind retracted skin). **c** Non-puerperal mastitis (*white star*, abscess; *black star*, solid portion). **d** Massive puerperal mastitis (*star*, abscess cavity)

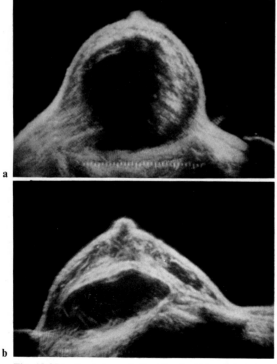

Fig. 18.25a, b. Augmentation implants. **a** Intramammary; **b** retromammary

Table 18.1. Detection of carcinoma: comparison of X-ray and (Octoson) ultrasound mammography

	(Sept. 1979 to Apr. 1985)	Ultrasound positive	Ultrasound negative
A. Carcinomas (total)			
	260 (100%)	245 (94%)	15 (6%)
X-ray positive	248 (95%)	235 (90%)	13 (5%)
X-ray negative	12 (5%)	10 (4%)	2 (1%)
B. Carcinomas (≦1 cm ⌀)			
	39 (100%)	32 (82%)	7 (18%)
X-ray positive	36 (92%)	30 (77%)	6 (15%)
X-ray negative	3 (8%)	2 (5%)	1 (3%)

available means of ultrasound imaging. With real-time equipment, only a linear or a sector scanning pattern is possible; a compound scan with lateral compounding, which will provide entirely different information, cannot be obtained. Thus, it is reasonable to assume that

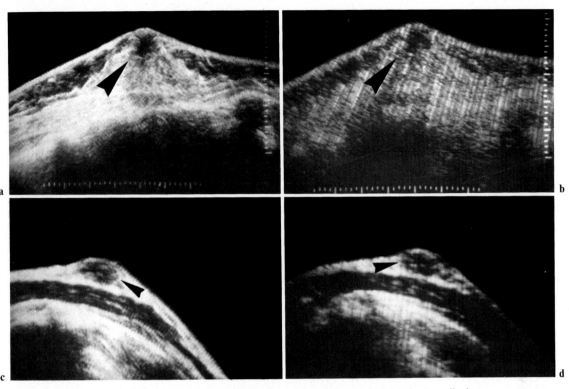

Fig. 18.26 a–d. Gynecomastias: compound and simple scans. **a, b** Diffuse type; **c, d** circumscribed type

different methods of imaging the same tissue area will yield different and complementary information, regardless of resolution.

For tissue differentiation, then, an instrument with the capability of real-time and compound imaging is preferred. If we recognize the limitations of real-time sonography of the breast, we should limit its application to specifically defined areas, i.e., the differentiation of cystic and solid masses and ultrasound-guided fine-needle aspiration.

18.4 Conclusions

There are several areas in which sonography seems superior to other noninvasive methods of breast diagnosis:

1. The diagnosis of cystic lesions, including simple breast cysts, suppurative mastitis, and duct ectasia
2. Evaluation of radiographically dense breasts
3. Short-term monitoring of histologically confirmed lesions (e.g., fibroadenoma)
4. Evaluation of mastopathic changes

In the diagnosis of carcinoma, ultrasound mammography is a useful adjunct to traditional diagnostic methods. Hitherto, ultrasound was unable to demonstrate microcalcifications and distinguish carcinoma from mastopathic lesions. The new "Computed Sonography" (Acuson) allows the visualization of microcalcifications (Fig. 18.29 a) and other small lesions (18.29 b) which could contribute to the early detection of carcinoma. As for future developments, it appears on the one hand that the increased availability of small, low-cost real-time scanners will greatly expand the basic diagnosis of breast disease (i.e., the differentiation of cystic and solid masses), especially in the office setting. Prerequisites are special transducers (e.g., 5–7 MHz) and experience.

On the other hand, detailed tissue differentiation will for the present remain confined to specialized centers, which must continually correlate their results with other diagnostic methods and with specialized mammary pathology. Despite its problems and unsuitability for screening, ultrasound mammography has become an established modality in the diagnosis of breast disease. Table 18.1 summarizes our experience in the detection of carcinomas using X-ray and ultrasound mammography (Lauth et al. 1984). X-rays were able to detect 95% of all carcino-

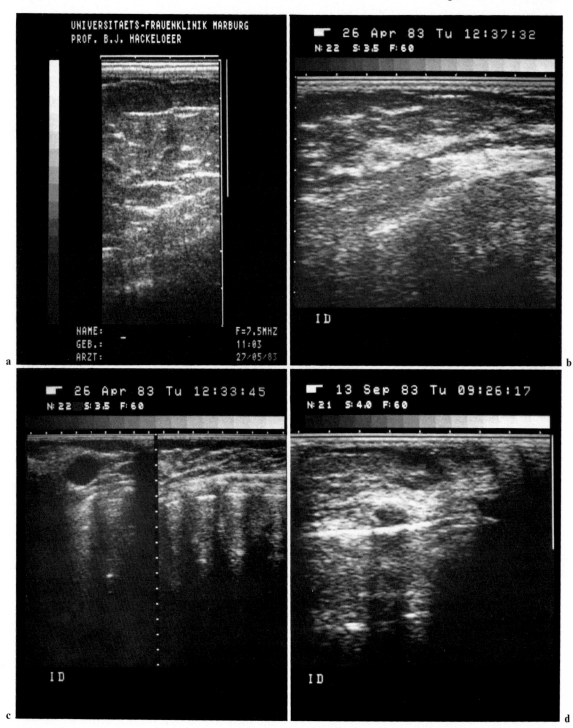

Fig. 18.27a–g. Real-time and Octoson ultrasound mammography. **a–d** Real-time scans; **a** 7.5 MHz, involuted breast; **b** 5 MHz, normal breast; **c** 5 MHz, cyst; **d** 5 MHz, carcinoma. **e, f** Comparisons of Octoson and real-time scans of carcinomas: **e** (1) and (2) show the carcinoma as a focal lesion (1) with acoustic shadowing, while two different real-time scanners, (3) and (4), show no shadows; **f** this solid carcinoma simplex appears as an inconspicuous focal lesion in the Octoson scans (1) and (2), and as a conspicuous mass in the real-time scans (3) and (4). **g** Comparison of Octoson and real-time scans in a patient with fibroadenoma (diameter 1.7 cm). The Octoson scans delineate the focal lesion (1) and show acoustic enhancement (2). The real-time scanner demonstrates the lesion well in one scan (3), but not in the other (4)

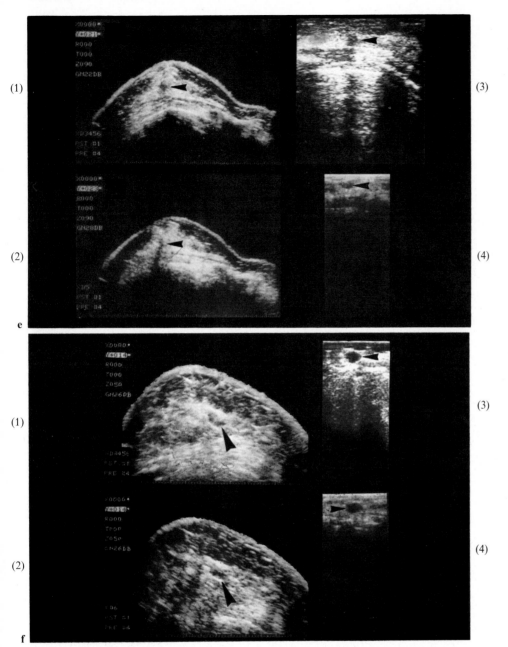

Fig. 18.27 e–f

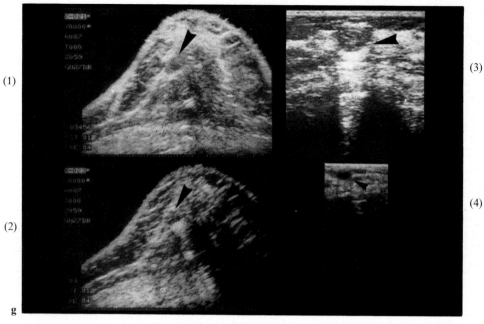

(1)

(3)

(2)

(4)

g

Fig. 18.27g

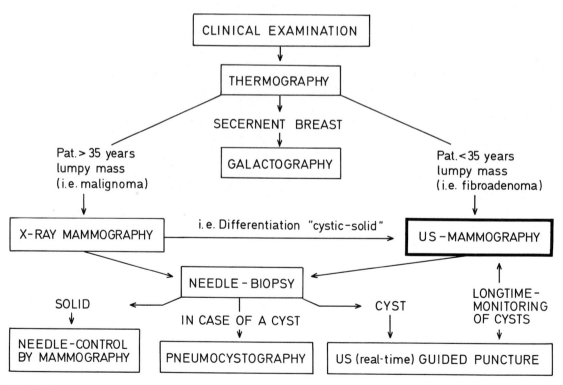

```
                    ┌─────────────────────────┐
                    │   CLINICAL EXAMINATION   │
                    └─────────────────────────┘
                                  │
                    ┌─────────────────────────┐
                    │       THERMOGRAPHY       │
                    └─────────────────────────┘
```

CLINICAL EXAMINATION

THERMOGRAPHY

SECERNENT BREAST

GALACTOGRAPHY

Pat. > 35 years
lumpy mass
(i.e. malignoma)

Pat. < 35 years
lumpy mass
(i.e. fibroadenoma)

X-RAY MAMMOGRAPHY   i.e. Differentiation "cystic-solid"   US-MAMMOGRAPHY

NEEDLE-BIOPSY

SOLID   CYST

IN CASE OF A CYST

LONGTIME-
MONITORING
OF CYSTS

NEEDLE-CONTROL
BY MAMMOGRAPHY

PNEUMOCYSTOGRAPHY

US (real-time) GUIDED PUNCTURE

Fig. 18.28

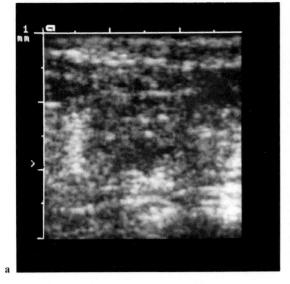

a b

Fig. 18.29. a Microcalcifications. Invasive carcinoma; **b** small axillary. Lymph node with hematoma following puncture

mas, while ultrasound detected 94% yielding a cumulative success rate of 99%. These results clearly emphasize the value of combining the two modalities (Fig. 18.28).

References

Bässler R (1978) Pathologie der Brustdrüse. In: Doerr W, Seifert G, Uehlinger E (eds) Spezielle pathologische Anatomie, Bd 11. Springer, Berlin Heidelberg New York

Cole-Beuglet C, Goldberg BB, Kurtz AB, Rubin CS, Patchefsky AS, Shaber GS (1981) Ultrasound mammography: A comparison with radiographic mammography. Radiology 139:693–698

Duda V (1982) Ultraschall-Mammographie: Das sonographische Erscheinungsbild physiologischer und pathologischer Strukturen der Mamma unter Anwendung eines Immersions scanners. Med Diss, Marburg

Hackelöer BJ, Lauth G, Duda V, Hüneke B, Buchholz R (1980) Neue Möglichkeiten der Ultraschallmammographie. Geburtshilfe Frauenheilkd 40:301–312

Hackelöer BJ, Lauth G, Duda V, Hüneke B, Buchholz R (1981a) Neue Aspekte der Ultraschall-Mammografie. Thieme, Stuttgart, S. 176–178 (Ultraschalldiagnostik in der Medizin)

Hackelöer BJ, Hüneke B, Duda V, Eulenburg R, Lauth G, Buchholz R (1981b) Sonographische Differentialdiagnose der Mammakarzinome. Ultraschall Med 2/3:129–134

Harper P, Kelly-Fry E (1980) Ultrasound visualization of the breast in symptomatic patients. Radiology 137/2:465–469

Hüneke B (1982) Ultraschall-Mammographie: Stellenwert und Bedeutung der Methode im Vergleich mit Röntgenmammographie, Thermographie und Feinnadelbiopsie. Med Diss, Marburg

Igl W, Lohe K, Eiermann W, Bassermann R, Lissner J (1980) Sonographische Carcinomdiagnostik der weiblichen Brust im Vergleich zur Mammographie. Tum Diagn 5:244–253

Jellins G, Kossoff G, Buddee FW, Reeve TS (1971) Ultrasonic visualization of the breast. Med J Aust 1:305–307

Jellins J, Kossoff G, Reeve TS, Barraclough BH (1975) Ultrasonic grey scale visualization of breast disease. Ultrasound Med Biol 1/4:393–404

Jellins J, Hughes C, Ryan J, Reeve TS, Kossoff G (1977a) A comparative evaluation of a case of cystosarcoma phylloides: ultrasound, xeroradiography and thermography. Radiology 124/3:803–804

Jellins J, Kossoff G, Reeve TS (1977b) Detection and classification of liquid-filled masses in the breast by grey scale echography. Radiology 125/1:205–212

Jellins J, Kossoff G, Barraclough BH, Reeve TS (1978) Comparative study of breast imaging by echography and xerography. Excerpta Medica 299–304

Kobayashi T (1974) Clinical evaluation of ultrasound techniques in breast and malignant abdominal tumors. Excerpta Medica 191–198

Kossoff G (1972) Improved techniques in ultrasonic sectional echography. Ultrasonics 10:221–227

Kossoff G, Carpenter DA, Radovanovich G, Robinson DE, Garrett WJ (1975) Octoson: A new rapid multitransducer general purpose water-coupling echoscope. Excerpta Medica 90–95

Kossoff G, Garrett WJ, Darpenter DA, Jellins J, Dadd MJ (1976) Principles and classification of soft tissues by grey scale echography. Ultrasound Med Biol 2:89–105

Kossoff G, Jellins J, Reeve TS (1978) Ultrasound in the detection of early breast cancer. Cancer Camp 1:149–158

Kratochwil A, Kolb S, Stöger H, Dahlberg BE, Brezina K, Czech (1975) Moderne Methoden der Mammadiagnostik. Wien Klin Wochenschr 87/2:47–52

Lambie RW, Hodgen D, Herman EM, Kopperman M (1983) Sonomammographic manifestations of mammographically detectable breast microcalcifications. J Ultrasound Med 2:509

Lauth G, Duda V, Eulenburg R, Hackelöer BJ, Hüneke B (1984) Möglichkeiten und Grenzen der Brustkrebs-Früherkennung mittels Ultraschall-Mammographie. Röntgenpraxis 37:62

Mulz D, Egger H, Knüpfer A, Althammer G (1981) Mikrokalk im Mammogramm und Darstellungsmöglichkeiten im Ultraschall. Geburtshilfe Frauenheilkd 41:255–258

Pluygers E, Rombaut M (1980) Ultrasonic diagnosis of breast diseases. Tum Diagn 4:187–194

Schmidt W, Teubner J, Kaick G van, Fournier D von, Kubli F (1981) Ultrasonographische Untersuchungsergebnisse bei der Mammadiagnostik. Geburtshilfe Frauenheilkd 41/8:533–539

Wagai T, Takahashi S, Ohashi H, Ishikawa H (1967) A trial for quantitative diagnosis of breast tumor by ultrasono-tomography. Med Ultrason 5:39–40

Wigley KD, Thomas JL, Bernardino ML, Rosenbaum JL (1981) Sonography of gynecomastia. Am J Roentgenol 136:927–930

Wild JJ, Neal D (1951) High-frequency ultrasonic waves for detecting changes of texture in living tissues. Lancet I:655–657

Wild JJ, Reid JM (1952) Further pilot echographic studies on the histological structure of tumors of the human breast. Am J Pathol 28:839–861

19 Appendix

In Cooperation with U. VOIGT, H. SCHUHMACHER, and P. JEANTY

Table 1. Synopsis of fetal biometric data (outer-outer, tissue velocity 1,540 m/s) for the second and third trimester (Bonn, 1984)

Week	BPD	OFD	HC	TTD	AC	Femur	CRL	Weight
12	2.0	—	—	1.7	5.3	—	4.7	—
13	2.4	—	—	2.0	6.3	1.0	6.0	14
14	2.8	3.1	10.6	2.4	7.5	1.2	7.3	25
15	3.2	3.8	11.5	2.7	8.5	1.6	8.6	50
16	3.5	4.1	12.7	3.1	9.7	1.8	9.7	80
17	3.8	4.6	14.0	3.4	10.7	2.2	11.0	100
18	4.2	5.0	15.2	3.7	11.6	2.5	12.0	150
19	4.6	5.4	16.4	4.0	12.6	2.8	13.0	200
20	4.9	5.8	17.6	4.4	13.5	3.1	14.0	250
21	5.2	6.3	19.0	4.7	14.5	3.4	CHL ▼	300
22	5.6	6.7	20.3	5.0	15.5	3.6		350
23	5.9	7.2	21.5	5.3	16.5	3.9	28	450
24	6.2	7.6	22.6	5.6	17.3	4.1		530
25	6.5	8.0	24.0	5.9	18.3	4.4	31	700
26	6.8	8.4	25.1	6.2	19.1	4.7		850
27	7.1	8.8	26.3	6.5	20.2	4.9	34	1,000
28	7.4	9.1	27.4	6.9	21.1	5.1		1,100
29	7.7	9.5	28.4	7.2	22.2	5.4	37	1,250
30	8.0	9.8	29.3	7.4	23.0	5.6		1,400
31	8.2	10.0	30.3	7.8	24.0	5.9	40	1,600
32	8.5	10.3	31.1	8.1	24.9	6.1		1,800
33	8.7	10.5	31.8	8.3	25.8	6.3	43	2,000
34	8.9	10.7	32.5	8.6	26.8	6.5		2,250
35	9.1	10.9	33.2	8.9	27.7	6.7	45	2,550
36	9.3	11.1	33.7	9.2	28.7	6.9		2,750
37	9.5	11.2	34.0	9.4	29.6	7.1	47	2,950
38	9.6	11.3	34.4	9.7	30.6	7.3		3,100
39	9.8	11.4	34.7	9.9	31.5	7.4	50	3,250
40	9.9	11.5	34.9	10.1	32.0	7.5		3,400

BPD

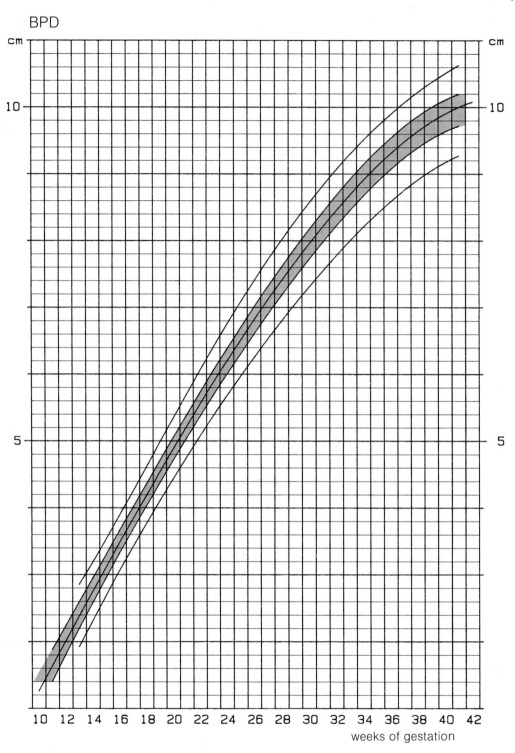

Fig. 1. Percentile growth curves (5-25-50-75-95) of BPD (outer-outer, tissue velocity 1540 m/s) (Bonn, 1984)

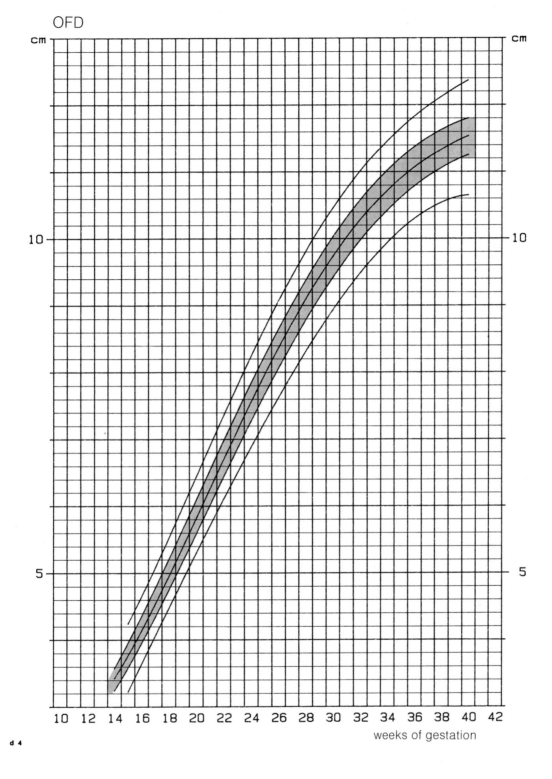

Fig. 2. Percentile growth curves (5-25-50-75-95) of OFD (outer-outer, tissue velocity 1540 m/s) (Bonn, 1984)

HC

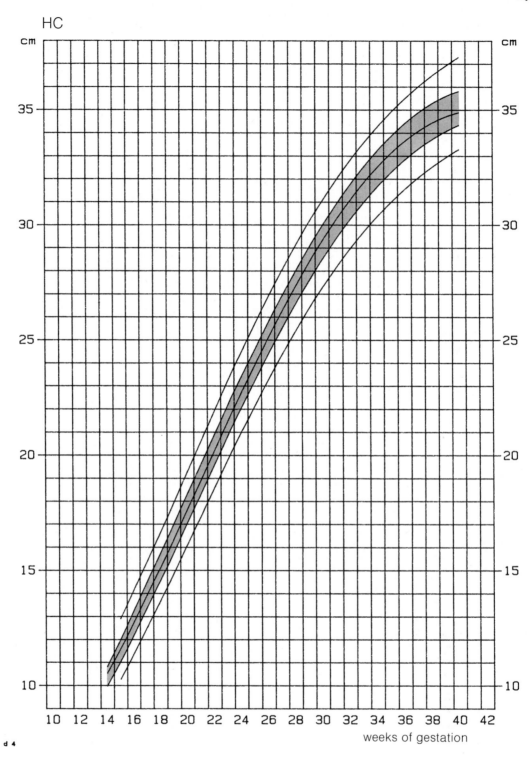

Fig. 3. Percentile growth curves (5-25-50-75-95) of HC (Bonn, 1984)

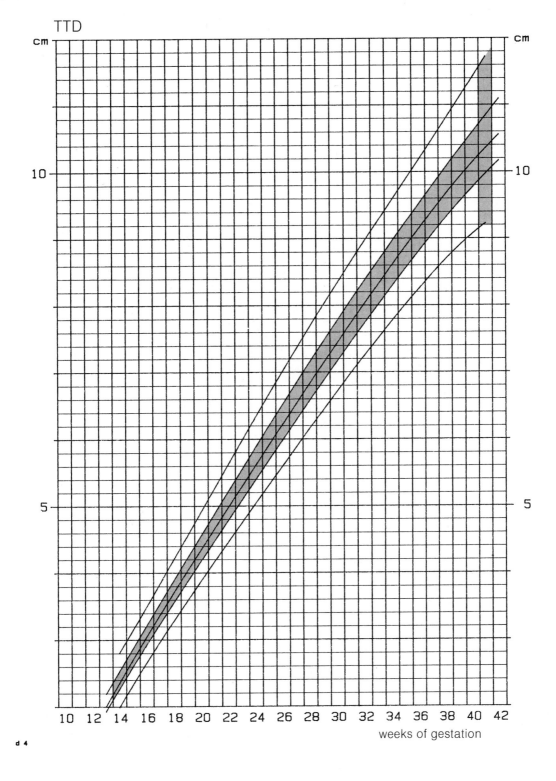

Fig. 4. Percentile growth curves of TTD (outer-outer, tissue velocity 1540 m/s) (Bonn, 1984)

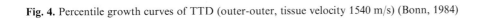

femur

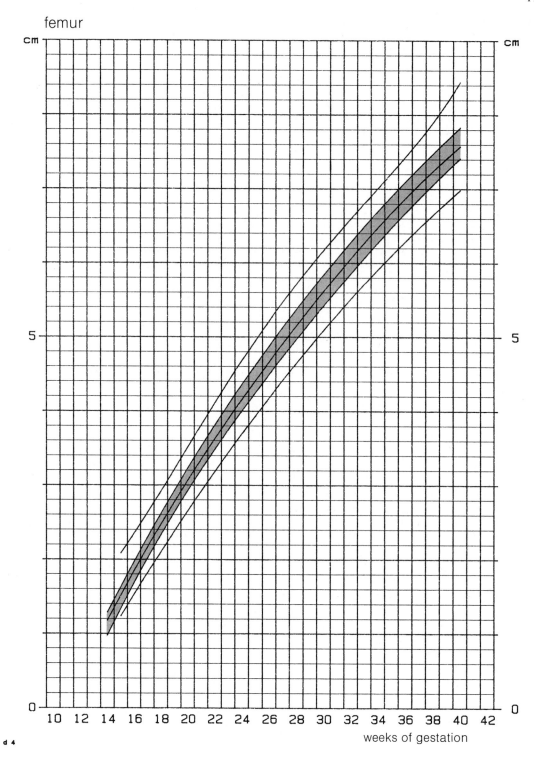

Fig. 5. Percentile growth curves (5-25-50-75-95) of femur diaphyseal length (Bonn, 1984)

CRL

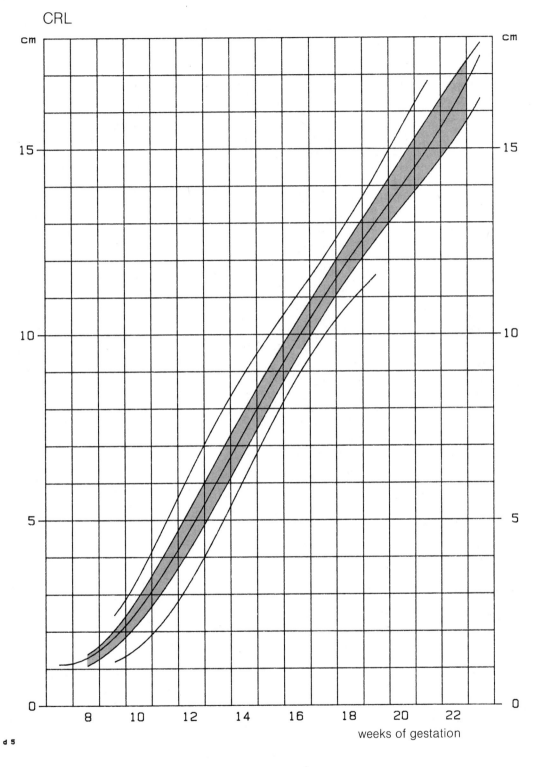

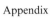

Fig. 6. Percentile growth curves (5-25-50-75-95) of CRL (Bonn, 1984)

Table 2. Normal ranges of CRL (mm) as a function of gestational age (A.M., arithmetic mean; s, standard deviation; p.m., postmenstrual). [From Hansmann M et al. (1979) Geburtshilfe. Frauenheilkd 39:656]

Gestational age (pm week)	Crown-rump length			Gestational age (pm week)	Crown-rump length		
	−2	AM	+2 s		−2	AM	+2 s
Day 1	2.3	6.9	11.5	Day 2	51.3	68.8	86.3
Day 2	2.8	7.6	12.5	Day 4	55.6	72.6	90.6
Day 3	3.2	8.3	13.4	Day 6	57.8	76.3	94.8
Day 4	3.6	9.0	14.3				
Day 5	3.9	9.6	15.2	Day 2	62.5	81.8	101.1
Day 6	4.3	10.2	16.1	Day 4	65.6	85.4	105.2
Day 7	4.7	10.8	16.9	Day 6	68.6	88.9	109.2
Day 1	5.0	11.4	17.8				
Day 2	5.4	12.1	18.7	Day 2	72.8	93.9	115.0
Day 3	5.8	12.7	19.6	Day 4	75.5	97.1	118.7
Day 4	6.2	13.3	20.5	Day 6	78.0	100.1	122.2
Day 5	6.6	14.0	21.4				
Day 6	7.0	14.7	22.4	Day 2	81.5	104.4	127.3
Day 7	7.5	15.4	23.4	Day 4	83.6	107.0	130.4
Day 1	8.0	16.2	24.4	Day 6	85.6	109.5	133.4
Day 3	9.1	17.8	26.5				
Day 5	10.3	19.6	28.8	Day 2	88.3	113.0	137.7
Day 7	11.7	21.5	31.2	Day 4	89.9	115.1	140.4
Day 2	13.3	23.6	33.9	Day 6	91.5	117.2	142.9
Day 4	15.1	25.9	36.6				
Day 6	17.0	28.3	39.6	Day 2	93.5	120.0	146.5
Day 2	20.3	32.4	44.4	Day 4	94.8	121.9	148.9
Day 4	22.7	35.3	47.9	Day 6	96.2	123.7	151.2
Day 6	25.2	38.3	51.4				
Day 2	29.3	43.2	57.1	Day 1	97.5	125.5	153.6
Day 4	32.2	46.6	61.3	Day 3	98.9	127.4	156.0
Day 6	35.3	50.2	65.1	Day 5	100.3	129.4	158.5
				Day 7	102.0	131.6	161.2
Day 2	40.0	55.6	71.3				
Day 4	43.2	59.4	75.5	Day 1	102.9	132.8	162.6
Day 6	46.4	63.1	79.8	Day 2	104.0	134.0	164.1

Table 3. Normal ranges for estimation of gestational age from CRL (A.M., arithmetic mean; s, standard deviation; p.m., postmenstrual). [From Hansmann M et al. (1979) Geburtshilfe. Frauenheilkd 39:656].

Measured CRL (mm)	Estimated gestational age (pm week/day)			Measured CRL (mm)	Estimated gestational age (pm week/day)		
	$-2 s$	A.M.	$+2 s$		$-2 s$	A.M.	$+2 s$
6	5–1	6–1	6–7	52	10–7	12–2	13–4
7	5–3	6–2	7–2	54	10–7	12–3	13–5
8	5–4	6–4	7–3	56	11–1	12–4	13–6
9	5–6	6–6	7–6	58	11–2	12–5	13–7
10	6–1	6–7	7–7	60	11–3	12–6	14–1
11	6–2	7–2	8–1	63	11–4	12–7	14–3
12	6–3	7–3	8–3	66	11–5	13–2	14–5
13	6–5	7–4	8–4	70	11–7	13–3	14–7
14	6–6	7–6	8–6	73	12–1	13–5	15–1
15	6–7	7–7	8–7	76	12–2	13–6	15–3
16	7–2	8–2	9–1	80	12–4	14–1	15–5
17	7–3	8–3	9–2				
18	7–4	8–4	9–4	83	12–5	14–2	15–7
19	7–5	8–5	9–5	86	12–6	14–4	16–2
20	7–6	8–6	9–6	90	13–1	14–6	16–4
21	7–7	8–7	9–7	93	13–3	15–1	16–6
22	8–1	9–1	10–1	96	13–4	15–3	17–1
23	8–2	9–2	10–2	100	13–6	15–5	17–3
24	8–3	9–3	10–3	103	14–1	15–7	17–6
26	8–5	9–5	10–5	106	14–3	16–2	18–1
28	8–6	9–7	11–1	110	14–5	16–4	18–4
30	9–1	10–2	11–2				
				113	14–7	16–7	18–7
32	9–2	10–3	11–4	116	15–2	17–2	19–2
34	9–4	10–5	11–5	120	15–4	17–4	19–4
36	9–5	10–6	11–7	123	15–7	17–7	19–7
38	9–6	11–1	12–2	126	16–2	18–2	20–3
40	10–1	11–2	12–3	130	16–5	18–6	20–6
				133	16–7	19–1	21–2
42	10–2	11–3	12–4	136	17–3	19–4	21–6
44	10–3	11–4	12–6	140	17–6	19–7	22–2
46	10–5	11–6	12–7	143	18–1	20–3	22–5
48	10–6	11–7	13–2	146	18–4	20–6	23–1
50	10–6	12–1	13–3	150	18–7	21–3	23–5

Table 4. Estimation of gestational age from BPD (*P*, percentile)

BPD (mm)	Day 5th P	Day/Week 50th P	Day 95th P	BPD (mm)	Day 5th P	Day/Week 50th P	Day 95th P
29	86	92, 93, 94	101	51	133	141, 142, 143	153
30	89	95, 96, 97	103	52	135	144, 145	155
31	90	98 *(wk 14)*	106	53	136	146, 147 *(wk 21)*	158
32	93	99, 100, 101	108	54	140	148, 149, 150	160
33	94	102, 103	111	55	142	151, 152	161
34	96	104, 105 *(wk 15)*	114	56	145	153, 154 *(wk 22)*	163
35	99	106, 107, 108	115	57	147	155, 156, 157	165
36	101	109, 110, 111	118	58	150	158, 159, 160	167
37	104	112 *(wk 16)*	120	59	151	161 *(wk 23)*	171
38	105	113, 114, 115	123	60	153	162, 163, 164	172
39	108	116, 117, 118	125	61	155	165, 166, 167	175
40	110	119 *(wk 17)*	127	62	158	168 *(wk 24)*	178
41	112	120, 121, 122	130	63	160	169, 170, 171	179
42	115	123, 124	132	64	162	172, 173	182
43	116	125, 126 *(wk 18)*	134	65	165	174, 175 *(wk 25)*	184
44	118	127, 128, 129	136	66	167	176, 177	187
45	121	130, 131	139	67	169	178, 179, 180	190
46	123	132, 133 *(wk 19)*	141	68	171	181, 182 *(wk 26)*	191
47	125	134, 135	144	69	174	183, 184	193
48	126	136, 137	146	70	175	185, 186	195
49	127	138, 139	148	71	177	187, 188, 189 *(wk 27)*	199
50	130	140 *(wk 20)*	148				

Table 4 (continued)

BPD (mm)	Day 5th P	Day/Week 50th P	Day 95th P
72	179	190, 191	200
73	182	192, 193, 194	205
74	183	195, 196 *(28)*	207
75	185	197, 198, 199	209
76	187	200, 201	212
77	190	202, 203 *(29)*	215
78	191	204, 205, 206, 207	220
79	192	208, 209	224
80	195	210 *(30)*	225
81	198	211, 212, 213, 214, 215, 216	228
82	202	217 *(31)*	232
83	203	218, 219, 220, 221, 222	236
84	206	223, 224 *(32)*	240
85	209	225, 226, 227, 228	242
86	211	229, 230, 231 *(33)*	246
87	212	232, 233, 234, 235	253
88	217	236, 237, 238 *(34)*	255
89	221	239, 240, 241, 242	259
90	224	243, 244, 245 *(35)*	262
91	225	246, 247, 248, 249, 250	271
92	233	251, 252 *(36)*	275
93	236	253, 254, 255, 256, 257, 258, 259 *(37)*	278
94	243	260, 261, 262, 263, 264, 265, 266 *(38)*	281
95	247	267, 268, 269, 270, 271	287
96	247	272	290
97	251	273 *(39)*	294
98	255	274	294
99	256	275	298
100	257	276	296
1	260	277	298
2	260	278	296
3	261	279, 280 *(40)*	296
4	262	281, 282	296
5	265	283, 284, 285, 286, 287 *(41)*	296

Table 5. Calculation of HC from BPD and OFD using the formula $HC = 2.325\sqrt{BPD + OFD}$ (Bonn, 1984)

OFD (mm) \ BPD (mm)	30	31	32	33	34	35	36	37	38	39	40	41	42	43	44	45	46	47	48	49	50
40	116	118	119	121	122	124	125	127	128	130	132	133	135	137	138	140	142	143	145	147	149
41	118	120	121	122	124	125	127	128	130	132	133	135	136	138	140	142	143	145	147	149	150
42	120	121	123	124	126	127	129	130	132	133	135	136	138	140	141	143	145	147	148	150	152
43	122	123	125	126	127	129	130	132	133	135	137	138	140	141	143	145	146	148	150	152	153
44	124	125	126	128	129	131	132	134	135	137	138	140	141	143	145	146	148	150	151	153	155
45	126	127	128	130	131	133	134	135	137	138	140	142	143	145	146	148	150	151	153	155	156
46	128	129	130	132	133	134	136	137	139	140	142	143	145	146	148	150	151	153	155	156	158
47	130	131	132	134	135	136	138	139	141	142	143	145	147	148	150	151	153	155	156	158	160
48	132	133	134	135	137	138	139	141	142	144	145	147	148	150	151	153	155	156	158	159	161
49	134	135	136	137	139	140	141	143	144	146	147	149	150	152	153	155	156	158	159	161	163
50	136	137	138	139	141	142	143	145	146	147	149	150	152	153	155	156	158	160	161	163	164
51	138	139	140	141	143	144	145	146	148	149	151	152	154	155	157	158	160	161	163	164	166
52	140	141	142	143	144	146	147	148	150	151	153	154	155	157	158	160	161	163	165	166	168
53	142	143	144	145	146	148	149	150	152	153	154	156	157	159	160	162	163	165	166	168	169
54	144	145	146	147	148	150	151	152	154	155	156	158	159	160	162	163	165	166	168	170	171
55	146	147	148	149	150	152	153	154	155	157	158	159	161	162	164	165	167	168	170	171	173
56	148	149	150	151	152	154	155	156	157	159	160	161	163	164	166	167	168	170	171	173	175
57	150	151	152	153	154	156	157	158	159	161	162	163	165	166	167	169	170	172	173	175	176
58	152	153	154	155	156	158	159	160	161	163	164	165	166	168	169	171	172	174	175	177	178
59	154	155	156	157	158	159	161	162	163	164	166	167	168	170	171	173	174	175	177	178	180
60	156	157	158	159	160	161	163	164	165	166	168	169	170	172	173	174	176	177	179	180	182
61	158	159	160	161	162	164	165	166	167	168	170	171	172	174	175	176	178	179	180	182	183
62	160	161	162	163	164	166	167	168	169	170	172	173	174	175	177	178	179	181	182	184	185
63	162	163	164	165	166	168	169	170	171	172	174	175	176	177	179	180	181	183	184	186	187
64	164	165	166	167	168	170	171	172	173	174	175	177	178	179	181	182	183	185	186	187	189
65	166	167	168	169	171	172	173	174	175	176	177	179	180	181	182	184	185	186	188	189	191
66	169	170	171	172	173	174	175	176	177	178	179	181	182	183	184	186	187	188	190	191	193
67	171	172	173	174	175	176	177	178	179	180	181	183	184	185	186	188	189	190	192	193	194
68	173	174	175	176	177	178	179	180	181	182	183	185	186	187	188	190	191	192	194	195	196
69	175	176	177	178	179	180	181	182	183	184	185	187	188	189	190	192	193	194	195	197	198
70	177	178	179	180	181	182	183	184	185	186	187	189	190	191	192	193	195	196	197	199	200
71	179	180	181	182	183	184	185	186	187	188	189	191	192	193	194	195	197	198	199	201	202
72	181	182	183	184	185	186	187	188	189	190	191	193	194	195	196	197	199	200	201	203	204
73	183	184	185	186	187	188	189	190	191	192	194	195	196	197	198	199	201	202	203	205	206
74	186	187	187	188	189	190	191	192	193	194	196	197	198	199	200	201	203	204	205	206	208
75	188	189	190	191	191	192	193	194	195	197	198	199	200	201	202	203	205	206	207	208	210
76	190	191	192	193	194	195	196	197	198	199	200	201	202	203	204	205	207	208	209	210	212
77	192	193	194	195	196	197	198	199	200	201	202	203	204	205	206	207	209	210	211	212	213
78	194	195	196	197	198	199	200	201	202	203	204	205	206	207	208	209	211	212	213	214	215
79	196	197	198	199	200	201	202	203	204	205	206	207	208	209	210	211	213	214	215	216	217
80	199	199	200	201	202	203	204	205	206	207	208	209	210	211	212	213	215	216	217	218	219

Table 5 (continued)

Appendix 443

BPD (mm)

OFD (mm)	90	91	92	93	94	95	96	97	98	99	100	101	102	103	104	105	106	107	108	109	110
100	313	314	316	318	319	321	322	324	326	327	329	330	332	334	335	337	339	341	342	344	346
101	315	316	318	319	321	322	324	326	327	329	330	332	334	335	337	339	340	342	344	345	347
102	316	318	319	321	322	324	326	327	329	330	332	334	335	337	339	340	342	344	345	347	349
103	318	320	321	323	324	326	327	329	331	332	334	335	337	339	340	342	344	345	347	349	350
104	320	321	323	324	326	327	329	331	332	334	335	337	339	340	342	344	345	347	349	350	352
105	322	323	325	326	328	329	331	332	334	336	337	339	340	342	344	345	347	349	350	352	354
106	323	325	326	328	329	331	332	334	336	337	339	340	342	344	345	347	349	350	352	353	355
107	325	327	328	330	331	333	334	336	337	339	341	342	344	345	347	349	350	352	353	355	357
108	327	328	330	331	333	334	336	338	339	341	342	344	345	347	349	350	352	353	355	357	358
109	329	330	332	333	335	336	338	339	341	342	344	345	347	349	350	352	353	355	357	358	360
110	330	332	333	335	336	338	339	341	343	344	346	347	349	350	352	354	355	357	358	360	362
111	332	334	335	337	338	340	341	343	344	346	347	349	350	352	354	355	357	358	360	362	363
112	334	336	337	338	340	341	343	344	346	348	349	351	352	354	355	357	359	360	362	363	365
113	336	337	339	340	342	343	345	346	348	349	351	352	354	355	357	359	360	362	363	365	367
114	338	339	341	342	344	345	347	348	350	351	353	354	356	357	359	360	362	364	365	367	368
115	340	341	342	344	345	347	348	350	351	353	354	356	357	359	360	362	364	365	367	368	370
116	341	343	344	346	347	349	350	352	353	355	356	358	359	361	362	364	365	367	368	370	372
117	343	345	346	347	349	350	352	353	355	356	358	359	361	362	364	366	367	369	370	372	373
118	345	346	348	349	351	352	354	355	357	358	360	361	363	364	366	367	369	370	372	373	375
119	347	348	350	351	353	354	355	357	358	360	361	363	364	366	367	369	371	372	374	375	377
120	349	350	352	353	354	356	357	359	360	362	363	365	366	368	369	371	372	374	375	377	378
121	351	352	353	355	356	358	359	361	362	363	365	366	368	369	371	372	374	376	377	379	380
122	352	354	355	357	358	360	361	362	364	365	367	368	370	371	373	374	376	377	379	380	382
123	354	356	357	359	360	361	363	364	366	367	369	370	372	373	374	376	378	379	381	382	384
124	356	358	359	360	362	363	365	366	367	369	370	372	373	375	376	378	379	381	382	384	385
125	358	359	361	362	364	365	366	368	369	371	372	374	375	377	378	380	381	383	384	386	387
126	360	361	363	364	365	367	368	370	371	373	374	375	377	378	380	381	383	384	386	387	389
127	362	363	365	366	367	369	370	372	373	374	376	377	379	380	382	383	385	386	388	389	391
128	364	365	366	368	369	371	372	373	375	376	378	379	381	382	383	385	386	388	389	391	392
129	366	367	368	370	371	372	374	375	377	378	379	381	382	384	385	387	388	390	391	393	394
130	368	369	370	372	373	374	376	377	379	380	381	383	384	386	387	389	390	391	393	394	396
131	370	371	372	374	375	376	378	379	380	382	383	385	386	387	389	390	392	393	395	396	398
132	371	373	374	375	377	378	379	381	382	384	385	386	388	389	391	392	394	395	397	398	399
133	373	375	376	377	379	380	381	383	384	385	387	388	390	391	393	394	395	397	398	400	401
134	375	377	378	379	381	382	383	385	386	387	389	390	392	393	394	396	397	399	400	402	403
135	377	379	380	381	382	384	385	386	388	389	391	392	393	395	396	398	399	401	402	403	405
136	379	380	382	383	384	386	387	388	390	391	392	394	395	397	398	399	401	402	404	405	407
137	381	382	384	385	386	388	389	390	392	393	394	396	397	399	400	401	403	404	406	407	408
138	383	384	386	387	388	390	391	392	394	395	396	398	399	400	402	403	405	406	407	409	410
139	385	386	388	389	390	391	393	394	395	397	398	399	401	402	404	405	406	408	409	411	412
140	387	388	389	391	392	393	395	396	397	399	400	401	403	404	405	407	408	410	411	413	414

Table 5 (continued)

OFD (mm)	BPD (mm) 70	71	72	73	74	75	76	77	78	79	80	81	82	83	84	85	86	87	88	89	90
80	247	249	250	252	253	255	257	258	260	261	263	265	266	268	270	271	273	275	277	279	280
81	249	250	252	254	255	257	258	260	261	263	265	266	268	270	271	273	275	276	279	280	282
82	251	252	254	255	257	258	260	262	263	265	266	268	270	271	273	275	276	278	280	281	283
83	252	254	255	257	259	260	262	263	265	266	268	270	271	273	275	276	278	280	281	283	285
84	254	256	257	259	260	262	263	265	267	268	270	271	273	275	276	278	280	281	283	285	286
85	256	257	259	261	262	264	265	267	268	270	271	273	275	276	278	279	281	283	284	286	288
86	258	259	261	262	264	265	267	268	270	272	273	275	276	278	280	281	283	284	286	288	289
87	260	261	263	264	266	267	269	270	272	273	275	276	278	280	281	283	284	286	288	289	291
88	261	263	264	266	267	269	270	272	273	275	277	278	280	281	283	284	286	288	289	291	293
89	263	265	266	268	269	271	272	274	275	277	278	280	281	283	285	286	288	289	291	293	294
90	265	267	268	269	271	272	274	275	277	278	280	282	283	285	286	288	289	291	293	294	296
91	267	268	270	271	273	274	276	277	279	280	282	283	285	286	288	290	291	293	294	296	298
92	269	270	272	273	275	276	277	279	280	282	283	285	287	288	290	291	293	294	296	298	299
93	271	272	273	275	276	278	279	281	282	284	285	287	288	290	291	293	295	296	298	299	301
94	272	274	275	277	278	280	281	283	284	285	287	288	290	292	293	295	296	298	299	301	303
95	274	276	277	279	280	281	283	284	286	287	289	290	292	293	295	296	298	300	301	303	304
96	276	278	279	280	282	283	285	286	288	289	291	292	294	295	297	298	300	301	303	304	306
97	278	279	281	282	284	285	287	288	289	291	292	294	295	297	298	300	301	303	305	306	308
98	280	281	283	284	285	287	288	290	291	293	294	296	297	299	300	302	303	305	306	308	309
99	282	283	285	286	287	289	290	292	293	294	296	297	299	300	302	303	305	306	308	310	311
100	284	285	286	288	289	291	292	293	295	296	298	299	301	302	304	305	307	308	310	311	313
101	286	287	288	290	291	292	294	295	297	298	300	301	302	304	305	307	308	310	311	313	315
102	288	289	290	292	293	294	296	297	299	300	301	303	304	306	307	309	310	312	313	315	316
103	290	291	292	294	295	296	298	299	300	302	303	305	306	308	309	310	312	313	315	316	318
104	291	293	294	295	297	298	299	301	302	304	305	306	308	309	311	312	314	315	317	319	320
105	293	295	296	297	299	300	301	303	304	306	307	308	310	311	313	314	316	317	319	320	322
106	295	297	298	299	301	302	303	305	306	307	309	310	312	313	314	316	317	319	320	322	323
107	297	299	300	301	302	304	305	306	308	309	311	312	313	315	316	318	319	321	322	324	325
108	299	301	302	303	304	306	307	308	310	311	312	314	315	317	318	320	321	322	324	325	327
109	301	302	304	305	306	308	309	310	312	313	314	316	317	319	320	321	323	324	326	327	329
110	303	304	306	307	308	310	311	312	314	315	316	318	319	320	322	323	325	326	328	329	330
111	305	306	308	309	310	311	313	314	315	317	318	319	321	322	324	325	326	328	329	331	332
112	307	308	310	311	312	313	315	316	317	319	320	321	323	324	325	327	328	330	331	333	334
113	309	310	312	313	314	315	317	318	319	321	322	323	325	326	327	329	330	332	333	334	336
114	311	312	313	315	316	317	319	320	321	322	324	325	326	328	329	331	332	333	335	336	338
115	313	314	315	317	318	319	320	322	323	324	326	327	328	330	331	332	334	335	337	339	340
116	315	316	317	319	320	321	322	324	325	326	328	329	330	332	333	334	336	337	339	340	341
117	317	318	319	321	322	323	324	326	327	328	330	331	332	334	335	336	338	339	340	342	343
118	319	320	321	323	324	325	326	328	329	330	331	333	334	335	337	338	339	341	342	344	345
119	321	322	323	325	326	327	328	330	331	332	333	335	336	337	339	340	341	343	344	345	347
120	323	324	325	327	328	329	330	331	333	334	335	337	338	339	341	342	343	345	346	347	349

Table 5 (continued)

OFD (mm)	\\ BPD (mm) →	50	51	52	53	54	55	56	57	58	59	60	61	62	63	64	65	66	67	68	69	70
60		182	183	185	186	188	189	191	192	194	196	197	199	201	202	204	206	207	209	211	213	214
61		183	185	186	188	189	191	193	194	196	197	199	201	202	204	206	207	209	211	212	214	216
62		185	187	188	190	191	193	194	196	197	199	201	202	204	206	207	209	211	212	214	216	217
63		187	188	190	191	193	194	196	198	199	201	202	204	206	207	209	210	212	214	216	217	219
64		189	190	192	193	195	196	198	199	201	202	204	206	207	209	210	212	214	215	217	219	221
65		191	192	194	195	196	198	199	201	203	204	206	207	209	210	212	214	215	217	219	220	222
66		193	194	195	197	198	200	201	203	204	206	207	209	211	212	214	215	217	219	220	222	224
67		194	196	197	199	200	202	203	205	206	208	209	211	212	214	215	217	219	220	222	224	225
68		196	198	199	200	202	203	205	206	208	209	211	212	214	216	217	219	220	222	224	225	227
69		198	199	201	202	204	205	207	208	210	211	213	214	216	217	219	220	222	224	225	227	229
70		200	201	203	204	206	207	208	210	211	213	214	216	217	219	221	222	224	225	227	229	230
71		202	203	205	206	207	209	210	212	213	215	216	218	219	221	222	224	225	227	229	230	232
72		204	205	206	208	209	211	212	214	215	216	218	219	221	222	224	226	227	229	230	232	233
73		206	207	208	210	211	213	214	215	217	218	220	221	223	224	226	227	229	230	232	234	235
74		208	209	210	212	213	214	216	217	219	220	221	223	224	226	227	229	231	232	234	235	237
75		210	211	212	214	215	216	218	219	220	222	223	225	226	228	229	231	232	234	235	237	239
76		212	213	214	215	217	218	219	221	222	224	225	227	228	230	231	233	234	236	237	239	240
77		213	215	216	217	219	220	221	223	224	226	227	228	230	231	233	234	236	237	239	240	242
78		215	217	218	219	221	222	223	225	226	227	229	230	232	233	235	236	238	239	241	242	244
79		217	219	220	221	222	224	225	226	228	229	231	232	233	235	236	238	239	241	242	244	245
80		219	221	222	223	224	226	227	228	230	231	232	234	235	237	238	240	241	243	244	246	247
81		221	223	224	225	226	228	229	230	232	233	234	236	237	239	240	241	243	244	246	247	249
82		223	225	226	227	228	230	231	232	234	235	236	238	239	240	242	243	245	246	248	249	251
83		225	226	228	229	230	231	233	234	235	237	238	239	241	242	244	245	247	248	249	251	252
84		227	228	230	231	232	233	235	236	237	239	240	241	243	244	246	247	248	250	251	253	254
85		229	230	232	233	234	235	237	238	239	241	242	243	245	246	247	249	250	252	253	255	256
86		231	232	234	235	236	237	239	240	241	242	244	245	246	248	249	251	252	253	255	256	258
87		233	234	236	237	238	239	241	242	243	244	246	247	248	250	251	252	254	255	257	258	260
88		235	236	238	239	240	241	243	244	245	246	248	249	250	252	253	254	256	257	259	260	261
89		237	238	240	241	242	243	244	246	247	248	250	251	252	254	255	256	258	259	260	262	263
90		239	241	242	243	244	245	246	248	249	250	251	253	254	255	257	258	259	261	262	264	265
91		241	243	244	245	246	247	248	250	251	252	253	255	256	257	259	260	261	263	264	266	267
92		243	245	246	247	248	249	250	252	253	254	255	257	258	259	261	262	263	265	266	267	269
93		245	247	248	249	250	251	252	254	255	256	257	259	260	261	262	264	265	266	268	269	271
94		248	249	250	251	252	253	254	256	257	258	259	261	262	263	264	266	267	268	270	271	272
95		250	251	252	253	254	255	256	258	259	260	261	262	264	265	266	268	269	270	272	273	274
96		252	253	254	255	256	257	258	260	261	262	263	264	266	267	268	270	271	272	274	275	276
97		254	255	256	257	258	259	260	262	263	264	265	266	268	269	270	271	273	274	275	277	278
98		256	257	258	259	260	261	262	264	265	266	267	268	270	271	272	273	275	276	277	279	280
99		258	259	260	261	262	263	264	266	267	268	269	270	272	273	274	275	277	278	279	281	282
100		260	261	262	263	264	265	266	268	269	270	271	272	274	275	276	277	279	280	281	282	284

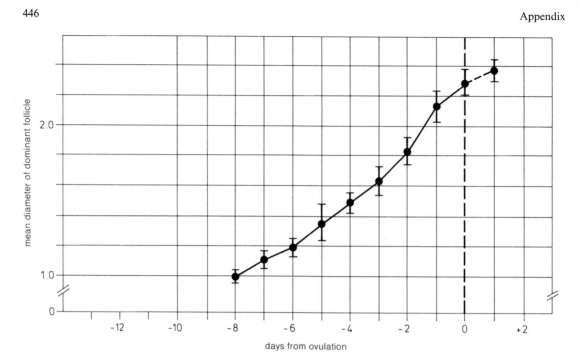

Fig. 7. Mean diameter of the dominant follicle as a function of ovulation. [From Wildt et al. (1983) "The pulsatile pattern of gonadotropin secretion and follicular development during the menstrual cycle and in women with hypothalamic and hyperandrogenemic amenorrhea". In: Leyendecker G, Stock H, Wildt L (eds), Brain and Pituitary Peptides, 2nd Ferring Symposium, Kiel, 1982. Karger, Basel, pp 28–57]

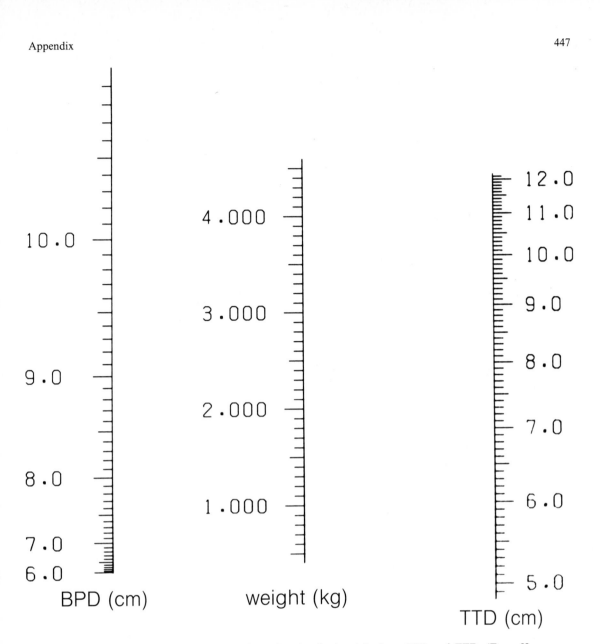

Fig. 8. Nomogram of Hansmann and Voigt for estimating fetal weight from BPD and TTD. (From Hansmann M (1976) Gynaekologe 9:133)

Table 6. Multiparametric nonlinear weight estimation by ultrasound with correction for gestational age: 29–41 weeks. [From Hansmann M, Schuhmacher H, Voigt U (1978). In: Kratochwil A, Reinold E (eds) Ultraschalldiagnostik. Thieme, Stuttgart, p 69]

Weight estimation for 29 weeks (middle of week = 30/4 = 207th postmenstrual day)

BPD↓/TTD/	66*	68*	70:	72:	74.	76.	78	80	82	84.	86.	88:	90:	92*	94*	BPD↓/TTD/
40*	211*	212*	222*	240*	267*	301*	343*	391*	446*	505*	570*	638*	711*	786*	863*	40*
42*	261*	262*	271*	290*	317*	351*	393*	441*	496*	555*	620*	688*	760*	836*	913*	42*
44*	312*	313*	323*	341*	368*	403*	444*	493*	547*	607*	671*	740*	812*	887*	965*	44*
46*	365*	366*	376*	394*	421*	456*	498*	546*	600*	660*	724*	793*	865*	940*	1018*	46*
48*	420*	421*	430*	449*	476*	510*	552*	600*	655*	714*	779*	847*	919*	995*	1072*	48*
50*	476*	477*	486*	505*	532*	566*	608*	656*	711*	770*	835*	903*	975*	1051*	1128*	50*
52:	533*	534*	544*	562*	589*	623*	665*	713*	768*	827*	892*	960*	1033*	1108*	1185*	52:
54:	591*	592*	602*	620*	647*	682*	724*	772*	826*	886*	950*	1019*	1091*	1166*	1244*	54:
56:	651*	652*	662*	680*	707*	741*	783*	831*	886*	945*	1010*	1078*	1151*	1226*	1303*	56:
58:	711*	713*	722*	741*	767*	802*	844*	892*	946*	1006*	1070*	1139*	1211*	1286*	1364*	58:
60.	773*	774*	784*	802*	829*	864.	905:	954:	1008:	1068*	1132*	1201*	1273*	1348*	1426*	60.
62.	836*	837*	846.	865:	892.	926.	968.	1016.	1071.	1130.	1195.	1263.	1335.	1411*	1488*	62.
64.	899*	900*	910:	928:	955.	990.	1031.	1080.	1134.	1194.	1258.	1327.	1399.	1474*	1552*	64.
66.	963*	964*	974:	992:	1019.	1054.	1095.	1144.	1198.	1258.	1322.	1391.	1463.	1538*	1616*	66.
68	1028*	1029*	1039:	1057:	1084.	1119.	1160.	1209.	1263.	1322.	1387.	1455.	1528.	1603*	1681*	68
70	1093*	1095*	1104:	1123:	1149.	1184.	1226.	1274.	1328.	1388.	1452.	1521.	1593.	1668*	1746*	70
72	1159*	1160*	1170:	1188:	1215.	1250.	1292.	1340.	1394.	1454.	1518.	1587.	1659.	1734*	1812*	72
74	1225*	1227*	1236:	1255:	1282.	1316.	1358.	1406.	1460.	1520.	1584.	1653.	1725:	1801*	1878*	74
76	1292*	1293*	1303:	1321:	1348.	1383.	1424.	1473.	1527.	1587.	1651.	1720.	1792:	1867*	1945*	76
78	1359*	1360*	1370:	1388:	1415.	1450.	1491.	1540.	1594.	1654.	1718.	1787.	1859:	1934*	2012*	78
80.	1426.	1427.	1437:	1455:	1482:	1517:	1559:	1607:	1661:	1721.	1785.	1854.	1926:	2001*	2079*	80.
82.	1493.	1495.	1504:	1523:	1550*	1584*	1626*	1674*	1728*	1788.	1852.	1921.	1993:	2068*	2146*	82.
84.	1561.	1562.	1571:	1590:	1617*	1651*	1693*	1741*	1796*	1855.	1920.	1988.	2060:	2136*	2213*	84.
86.	1628.	1629.	1639:	1657:	1684*	1718*	1760*	1809*	1863:	1922.	1987.	2055.	2128:	2203*	2281*	86.
88:	1695.	1696.	1706:	1724:	1751*	1786*	1827*	1876*	1930:	1989.	2054.	2122.	2195:	2270*	2348*	88:
90:	1762.	1763.	1773:	1791:	1818*	1852*	1894*	1943*	1997:	2056.	2121.	2189:	2262:	2337*	2415*	90:
92*	1828*	1830*	1839:	1858:	1884*	1919*	1961*	2009*	2063:	2123.	2187.	2256:	2328:	2403*	2481*	92*
94*	1895*	1896*	1905:	1924:	1951*	1985*	2027*	2075*	2129:	2189.	2254.	2322:	2394:	2470*	2547*	94*
96*	1960*	1962*	1971:	1990:	2016*	2051*	2093*	2141*	2195:	2255.	2319.	2388:	2460:	2535*	2613*	96*
98*	2025*	2027*	2036:	2055:	2082*	2116*	2158*	2206*	2260:	2320.	2384.	2453:	2525:	2601*	2678*	98*
100*	2090*	2091*	2101:	2119:	2146*	2181*	2223*	2271*	2325:	2385.	2449.	2518:	2590:	2665*	2743*	100*

Explanation of symbols . ∖: ∖* = at least one ultrasound parameter outside the 1st∖2nd∖3rd standard deviation. Ultrasound parameters at 29 weeks

	-3STD	-2STD	-1STD	AM	1STD	2STD	3STD
Normal range Percentiles	0.13%	2.28%	15.87%	50.00%	84.13%	97.72%	99.87%
Biparietal diameter = BPD (mm)	68.0*	72.0*	76.0*	80.0	84.0*	88.0*	92.0*
Transverse trunk diameter = TTD (mm)	51.0*	58.0*	65.0*	72.0	79.0.	86.0*	93.0*
Head-to-trunk ratio = BPD/TTD	0.9097*	0.9819:	1.0541:	1.1262	1.1984.	1.2706:	1.3428*
Fetal weight = WT (grams)	480*	770:	1060.	1350	1640.	1930:	2220*

Table 6 (continued)

Weight estimation for 30 weeks (middle of week = 31/4 = 214th postmenstrual day)

BPD↓/TTD→	68*	70*	72:	74:	76.	78.	80	82	84	86	88.	90.	92:	94:	96*	BPD↓/TTD→
40*	183*	193*	211*	238*	273*	314*	363*	417*	477*	541*	610*	682*	757*	835*	914*	40*
42*	233*	243*	261*	288*	322*	364*	413*	467*	526*	591*	659*	732*	807*	885*	964*	42*
44*	285*	294*	313*	339*	374*	416*	464*	518*	578*	642*	711*	783*	858*	936*	1015*	44*
46*	338*	347*	366*	392*	427*	469*	517*	571*	631*	695*	764*	836*	911*	989*	1069*	46*
48*	392*	402*	420*	447*	481*	523*	572*	626*	685*	750*	818*	891*	966*	1044*	1123*	48*
50*	448*	458*	476*	503*	537*	579*	627*	682*	741*	806*	874*	947*	1022*	1099*	1179*	50*
52*	505*	515*	533*	560*	595*	636*	685*	739*	798*	863*	931*	1004*	1079*	1157*	1236*	52*
54:	564*	573*	592*	618*	653*	695*	743*	797*	857*	921*	990*	1062*	1137*	1215*	1295*	54:
56:	623*	633*	651:	678:	713*	754*	803*	857:	916*	981*	1049*	1122*	1197*	1275*	1354*	56:
58:	684*	693*	712:	739:	773:	815*	863*	917:	977*	1042*	1110*	1182*	1258*	1335*	1415*	58:
60:	746*	755*	774:	800:	835:	877:	925*	979*	1039*	1103*	1172*	1244*	1319*	1397*	1476*	60.
62.	808*	818*	836:	863:	897:	939:	987:	1042:	1101*	1166*	1234*	1307*	1382*	1459*	1539*	62.
64.	871*	881*	899:	926:	961:	1003:	1051:	1105:	1165:	1229*	1298*	1370*	1445*	1523*	1602*	64.
66.	935*	945:	964:	990:	1025:	1067:	1115:	1169:	1229:	1293:	1362*	1434*	1509*	1587*	1666*	66.
68	1000*	1010:	1028:	1055:	1090:	1131:	1180:	1234:	1294:	1358:	1427:	1499:	1574*	1652*	1731*	68
70	1066*	1075:	1094:	1121:	1155:	1197:	1245:	1299:	1359:	1423:	1492:	1564:	1640:	1717*	1797*	70
72	1132*	1141:	1160:	1186:	1221:	1263:	1311:	1365:	1425:	1489:	1558:	1630:	1705:	1783:	1863*	72
74	1198*	1207:	1226:	1253:	1287:	1329:	1377:	1432:	1491:	1556:	1624:	1696:	1772:	1849:	1929*	74
76	1265*	1274:	1293:	1319:	1354:	1396:	1444:	1498:	1558:	1622:	1691:	1763:	1838:	1916:	1995*	76
78	1331*	1341:	1359:	1386:	1421:	1463:	1511:	1565:	1625:	1689:	1758:	1830:	1905:	1983:	2062*	78
80	1399*	1408:	1427:	1453:	1488:	1530:	1578:	1632:	1692:	1756:	1825:	1897:	1972:	2050:	2130*	80
82	1466*	1475:	1494:	1521:	1555:	1597:	1645:	1700:	1759:	1824:	1892:	1964:	2040:	2117:	2197*	82
84	1533*	1543:	1561:	1588:	1622:	1664:	1713:	1767:	1826:	1891:	1959:	2032:	2107:	2185:	2264*	84.
86	1600*	1610:	1628:	1655:	1690*	1731:	1780:	1834:	1894:	1958:	2027:	2099:	2174:	2252:	2331*	86.
88	1667*	1677:	1695:	1722:	1757:	1798:	1847:	1901:	1961:	2025:	2094:	2166:	2241:	2319:	2398*	88.
90	1734*	1744:	1762:	1789:	1824:	1865:	1914*	1968:	2028:	2092:	2161:	2233:	2308:	2386:	2465*	90:
92	1801*	1810:	1829:	1856:	1890*	1932:	1980*	2034:	2094:	2159:	2227:	2299:	2375:	2452:	2532*	92:
94	1867*	1877:	1895:	1922:	1956:	1998:	2046:	2101:	2160:	2225:	2293:	2366:	2441:	2518:	2598*	94:
96	1933*	1942:	1961:	1988:	2022:	2064:	2112:	2166:	2226:	2290:	2359:	2431:	2507:	2584:	2664*	96:
98	1998*	2007:	2026:	2053:	2087:	2129:	2177:	2232:	2291:	2356:	2424:	2497:	2572:	2649:	2729*	98*
100*	2063*	2072:	2091:	2117:	2152:	2194:	2242:	2296:	2356:	2420:	2489:	2561:	2636:	2714:	2794*	100*
102*	2126*	2136:	2155:	2181:	2216:	2258:	2306:	2360:	2420:	2484:	2553:	2625:	2700:	2778:	2857*	102*
104*	2190*	2199:	2218:	2244:	2279:	2321:	2369:	2423:	2483:	2547:	2616:	2688:	2763:	2841:	2921*	104*
106*	2252*	2261:	2280:	2307:	2341:	2383:	2431:	2486:	2545:	2610:	2678:	2750:	2826:	2903:	2983*	106*
108*	2313*	2323:	2341:	2368:	2403:	2444:	2493:	2547:	2607:	2671:	2740:	2812:	2887:	2965:	3044*	108*

Explanation of symbols . \ : \ * = at least one ultrasound parameter outside the 1st\2nd\3rd standard deviation. Ultrasound parameters at 30 weeks

	-3STD:	-2STD:	-1STD.	AM	1STD.	2STD:	3STD*
Normal range							
Percentiles	0.13%	2.28%	15.87%	50.00%	84.13%	97.72%	99.87%
Biparietal diameter = BPD (mm)	70.5*	74.5:	78.5.	82.5	86.5.	90.5:	94.5*
Transverse trunk diameter = TTD (mm)	53.2*	60.5:	67.7.	75.0	82.2:	89.5:	96.7*
Head-to-trunk ratio = BPD/TTD	0.8990*	0.9702:	1.0413.	1.1125	1.1837.	1.2548:	1.3260*
Fetal weight = WT (grams)	600*	900:	1200.	1500	1800.	2100:	2400*

Table 6 (continued)

Weight estimation for 31 weeks (middle of week = 32/4 = 221th postmenstrual day)

BPD↓ TTD→	70*	72*	74:	76:	78.	80.	82.	84.	86	88	90.	92.	94:	96:	98*	100*	102*	BPD↓ TTD→
40*	183*	202*	228*	263*	305*	353*	407*	467*	531*	600*	672*	747*	825*	905*	985*	1067*	1148*	40*
42*	233*	252*	278*	313*	355*	403*	457*	517*	581*	650*	722*	797*	875*	954*	1035*	1117*	1198*	42*
44*	285*	303*	330*	364*	406*	454*	509*	568*	633*	701*	774*	849*	926*	1006*	1087*	1168*	1250*	44*
46*	338*	356*	383*	417*	459*	507*	562*	621*	686*	754*	827*	902*	979*	1059*	1140*	1221*	1303*	46*
48*	392*	411*	437*	472*	514*	562*	616*	676*	740*	809*	881*	956*	1034*	1113*	1194*	1276*	1357*	48*
50*	448*	466*	493*	528*	570*	618*	672*	732*	796*	865*	937*	1012*	1090*	1169*	1250*	1332*	1413*	50*
52*	505*	524*	550*	585*	627*	675*	729*	789*	853*	922*	994*	1069*	1147*	1227*	1307*	1389*	1470*	52*
54*	564*	582*	609*	643*	685*	733*	788*	847*	912*	980*	1053*	1128*	1206*	1285*	1366*	1447*	1529*	54*
56:	623*	642*	668*	703*	745*	793*	847*	907*	971*	1040*	1113*	1188*	1265*	1345*	1425*	1507*	1588*	56:
58:	684*	702*	729.	764*	805*	854*	908*	968*	1032*	1101*	1173*	1248*	1326*	1405*	1486*	1567*	1649*	58:
60:	745*	764*	791:	825:	867:	915*	970*	1029*	1094*	1162*	1235*	1310*	1387*	1467*	1548*	1629*	1710*	60:
62:	808*	827*	853:	888:	930:	978:	1032*	1092*	1156*	1225*	1297*	1372*	1450*	1529*	1610*	1692*	1773*	62:
64.	871*	890*	917.	951.	993.	1041.	1096.	1155*	1220*	1288*	1360*	1436*	1513*	1593*	1673*	1755*	1836*	64.
66.	935*	954*	981.	1015.	1057.	1105.	1160.	1219.	1284.	1352*	1425*	1500*	1577*	1657*	1738*	1819*	1900*	66.
68.	1000*	1019*	1046.	1080.	1122.	1170.	1224.	1284.	1348.	1417.	1489*	1565*	1642*	1722*	1802*	1884*	1965*	68.
70.	1066*	1084*	1111.	1146.	1187.	1236.	1290.	1349.	1414.	1482.	1555.	1630*	1708*	1787*	1868*	1949*	2031*	70.
72	1132*	1150*	1177.	1211.	1253.	1301.	1356.	1415.	1480.	1548.	1621.	1696:	1773*	1853*	1934*	2015*	2097*	72
74	1198*	1216*	1243.	1278.	1319.	1368.	1422.	1482.	1546.	1615.	1687.	1762.	1840*	1919:	2000*	2081*	2163*	74
76	1265*	1283*	1310.	1344.	1386.	1434.	1489.	1548.	1613.	1681.	1754.	1829.	1906*	1986:	2067*	2148*	2230*	76
78	1331*	1350*	1377.	1411.	1453.	1501.	1556.	1615.	1680.	1748.	1820.	1896.	1973*	2053:	2134*	2215*	2296*	78
80	1399*	1417*	1444.	1478.	1520.	1568.	1623.	1682.	1747.	1815.	1888.	1963.	2041*	2120:	2201*	2282*	2364*	80
82	1466*	1484*	1511.	1546.	1587.	1636.	1690.	1750.	1814.	1883.	1955.	2030.	2108*	2187:	2268*	2349*	2431*	82
84	1533*	1552*	1578.	1613.	1655.	1703.	1757.	1817.	1881.	1950.	2022.	2097.	2175*	2254:	2335*	2417*	2498*	84
86.	1600*	1619*	1646.	1680:	1722.	1770.	1824.	1884.	1948.	2017.	2089.	2165.	2242*	2322:	2402*	2484*	2565*	86.
88:	1667*	1686*	1713.	1747:	1789.	1837.	1891.	1951.	2015.	2084.	2156.	2232.	2309*	2389:	2469*	2551*	2632*	88:
90:	1734*	1753*	1780.	1814:	1856.	1904*	1958.	2018.	2082.	2151.	2223.	2298.	2376*	2456:	2536*	2618*	2699*	90:
92:	1801*	1819*	1846.	1881:	1922.	1971*	2025.	2085.	2149.	2218.	2290.	2365.	2443*	2522:	2603*	2684*	2766*	92:
94*	1867*	1885*	1912.	1947:	1989.	2037*	2091*	2151.	2215.	2284.	2356.	2431.	2509*	2588:	2669*	2751*	2832*	94*
96*	1933*	1951*	1978.	2013:	2054.	2103*	2157*	2216.	2281.	2349.	2422.	2497.	2575*	2654:	2735*	2816*	2898*	96*
98*	1998*	2016*	2043.	2078:	2119.	2168*	2222*	2282.	2346.	2415.	2487.	2562.	2640*	2719:	2800*	2881*	2963*	98*
100*	2063*	2081*	2108.	2142:	2184.	2232*	2287*	2346.	2411.	2479.	2552.	2627.	2704*	2784:	2865*	2946*	3028*	100*
102*	2126*	2145*	2172.	2206:	2248.	2296*	2351*	2410.	2475.	2543.	2616.	2691.	2768*	2848:	2929*	3010*	3091*	102*
104*	2190*	2208*	2235.	2269:	2311.	2359*	2414*	2473.	2538.	2606.	2679.	2754.	2831*	2911:	2992*	3073*	3155*	104*
106*	2252*	2270*	2297.	2332:	2373.	2422*	2476*	2536.	2600.	2669.	2741.	2816.	2894*	2973:	3054*	3135*	3217*	106*
108*	2313*	2332*	2359.	2393:	2435.	2483*	2537*	2597.	2661.	2730.	2802.	2877.	2955*	3035:	3116*	3197*	3278*	108*
110*	2374*	2392*	2419.	2453:	2495.	2544*	2598*	2657.	2722.	2790.	2863.	2938.	3016*	3095:	3176*	3257*	3339*	110*
112*	2433*	2451*	2478.	2513:	2554.	2603*	2657*	2717.	2781.	2850.	2922.	2997.	3075*	3154:	3235*	3316*	3398*	112*
114*	2491*	2509*	2536.	2571:	2612.	2661*	2715*	2771.	2839.	2908.	2980.	3055.	3133*	3212:	3293*	3375*	3456*	114*
116*	2548*	2566*	2593.	2628:	2669.	2718*	2772*	2831.	2896.	2964.	3037.	3112.	3190*	3269:	3350*	3431*	3513*	116*

Explanation of symbols . \ : \ * = at least one ultrasound parameter outside the 1st \ 2nd \ 3rd standard deviation. Ultrasound parameters at 31 weeks

Normal range							
Percentiles	-3STD: 0,13%	-2STD: 2,28%	-1STD: 15,87%	AM 50,00%	1STD: 84,13%	2STD: 97,72%	3STD: 99,87%
Biparietal diameter = BPD (mm)	73,0*	77,0*	81,0*	85,0*	89,0*	93,0*	97,0*
Transverse trunk diameter = TTD (mm)	55,0*	62,5*	70,0*	77,5*	85,0*	92,5*	100,0*
Head-to-trunk ratio = BPD/TTD	0,8901*	0,9592*	1,0284*	1,0975*	1,1666*	1,2358*	1,3049*
Fetal weight = WT (grams)	600*	950.	1300.	1650.	2000.	2350.	2700.

Table 6 (continued)

Weight estimation for 32 weeks (middle of week = 33/4 = 228th postmenstrual day)

BPD↓\TTD→	70*	72*	74*	76:	78:	80.	82.	84	86	88	90	92.	94.	96*	98:	100*	102*	104*	106*
42*	239*	257*	284*	318*	360*	408*	463*	522*	587*	655*	728*	803*	880*	960*	1041*	1122*	1204*	1284*	1364*
44*	290*	309*	335*	370*	412*	460*	514*	574*	638*	707*	779*	854*	932*	1011*	1092*	1174*	1255*	1336*	1416*
46*	343*	362*	388*	423*	465*	513*	567*	627*	691*	760*	832*	907*	985*	1064*	1145*	1227*	1308*	1389*	1469*
48*	398*	416*	443*	477*	519*	567*	622*	681*	746*	814*	887*	962*	1039*	1119*	1200*	1281*	1363*	1443*	1523*
50*	454*	472*	499*	533*	575*	623*	678*	737*	802*	870*	943*	1018*	1095*	1175*	1256*	1337*	1419*	1499*	1579*
52*	511*	529*	556*	591*	632*	681*	735*	794*	859*	927*	1000*	1075*	1153*	1232*	1313*	1394*	1476*	1557*	1636*
54*	569*	588*	614*	649*	691*	739*	793*	853*	917*	986*	1058*	1133*	1211*	1291*	1371*	1453*	1534*	1615*	1695*
56*	629*	647*	674*	709*	750*	799*	853*	912*	977*	1045*	1118*	1193*	1271*	1350*	1431*	1512*	1594*	1675*	1754*
58*	689*	708*	735*	769*	811*	859*	913*	973*	1037*	1106*	1178*	1254*	1331*	1411*	1491*	1573*	1654*	1735*	1815*
60:	751*	770*	796*	831*	873*	921*	975*	1035*	1099*	1168*	1240*	1315*	1393*	1472*	1553*	1635*	1716*	1797*	1877*
62:	814*	832*	859*	893*	935*	983*	1038*	1097*	1162*	1230*	1303*	1378*	1455*	1535*	1616*	1697*	1779*	1859*	1939*
64:	877*	895*	922*	957*	998*	1047*	1101*	1161*	1225*	1294*	1366*	1441*	1519*	1598*	1679*	1760*	1842*	1923*	2003*
66:	941*	960*	986*	1021*	1063:	1111:	1165:	1225:	1289*	1358*	1430*	1505*	1583*	1662*	1743*	1825*	1906*	1987*	2067*
68.	1006*	1024*	1051*	1086:	1127:	1176.	1230:	1290:	1354:	1423*	1495*	1570*	1648*	1727*	1808*	1889*	1971*	2052*	2131*
70.	1071*	1090*	1117:	1151:	1193:	1241:	1295.	1355.	1419.	1488:	1560*	1635*	1713*	1793*	1873*	1955*	2036*	2117*	2197*
72.	1137*	1156*	1182:	1217:	1259:	1307.	1361.	1421.	1485.	1554:	1626*	1701*	1779*	1858*	1939*	2021*	2102*	2183*	2263*
74.	1203*	1222*	1249:	1283:	1325:	1373.	1428.	1487.	1552.	1620.	1692*	1768*	1845*	1925*	2005*	2087*	2168*	2249*	2329*
76	1270*	1289*	1315:	1350:	1392.	1440.	1494.	1554.	1618.	1687.	1759.	1834*	1912*	1991:	2072*	2154*	2235*	2316*	2396*
78	1337*	1355*	1382:	1417:	1459.	1507.	1561.	1621.	1685.	1754.	1826.	1901.	1968:	2058:	2139:	2221*	2302*	2383*	2463*
80	1404*	1422*	1449:	1484.	1526.	1574.	1628.	1688.	1752.	1821.	1893.	1968.	2046.	2126.	2206:	2288:	2369*	2450*	2530*
82	1471*	1490*	1517:	1551.	1593.	1641.	1695.	1755.	1819.	1888.	1960.	2036.	2113.	2193.	2273:	2355:	2436*	2517*	2597*
84	1539*	1557*	1584.	1618.	1660.	1708.	1763.	1822.	1887.	1955.	2028.	2103.	2180.	2260.	2341.	2422:	2504:	2584*	2664*
86	1606*	1624*	1651.	1686.	1727.	1776.	1830.	1890.	1954.	2023.	2095.	2170.	2248.	2327.	2408.	2489:	2571:	2652*	2731*
88	1673*	1691*	1718.	1753.	1794.	1843.	1897.	1957.	2021.	2090.	2162.	2237.	2315.	2394.	2475:	2556:	2638:	2719*	2799*
90.	1740*	1758*	1785.	1820:	1861:	1910.	1964.	2024.	2088.	2157.	2229.	2304.	2382.	2461.	2542:	2623:	2704:	2786*	2865*
92.	1806*	1825*	1852.	1886:	1928:	1976:	2030.	2090.	2154.	2223.	2295.	2371.	2448.	2528.	2608.	2690:	2771:	2852*	2932*
94.	1873*	1891*	1918.	1952:	1994:	2042:	2097:	2156.	2221.	2289:	2362.	2437.	2514.	2594.	2675.	2756:	2838.	2918*	2998*
96.	1938*	1957*	1984.	2018:	2060:	2108:	2162:	2222:	2286:	2355:	2427.	2502.	2580.	2660.	2740.	2822*	2903.	2984*	3064*
98*	2003*	2022*	2049*	2083:	2125:	2173:	2228:	2287:	2352*	2420:	2492:	2568:	2645.	2725.	2806.	2887*	2968.	3049*	3129*
100:	2068*	2087*	2113:	2148:	2190:	2238:	2292:	2352:	2416*	2485*	2557:	2632.	2710.	2789.	2870.	2952*	3033.	3114*	3194*
102:	2132*	2150*	2177:	2212:	2254:	2302:	2356:	2419*	2480*	2549*	2621*	2696.	2774.	2853.	2934.	3016*	3097.	3178*	3258*
104:	2195*	2214*	2240*	2275:	2317:	2365:	2419:	2482*	2543*	2612*	2684*	2759.	2837.	2917.	2997:	3079*	3160.	3241*	3321*
106*	2257*	2276*	2303*	2337*	2379*	2427*	2482*	2541*	2606*	2674*	2746*	2822*	2899*	2979*	3060*	3141*	3222*	3303*	3383*
108*	2319*	2337*	2364*	2398*	2440*	2489*	2543*	2603*	2667*	2735*	2808*	2883*	2961*	3040*	3121*	3202*	3284*	3365*	3444*
110*	2379*	2398*	2424*	2459*	2501*	2549*	2603*	2663*	2727*	2796*	2868*	2943*	3021*	3101*	3181*	3263*	3344*	3425*	3505*
112*	2438*	2457*	2484*	2518*	2560*	2608*	2663*	2722*	2787*	2855*	2927*	3003*	3080*	3160*	3240*	3322*	3403*	3484*	3564*
114*	2496*	2515*	2542*	2576*	2618*	2666*	2721*	2780*	2845*	2913*	2986*	3061*	3138*	3218*	3299*	3380*	3461*	3542*	3622*
116*	2553*	2572*	2599*	2633*	2675*	2723*	2777*	2837*	2901*	2970*	3042*	3118*	3195*	3275*	3355*	3437*	3518*	3599*	3679*
118*	2609*	2627*	2654*	2689*	2730*	2779*	2833*	2893*	2957*	3026*	3098*	3173*	3251*	3330*	3411*	3492*	3574*	3655*	3734*
120*	2663*	2681*	2708*	2743*	2784*	2833*	2887*	2947*	3011*	3080*	3152*	3227*	3305*	3384*	3465*	3546*	3628*	3709*	3789*
122*	2716*	2734*	2761*	2795*	2837*	2885*	2940*	2999*	3064*	3132*	3205*	3280*	3357*	3437*	3518*	3599*	3681*	3761*	3841*

Explanation of symbols . \: * = at least one ultrasound parameter outside the 1st\2nd\3rd standard deviation. Ultrasound parameters at 32 weeks

Normal range	-3STD	-2STD	-1STD	AM	1STD	2STD	3STD
Percentiles	0.13%	2.28%	15.87%	50.00%	84.13%	97.72%	99.87%
Biparietal diameter = BPD (mm)	75.5	79.5	83.5	87.5	91.5	95.5	99.5
Transverse trunk diameter = TTD (mm)	58.7	66.5	74.2	82.0	89.7	97.5	105.2
Head-to-trunk ratio = BPD/TTD	0.8830	0.9491	1.0152	1.0812	1.1473	1.2134	1.2795
Fetal weight = WT (grams)	590	1000	1410	1820	2230	2640	3050

Table 6 (continued)

Weight estimation for 33 weeks (middle of week = 33/4 = 228th postmenstrual day)

BPD↓/TTD→	72*	74*	76*	78:	80:	82.	84.	86	88	90	92*	94*	96*	98:	100:	102*	104*	106*	108*	BPD↓/TTD→
36*	171*	198*	232*	274*	322*	376*	436*	500*	569*	641*	717*	794*	874*	954*	1036:	1117*	1198*	1278*	1356*	36*
38*	217*	244*	279*	320*	369*	423*	482*	547*	615*	688*	763*	841*	920*	1001*	1082*	1164*	1245*	1324*	1402*	38*
40*	265*	292*	327*	368*	417*	471*	531*	595*	664*	736*	811*	889*	968*	1049*	1130*	1212*	1293*	1373*	1451*	40*
42*	315*	342*	377*	418*	467*	521*	580*	645*	713*	786*	861*	939*	1018*	1099*	1180*	1262*	1343*	1422*	1500*	42*
44*	367*	393*	428*	470*	518*	572*	632*	696*	765*	837*	912*	990*	1070*	1150*	1232*	1313*	1394*	1474*	1552*	44*
46*	420*	447*	481*	523*	571*	625*	685*	749*	818*	890*	965*	1043*	1123*	1203*	1285*	1366*	1447*	1527*	1605*	46*
48*	474*	501*	536*	577*	626*	680*	739*	804*	872*	945*	1020*	1098*	1177*	1258*	1339*	1421*	1502*	1581*	1659*	48*
50*	530*	557*	592*	633*	682*	736*	795*	860*	928*	1001*	1076*	1154*	1233*	1314*	1395*	1477*	1558*	1637*	1715*	50*
52*	587*	614*	649*	690*	739*	793*	853*	917*	986*	1058*	1133*	1211*	1290*	1371*	1452*	1534*	1615*	1695*	1773*	52*
54*	646*	673*	707*	749*	797*	851*	911*	975*	1044*	1116*	1192*	1269*	1349*	1429*	1511*	1592*	1673*	1753*	1831*	54*
56*	705*	732*	767*	808*	857*	911*	971*	1035*	1104*	1176*	1251*	1329*	1408*	1489*	1570*	1652*	1733*	1812*	1891*	56*
58*	766*	793*	827*	869*	917*	972*	1031*	1096*	1164*	1236*	1312*	1389*	1469*	1550*	1631*	1712*	1793*	1873*	1951*	58*
60:	828*	854*	889*	931*	979*	1033*	1093*	1157*	1226*	1298*	1373*	1451*	1531*	1611*	1693*	1774*	1855*	1935*	2013*	60:
62:	890*	917*	952*	993:	1042*	1096*	1155*	1220*	1288*	1361*	1436*	1514*	1593*	1674*	1755:	1837*	1918*	1997*	2075*	62:
64:	954*	980*	1015*	1057:	1105*	1159*	1219*	1283*	1352*	1424*	1499*	1577*	1656*	1737*	1819*	1900*	1981*	2061*	2139*	64:
66:	1018*	1044*	1079*	1121*	1169:	1223*	1283*	1347*	1416*	1488*	1563*	1641*	1721*	1801*	1883*	1964*	2045*	2125*	2203*	66:
68:	1082*	1109*	1144*	1185*	1234*	1288*	1348*	1412*	1481*	1553*	1628*	1706*	1785*	1866*	1947*	2029*	2110*	2190*	2268*	68:
70.	1148*	1175*	1209*	1251*	1299*	1353*	1413*	1477*	1546*	1618*	1694*	1771*	1851*	1931*	2013*	2094*	2175*	2255*	2333*	70.
72.	1214*	1241*	1275*	1317*	1365*	1419*	1479*	1543*	1612*	1684*	1759*	1837*	1917*	1997*	2079*	2160*	2241*	2321*	2399*	72.
74.	1280*	1307*	1341*	1383*	1432*	1486*	1545*	1610*	1678*	1751*	1826*	1903*	1983*	2064*	2145*	2227*	2307*	2387*	2465*	74.
76.	1347*	1373*	1408*	1450*	1498*	1552*	1612*	1676*	1745*	1817*	1892*	1970:	2050*	2130:	2212*	2293*	2374*	2454*	2532*	76.
78	1414*	1440*	1475*	1517*	1565*	1619*	1679*	1743*	1812*	1884*	1959*	2037:	2116*	2197:	2279*	2360*	2441*	2521*	2599*	78
80	1481*	1508*	1542*	1584*	1632*	1686*	1746*	1810*	1879*	1951*	2027*	2104*	2184*	2264:	2346:	2427*	2508*	2588*	2666*	80
82	1548*	1575*	1609*	1651*	1699*	1754*	1813*	1878*	1946*	2019*	2094*	2171*	2251*	2332:	2413:	2494*	2575*	2655*	2733*	82
84	1615*	1642*	1677*	1718*	1767*	1821*	1880*	1945*	2013*	2086*	2161*	2239*	2318*	2399:	2480:	2562*	2643*	2722*	2800*	84
86	1682*	1709*	1744*	1785*	1834*	1888*	1948*	2012*	2081*	2153*	2228*	2306*	2385*	2466*	2547:	2629*	2710*	2790*	2868*	86
88	1749*	1776*	1811*	1853*	1901*	1955*	2015*	2079*	2148.	2220*	2295*	2373*	2452*	2533*	2615:	2696*	2777*	2857*	2935*	88
90	1816*	1843*	1878*	1919*	1968*	2022*	2082*	2146.	2215*	2287*	2362*	2440*	2519*	2600*	2681:	2763*	2844*	2924*	3002*	90
92	1883*	1910*	1944*	1986*	2034*	2089.	2148.	2213*	2281*	2353*	2429*	2506*	2586*	2667*	2748:	2829*	2910*	2990*	3068*	92
94	1949*	1976*	2010*	2052*	2101*	2155.	2214.	2279*	2347*	2420*	2495*	2573*	2652*	2733*	2814*	2896*	2977*	3056*	3134*	94
96	2015*	2042*	2076*	2118*	2166*	2220*	2280*	2345*	2413*	2485*	2561*	2638*	2718*	2798*	2880*	2961*	3042*	3122*	3200*	96
98	2080*	2107*	2141*	2183*	2231*	2286*	2345*	2410*	2478*	2551*	2626*	2703*	2783*	2864*	2945:	3027*	3107*	3187*	3265*	98
100:	2145*	2172*	2206*	2248*	2296*	2350*	2410*	2474*	2543*	2615*	2690*	2768*	2848*	2928*	3010:	3091*	3172*	3252*	3330*	100:
102:	2209*	2235*	2270*	2312*	2360*	2414*	2474*	2538*	2607*	2679*	2754*	2832*	2912*	2992*	3074*	3155*	3236*	3316*	3394*	102:
104:	2272*	2299*	2333*	2375*	2423*	2477*	2537*	2601*	2670*	2743*	2818*	2895*	2975*	3055*	3137:	3218*	3299*	3379*	3457*	104:
106:	2334*	2361*	2395*	2437*	2485*	2540*	2599*	2664*	2732*	2805*	2880*	2957*	3037*	3118*	3199:	3281*	3361*	3441*	3519*	106:
108:	2395*	2422*	2457*	2498*	2547*	2601*	2661*	2725*	2794*	2866*	2941*	3019*	3098*	3179*	3260:	3342*	3423*	3503*	3581*	108:
110:	2456*	2483*	2517*	2559*	2607*	2661*	2721*	2785*	2854*	2926*	3002*	3079*	3159*	3239*	3321*	3402*	3483*	3563*	3641*	110:
112*	2515*	2542*	2576*	2618*	2666*	2721*	2780*	2845*	2913*	2986*	3061*	3138*	3218*	3299*	3380*	3462*	3542*	3622*	3700*	112*
114*	2573*	2600*	2634*	2676*	2724*	2779*	2838*	2903*	2971*	3044*	3119*	3196*	3276*	3357*	3438*	3520*	3600*	3680*	3758*	114*
116*	2630*	2657*	2691*	2733*	2781*	2836*	2895*	2960*	3028*	3100*	3176*	3253*	3333*	3414*	3495*	3576*	3657*	3737*	3815*	116*
118*	2685*	2712*	2747*	2788*	2837*	2891*	2951*	3015*	3084*	3156*	3231*	3309*	3388*	3469*	3550*	3632*	3713*	3793*	3871*	118*
120*	2740*	2766*	2801*	2843*	2891*	2945*	3005*	3069*	3138*	3210*	3285*	3363*	3442*	3523*	3605*	3686*	3767*	3847*	3925*	120*
122*	2792*	2819*	2853*	2895*	2944*	2998*	3057*	3122*	3190*	3263*	3338*	3416*	3495*	3576*	3657*	3739*	3820*	3899*	3977*	122*
124*	2843*	2870*	2905*	2946*	2995*	3049*	3108*	3173*	3241*	3314*	3389*	3467*	3546*	3627*	3708*	3790*	3871*	3950*	4028*	124*
126*	2893*	2919*	2954*	2996*	3044*	3098*	3158*	3222*	3291*	3363*	3438*	3516*	3595*	3676*	3758*	3839*	3920*	4000*	4078*	126*
128*	2940*	2967*	3002*	3043*	3092*	3146*	3205*	3270*	3338*	3411*	3486*	3564*	3643*	3724*	3805*	3887*	3968*	4047*	4125*	128*
130*	2986*	3013*	3048*	3089*	3137*	3192*	3251*	3316*	3384*	3457*	3532*	3609*	3689*	3770*	3851*	3933*	4013*	4093*	4171*	130*
132*	3030*	3057*	3091*	3133*	3181*	3236*	3295*	3360*	3428*	3500*	3576*	3653*	3733*	3814*	3895*	3976*	4057*	4137*	4215*	132*

Explanation of symbols . \ : \ * = at least one ultrasound parameter outside the 1st \ 2nd \ 3rd standard deviation. Ultrasound parameters at 33 weeks

Normal range	-3STD*	-2STD:	-1STD.	AM	1STD.	2STD:	3STD*
Percentiles	0.13%	2.28%	15.87%	50.00%	84.13%	97.72%	99.87%
Biparietal diameter = BPD (mm)	77.5*	81.5:	85.5.	89.5	93.5.	97.5:	101.5*
Transverse trunk diameter = TTD (mm)	59.7*	68.0:	76.2.	84.5	92.7.	101.0:	109.2*
Head-to-trunk ratio = BPD/TTD	0.8717*	0.9370:	1.0022.	1.0675	1.1328.	1.1980:	1.2633*
Fetal weight = WT (grams)	760*	1180:	1600.	2020	2440.	2860:	3280*

Table 6 (continued)

Weight estimation for 34 weeks (middle of week = 35/4 = 242th postmenstrual day)

BPD↓/TTD→	74*	76*	78*	80*	82:	84:	86.	88.	90	92	94	96*	98.	100:	102:	104*	106*	108*	110*	BPD↓/TTD→
40*	360*	394*	436*	485*	539*	598*	663*	731*	804*	879*	957*	1036*	1117*	1198*	1280*	1361*	1440*	1518*	1594*	40*
42*	410*	444*	486*	534*	589*	648*	713*	781*	854*	929*	1006*	1086*	1167*	1248*	1329*	1410*	1490*	1568*	1644*	42*
44*	461*	496*	538*	586*	640*	700*	764*	833*	905*	980*	1058*	1137*	1218*	1300*	1381*	1462*	1542*	1620*	1696*	44*
46*	514*	549*	591*	639*	693*	753*	817*	886*	958*	1033*	1111*	1190*	1271*	1353*	1434*	1515*	1595*	1673*	1749*	46*
48*	569*	603*	645*	693*	748*	807*	872*	940*	1013*	1088*	1165*	1245*	1326*	1407*	1488*	1569*	1649*	1727*	1803*	48*
50*	625*	659*	701*	749*	804*	863*	928*	996*	1068*	1144*	1221*	1301*	1382*	1463*	1544*	1625*	1705*	1783*	1859*	50*
52*	682*	716*	758*	807*	861*	920*	985*	1053*	1126*	1201*	1279*	1358*	1439*	1520*	1602*	1683*	1762*	1840*	1916*	52*
54*	740*	775*	817*	865*	919*	979*	1043*	1112*	1184*	1259*	1337*	1416*	1497*	1579*	1660*	1741*	1821*	1899*	1975*	54*
56*	800*	834*	876*	924*	979*	1038*	1103*	1171*	1244*	1319*	1397*	1476*	1557*	1638*	1720*	1801*	1880*	1958*	2034*	56*
58*	861*	895*	937*	985*	1039*	1099*	1163*	1232*	1304*	1379*	1457*	1537*	1617*	1699*	1780*	1861*	1941*	2019*	2095*	58*
60*	922*	957*	998*	1047*	1101*	1161*	1225*	1294*	1366*	1441*	1519*	1598*	1679*	1761*	1842*	1923*	2003*	2081*	2157*	60*
62:	985*	1019*	1061*	1109*	1164*	1223*	1288*	1356*	1428*	1504*	1581*	1661*	1742*	1823*	1904*	1985*	2065*	2143*	2219*	62:
64:	1048*	1083*	1124*	1173*	1227*	1287*	1351*	1420*	1492*	1567*	1645*	1724*	1805*	1886*	1968*	2049*	2128*	2207*	2282*	64:
66:	1112*	1147*	1188*	1237*	1291*	1351*	1415*	1484*	1556*	1631*	1709*	1788*	1869*	1950*	2032*	2113*	2193*	2271*	2347*	66:
68:	1177*	1212*	1253*	1302*	1356*	1415*	1480*	1548*	1621*	1696*	1774*	1853*	1934*	2015*	2097*	2178*	2257*	2335*	2411*	68:
70.	1242*	1277*	1319*	1367*	1421*	1481*	1545*	1614*	1686*	1761*	1839*	1919*	1999*	2081*	2162*	2243*	2323*	2401*	2477*	70.
72.	1308*	1343*	1385*	1433*	1487*	1547*	1611*	1680*	1752*	1827*	1905*	1984*	2065*	2146*	2228*	2309*	2389*	2467*	2543*	72.
74.	1375*	1409*	1451*	1499*	1553*	1613*	1677*	1746*	1818*	1894*	1971*	2051*	2131*	2213*	2294*	2375*	2455*	2533*	2609*	74.
76.	1441*	1476*	1518*	1566*	1620*	1680*	1744*	1813*	1885*	1960*	2038*	2117*	2198*	2280*	2361*	2442*	2522*	2600*	2676*	76.
78.	1508*	1543*	1584*	1633*	1687*	1747*	1811*	1880*	1952*	2027*	2105*	2184*	2265*	2346*	2428*	2509*	2589*	2667*	2742*	78.
80.	1575*	1610*	1652*	1700*	1754*	1814*	1878*	1947*	2019*	2094*	2172*	2251*	2332*	2414*	2495*	2576*	2656*	2734*	2810*	80.
82.	1643*	1677*	1719*	1767*	1821*	1881*	1945*	2014*	2086*	2162*	2239*	2319*	2399.	2481*	2562*	2643*	2723*	2801*	2877*	82.
84.	1710*	1744*	1786*	1834*	1889*	1948*	2013*	2081*	2154*	2229*	2306*	2386*	2467*	2548*	2630*	2710*	2790*	2868*	2944*	84.
86.	1777*	1812*	1853*	1902*	1956*	2015*	2080*	2148*	2221*	2296*	2374*	2453*	2534*	2615*	2697*	2778*	2857*	2935*	3011*	86.
88.	1844*	1879*	1920*	1969*	2023*	2082*	2147*	2215*	2288*	2363*	2441*	2520*	2601*	2682*	2764*	2845*	2924*	3002*	3078*	88.
90.	1911*	1946*	1987*	2036*	2090*	2149*	2214*	2282*	2355*	2430*	2508*	2587*	2668*	2749*	2831*	2912*	2991*	3069*	3145*	90.
92.	1978*	2012*	2054*	2102*	2156*	2216*	2280*	2349*	2421*	2496*	2574*	2654*	2734*	2816*	2897*	2978*	3058*	3136*	3212*	92.
94.	2044*	2078*	2120*	2168*	2222*	2282*	2347*	2415*	2487*	2563*	2640*	2720*	2801*	2882*	2963*	3044*	3124*	3202*	3278*	94.
96.	2109*	2144*	2186*	2234*	2288*	2348*	2412*	2481*	2553*	2628*	2706*	2786*	2866*	2948*	3029*	3110*	3190*	3268*	3344*	96.
98.	2175*	2209*	2251*	2299*	2353*	2413*	2477*	2546*	2618*	2694*	2771*	2851*	2931*	3013*	3094*	3175*	3255*	3333*	3409*	98.
100.	2239*	2274*	2316*	2364*	2418*	2478*	2542*	2611*	2683*	2758*	2836*	2915*	2996*	3078*	3159*	3240*	3320*	3398*	3474*	100.
102.	2303*	2338*	2379*	2428*	2482*	2542*	2606*	2675*	2747*	2822*	2900*	2979*	3060*	3141*	3223*	3304*	3384*	3462*	3538*	102.
104.	2366*	2401*	2443*	2491*	2545*	2605*	2669*	2738*	2810*	2885*	2963*	3042*	3123*	3205*	3286*	3367*	3447*	3525*	3601*	104.
106.	2429*	2463*	2505*	2553*	2607*	2667*	2731*	2800*	2872*	2948*	3025*	3105*	3185*	3267*	3348*	3429*	3509*	3587*	3663*	106.
108.	2490*	2525*	2566*	2615*	2669*	2728*	2793*	2861*	2934*	3009*	3087*	3166*	3247*	3328*	3410*	3491*	3570*	3648*	3724*	108.
110.	2550*	2585*	2627*	2675*	2729*	2789*	2853*	2922*	2994*	3069*	3147*	3226*	3307*	3389*	3470*	3551*	3631*	3709*	3785*	110.
112.	2610*	2644*	2686*	2734*	2788*	2848*	2912*	2981*	3053*	3129*	3206*	3286*	3366*	3448*	3529*	3610*	3690*	3768*	3844*	112.
114*	2668*	2702*	2744*	2792*	2846*	2906*	2971*	3039*	3111*	3187*	3264*	3344*	3424*	3506*	3587*	3668*	3748*	3826*	3902*	114*
116*	2724*	2759*	2801*	2849*	2903*	2963*	3027*	3096*	3168*	3243*	3321*	3401*	3481*	3563*	3644*	3725*	3805*	3883*	3959*	116*
118*	2780*	2815*	2856*	2905*	2959*	3018*	3083*	3151*	3224*	3299*	3377*	3456*	3537*	3618*	3700*	3781*	3860*	3938*	4014*	118*
120*	2834*	2869*	2910*	2959*	3013*	3073*	3137*	3206*	3278*	3353*	3431*	3510*	3591*	3672*	3754*	3835*	3915*	3993*	4069*	120*
122*	2887*	2922*	2963*	3011*	3066*	3125*	3190*	3258*	3330*	3406*	3483*	3563*	3644*	3725*	3806*	3887*	3967*	4045*	4121*	122*
124*	2938*	2972*	3014*	3062*	3117*	3176*	3241*	3309*	3381*	3457*	3534*	3614*	3695*	3776*	3857*	3938*	4018*	4096*	4172*	124*
126*	2987*	3022*	3063*	3112*	3166*	3226*	3290*	3359*	3431*	3506*	3584*	3663*	3744*	3825*	3907*	3988*	4067*	4146*	4221*	126*
128*	3035*	3069*	3111*	3159*	3214*	3273*	3338*	3406*	3478*	3554*	3631*	3711*	3792*	3873*	3954*	4035*	4115*	4193*	4269*	128*
130*	3081*	3115*	3157*	3205*	3259*	3319*	3383*	3452*	3524*	3600*	3677*	3757*	3837*	3919*	4000*	4081*	4161*	4239*	4315*	130*
132*	3125*	3159*	3201*	3249*	3303*	3363*	3427*	3496*	3568*	3644*	3721*	3801*	3881*	3963*	4044*	4125*	4205*	4283*	4359*	132*
134*	3167*	3201*	3243*	3291*	3345*	3405*	3469*	3538*	3610*	3685*	3763*	3843*	3923*	4005*	4086*	4167*	4247*	4325*	4401*	134*
136*	3206*	3241*	3283*	3331*	3385*	3445*	3509*	3578*	3650*	3725*	3803*	3883*	3963*	4045*	4126*	4207*	4287*	4365*	4441*	136*

Explanation of symbols . \ : \ * ; * = at least one ultrasound parameter outside the 1st\(2nd)\3rd standard deviation. Ultrasound parameters at 34 weeks

	-3STD: 0.13%	-2STD: 2.28%	-1STD: 15.87%	AM 50.00%	1STD: 84.13%	2STD: 97.72%	3STD: 99.87%
Normal range / Percentiles							
Biparietal diameter = BPD (mm)	80.0*	84.0*	88.0*	92.0	96.0*	100.0*	104.0*
Transverse trunk diameter = TTD (mm)	61.5*	70.0*	78.5*	87.0	95.5*	104.0*	112.5*
Head-to-trunk ratio = BPD/TTD	0.8634*	0.9264*	0.9895*	1.0525	1.1155*	1.1786*	1.2416*
Fetal weight = WT (grams)	890*	1345*	1800*	2255	2710	3165	3620*

Biparietal diameter = BPD (mm)
Transverse trunk diameter = TTD (mm)
Head-to-trunk ratio = BPD/TTD
Fetal weight = WT (grams)

Table 6 (continued)

Weight estimation for 35 weeks (middle of week = 36/4 = 249th postmenstrual day)

BPD↓/TTD→	74*	76*	78*	80*	82:	84:	86.	88.	90.	92	94	96	98	100.	102:	104:	106*	108*	110*	BPD/TTD
42*	484	519	561	609	663	723	787	856	928	1003	1081	1160	1241	1323	1404	1485	1565	1643	1719	42*
44*	536	570	612	660	715	774	839	907	980	1055	1132	1212	1293	1374	1455	1536	1616	1694	1770	44*
46*	589	623	665	713	768	827	892	960	1033	1108	1185	1265	1346	1427	1509	1589	1669	1747	1823	46*
48*	643	678	720	768	822	882	946	1015	1087	1162	1240	1319	1400	1482	1563	1644	1724	1802	1878	48*
50*	699	734	776	824	878	938	1002	1071	1143	1218	1296	1375	1456	1538	1619	1700	1780	1858	1934	50*
52*	756	791	833	881	935	995	1059	1128	1200	1275	1353	1433	1513	1595	1676	1757	1837	1915	1991	52*
54*	815	849	891	939	993	1053	1118	1186	1259	1334	1411	1491	1572	1653	1735	1815	1895	1973	2049	54*
56*	874	909	951	999	1053	1113	1177	1246	1318	1393	1471	1551	1631	1713	1794	1875	1955	2033	2109	56*
58*	935	970	1011	1060	1114	1173	1238	1306	1379	1454	1532	1611	1692	1773	1855	1936	2015	2094	2169	58*
60*	997	1031	1073	1121	1176	1235	1300	1368	1440	1516	1593	1673	1754	1835	1916	1997	2077	2155	2231	60*
62*	1059	1094	1136	1184	1238	1298	1362	1431	1503	1578	1656	1735	1816	1897	1979	2060	2140	2218	2294	62*
64.	1123	1157	1199	1247	1301	1361	1425	1494	1566	1642	1719	1799	1879	1961	2042	2123	2203	2281	2357	64.
66.	1187	1221	1263	1311	1366	1425	1490	1558	1630	1706	1783	1863	1944	2025	2106	2187	2267	2345	2421	66:
68.	1252	1286	1328	1376	1430	1490	1554	1623	1695	1770	1848	1928	2008	2090	2171	2252	2332	2410	2486	68:
70.	1317	1352	1393	1442	1496	1555	1620	1688	1761	1836	1914	1993	2074	2155	2237	2318	2397	2475	2551	70.
72.	1383	1417	1459	1507	1562	1621	1686	1754	1827	1902	1979	2059	2140	2221	2303	2383	2463	2541	2617	72.
74.	1449	1484	1525	1574	1628	1688	1752	1821	1893	1968	2046	2125	2206	2287	2369	2450	2530	2608	2683	74.
76.	1516	1550	1592	1640	1695	1754	1819	1887	1960	2035	2112	2192	2273	2354	2435	2516	2596	2674	2750	76.
78.	1583	1617	1659	1707	1762	1821	1886	1954	2026	2102	2179	2259	2339	2421	2502	2583	2663	2741	2817	78.
80.	1650	1684	1726	1774	1829	1888	1953	2021	2094	2169	2246	2326	2407	2488	2570	2650	2730	2808	2884	80.
82.	1717	1752	1793	1842	1896	1956	2020	2089	2161	2236	2314	2393	2474	2555	2637	2718	2797	2876	2951	82.
84.	1784	1819	1861	1909	1963	2023	2087	2156	2228	2303	2381	2460	2541	2623	2704	2785	2865	2943	3019	84.
86.	1852	1886	1928	1976	2030	2090	2154	2223	2295	2370	2448	2528	2608	2690	2771	2852	2932	3010	3086	86.
88.	1919	1953	1995	2043	2097	2156	2221	2290	2362	2438	2515	2595	2675	2757	2838	2919	2999	3077	3153	88.
90.	1985	2020	2062	2110	2164	2224	2288	2357	2430	2504	2582	2662	2742	2824	2905	2986	3066	3144	3220	90.
92.	2052	2087	2128	2177	2231	2290	2355	2423	2496	2571	2649	2728	2809	2890	2972	3053	3132	3210	3286	92.
94.	2118	2153	2194	2243	2297	2357	2421	2490	2562	2637	2715	2794	2875	2957	3038	3119	3199	3277	3353	94.
96.	2184	2219	2260	2309	2363	2422	2487	2555	2628	2703	2781	2860	2941	3022	3104	3185	3264	3342	3418	96.
98.	2249	2284	2325	2374	2428	2488	2552	2621	2693	2768	2846	2925	3006	3087	3169	3250	3330	3408	3483	98.
100.	2314	2349	2390	2438	2493	2552	2617	2685	2758	2833	2910	2990	3071	3152	3234	3314	3394	3472	3548	100.
102.	2378	2412	2454	2502	2557	2616	2681	2749	2821	2897	2974	3054	3135	3216	3297	3378	3458	3536	3612	102.
104.	2441	2475	2517	2565	2620	2679	2744	2812	2885	2960	3038	3117	3198	3279	3361	3441	3521	3599	3675	104.
106.	2503	2538	2579	2628	2682	2742	2806	2875	2947	3022	3100	3179	3260	3341	3423	3504	3584	3662	3737	106.
108.	2564	2599	2641	2689	2743	2803	2867	2936	3008	3083	3161	3240	3321	3403	3484	3565	3645	3723	3799	108:
110.	2625	2659	2701	2749	2804	2863	2928	2996	3069	3144	3221	3301	3382	3463	3545	3625	3705	3783	3859	110:
112.	2684	2719	2760	2809	2863	2923	2987	3056	3128	3203	3281	3360	3441	3522	3604	3685	3765	3843	3918	112:
114.	2742	2777	2818	2867	2921	2981	3045	3114	3186	3261	3339	3418	3499	3580	3662	3743	3823	3901	3976	114:
116.	2799	2834	2875	2924	2978	3037	3102	3170	3243	3318	3396	3475	3556	3637	3719	3800	3879	3957	4033	116:
118*	2855	2889	2931	2979	3033	3093	3157	3226	3298	3373	3451	3531	3611	3693	3774	3855	3935	4013	4089	118*
120*	2909	2943	2985	3033	3087	3147	3211	3280	3352	3428	3505	3585	3665	3747	3828	3909	3989	4067	4143	120*
122*	2961	2996	3037	3086	3140	3200	3264	3333	3405	3480	3558	3637	3718	3800	3881	3962	4042	4120	4196	122*
124*	3012	3047	3089	3137	3191	3251	3315	3384	3456	3531	3609	3688	3769	3851	3932	4013	4093	4171	4247	124*
126*	3062	3096	3138	3186	3240	3300	3364	3433	3505	3581	3658	3738	3818	3900	3981	4062	4142	4220	4296	126*
128*	3109	3144	3186	3234	3288	3348	3412	3481	3553	3628	3706	3785	3866	3948	4029	4110	4190	4268	4344	128*
130*	3155	3190	3231	3280	3334	3394	3458	3527	3599	3674	3752	3831	3912	3993	4075	4156	4236	4314	4389	130*
132*	3199	3234	3275	3324	3378	3438	3502	3571	3643	3718	3796	3875	3956	4037	4119	4200	4279	4358	4433	132*
134*	3241	3276	3317	3366	3420	3479	3544	3612	3685	3760	3838	3917	3998	4079	4161	4242	4321	4399	4475	134*
136*	3281	3315	3357	3406	3460	3519	3584	3652	3725	3800	3878	3957	4038	4119	4201	4282	4361	4439	4515	136*
138*	3319	3353	3395	3443	3498	3557	3622	3690	3762	3838	3915	3995	4076	4157	4238	4319	4399	4477	4553	138*

Explanation of symbols . \ : \ * = at least one ultrasound parameter outside the 1st \ 2nd \ 3rd standard deviation. Ultrasound parameters at 35 weeks

	-3STD*	-2STD:	-1STD.	AM	1STD.	2STD:	3STD*
Normal range Percentiles	0.13%	2.28%	15.87%	50.00%	84.13%	97.72%	99.87%
Biparietal diameter=BPD (mm)	81.0*	85.0*	89.0*	93.0	97.0	101.0*	105.0*
Transverse trunk diameter=TTD (mm)	63.8*	72.5*	81.3*	90.0	98.8	107.5*	116.3*
Head-to-trunk ratio=BPD/TTD	0.8527*	0.9147*	0.9767.	1.0387	1.1008	1.1628:	1.2248*
Fetal weight=WT (grams)	1000*	1500.	2000.	2500	3000.	3500.	4000*

Table 6 (continued)   Weight estimation for 36 weeks (middle of week = 37/4 = 256th postmenstrual day)

BPD↓/TTD→	76x	78x	80x	82x	84:	86:	88.	90.	92	94	96	98	100.	102.	104:	106:	108:	110:	112x	BPD↓/TTD→
44x	650	692	740	794	854	919	987	1059	1135	1212	1292	1372	1454	1535	1616	1696	1774	1850	1923	44x
46x	703	745	793	848	907	972	1040	1112	1188	1265	1345	1425	1507	1588	1669	1749	1827	1903	1976	46x
48x	758	799	848	902	962	1026	1095	1167	1242	1320	1399	1480	1561	1643	1724	1804	1882	1957	2030	48x
50x	814	855	904	958	1018	1082	1151	1223	1298	1376	1455	1536	1617	1699	1780	1860	1938	2013	2086	50x
52x	871	913	961	1015	1075	1139	1208	1280	1355	1433	1512	1593	1675	1756	1837	1917	1995	2071	2143	52x
54x	929	971	1019	1074	1133	1198	1266	1338	1414	1491	1571	1652	1733	1814	1895	1975	2053	2129	2202	54x
56x	989	1031	1079	1133	1193	1257	1326	1398	1473	1551	1630	1711	1793	1874	1955	2035	2113	2189	2261	56x
58x	1049	1091	1140	1194	1253	1318	1386	1459	1534	1612	1691	1772	1853	1935	2016	2095	2173	2249	2322	58x
60x	1111	1153	1201	1255	1315	1379	1448	1520	1596	1673	1753	1833	1915	1996	2077	2157	2235	2311	2384	60x
62x	1174	1215	1264	1318	1378	1442	1511	1583	1658	1736	1815	1896	1977	2059	2140	2220	2298	2373	2446	62x
64x	1237	1279	1327	1381	1441	1505	1574	1646	1721	1799	1879	1959	2041	2122	2203	2283	2361	2437	2510	64x
66:	1301	1343	1391	1445	1505	1569	1638	1710	1785	1863	1943	2023	2105	2186	2267	2347	2425	2501	2574	66:
68:	1366	1408	1456	1510	1570	1634	1703	1775	1850	1928	2007	2088	2170	2251	2332	2412	2490	2566	2639	68:
70:	1431	1473	1521	1576	1635	1700	1768	1841	1916	1993	2073	2154	2235	2317	2397	2477	2555	2631	2704	70:
72:	1497	1539	1587	1642	1701	1766	1834	1906	1982	2059	2139	2220	2301	2382	2463	2543	2621	2697	2770	72:
74:	1564	1605	1654	1708	1767	1832	1901	1973	2048	2126	2205	2286	2367	2449	2530	2609	2687	2763	2836	74:
76:	1630	1672	1720	1774	1834	1898	1965	2039	2114	2192	2272	2352	2434	2515	2596	2676	2754	2830	2903	76:
78.	1697	1739	1787	1841	1901	1965	2034	2106	2182	2259	2339	2419	2501	2582	2663	2743	2821	2897	2970	78.
80.	1764	1806	1854	1909	1968	2033	2101	2173	2249	2326	2406	2487	2568	2649	2730	2810	2888	2964	3037	80.
82.	1832	1873	1922	1976	2036	2101	2168	2241	2316	2394	2473	2554	2635	2717	2797	2877	2955	3031	3104	82.
84	1899	1940	1989	2043	2103	2167	2236	2308	2383	2461	2540	2621	2702	2784	2865	2945	3023	3099	3171	84
86	1966	2008	2056	2110	2170	2234	2303	2375	2450	2528	2607	2688	2770	2851	2932	3012	3090	3166	3239	86
88	2033	2075	2123	2177	2237	2301	2370	2442	2517	2595	2675	2755	2837	2918	2999	3079	3157	3233	3306	88
90	2100	2142	2190	2244	2304	2368	2437	2509	2584	2662	2741	2822	2903	2985	3066	3146	3224	3300	3373	90
92	2166	2208	2257	2311	2370	2435	2503	2576	2651	2729	2808	2889	2970	3052	3133	3212	3290	3366	3439	92
94	2233	2275	2323	2377	2437	2501	2570	2642	2717	2795	2874	2955	3036	3117	3199	3278	3356	3432	3505	94
96	2298	2340	2388	2443	2502	2567	2635	2708	2783	2860	2940	3021	3102	3184	3264	3344	3422	3498	3571	96
98	2364	2405	2454	2508	2567	2632	2700	2773	2848	2926	3005	3086	3167	3249	3330	3409	3487	3563	3636	98
100	2428	2470	2518	2573	2632	2697	2765	2837	2913	2990	3070	3151	3232	3313	3394	3474	3552	3628	3701	100
102x	2492	2534	2582	2636	2696	2760	2829	2901	2977	3054	3134	3214	3296	3377	3458	3538	3616	3692	3765	102x
104x	2555	2597	2645	2700	2759	2824	2892	2964	3040	3117	3197	3278	3359	3440	3521	3601	3679	3755	3828	104x
106x	2618	2659	2708	2762	2821	2886	2954	3027	3102	3180	3259	3340	3421	3503	3584	3663	3741	3817	3890	106x
108x	2679	2721	2769	2823	2883	2947	3016	3088	3163	3241	3320	3401	3483	3564	3645	3725	3803	3879	3952	108x
110x	2739	2781	2829	2884	2943	3008	3076	3149	3224	3301	3380	3462	3543	3624	3705	3785	3863	3939	4012	110x
112x	2799	2840	2889	2943	3002	3067	3135	3208	3283	3361	3440	3521	3602	3684	3765	3844	3922	3998	4071	112x
114x	2857	2898	2947	3001	3061	3125	3194	3266	3341	3419	3498	3579	3660	3742	3823	3902	3981	4056	4129	114x
116x	2913	2955	3003	3058	3117	3182	3250	3323	3398	3476	3555	3636	3717	3799	3880	3959	4037	4113	4186	116x
118x	2969	3011	3059	3113	3173	3237	3306	3378	3453	3531	3610	3691	3773	3854	3935	4015	4093	4169	4242	118x
120x	3023	3065	3113	3167	3227	3291	3360	3432	3507	3585	3665	3745	3827	3908	3989	4069	4147	4223	4296	120x
122x	3076	3117	3166	3220	3280	3344	3413	3485	3560	3638	3717	3798	3879	3961	4042	4122	4200	4275	4348	122x
124x	3127	3168	3217	3271	3331	3395	3464	3536	3611	3689	3768	3849	3930	4012	4093	4173	4251	4326	4399	124x
126x	3176	3218	3266	3320	3380	3444	3513	3585	3660	3738	3818	3898	3980	4061	4142	4222	4300	4376	4449	126x
128x	3224	3265	3314	3368	3428	3492	3561	3633	3708	3786	3865	3946	4027	4109	4190	4270	4348	4423	4496	128x
130x	3270	3311	3360	3414	3473	3538	3606	3679	3754	3832	3911	3992	4073	4155	4236	4315	4393	4469	4542	130x
132x	3314	3355	3404	3458	3517	3582	3650	3723	3798	3876	3955	4036	4117	4199	4280	4359	4437	4513	4586	132x
134x	3355	3397	3445	3499	3559	3624	3692	3765	3840	3918	3997	4078	4159	4241	4322	4401	4479	4555	4628	134x
136x	3395	3437	3485	3540	3599	3664	3732	3805	3880	3957	4037	4118	4199	4281	4361	4441	4519	4595	4668	136x
138x	3433	3475	3523	3577	3637	3701	3770	3842	3918	3995	4075	4155	4237	4318	4399	4479	4557	4633	4706	138x
140x	3469	3510	3559	3613	3673	3737	3806	3878	3953	4031	4110	4191	4272	4354	4435	4515	4593	4669	4741	140x

Explanation of symbols . \: \: /* = at least one ultrasound parameter outside the 1st\ 2nd\ 3rd standard deviation. Ultrasound parameters at 36 weeks

Normal range Percentiles	-3STD 0.13%	-2STD 2.28%	-1STD 15.87%	AM 50.00%	1STD 84.13%	2STD 97.72%	3STD 99.87%
Biparietal diameter = BPD (mm)	82.5	86.5	90.5	94.5	98.5	102.5	106.5
Transverse trunk diameter = TTD (mm)	65.0	74.0	83.0	92.0	101.0	110.0	119.0
Head-to-trunk ratio = BPD/TTD	0.8420	0.9030	0.9640	1.0250	1.0860	1.1470	1.2080
Fetal weight = WT (grams)	1160	1680	2200	2720	3240	3760	4280

Table 6 (continued)

Weight estimation for 37 weeks (middle of week = 38/4 = 263th postmenstrual day)

BPD→ TTD↓	78*	80*	82*	84*	86:	88:	90.	92.	94	96	98	100.	102.	104:	106:	108*	110*	112*	114*	BPD→ TTD↓
46*	824*	872*	927*	986*	1051*	1119*	1192*	1267*	1344*	1424*	1505*	1586*	1668*	1748*	1828*	1906*	1982*	2055*	2124*	46*
48*	879*	927*	981*	1041*	1105*	1174*	1246*	1321*	1399*	1478*	1559*	1641*	1722*	1803*	1883*	1961*	2037*	2110*	2179*	48*
50*	935*	983*	1037*	1097*	1161*	1230*	1302*	1377*	1455*	1534*	1615*	1697*	1778*	1859*	1939*	2017*	2093*	2166*	2235*	50*
52*	992*	1040*	1094*	1154*	1218*	1287*	1359*	1434*	1512*	1592*	1672*	1754*	1835*	1916*	1996*	2074*	2150*	2223*	2292*	52*
54*	1050*	1099*	1153*	1212*	1277*	1345*	1418*	1493*	1571*	1650*	1731*	1812*	1894*	1975*	2054*	2132*	2208*	2281*	2350*	54*
56*	1110*	1158*	1212*	1272*	1336*	1405*	1477*	1552*	1630*	1710*	1790*	1872*	1953*	2034*	2114*	2192*	2268*	2341*	2410*	56*
58*	1170*	1219*	1273*	1333*	1397*	1466*	1538*	1613*	1691*	1770*	1851*	1932*	2014*	2095*	2175*	2253*	2328*	2401*	2471*	58*
60*	1232*	1280*	1335*	1394*	1459*	1527*	1600*	1675*	1752*	1832*	1913*	1994*	2076*	2156*	2236*	2314*	2390*	2463*	2532*	60*
62*	1295*	1343*	1397*	1457*	1521*	1590*	1662*	1737*	1815*	1894*	1975*	2057*	2138*	2219*	2299*	2377*	2453*	2526*	2595*	62*
64*	1358*	1406*	1461*	1520*	1585*	1653*	1725*	1801*	1878*	1958*	2039*	2120*	2201*	2282*	2362*	2440*	2516*	2589*	2658*	64*
66:	1422*	1470*	1525*	1584*	1649*	1717*	1790*	1865*	1942*	2022*	2103*	2184*	2266*	2346*	2426*	2504*	2580*	2653*	2722*	66:
68:	1487*	1535*	1589*	1649*	1713*	1782*	1854*	1930*	2007*	2087*	2167*	2249*	2330*	2411*	2491*	2569*	2645*	2718*	2787*	68:
70:	1552*	1601*	1655*	1714*	1779*	1847*	1920*	1995*	2073*	2152*	2233*	2314*	2396*	2477*	2556*	2634*	2710*	2783*	2853*	70:
72:	1618*	1666*	1721*	1780*	1845*	1913*	1986*	2061*	2139*	2218*	2299*	2380*	2462*	2543*	2622*	2700*	2776*	2849*	2918*	72:
74:	1684*	1733*	1787*	1847*	1911*	1980*	2052*	2127*	2205*	2284*	2365*	2446*	2528*	2609*	2689*	2767*	2843*	2915*	2985*	74:
76:	1751*	1799*	1854*	1913*	1978*	2046*	2119*	2194*	2271*	2351*	2432*	2513*	2595*	2675*	2755*	2833*	2909*	2982*	3051*	76:
78:	1818*	1866*	1921*	1980*	2045*	2113*	2186*	2261*	2338*	2418*	2499*	2580*	2661*	2742*	2822*	2900*	2976*	3049*	3118*	78:
80.	1885*	1934*	1988*	2047*	2112*	2180*	2253:	2328*	2406*	2485*	2566*	2647*	2729*	2810*	2889*	2967*	3043*	3116*	3186*	80.
82.	1952*	2001*	2055*	2115*	2179*	2248*	2320:	2395.	2473*	2552:	2633:	2714:	2796:	2877:	2957:	3035*	3110*	3183*	3253*	82.
84.	2020*	2068*	2122*	2182*	2246*	2315*	2387:	2462.	2540.	2619.	2700.	2782.	2863.	2944.	3024.	3102*	3178*	3251*	3320*	84.
86	2087*	2135*	2189*	2249*	2313*	2382*	2454:	2530.	2607.	2687	2767	2849	2930	3011	3091	3169*	3245*	3318*	3387*	86
88	2154*	2202*	2256*	2316*	2381*	2449*	2521:	2588.	2674.	2754	2834	2916	2997	3078	3158	3236:	3312	3385	3454*	88
90	2221*	2269*	2323*	2383*	2447*	2516:	2588.	2664.	2741.	2821	2901	2983	3064	3145	3225	3303:	3379	3452	3521*	90
92	2287*	2336*	2390*	2450*	2514:	2583.	2655.	2730.	2808	2887	2968	3049	3131	3212	3292	3370:	3445	3518	3588*	92
94	2354*	2402*	2456*	2516*	2580:	2649.	2721.	2796.	2874	2953	3034	3116	3197	3278	3358	3436:	3512	3584	3654*	94
96	2419*	2468*	2522*	2581*	2646:	2714.	2786.	2862.	2940	3019	3100	3181	3263	3344	3423	3501:	3577	3650	3720*	96
98	2485*	2533*	2587*	2647*	2711:	2780:	2852.	2927.	3005	3084	3165	3247	3328	3409	3489	3567:	3643	3715	3785*	98
100.	2549*	2597*	2652*	2711*	2776:	2844:	2917.	2992.	3070	3149	3230	3311	3393	3474	3553	3631:	3707	3780	3849*	100.
102.	2613*	2661*	2716*	2775*	2840:	2908:	2981.	3056.	3133	3213	3294	3375	3457	3537	3617	3695:	3771	3844	3913*	102.
104.	2676*	2725*	2779*	2838*	2903:	2971:	3044.	3119.	3197	3276	3357	3438	3520	3601	3680	3758:	3834	3907	3976*	104.
106.	2738*	2787*	2841*	2901*	2965:	3034:	3106.	3181.	3259	3338	3419	3500	3582	3663	3743	3821:	3897	3969	4039*	106.
108.	2800*	2849*	2903*	2962*	3026:	3095:	3167.	3243.	3320	3400	3480	3562	3643	3724	3804	3882:	3958	4031	4100*	108.
110.	2860*	2909*	2963*	3022*	3087:	3155:	3228.	3303.	3381	3460	3541	3622	3704	3785	3864	3942:	4018	4091	4161*	110.
112.	2919*	2968*	3022*	3082*	3146:	3215:	3287.	3362.	3440	3519	3600	3681	3763	3844	3924	4002:	4078	4150	4220*	112.
114:	2978*	3026*	3080*	3140*	3204:	3273:	3345.	3420.	3498	3577	3658	3740	3821	3902	3982	4060*	4136	4208	4278*	114:
116:	3034*	3083*	3137*	3197*	3261:	3330:	3402.	3477.	3555	3634	3715	3796	3878	3959	4038	4117*	4192	4265	4335*	116:
118:	3090*	3138*	3192*	3252*	3316:	3385:	3457.	3533.	3610	3690	3770	3852	3933	4014	4094	4172*	4248	4321	4390*	118:
120:	3144*	3192*	3247*	3306*	3371:	3439:	3511.	3587.	3664	3744	3825	3906	3987	4068	4148	4226*	4302	4375	4444*	120:
122:	3197*	3245*	3299*	3359*	3423:	3492:	3564.	3639.	3717	3796	3877	3958	4040	4121	4201	4279*	4355	4427	4497*	122:
124*	3248*	3296*	3350*	3410*	3474:	3543:	3615.	3690.	3768	3847	3928	4010	4091	4172	4252	4330*	4406	4479	4548*	124*
126*	3297*	3345*	3400*	3459*	3524:	3592:	3664.	3740.	3817	3897	3978	4059	4140	4221	4301	4379*	4455	4528	4597*	126*
128*	3345*	3393*	3447*	3507*	3571:	3640:	3712.	3787.	3865	3944	4025	4107	4188	4269	4349	4427*	4503	4576	4645*	128*
130*	3390*	3439*	3493*	3553*	3617*	3686:	3758.	3833.	3911	3990	4071	4152	4234	4315	4395	4473*	4549	4621	4691*	130*
132*	3434*	3483*	3537*	3597*	3661*	3730:	3802.	3877.	3955	4034	4115	4196	4278	4359	4439	4517*	4592	4665	4735*	132*
134*	3476*	3525*	3579*	3638*	3703*	3772:	3844.	3919.	3997	4076	4157	4238	4320	4401	4480	4559*	4634	4707	4777*	134*
136*	3516*	3565*	3619*	3678*	3743*	3811*	3884.	3959.	4037	4116	4196	4278	4360	4441	4520	4598*	4674	4747	4817*	136*
138*	3554*	3602*	3657*	3716*	3781*	3849*	3922.	3997.	4074	4154	4235	4316	4398	4478	4558	4636*	4712	4785	4854*	138*
140*	3590*	3638*	3692*	3752*	3816*	3885*	3957.	4032.	4110	4190	4270	4352	4433	4514	4594	4672*	4748	4821	4890*	140*
142*	3623*	3671*	3726*	3785*	3850*	3918*	3990*	4066*	4143	4223	4304	4385	4466	4547	4627	4705*	4781	4854	4923*	142*

Explanation of symbols . \ : * = at least one ultrasound parameter outside the 1st\2nd\3rd standard deviation. Ultrasound parameters at 37 weeks

Normal range Percentiles	-3STD: 0.13%	-2STD: 2.28%	-1STD: 15.87%	AM: 50.00%	1STD: 84.13%	2STD: 97.72%	3STD: 99.87%
Biparietal diameter = BPD (mm)	84.0	88.0	92.0	96.0	100.0	104.0	108.0
Transverse trunk diameter = TTD (mm)	65.5	75.0	84.5	96.0	103.5	113.0	122.5
Head-to-trunk ratio = BPD/TTD	0.8320	0.8930	0.9540	1.0150	1.0760	1.1370	1.1980
Fetal weight = WT (grams)	1380	1910	2440	2970	3500	4030	4560

Table 6 (continued)   Weight estimation for 38 weeks (middle of week = 39/4 = 270th postmenstrual day)

BPD↓/TTD\	78*	80*	82*	84*	86:	88:	90.	92*	94	96*	98*	100	102*	104.	106:	108:	110*	112*	114*	BPD↓/TTD\
48*	956*	1004*	1058*	1118*	1182*	1251*	1323*	1398*	1476*	1556*	1636*	1718*	1799*	1880*	1960.	2038*	2114*	2187*	2256*	48*
50*	1012*	1060*	1114*	1174*	1238*	1307*	1379*	1454*	1532*	1612*	1692*	1774*	1855*	1936*	2016.	2094*	2170*	2243*	2312*	50*
52*	1069*	1117*	1171*	1231*	1295*	1364*	1436*	1510*	1589*	1669*	1749*	1831*	1912*	1993*	2073.	2151*	2227*	2300*	2369*	52*
54*	1127*	1176*	1230*	1289*	1354*	1422*	1495*	1570*	1648*	1727*	1808*	1889*	1971*	2052*	2131.	2209*	2285*	2358*	2428*	54*
56*	1187*	1235*	1289*	1349*	1413*	1482*	1554*	1630*	1707*	1787*	1867*	1949*	2030*	2111*	2191.	2269*	2345*	2418*	2487*	56*
58*	1247*	1296*	1350*	1410*	1474*	1543*	1615*	1690*	1768*	1847*	1928*	2010*	2091*	2172*	2252.	2330*	2406*	2478*	2548*	58*
60*	1309*	1358*	1412*	1471*	1536*	1604*	1677*	1752*	1830*	1909*	1990*	2071*	2153*	2234*	2313.	2391*	2467*	2540*	2609*	60*
62*	1372*	1420*	1474*	1534*	1598*	1667*	1739*	1814*	1892*	1972*	2052*	2134*	2215*	2296*	2376.	2454*	2530*	2603*	2672*	62*
64*	1435*	1483*	1538*	1597*	1662*	1730*	1803*	1878*	1955*	2035*	2116*	2197*	2279*	2359*	2439.	2517*	2593*	2666*	2735*	64*
66*	1499*	1548*	1602*	1661*	1726*	1794*	1867*	1942*	2020*	2099*	2180*	2261*	2343*	2424*	2503.	2581*	2657*	2730*	2799*	66*
68*	1564*	1612*	1667*	1726*	1791*	1859*	1931*	2007*	2084*	2164*	2244*	2326*	2407*	2488*	2568.	2646*	2722*	2795*	2864*	68*
70:	1629*	1678*	1732*	1792*	1856*	1925*	1997*	2072*	2150*	2229*	2310*	2391*	2473*	2554*	2634.	2712*	2787*	2860*	2930*	70:
72:	1695*	1744*	1798*	1857*	1922*	1990*	2063*	2138*	2216*	2295*	2376*	2457*	2539*	2620*	2699.	2777*	2853*	2926*	2996*	72:
74:	1762*	1810*	1864*	1924*	1988*	2057*	2129*	2204*	2282*	2361*	2442*	2524*	2605*	2686*	2766.	2844*	2920*	2993*	3062*	74:
76:	1828*	1877*	1931*	1990*	2055*	2123:	2196:	2271*	2349*	2428*	2509*	2590*	2672*	2753*	2832.	2910*	2986*	3059*	3128*	76:
78:	1895*	1943*	1998*	2057*	2123*	2190:	2263:	2338*	2415*	2495*	2576*	2657*	2739*	2819*	2899.	2977*	3053*	3126*	3195*	78:
80.	1962*	2010*	2065*	2124*	2189:	2257:	2330.	2405*	2483*	2562*	2643*	2724*	2806*	2887*	2966.	3044*	3120*	3193*	3263*	80.
82.	2030*	2078*	2132*	2192*	2256:	2325:	2397.	2472*	2550*	2629:	2710*	2792*	2873*	2954*	3034.	3112*	3188*	3261*	3330*	82.
84.	2097*	2145*	2199*	2259*	2323*	2392:	2464.	2539*	2617*	2697:	2777*	2859*	2940*	3021*	3101.	3179*	3255*	3328*	3397*	84.
86.	2164*	2212*	2267*	2326*	2391*	2459:	2531.	2607*	2684:	2764:	2844*	2926*	3007*	3088*	3168.	3246*	3322*	3395*	3464*	86.
88	2231*	2279*	2334*	2393*	2458*	2526:	2598:	2674*	2751:	2831:	2912*	2993*	3074*	3155:	3235:	3313*	3389*	3462*	3531*	88
90	2298*	2346*	2400*	2460*	2525*	2593:	2665:	2741*	2818*	2898:	2978*	3060*	3141:	3222:	3302:	3380*	3456*	3529*	3598*	90
92	2364*	2413*	2467*	2527*	2591*	2660:	2732:	2807*	2885*	2964:	3045*	3126*	3208:	3289:	3369:	3447*	3523*	3595*	3665*	92
94	2431*	2479*	2533*	2593*	2657*	2726:	2798:	2873*	2951*	3030*	3111*	3193*	3274:	3355:	3435:	3513*	3589*	3662*	3731*	94
96	2496*	2545*	2599*	2659*	2723*	2792:	2864:	2939*	3017*	3096*	3177*	3258*	3340:	3421:	3501:	3579*	3654*	3727*	3797*	96
98	2562*	2610*	2664*	2724*	2788*	2857:	2929:	3004*	3082*	3161*	3242*	3324*	3405:	3486:	3566:	3644*	3720*	3793*	3862*	98
100	2626*	2675*	2729*	2788*	2853*	2921:	2994:	3069*	3147*	3226*	3307*	3388*	3470:	3551:	3630:	3708:	3784*	3857*	3927*	100
102	2690*	2738*	2793*	2852*	2917*	2985:	3058:	3133*	3211*	3290*	3371*	3452*	3534:	3615:	3694:	3772:	3848*	3921*	3990*	102
104	2753*	2802*	2856*	2915*	2980*	3048:	3121:	3196*	3274*	3353*	3434*	3515*	3597:	3678:	3757:	3835:	3911*	3984*	4054*	104
106	2816*	2864*	2918*	2978*	3042*	3111:	3183:	3258*	3336*	3415*	3496*	3578*	3659:	3740:	3820:	3898:	3974*	4046*	4116*	106
108	2877*	2925*	2979*	3039*	3103*	3172:	3244:	3320*	3397*	3477*	3557*	3639*	3720:	3801:	3881:	3959:	4035*	4108*	4177*	108
110	2937*	2986*	3040*	3099*	3164*	3232:	3305:	3380*	3458*	3537*	3618*	3699*	3781:	3862:	3941:	4020:	4095*	4168*	4238*	110
112	2997*	3045*	3099*	3159*	3223*	3292:	3364:	3439*	3517*	3596*	3677*	3759*	3840:	3921:	4001:	4079:	4155*	4227*	4297*	112
114	3055*	3103*	3157*	3217*	3281*	3350:	3422:	3497*	3575*	3654*	3735*	3817*	3898:	3979:	4059:	4137:	4213*	4286*	4355*	114
116	3111*	3160*	3214*	3274*	3338*	3407:	3479:	3554*	3632*	3711*	3792*	3873*	3955:	4036:	4116:	4194:	4269*	4342*	4412*	116
118	3167*	3215*	3270*	3329*	3394*	3462:	3534:	3610*	3687*	3767*	3847*	3929*	4010:	4091:	4171:	4249:	4325*	4398*	4467*	118
120	3221*	3269*	3324*	3383*	3448*	3516:	3589:	3664*	3741*	3821*	3902*	3983*	4065:	4145:	4225:	4303:	4379*	4452*	4521*	120
122	3274*	3322*	3377*	3436*	3500*	3569:	3641:	3716*	3794*	3873*	3954*	4036*	4117:	4198:	4278:	4356:	4432*	4505*	4574*	122
124	3325*	3373*	3427*	3487*	3551*	3620:	3692:	3767*	3845*	3925*	4005*	4087*	4168:	4249:	4329:	4407:	4483*	4556*	4625*	124
126	3374*	3422*	3477*	3536*	3601*	3669:	3742:	3817*	3894*	3974*	4055*	4136*	4217:	4298:	4378:	4456:	4532*	4605*	4674*	126
128	3422*	3470*	3524*	3584*	3648*	3717:	3789:	3864*	3942*	4022*	4102*	4184*	4265:	4346:	4426:	4504:	4580*	4653*	4722*	128
130	3468*	3516*	3570*	3630*	3694*	3763:	3835:	3910*	3988*	4067*	4148*	4230*	4311:	4392:	4472:	4550:	4626*	4698*	4768*	130
132	3512*	3560*	3614*	3674*	3738*	3807:	3879:	3954*	4032*	4111*	4192*	4274*	4355:	4436:	4516:	4594:	4670*	4742*	4812*	132
134	3553*	3602*	3656*	3716*	3780*	3849:	3921:	3996*	4074*	4153*	4234*	4315*	4397:	4478:	4558:	4636:	4712*	4784*	4854*	134
136	3593*	3642*	3696*	3756*	3820*	3889:	3961:	4036*	4114*	4193*	4274*	4355*	4437:	4518:	4598:	4676:	4751*	4824*	4894*	136
138	3631*	3679*	3734*	3793*	3858*	3926:	3999:	4074*	4152*	4231*	4312*	4393*	4475:	4556:	4635:	4713:	4789*	4862*	4931*	138
140	3667*	3715*	3769*	3829*	3893*	3962:	4034:	4109*	4187*	4267*	4347*	4429*	4510:	4591:	4671:	4749:	4825*	4898*	4967*	140
142	3700*	3748*	3803*	3862*	3927*	3995:	4068:	4143*	4220*	4300*	4381*	4462*	4543:	4624:	4704:	4782:	4858*	4931*	5000*	142
144	3731*	3779*	3834*	3893*	3958*	4026:	4098:	4174*	4251*	4331*	4413*	4494*	4574:	4655:	4735:	4813:	4889*	4962*	5031*	144

Explanation of symbols . \: : \ * = at least one ultrasound parameter outside the 1st \ 2nd \ 3rd standard deviation. Ultrasound parameters at 38 weeks

Normal range Percentiles	-3STD 0.13%	-2STD 2.28%	-1STD 15.87%	AM 50.00%	1STD 84.13%	2STD 97.72%	3STD 99.87%
Biparietal diameter=BPD (mm)	85.0*	89.0	93.0	97.0	101.0	105.0	109.0*
Transverse trunk diameter=TTD (mm)	66.5*	76.5	86.5	96.5	106.5	116.5	126.5*
Head-to-trunk ratio=BPD/TTD	0.8220*	0.8830	0.9440	1.0050	1.0660	1.1270	1.1880*
Fetal weight=WT (grams)	1660*	2190	2720	3250	3780	4310	4840*

Table 6 (continued)   Weight estimation for 39 weeks (middle of week = 40/4 = 277th postmenstrual day)

BPD↓/TTD→	80*	82*	84*	86:	88:	90.	92.	94	96	98	100	102.	104.	106:	108:	110:	112*	114*	116*	BPD↓/TTD→
50*	1132*	1186*	1246*	1310*	1379*	1451*	1526*	1604*	1684*	1764*	1846*	1927*	2008*	2088*	2166*	2242*	2315*	2384*	2449*	50*
52*	1199*	1244*	1303*	1368*	1436*	1508*	1584*	1661*	1741*	1821*	1903*	1984*	2065*	2145*	2223*	2299*	2372*	2441*	2507*	52*
54*	1248*	1302*	1362*	1426*	1495*	1567*	1642*	1720*	1799*	1880*	1961*	2043*	2124*	2203*	2282*	2357*	2430*	2500*	2565*	54*
56*	1307*	1361*	1421*	1486*	1554*	1626*	1702*	1779*	1859*	1939*	2021*	2103*	2184*	2263*	2341*	2417*	2490*	2560*	2625*	56*
58*	1358*	1422*	1482*	1546*	1615*	1687*	1762*	1840*	1919*	2000*	2082*	2163*	2244*	2324*	2402*	2478*	2550*	2620*	2685*	58*
60*	1430*	1484*	1543*	1608*	1676*	1749*	1824*	1902*	1981*	2062*	2143*	2225*	2306*	2385*	2463*	2539*	2612*	2682*	2747*	60*
62*	1492*	1546*	1606*	1670*	1739*	1811*	1886*	1964*	2044*	2124*	2206*	2287*	2368*	2448*	2526*	2602*	2675*	2744*	2809*	62*
64*	1555*	1610*	1669*	1734*	1802*	1875*	1950*	2028*	2107*	2188*	2269*	2351*	2431*	2511*	2589*	2665*	2738*	2807*	2873*	64*
66:	1620*	1674*	1733*	1798*	1866*	1939*	2014*	2092*	2171*	2252*	2333*	2415*	2496*	2575*	2653*	2729*	2802*	2871*	2937*	66:
68:	1684*	1739*	1798*	1863*	1931*	2003*	2079*	2156*	2236*	2317*	2398*	2479*	2560*	2640*	2718*	2794*	2867*	2936*	3002*	68:
70:	1750*	1804*	1864*	1928*	1997*	2069*	2144*	2222*	2301*	2382*	2463*	2545*	2626*	2706*	2784*	2859*	2932*	3002*	3067*	70:
72:	1816*	1870*	1930*	1994*	2063*	2135*	2210*	2288*	2367*	2448*	2529*	2611*	2692*	2771*	2849*	2925*	2998*	3068*	3133*	72:
74:	1882*	1936*	1996*	2060:	2129*	2201*	2276*	2354*	2433*	2514*	2596*	2677*	2758*	2838*	2916*	2992*	3065*	3134*	3199*	74:
76:	1949*	2003*	2062*	2127:	2195:	2268*	2343*	2421*	2500*	2581*	2662*	2744*	2825*	2904*	2982*	3058*	3131*	3201*	3266*	76:
78:	2016*	2070*	2129*	2194:	2262:	2335*	2410:	2488*	2567*	2648*	2729*	2811*	2892*	2971*	3049*	3125*	3198*	3267*	3333*	78:
80:	2083*	2137*	2197*	2261:	2330:	2402:	2477:	2555*	2634*	2715*	2796*	2878*	2959*	3038*	3117*	3192*	3265*	3335*	3400*	80:
82:	2150*	2204*	2264*	2328:	2397:	2469:	2544:	2622*	2701:	2782*	2864*	2945*	3026*	3106*	3184*	3260*	3332*	3400*	3467*	82:
84:	2217*	2271*	2331*	2395:	2464:	2536:	2612:	2689:	2769:	2849:	2931*	3012*	3093*	3173*	3251*	3327*	3400*	3469*	3534*	84:
86:	2284*	2339*	2398*	2463:	2531:	2603:	2679:	2756:	2836:	2917:	2998:	3079*	3160*	3240*	3318*	3394*	3467*	3536*	3602*	86:
88:	2351*	2406*	2465*	2530:	2598:	2671:	2746:	2823:	2903:	2984:	3065:	3147*	3227*	3307*	3385*	3461*	3534*	3603*	3669*	88:
90	2418*	2473*	2532*	2597:	2665:	2737:	2813:	2890:	2970:	3051:	3132:	3213:	3294:	3374:	3452:	3528*	3601*	3670*	3736*	90
92	2485*	2539*	2599*	2663:	2732:	2804:	2879:	2957:	3036:	3117:	3199:	3280:	3361:	3441:	3519:	3595*	3667*	3737*	3802*	92
94	2551*	2605*	2665*	2729:	2798:	2870:	2945:	3023:	3103:	3183:	3265:	3346:	3427:	3507:	3585:	3661*	3734*	3803*	3868*	94
96	2617*	2671*	2731*	2795:	2864:	2936:	3011:	3089:	3168:	3249:	3330:	3412:	3493:	3573:	3651:	3727*	3799*	3869*	3934*	96
98	2682*	2736*	2795*	2860:	2929:	3001:	3076:	3154:	3233:	3314:	3396:	3477:	3558:	3638:	3716:	3792*	3865*	3934*	3999*	98
100	2747*	2801*	2861*	2925:	2994:	3066:	3141:	3219:	3298:	3379:	3460:	3542:	3623:	3702:	3781:	3856*	3929*	3999*	4064*	100
102	2811*	2865*	2924*	2989:	3057:	3130:	3205:	3283:	3362:	3443:	3524:	3606:	3687:	3766:	3844:	3920*	3993*	4063*	4128*	102
104	2874*	2928*	2988*	3052:	3121:	3193:	3268:	3346:	3425:	3506:	3587:	3669:	3750:	3829:	3908:	3983*	4056*	4126*	4191*	104
106	2936*	2990*	3050*	3114*	3183:	3255:	3330:	3408:	3487:	3568:	3650:	3731:	3812:	3892:	3970:	4046*	4119*	4188*	4253*	106
108	2997*	3052*	3111*	3176*	3244:	3316:	3392:	3469:	3549:	3630:	3711:	3792:	3873:	3953:	4031:	4107*	4180*	4249*	4315*	108
110	3058*	3112*	3172*	3236*	3305:	3377:	3452:	3530:	3609:	3690:	3771:	3853:	3934:	4014:	4092:	4167*	4240*	4310*	4375*	110
112	3117*	3171*	3231*	3295*	3364:	3436:	3511:	3589:	3668:	3749:	3831:	3912:	3993:	4073:	4151:	4227*	4300*	4369*	4434*	112
114	3175*	3229*	3289*	3353*	3422:	3494:	3569:	3647:	3727:	3807:	3889:	3970:	4051:	4131:	4209:	4285*	4358*	4427*	4492*	114
116	3232*	3286*	3346*	3410*	3479:	3551:	3626:	3704:	3783:	3864:	3946:	4027:	4108:	4188:	4266:	4342*	4414*	4484*	4549*	116
118	3287*	3342*	3401*	3466*	3534:	3606:	3682:	3759:	3839:	3920:	4001:	4082:	4163:	4243:	4321:	4397*	4470*	4539*	4605*	118
120	3341*	3396*	3455*	3520:	3588:	3661:	3736:	3813:	3893:	3974:	4055:	4137:	4217:	4297:	4375:	4451*	4524*	4593*	4659*	120
122	3394*	3448*	3508*	3572:	3641:	3713:	3788:	3866:	3946:	4026:	4108:	4189:	4270:	4350:	4428:	4504*	4577*	4646*	4711*	122
124	3445*	3499*	3559*	3623:	3692:	3764:	3839:	3917:	3997:	4077:	4159:	4240:	4321:	4401:	4479:	4555*	4628*	4697*	4762*	124
126	3494*	3549*	3608*	3673:	3741:	3814:	3889:	3966:	4046:	4127:	4208:	4290:	4370:	4450:	4528:	4604*	4677*	4746*	4812*	126
128	3542*	3596*	3656*	3720:	3789:	3861:	3936:	4014:	4094:	4174:	4256:	4337:	4418:	4498:	4576:	4652*	4725*	4794*	4859*	128
130	3588*	3642*	3702*	3766:	3835:	3907:	3982:	4060:	4139:	4220:	4302:	4383:	4464:	4544:	4622:	4698*	4771*	4840*	4905*	130
132	3632*	3686*	3746*	3810:	3879:	3951:	4026:	4104:	4183:	4264:	4346:	4427:	4508:	4588:	4666:	4742*	4814*	4884*	4949*	132
134	3674*	3728*	3788*	3852:	3921:	3993:	4068:	4146:	4225:	4306:	4388:	4469:	4550:	4630:	4708:	4784*	4856*	4926*	4991*	134
136	3714*	3768*	3828*	3892:	3961:	4033:	4108:	4186:	4265:	4346:	4427:	4509:	4590:	4670:	4748:	4823*	4896*	4966*	5031*	136
138	3752*	3806*	3865*	3930:	3998:	4071:	4146:	4224:	4303:	4384:	4465:	4547:	4628:	4707:	4785:	4861*	4934*	5004*	5069*	138
140	3787*	3841*	3901*	3965:	4034:	4106:	4182:	4259:	4339:	4419:	4501:	4582:	4663:	4743:	4821:	4897*	4970*	5039*	5104*	140
142	3820*	3875*	3934*	3999:	4067:	4140:	4215:	4292:	4372:	4453:	4534:	4616:	4696:	4776:	4854:	4930*	5003*	5072*	5138*	142
144	3851*	3906*	3965*	4030:	4098:	4171:	4246:	4323:	4403:	4484:	4565:	4646:	4727:	4807:	4885:	4961*	5034*	5103*	5169*	144
146	3880*	3934*	3994*	4058:	4127:	4199:	4274:	4352:	4431:	4512:	4594:	4675:	4756:	4836:	4914*	4990*	5062*	5132*	5197*	146

Explanation of symbols . \:* = at least one ultrasound parameter outside the 1st\2nd\3rd standard deviation. Ultrasound parameters at 39 weeks

Normal range
Percentiles

	-3STD: 0.13%	-2STD: 2.28%	-1STD: 15.87%	AM 50.00%	1STD: 84.13%	2STD: 97.72%	3STD: 99.87%
Biparietal diameter=BPD (mm)	85.5*	89.5:	93.5.	97.5	101.5:	105.5:	109.5*
Transverse trunk diameter=TTD (mm)	66.1*	76.6:	87.1.	97.6	108.1:	118.6:	129.1*
Head-to-trunk ratio=BPD/TTD	0.8150*	0.8760:	0.9370.	0.9980	1.0590:	1.1200:	1.1810*
Fetal weight=WT (grams)	1840:	2370:	2900:	3430:	3960:	4490:	5020*

Table 6 (continued)

Weight estimation for 40 weeks (middle of week = 41/4 = 284th postmenstrual day)

BPD↓/TTD	80*	82*	84*	86:	88:	90.	92.	94	96	98	100	102.	104.	106:	108:	110:	112*	114*	116*	BPD↓/TTD
52*	1253	1308	1367	1432	1500	1573	1648	1725	1805	1886	1967	2048	2129	2209	2287	2363	2436	2505	2571	52*
54*	1312	1366	1426	1490	1559	1631	1706	1784	1863	1944	2025	2107	2188	2268	2346	2422	2494	2564	2629	54*
56*	1371	1426	1485	1550	1618	1691	1766	1843	1923	2004	2085	2166	2247	2327	2405	2481	2554	2623	2689	56*
58*	1432	1486	1546	1610	1679	1751	1826	1904	1983	2064	2146	2227	2308	2388	2466	2542	2615	2684	2749	58*
60*	1494	1548	1608	1672	1741	1813	1888	1966	2045	2126	2207	2289	2370	2449	2528	2603	2676	2746	2811	60*
62*	1556	1610	1670	1734	1803	1875	1951	2028	2108	2188	2270	2351	2432	2512	2590	2666	2739	2808	2873	62*
64*	1620	1674	1733	1798	1866	1939	2014	2092	2171	2252	2333	2415	2496	2575	2653	2729	2802	2872	2937	64*
66*	1684	1738	1798	1862	1931	2003	2078	2156	2235	2316	2397	2479	2560	2639	2718	2793	2866	2936	3001	66*
68:	1748	1803	1862	1927	1995	2068	2143	2221	2300	2381	2462	2544	2624	2704	2782	2858	2931	3000	3066	68:
70:	1814	1868	1928	1992	2061	2133	2208	2286	2365	2446	2528	2609	2690	2770	2848	2924	2996	3066	3131	70:
72:	1880	1934	1994	2058	2127	2199	2274	2352	2431	2512	2593	2675	2756	2836	2914	2989	3062	3132	3197	72:
74:	1946	2000	2060	2124	2193	2265	2340	2418	2498	2578	2660	2741	2822	2902	2980	3056	3129	3198	3263	74:
76:	2013	2067	2127	2191	2260	2332	2407	2485	2564	2645	2726	2808	2889	2968	3047	3122	3195	3265	3330	76:
78:	2080	2134	2193	2258	2326	2399	2474	2552	2631	2712	2793	2875	2956	3035	3113	3189	3262	3332	3397	78:
80.	2147	2201	2261	2325	2394	2466	2541	2619	2698	2779	2860	2942	3023	3103	3181	3257	3329	3399	3464	80.
82.	2214	2268	2328	2392	2461	2533	2608	2686	2766	2846	2928	3009	3090	3170	3248	3324	3397	3466	3531	82.
84.	2281	2335	2395	2461	2528	2600	2676	2753	2833	2913	2995	3076	3157	3237	3315	3391	3464	3533	3599	84.
86.	2348	2403	2462	2527	2595	2668	2743	2820	2900	2981	3062	3144	3224	3304	3382	3458	3531	3600	3666	86.
88.	2415	2470	2529	2594	2662	2735	2810	2888	2967	3048	3129	3211	3292	3371	3449	3525	3598	3667	3733	88.
90	2482	2537	2596	2661	2729	2802	2877	2954	3034	3115	3196	3278	3358	3438	3516	3592	3665	3734	3800	90
92	2549	2603	2663	2727	2796	2868	2943	3021	3100	3181	3263	3344	3425	3505	3583	3659	3732	3801	3866	92
94	2615	2669	2729	2793	2862	2934	3010	3087	3167	3247	3329	3410	3491	3571	3649	3725	3798	3867	3932	94
96	2681	2735	2795	2859	2928	3000	3075	3153	3232	3313	3395	3476	3557	3637	3715	3791	3863	3933	3998	96
98	2746	2800	2860	2924	2993	3065	3140	3218	3298	3378	3460	3541	3622	3702	3780	3856	3929	3998	4063	98
100	2811	2865	2925	2989	3058	3130	3205	3283	3362	3443	3524	3606	3687	3767	3845	3920	3993	4063	4128	100
102	2875	2929	2989	3053	3122	3194	3269	3347	3426	3507	3588	3670	3751	3830	3909	3984	4057	4127	4192	102
104	2938	2992	3052	3116	3185	3257	3332	3410	3489	3570	3651	3733	3814	3894	3972	4048	4120	4190	4255	104
106	3000	3054	3114	3178	3247	3319	3394	3472	3552	3632	3714	3795	3876	3956	4034	4110	4183	4252	4317	106
108	3061	3116	3175	3240	3308	3381	3456	3533	3613	3694	3775	3857	3937	4017	4095	4171	4244	4313	4379	108
110.	3122	3176	3236	3300	3369	3441	3516	3593	3673	3754	3835	3917	3998	4078	4156	4232	4304	4374	4439	110.
112.	3181	3235	3295	3359	3428	3500	3575	3653	3733	3813	3895	3976	4057	4137	4215	4291	4364	4433	4498	112.
114.	3239	3293	3353	3417	3486	3558	3633	3711	3791	3871	3953	4034	4115	4195	4273	4349	4422	4491	4556	114.
116.	3296	3350	3410	3474	3543	3615	3690	3768	3847	3928	4010	4091	4172	4252	4330	4406	4479	4548	4613	116.
118.	3351	3406	3465	3530	3598	3671	3746	3823	3903	3984	4065	4147	4227	4307	4385	4461	4534	4603	4669	118.
120.	3406	3460	3519	3584	3652	3725	3800	3878	3957	4038	4119	4201	4282	4361	4439	4515	4588	4658	4723	120.
122:	3458	3512	3572	3636	3705	3777	3853	3930	4010	4090	4172	4253	4334	4414	4492	4568	4641	4710	4775	122:
124:	3509	3563	3623	3687	3756	3828	3904	3981	4061	4141	4223	4304	4385	4465	4543	4619	4692	4761	4826	124:
126:	3559	3613	3672	3737	3805	3878	3953	4031	4110	4191	4272	4354	4435	4514	4592	4668	4741	4811	4876	126:
128:	3606	3660	3720	3784	3853	3925	4001	4078	4158	4238	4320	4401	4482	4562	4640	4716	4789	4858	4923	128:
130:	3652	3706	3766	3830	3899	3971	4046	4124	4204	4284	4366	4447	4528	4608	4686	4762	4835	4904	4969	130:
132*	3696	3750	3810	3874	3943	4015	4090	4168	4247	4328	4410	4491	4572	4652	4730	4806	4879	4948	5013	132*
134*	3738	3792	3852	3916	3985	4057	4132	4210	4289	4370	4452	4533	4614	4694	4772	4848	4921	4990	5055	134*
136*	3778	3832	3892	3956	4025	4097	4172	4250	4329	4410	4492	4573	4654	4734	4812	4888	4960	5030	5095	136*
138*	3816	3870	3930	3994	4063	4135	4210	4288	4367	4448	4529	4611	4692	4771	4850	4925	4998	5068	5133	138*
140*	3851	3906	3965	4030	4098	4170	4246	4323	4403	4483	4565	4646	4727	4807	4885	4961	5034	5103	5169	140*
142*	3885	3939	3998	4063	4131	4204	4279	4357	4436	4517	4598	4680	4761	4840	4918	4994	5067	5137	5202	142*
144*	3915	3970	4029	4094	4162	4235	4310	4387	4467	4548	4629	4711	4791	4871	4949	5025	5098	5167	5233	144*
146*	3944	3998	4058	4122	4191	4263	4338	4416	4495	4576	4658	4739	4820	4900	4978	5054	5127	5196	5261	146*
148*	3970	4024	4084	4148	4217	4289	4364	4442	4521	4602	4684	4765	4846	4926	5004	5080	5152	5222	5287	148*

Explanation of symbols . \ : \ * = at least one ultrasound parameter outside the 1st \ 2nd \ 3rd standard deviation. Ultrasound parameters at 40 weeks

Normal range Percentiles	-3STD: 0.13%	-2STD: 2.28%	-1STD: 15.87%	AM 50.00%	1STD: 84.13%	2STD: 97.72%	3STD: 99.87%
Biparietal diameter = BPD (mm)	85.6*	89.6:	93.6.	97.6	101.6.	105.6:	109.6*
Transverse trunk diameter = TTD (mm)	67.1*	78.1:	89.1.	100.1	111.1.	122.1:	133.1*
Head-to-trunk ratio = BPD/TTD	0.8108*	0.8718:	0.9328.	0.9938	1.0548.	1.1158:	1.1768*
Fetal weight = WT (grams)	2000*	2510:	3020.	3530	4040.	4550:	5060*

Table 6 (continued)

Weight estimation for 41 weeks (middle of week = 42/4 = 291th postmenstrual day)

BPD/TTD	80*	82*	84*	86:	88:	90.	92	94	96	98	100	102	104.	106.	108:	110:	112:	114*	116*	BPD/TTD
54*	1366*	1420*	1480*	1544*	1613*	1685*	1760*	1838*	1919*	1998*	2080*	2161*	2242*	2322*	2400*	2476*	2549*	2618*	2683*	54*
56*	1425*	1480*	1539*	1604*	1672*	1745*	1820*	1898*	1977*	2058*	2139*	2221*	2302*	2381*	2459*	2535*	2608*	2677*	2743*	56*
58*	1486*	1540*	1600*	1664*	1733*	1805*	1880*	1958*	2038*	2118*	2200*	2281*	2362*	2442*	2520*	2596*	2669*	2738*	2803*	58*
60*	1548*	1602*	1662*	1726*	1795*	1867*	1942*	2020*	2099*	2180*	2261*	2343*	2424*	2504*	2582*	2658*	2730*	2800*	2865*	60*
62*	1610*	1665*	1724*	1789*	1857*	1929*	2005*	2082*	2162*	2243*	2324*	2405*	2486*	2566*	2644*	2720*	2793*	2862*	2928*	62*
64*	1674*	1728*	1788*	1852*	1921*	1993*	2068*	2146*	2225*	2306*	2387*	2469*	2550*	2629*	2708*	2783*	2856*	2926*	2991*	64*
66*	1738*	1792*	1852*	1916*	1985*	2057*	2132*	2210*	2289*	2370*	2451*	2533*	2614*	2694*	2772*	2848*	2920*	2990*	3055*	66:
68:	1803*	1857*	1916*	1981*	2049*	2122*	2197*	2275*	2354*	2435*	2516*	2598*	2679*	2758*	2836*	2912*	2985*	3055*	3120*	68:
70:	1868*	1922*	1982*	2046*	2115*	2187*	2262*	2340*	2420*	2500*	2582*	2663*	2744*	2824*	2902*	2978*	3051*	3120*	3185*	70:
72:	1934*	1988*	2048*	2112*	2181*	2253*	2328*	2406*	2485*	2566*	2648*	2729*	2810*	2890*	2968*	3044*	3116*	3186*	3251*	72:
74:	2000*	2054*	2114*	2178*	2247*	2319*	2395*	2472*	2552*	2632*	2714*	2795*	2876*	2956*	3034*	3110*	3183*	3252*	3317*	74:
76:	2067*	2121*	2181*	2245*	2314*	2386*	2461*	2539*	2618*	2699*	2781*	2862*	2943*	3023*	3101*	3177*	3249*	3319*	3384*	76:
78:	2134*	2188*	2248*	2312*	2381*	2453*	2528*	2606*	2685*	2766*	2847*	2929*	3010*	3090*	3168*	3243*	3316*	3386*	3451*	78:
80.	2201*	2255*	2315*	2379*	2448*	2520*	2595*	2673*	2752*	2833*	2915*	2996*	3077*	3157*	3235*	3311*	3384*	3453*	3518*	80.
82.	2268*	2322*	2382*	2446*	2515*	2587*	2663*	2740*	2820*	2900*	2982*	3063*	3144*	3224*	3302*	3378*	3451*	3520*	3585*	82.
84.	2335*	2390*	2449*	2514*	2582*	2655*	2730*	2807*	2887*	2968*	3049*	3130*	3211*	3291*	3369*	3445*	3518*	3587*	3653*	84.
86.	2403*	2457*	2516*	2581*	2649*	2722*	2797*	2875*	2954*	3035*	3116*	3198*	3279*	3358*	3436*	3512*	3585*	3655*	3720*	86.
88.	2470*	2524*	2583*	2648*	2716*	2789*	2864*	2942*	3021*	3102*	3183*	3265*	3346*	3425*	3503*	3579*	3652*	3722*	3787*	88.
90.	2537*	2591*	2650*	2715*	2783*	2856*	2931*	3009*	3088*	3169*	3250*	3332*	3413*	3492*	3570*	3646*	3719*	3789*	3854*	90.
92.	2603*	2657*	2717*	2781*	2850*	2922*	2997*	3075*	3155*	3235*	3317*	3398*	3479*	3559*	3637*	3713*	3786*	3855*	3920*	92.
94	2669*	2724*	2783*	2848*	2916*	2988*	3064*	3141*	3221*	3302*	3383*	3464*	3545*	3625*	3703*	3779*	3852*	3921*	3987*	94
96	2735*	2789*	2849*	2913*	2982*	3054*	3129*	3207*	3287*	3367*	3449*	3530*	3611*	3691*	3769*	3845*	3918*	3987*	4052*	96
98	2800*	2854*	2914*	2978*	3047*	3119*	3195*	3272*	3352*	3432*	3514*	3595*	3676*	3756*	3834*	3910*	3983*	4052*	4118*	98
100	2865*	2919*	2979*	3043*	3112*	3184*	3259*	3337*	3416*	3497*	3579*	3660*	3741*	3821*	3899*	3975*	4047*	4117*	4182*	100
102	2929*	2983*	3043*	3107*	3176*	3248*	3323*	3401*	3480*	3561*	3642*	3724*	3805*	3885*	3963*	4039*	4111*	4181*	4246*	102
104.	2992*	3046*	3106*	3170*	3239*	3311*	3386*	3464*	3543*	3624*	3706*	3787*	3868*	3948*	4026*	4102*	4175*	4244*	4309*	104.
106.	3054*	3108*	3168*	3232*	3301*	3373*	3449*	3526*	3606*	3686*	3768*	3849*	3930*	4010*	4088*	4164*	4237*	4306*	4371*	106.
108:	3116*	3170*	3229*	3294*	3362*	3435*	3510*	3588*	3667*	3748*	3829*	3911*	3992*	4071*	4149*	4225*	4298*	4367*	4433*	108:
110:	3176*	3230*	3290*	3354*	3423*	3495*	3570*	3648*	3727*	3808*	3890*	3971*	4052*	4132*	4210*	4286*	4359*	4428*	4493*	110.
112:	3235*	3289*	3349*	3413*	3482*	3554*	3630*	3707*	3787*	3867*	3949*	4030*	4111*	4191*	4269*	4345*	4418*	4487*	4552*	112.
114:	3293*	3347*	3407*	3472*	3540*	3612*	3688*	3765*	3845*	3925*	4007*	4088*	4169*	4249*	4327*	4403*	4476*	4545*	4611*	114.
116:	3350*	3404*	3464*	3528*	3597*	3669*	3744*	3822*	3902*	3982*	4064*	4145*	4226*	4306*	4384*	4460*	4533*	4602*	4667*	116.
118.	3406*	3460*	3519*	3584*	3652*	3725*	3800*	3878*	3957*	4038*	4119*	4201*	4282*	4361*	4439*	4515*	4588*	4658*	4723*	118.
120.	3460*	3514*	3574*	3638*	3707*	3779*	3854*	3932*	4011*	4092*	4173*	4255*	4336*	4416*	4494*	4569*	4642*	4712*	4777*	120.
122.	3512*	3567*	3626*	3691*	3759*	3831*	3907*	3984*	4064*	4145*	4226*	4307*	4388*	4468*	4546*	4622*	4695*	4764*	4830*	122.
124.	3563*	3618*	3677*	3742*	3810*	3882*	3958*	4035*	4115*	4196*	4277*	4358*	4439*	4519*	4597*	4673*	4746*	4815*	4881*	124.
126.	3613*	3667*	3727*	3791*	3860*	3932*	4007*	4085*	4164*	4245*	4326*	4408*	4489*	4568*	4647*	4722*	4795*	4865*	4930*	126.
128.	3660*	3715*	3774*	3839*	3907*	3979*	4055*	4132*	4212*	4293*	4374*	4455*	4536*	4616*	4694*	4770*	4843*	4912*	4978*	128.
130:	3706*	3760*	3820*	3884*	3953*	4025*	4101*	4178*	4258*	4338*	4420*	4501*	4582*	4662*	4740*	4816*	4889*	4958*	5023*	130.
132:	3750*	3804*	3864*	3928*	3997*	4069*	4145*	4222*	4302*	4382*	4464*	4545*	4626*	4706*	4784*	4860*	4933*	5002*	5067*	132:
134:	3792*	3846*	3906*	3970*	4039*	4111*	4186*	4264*	4344*	4424*	4506*	4587*	4668*	4748*	4826*	4902*	4975*	5044*	5109*	134:
136*	3832*	3886*	3946*	4010*	4079*	4151*	4226*	4304*	4384*	4464*	4546*	4627*	4708*	4788*	4866*	4942*	5015*	5084*	5149*	136*
138*	3870*	3924*	3984*	4048*	4117*	4189*	4264*	4342*	4421*	4502*	4583*	4665*	4746*	4826*	4904*	4980*	5052*	5122*	5187*	138*
140*	3905*	3960*	4019*	4084*	4152*	4225*	4300*	4377*	4457*	4538*	4619*	4701*	4781*	4861*	4939*	5015*	5088*	5157*	5223*	140*
142*	3939*	3993*	4053*	4117*	4186*	4258*	4333*	4411*	4490*	4571*	4652*	4734*	4815*	4894*	4973*	5048*	5121*	5191*	5256*	142*
144*	3970*	4024*	4083*	4148*	4217*	4289*	4364*	4442*	4522*	4602*	4684*	4765*	4846*	4925*	5004*	5079*	5152*	5222*	5287*	144.
146*	3998*	4052*	4112*	4176*	4245*	4317*	4392*	4470*	4550*	4630*	4712*	4793*	4874*	4954*	5032*	5108*	5181*	5250*	5315*	146*
148*	4024*	4078*	4138*	4202*	4271*	4343*	4418*	4496*	4575*	4656*	4738*	4819*	4900*	4980*	5058*	5134*	5207*	5276*	5341*	148*
150*	4047*	4102*	4161*	4226*	4294*	4366*	4442*	4519*	4599*	4680*	4761*	4842*	4923*	5003*	5081*	5157*	5230*	5299*	5365*	150*

Explanation of symbols .\:* = at least one ultrasound parameter outside the 1st\2nd\3rd standard deviation. Ultrasound parameters at 41 weeks

Normal range Percentiles	-3STD. 0.13%	-2STD. 2.28%	-1STD. 15.87%	AM 50.00%	1STD. 84.13%	2STD. 97.72%	3STD* 99.87%
Biparietal diameter=BPD (mm)	84.2*	88.7:	93.2	97.7	102.2	106.7:	111.2*
Transverse trunk diameter=TTD (mm)	67.8*	79.1:	90.3	101.6	112.8	124.1:	135.3*
Head-to-trunk ratio=BPD/TTD	0.8045*	0.8655:	0.9265.	0.9875	1.0485	1.1095:	1.1705*
Fetal weight=WT (grams)	2100*	2600:	3100.	3600	4100	4600:	5100*

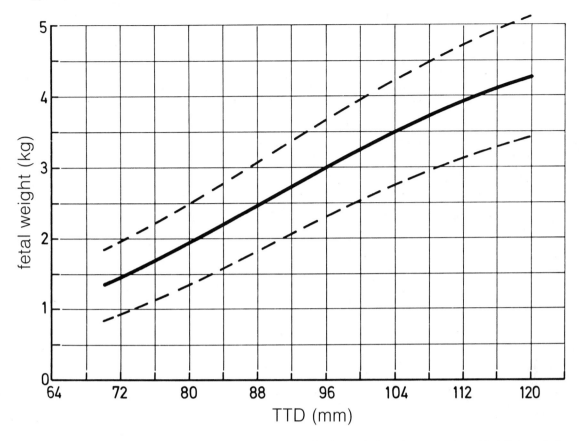

Fig. 9. Estimating fetal weight from TTD (particularly suited for fetuses in breech presentation with dolichocephalic head) (Bonn, 1976)

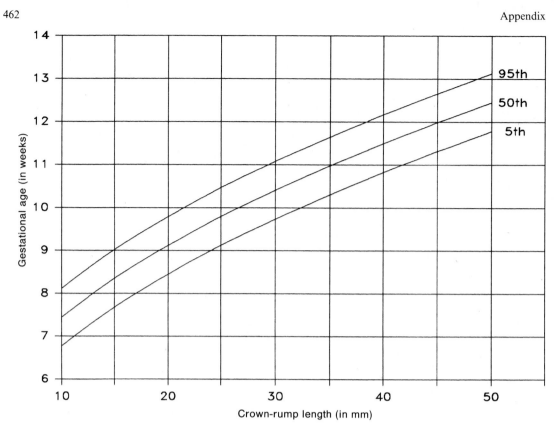

Fig. 10. Age from CRL. [From Robinson HP et al. (1975) Br J Obstet Gynecol 82:702]

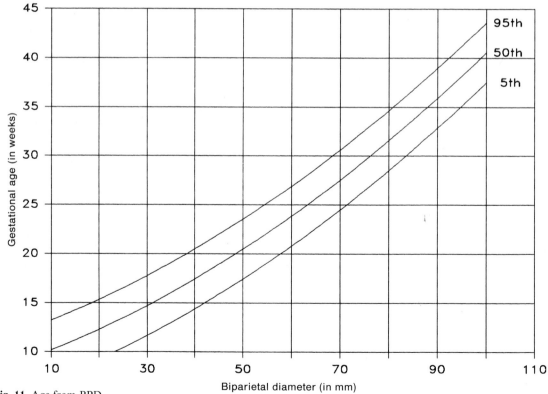

Fig. 11. Age from BPD

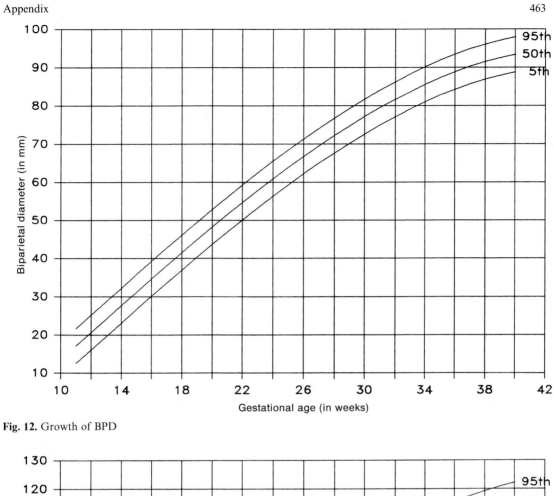

Fig. 12. Growth of BPD

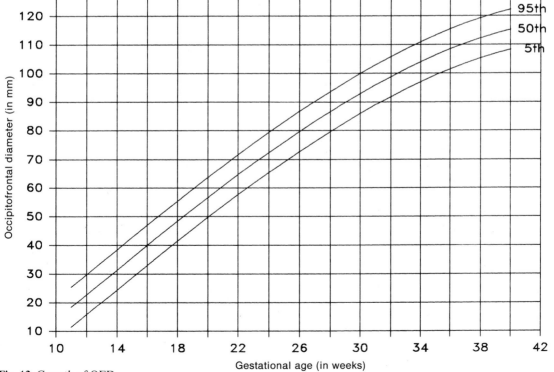

Fig. 13. Growth of OFD

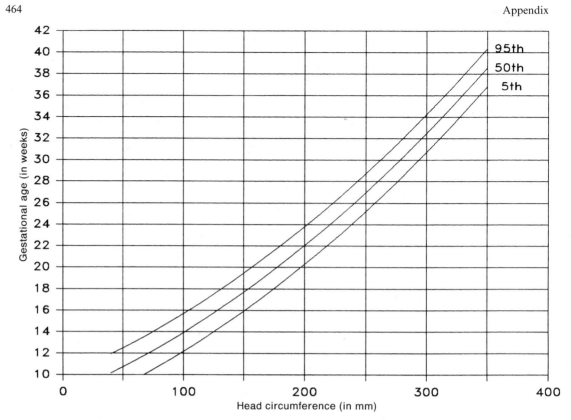

Fig. 14. Age from HC

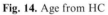

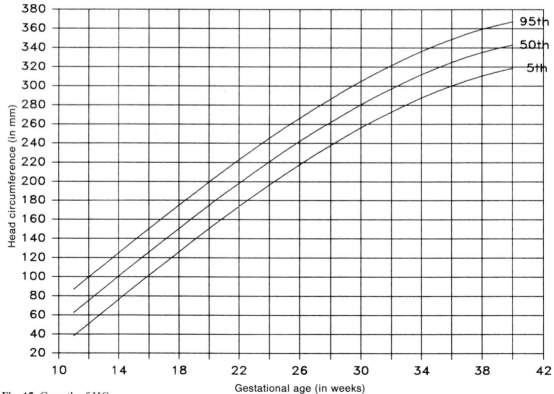

Fig. 15. Growth of HC

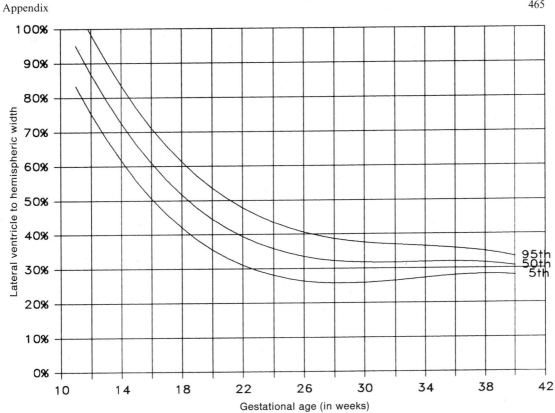

Fig. 16. Lateral ventricle to hemispheric width

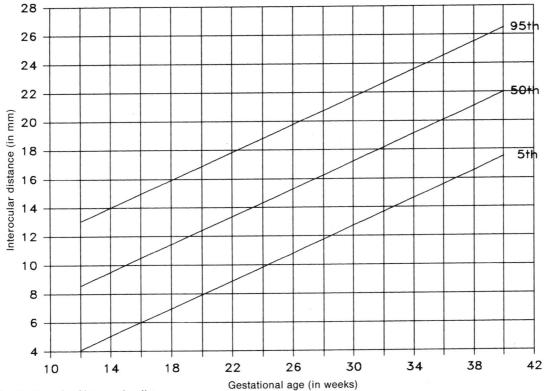

Fig. 17. Growth of interocular distance

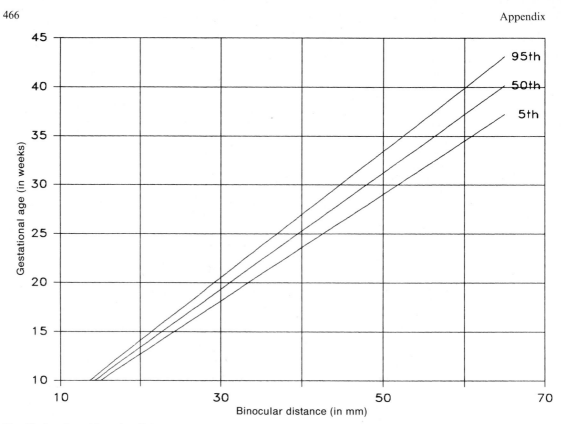

Fig. 18. Age from binocular distance

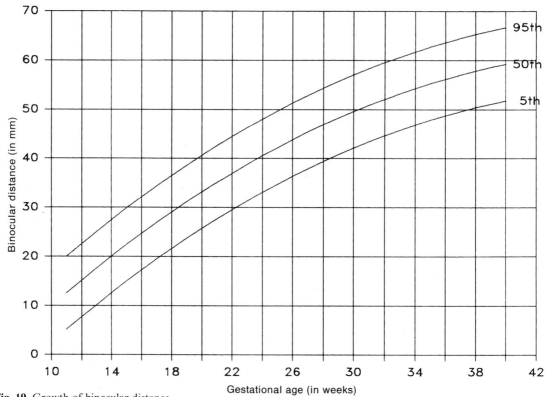

Fig. 19. Growth of binocular distance

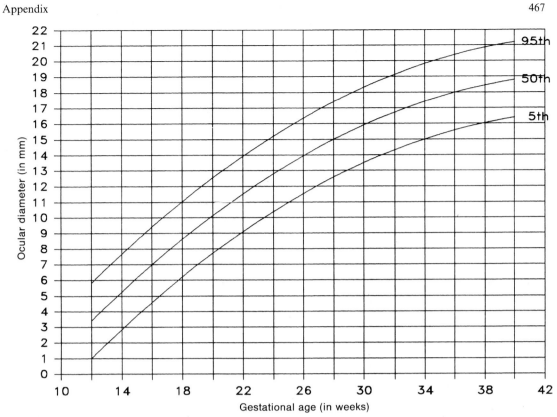

Fig. 20. Growth of ocular diameter

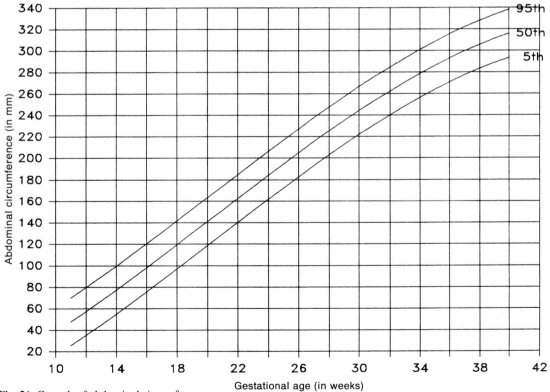

Fig. 21. Growth of abdominal circumference

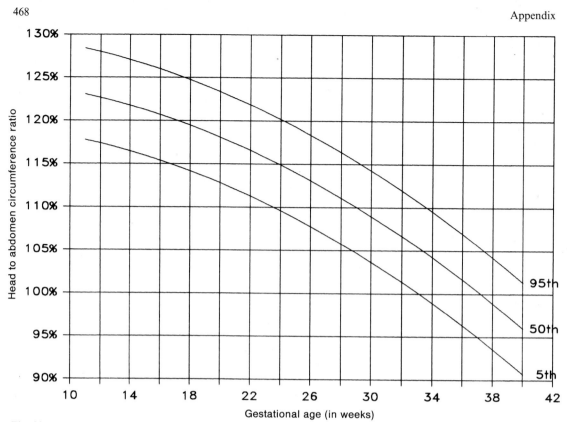

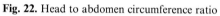

Fig. 22. Head to abdomen circumference ratio

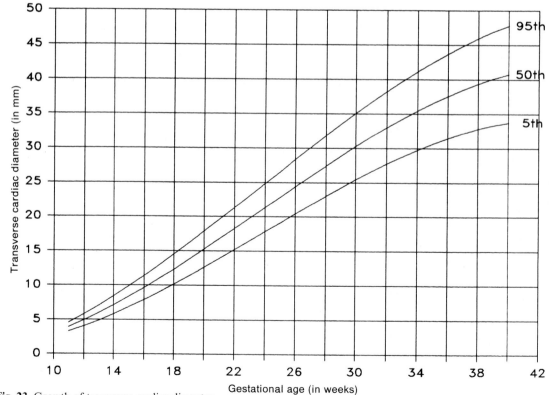

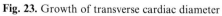

Fig. 23. Growth of transverse cardiac diameter

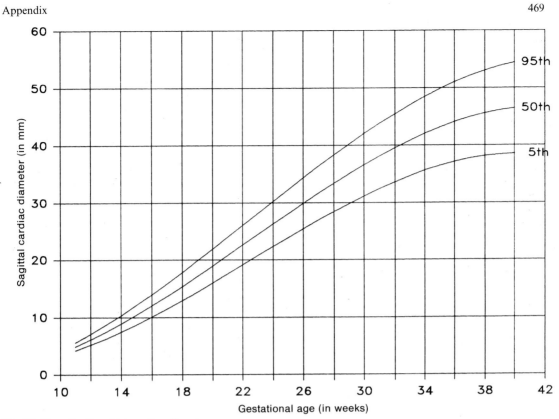

Fig. 24. Growth of sagittal cardiac diameter

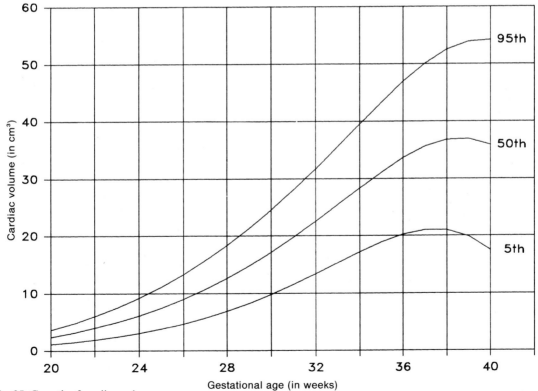

Fig. 25. Growth of cardiac volume

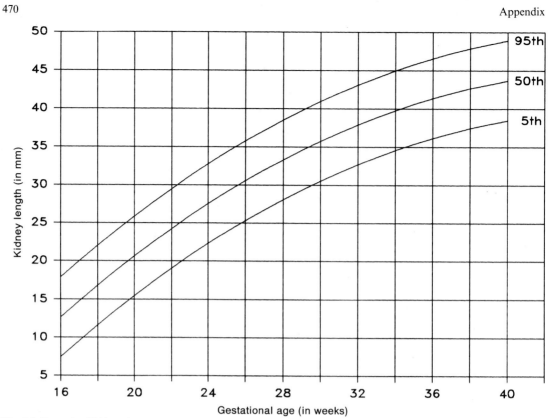

Fig. 26. Growth of kidney length

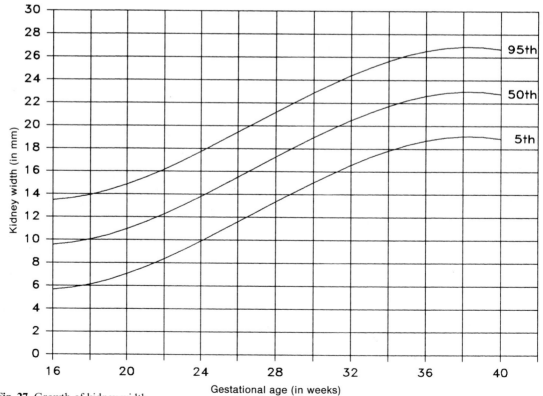

Fig. 27. Growth of kidney width

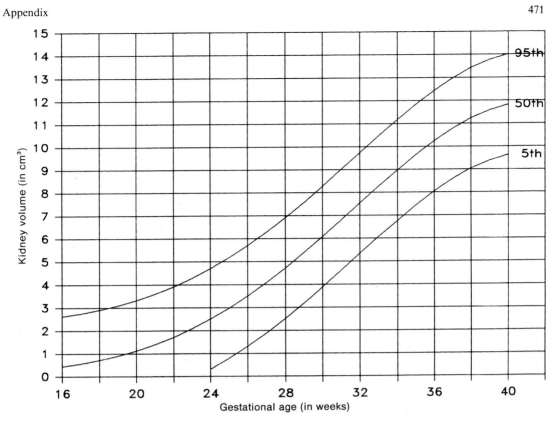

Fig. 28. Growth of kidney volume

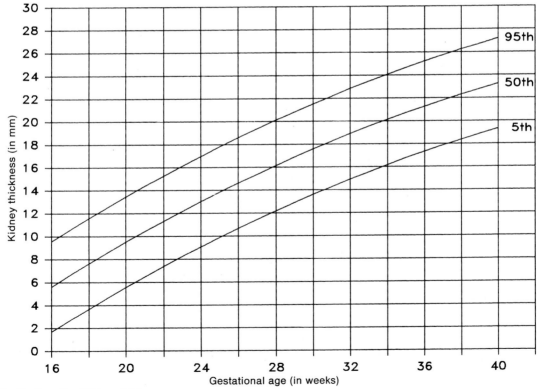

Fig. 29. Growth of kidney thickness

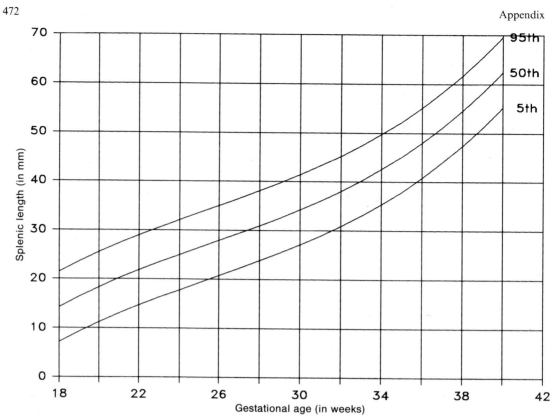

Fig. 30. Growth of splenic length

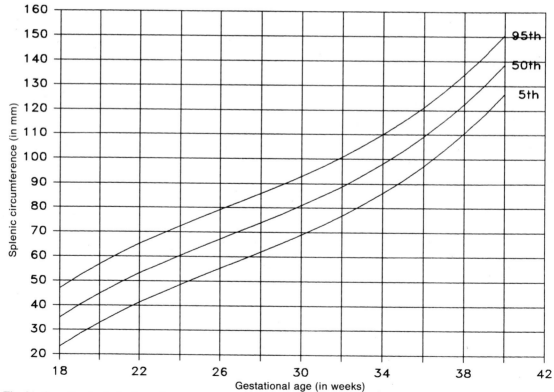

Fig. 31. Growth of splenic circumference

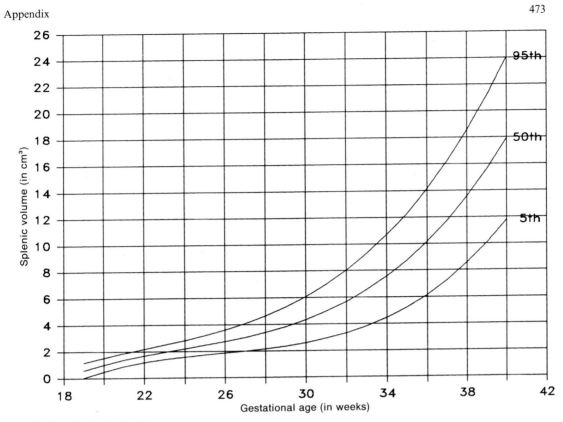

Fig. 32. Growth of splenic volume

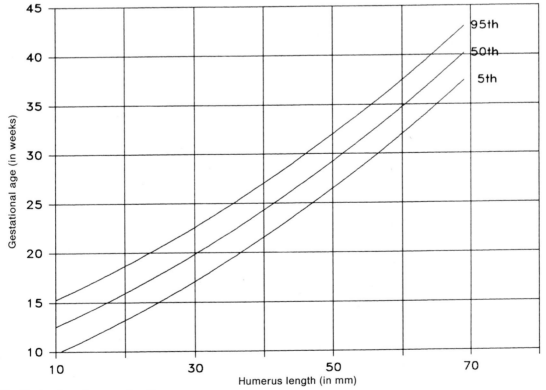

Fig. 33. Age from humerus length

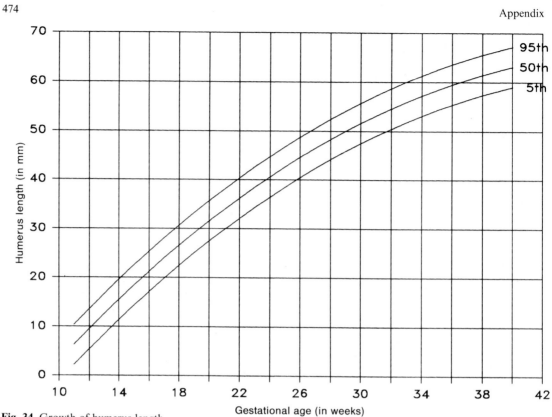

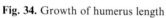

Fig. 34. Growth of humerus length

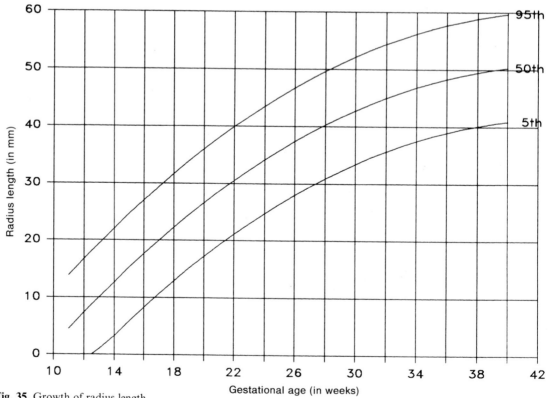

Fig. 35. Growth of radius length

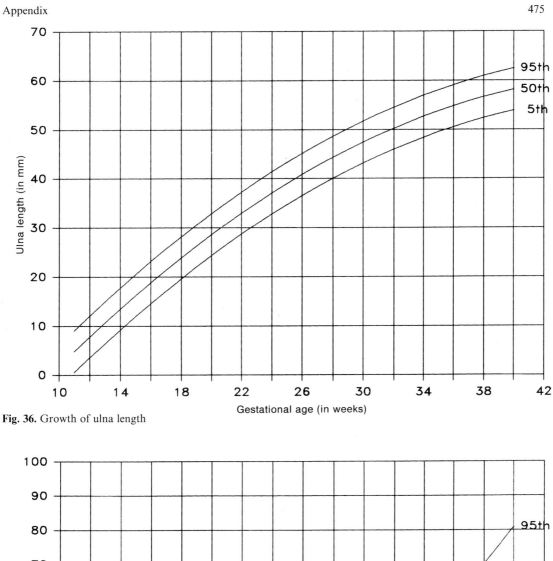

Fig. 36. Growth of ulna length

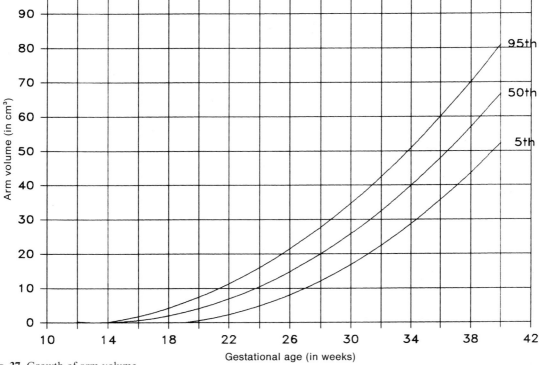

Fig. 37. Growth of arm volume

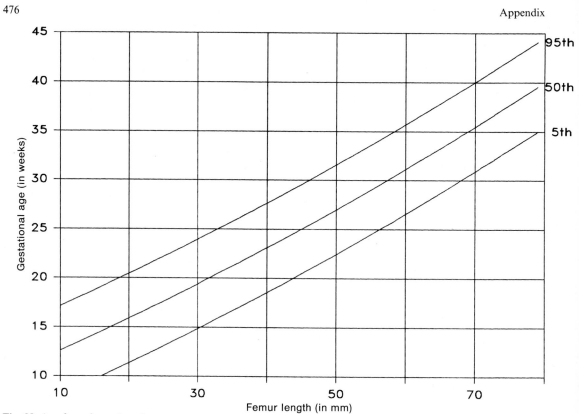

Fig. 38. Age from femur length

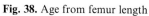

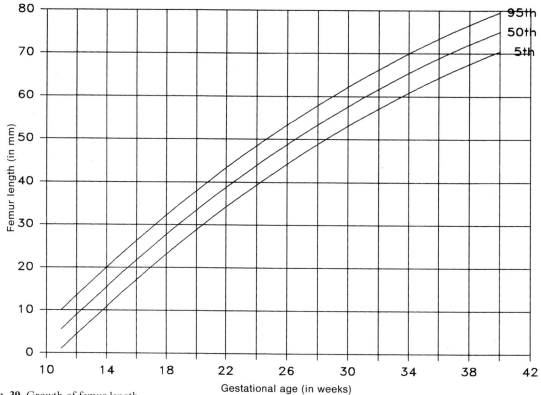

Fig. 39. Growth of femur length

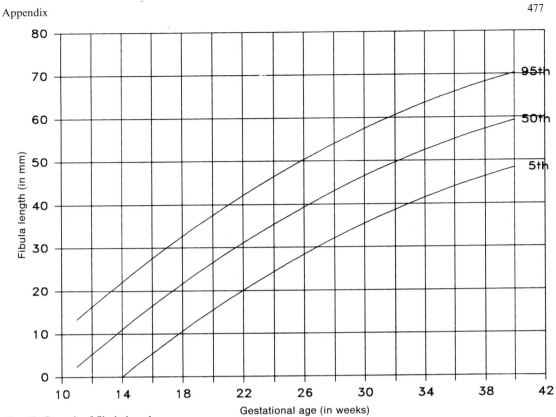

Fig. 40. Growth of fibula length

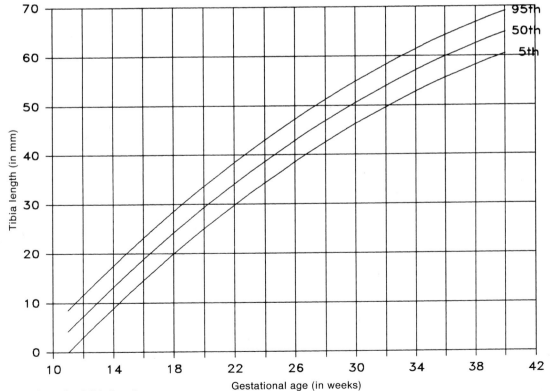

Fig. 41. Growth of tibia length

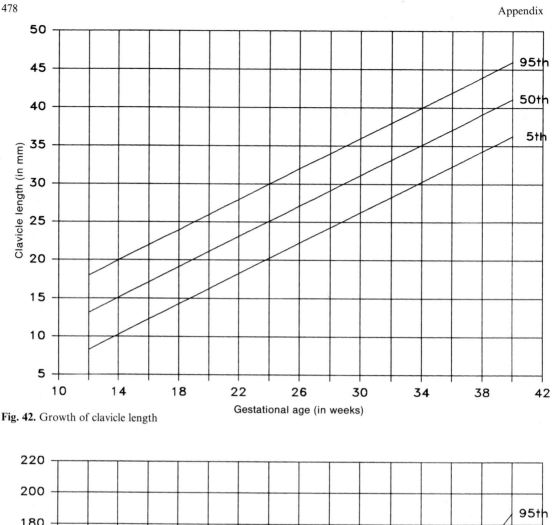

Fig. 42. Growth of clavicle length

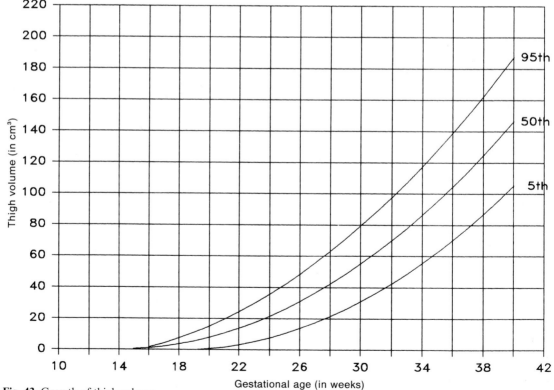

Fig. 43. Growth of thigh volume

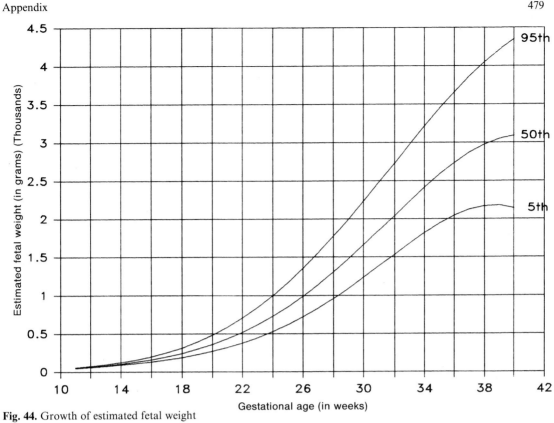

Fig. 44. Growth of estimated fetal weight

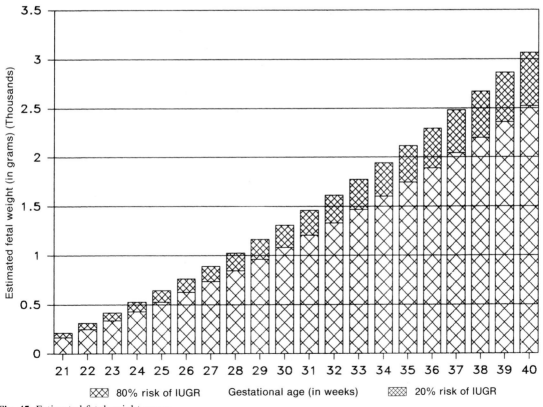

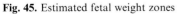

Fig. 45. Estimated fetal weight zones

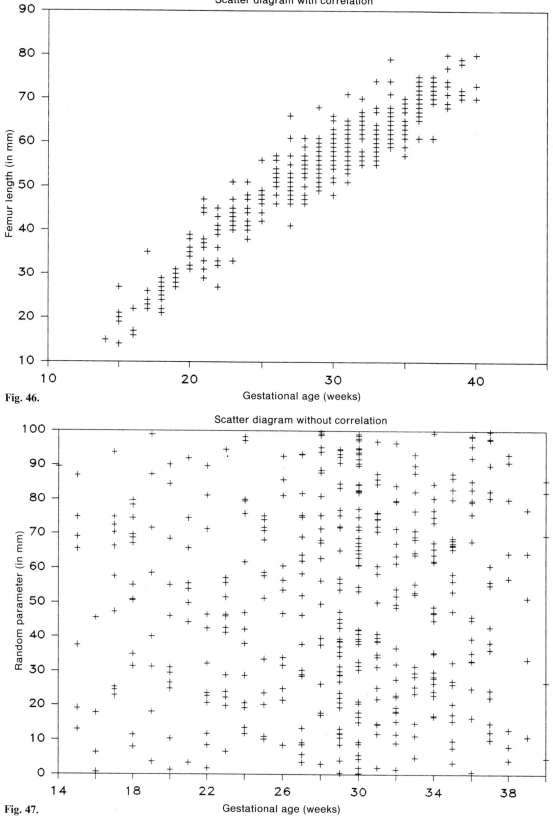

Fig. 46.

Fig. 47.

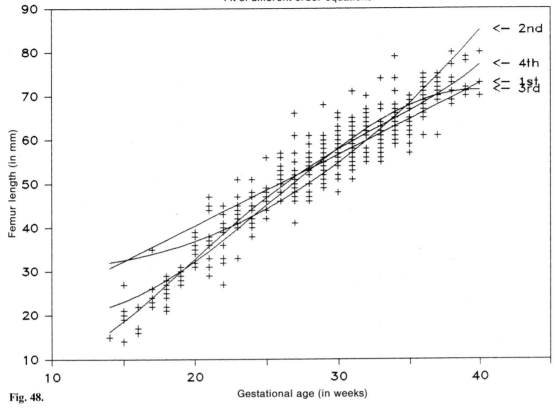

Fig. 48.

Subject Index

A Simple Reporting Program for Obstetrical Ultrasound

PHILIPPE JEANTY

Software Required

The "Obstetrical Ultrasound Reporting Software" (OURS) is a worksheet that is loaded into a more general program: Lotus 1–2–3 (TM) version 1A or 2. Lotus 1–2–3 (TM) is a spreadsheet software developed by Lotus Corporation of Cambridge, Massachusetts. This software was selected because it has been a very successful program and is fast and inexpensive. There is a large body of knowledge about it, and training is available under any desirable form. The equations that are used were all derived from our own data, except for the equation to predict the fetal weight, which is derived from the paper by Shepard et al. (Shepard MJ, Richards VA, Berkowitz RL et al., 1982: An evaluation of two equations for predicting fetal weight by ultrasound. Am J Obstet Gynecol 142:42–54) and that for the crown-rump length, which is the one developed by Robinson and Fleming (Robinson HP, Fleming JEE, 1975: A critical evaluation of sonar crown-rump length measurements. Br J Obstet Gynaecol 82:702–710). The equation to predict IUGR from the estimated fetal weight was derived from the original data, used in the paper of Chervenak et al. (Chervenak FA, Romero R, Berkowitz RL et al., 1984: The use of sonographic estimated fetal weight in the prediction of intrauterine growth retardation. Am J Perinatol 1:298–301).

Functions

The program is a series of instructions, called "macro", which are included in the worksheet and can be studied by the interested user. Since the 1–2–3 language is very simple, and contains only a couple of dozen instructions and formulas, it is easy to master, and the program can therefore easily be modified to be adapted by the user.

The program allows the entering of *"administrative" information* such as the name and address of the patient and physician, the reason for the scan [one of the 28 reasons suggested by the NIH guidelines (Diagnostic Ultrasound Imaging in Pregnancy, 1984: NIH publication 84–667) or free text], and the LMP. If the LMP is unknown, the program can work either on the "best estimate" of the number of weeks of gestation (as derived from an early physical examination) or even an approximate of the number of months (which the patient often knows).

The Measurements. A series of data collection forms are then proposed which cover virtually all the biometry covered above.

Establishment of the Gestational Age. Any combination of the LMP, crown-rump length, biparietal diameter, binocular distance, head perimeter, femur, and humerus.

Graphic Display of the Data. Graphs demonstrating the growth of the biparietal diameter, head perimeter, femur, abdominal perimeter, and estimated fetal weight are automatically provided. Graphs that summarize the evolution of a same patient over up to eight examinations can be produced too.

The Report. Finally, a report is composed and printed entirely by automatic wordprocessing. As many copies as necessary can be printed. The data can then be saved for archival purposes. They can later be restored, should a copy of an old report be needed. A sample report is provided for illustration below.

Procedures. The user is guided from one task to the next by a series of menus covering the whole series of tasks. The user never has to be involved with "computer instructions." The system of menus allow for very rapid movement between the different aspects of the program. It also permits return to a previous task, should an error have been introduced. More fluent use of the computer is therefore possible.

Hardware

OURS works on IBM Personal Computer (TM) and 100% IBM-compatible computers such as the Compaq (TM). The amount of memory required is at least 256 K of RAM. The use of a hard disk is recommended for speed. A printer (either dot matrix or letter quality) is needed to print the reports. The price of the whole equipment is estimated to be between $ 3000 and $ 7000.

Availability

The program is distributed as "user-supported": the user only pays a small contribution for a copy of the program and sends a donation if he feels satisfied with it. The user is allowed to distribute his copy of the program but has to do it free (he is not allowed to sell it). The user is also allowed to make whatever modification he wants in the program, but is not authorized to distribute this modified copy, in order that potential bugs do not creep into the program, rendering it potentially incorrect or misleading.

Order Instruction

Please send your informal order plus a cheque (or money order) for $ 40 to

Springer-Verlag
175 Fifth Avenue
New York, NY 10010
Attn.: Mrs. I. Cunningham
Tel. 212-460-1500

You will receive the software program directly from the author, Dr. Philippe Jeanty. It is therefore mandatory that the cheque be made out to Dr. P. Jeanty.

GESTATIONAL AGE ASSESSMENT
===========================

LMP (MM-DD-YY):   7 /19 / 85

```
                   Due Date (from LMP) : 25-Apr-86
Lower limit of Due Date from exam :      09-Apr-86
Most probable Due Date from exam :       25-Apr-86
Upper limit of Due Date from exam :      08-May-86
```

Predicted gestational age based on various parameters (in weeks & days)

```
                        LMP       21 + 6   <----
         Biparietal diameter      22 + 0   <----
         Binocular distance       22 + 2
              Head Perimeter      21 + 3   <----
                       Femur      21 + 6   <----
                     Humerus      22 + 3   <----

                Selected age      21 + 6
```

MISCELLANEOUS
=============

```
Placental Position : posterior
   Amount of Fluid : normal
    3 vessels cord : yes
 Number of fetuses : one
    Fetal position : vertex
               Sex : male
Fetal heart activity: regular
 Tape #, counter #:
```

NOTE: On the following pages you will see the detail of the measurements obtained during the examination. On the right of each parameter are the value(s) that have been obtained, and their mean. The three columns on the right represent the "estimated gestational age" from the parameter. The next set of three columns represents the predicted size of the parameter for the gestational age that has been selected. Finally the last column on the right checks whether or not a parameter is within limits (marked by a 0) or outside limits (marked by a 1). Please remember that since for most of the parameters used the confidence limits are the 5th and 95th percentile, it will NOT be unusual for one or two measurements to be outside the confidence limits. Please interpret these measurements in their clinical context.

OURS 1.

Your office, street, and phone number

Examination performed on December 19, 1985.

```
Re: Smith
    Bonnie
    29 years old
    (203) 832-3414
    54 East Main Street
    Any Town, USA
    85-32344
    1234-567-890
```

Dr Herodote

65 West Main Street
Another Town, USA

Dear Dr Herodote,

Thank you for refering to us Ms Bonnie Smith who is currently 21 weeks by dates. Her LMP occured on July 19, 1985. As you recall the reason for the examination was: Stage 1 examination (dating, placenta, screening for gross malformations...).

The estimated gestational age is 21 weeks and 6 days, based on an average of the last menstrual periods, biparietal diameter, head perimeter, femur length, and humerus length. The expected due date based on this gestational age is April 25, 1986. The 5th and 95th limits on this prediction of the due date are from April 9, 1986 to May 8, 1986.

The BPD measures 55 mm, which corresponds to 22 weeks and 0 day(s). The femur measures 37 mm (corresponding to 21 weeks and 6 day(s)). The estimated fetal weight (EFW) is 420 grams (which is about 0 pounds and 15 ounces). The EFW is within the normal range for this gestational age. The placenta is posterior, and the amount of fluid is normal.

This is where you can enter free form comments, such as: This kid looks great ! or whatever you wish !

You will find in the following pages a list of the parameters that have been obtained.

If you have any further questions, please call us.

Sincerely yours,

Your Name, M.D.

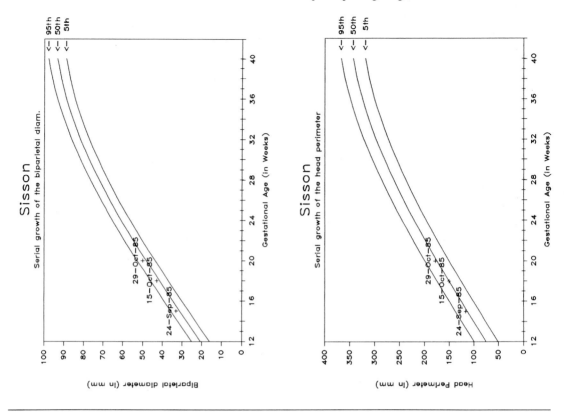

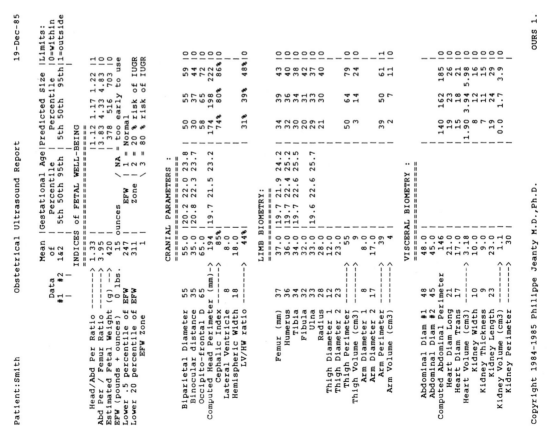

Patient:Smith   Obstetrical Ultrasound Report   19-Dec-85

	Data	Mean of	Gestational Age Percentile		Predicted Size Percentile			Limits: 0=within
	#1 #2	1&2	5th 50th 95th		5th 50th 95th			1=outside

INDICES of FETAL WELL-BEING
===============================

Head/Abd Per Ratio ------>	1.33	1.12 1.17 1.22	1
Abd Per / Femur Ratio ---->	3.95	3.83 4.33 4.83	0
Estimated Fetal Weight (g) -->	420	378 516 703	0
EFW (pounds + ounces)	0 lbs. 15 ounces		
Lower .5 percentile of EFW	247	EFW / NA = too early to use	
Lower 20 percentile of EFW	311	Zone	1 = Normal	
EFW Zone	1		2 = 20 % risk of IUGR	
			3 = 80 % risk of IUGR	

CRANIAL PARAMETERS :
==========================

Biparietal Diameter	55	55.0	20.2 22.0 23.8	50	55	59	0
Binocular distance	35	35.0	20.8 22.3 23.7	30	37	44	0
Occipito-frontal D	65	65.0		58	65	72	0
Computed Head Perimeter (mm)-->	194	19.7 21.5 23.2	174	198	222	0
Cephalic Index ------>	85%		74%	80%	86%	0
Lateral Ventricle	8	8.0					
Hemispheric Width	18	18.0					
LV/HW ratio ------>	44%		31%	39%	48%	0

LIMB BIOMETRY:
==============

Femur (mm)	37	37.0	19.7 21.9 24.2	34	39	43	0
Humerus	36	36.0	19.7 22.4 25.2	32	36	40	0
Tibia	34	34.0	19.7 22.6 25.5	30	34	38	0
Fibula	32	32.0		20	31	42	0
Ulna	33	33.0	19.6 22.6 25.7	29	33	37	0
Radius	28	28.0		21	30	40	0
Thigh Diameter 1	12	12.0					
Thigh Diameter 2	23	23.0					
Thigh Perimeter ------>	55		50	64	79	0
Thigh Volume (cm3) ------>	9		3	14	24	0
Arm Diameter 1	8	8.0					
Arm Diameter 2	17	17.0					
Arm Perimeter ------>	39		39	50	61	1
Arm Volume (cm3) ------>	4		2	7	11	0

VISCERAL BIOMETRY :
===================

Abdominal Diam #1	48	48.0					
Abdominal Diam #2	45	45.0					
Computed Abdominal Perimeter	146		140	162	185	0
Heart Diam Long	21	21.0		19	23	26	0
Heart Diam Trans	17	17.0		15	18	21	0
Heart Volume (cm3) ------>	3.18		1.90 3.94 5.98	0
Kidney Width	10	10.0		8	12	16	0
Kidney Thickness	9	9.0		7	11	15	0
Kidney Length	23	23.0		19	24	29	0
Kidney Volume (cm3) ------>	1.1		0.0 1.7 3.9	0
Kidney Perimeter ------>	30					

Copyright 1984-1985 Philippe Jeanty M.D.,Ph.D.   OURS 1.

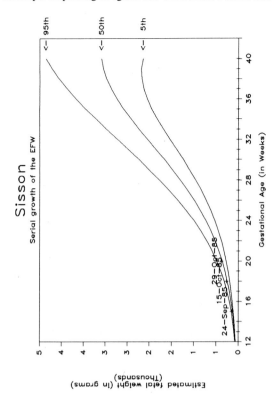

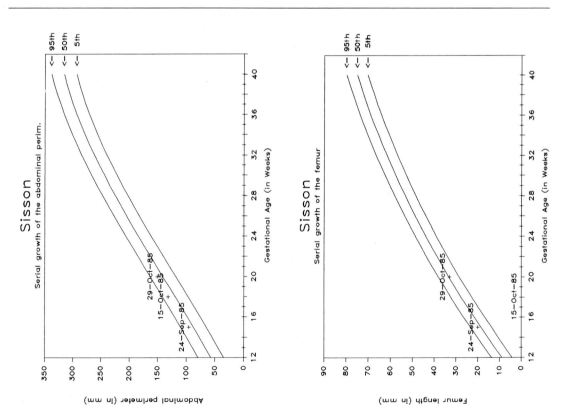